# THE DIABETIC FOOT

**Fifth Edition**

# The Diabetic Foot

**Fifth Edition**

## Marvin E. Levin, M.D.

*Professor of Clinical Medicine*
*Washington University School of Medicine*
*Associate Director*
*Diabetes Metabolism Clinic*
*St. Louis, Missouri*


## Lawrence W. O'Neal, M.D.

*Professor Emeritus*
*Clinical Surgery*
*St. Louis University School of Medicine*
*St. Louis, Missouri*


## John H. Bowker, M.D.

*Professor and Associate Chairman*
*Department of Orthopaedics and Rehabilitation*
*University of Miami School of Medicine*
*Director, Amputee and Diabetic Foot Services*
*Jackson Memorial Medical Center*
*Miami, Florida*

*With forewords by:*
*Paul W. Brand, M.D.*
*Gary W. Gibbons, M.D.*
*Harold Rifkin, M.D.*

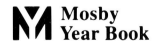

**Mosby**
**Year Book**

St. Louis    Baltimore    Boston    Chicago    London    Philadelphia    Sydney    Toronto

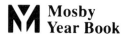

Sponsoring Editor: James D. Ryan/Joyce-Rachel John
Assistant Managing Editor, Text and Reference:
  George Mary Gardner
Production Supervisor: Karen Halm
Proofroom Manager: Barbara M. Kelly

1  2  3  4  5  6  7  8  9  0  97  96  95  94  93

**Library of Congress Cataloging-in-Publication
Data**
The diabetic foot / [edited by] Marvin E. Levin,
Lawrence W. O'Neal,
   John H. Bowker.—5th ed.
      p.   cm.
   Includes bibliographical references and index.
   ISBN 0-8016-6878-6
   1. Foot—Diseases.  2. Diabetes—
Complications.  3. Foot—Surgery.
   I. Levin, Marvin E., 1924–  .  II. O'Neal,
   Lawrence W., 1923—  .  III. Bowker, John H.
      [DNLM: 1. Diabetes Mellitus—
complications.  2. Foot Diseases—etiology.  3. Foot
Diseases—therapy.   WK 835 D535]
   RC951.D53   1992                    92-49437
   617.5'85—dc20                       CIP
   DNLM/DLC
   for Library of Congress

Dedicated to our children:
Lynn, Judith, and Michael
Patricia, Kathleen, Janet, and Laura
Thomas

# CONTRIBUTORS

**Brent T. Allen, M.D.**
*Assistant Professor of Surgery*
*Washington University School of Medicine*
*Attending Surgeon*
*Barnes Hospital*
*St. Louis, Missouri*

**Oscar M. Alvarez, Ph.D., M.D.**
*Director, University Wound Healing Clinic*
*New Brunswick, New Jersey*

**Charles B. Anderson, M.D.**
*Professor of Surgery*
*Washington University School of Medicine*
*Vascular Surgeon*
*Barnes Hospital*
*St. Louis, Missouri*

**Michael J. Auletta, M.D.**
*Assistant Clinical Professor of Dermatology*
*Director, Dermatologic Surgery*
*Robert Wood Johnson Medical School*
*New Brunswick, New Jersey*

**Thomas C. Bailey, M.D.**
*Instructor of Medicine*
*Washington University School of Medicine*
*Medical Director*
*Pharmacokinetics Service*
*The Jewish Hospital of St. Louis*
*St. Louis, Missouri*

**Andrew J.M. Boulton, M.D., F.R.C.P.**
*Reader in Medicine*
*Manchester University*
*Consultant Physician*
*Manchester Royal Infirmary*
*Manchester, United Kingdom*

**John H. Bowker, M.D.**
*Professor and Associate Chairman*
*Department of Orthopaedics and*
*    Rehabilitation*
*University of Miami School of Medicine*
*Director, Amputee and Diabetic Foot*
*    Services*
*Jackson Memorial Medical Center*
*Miami, Florida*

**Peter R. Cavanagh, Ph.D.**
*Professor and Director*
*Center for Locomotion Studies*
*Pennsylvania State University*
*University Park, Pennsylvania*

**Paul Cianci, M.D.**
*Professor of Medicine*
*University of California at Davis*
*Director, Department of Diving and*
*    Hyperbaric Medicine*
*Davis, California*

**William C. Coleman, D.P.M.**
*Ochsner Clinic*
*New Orleans, Louisiana*

**John A. Colwell, M.D., Ph.D.**
*Professor of Medicine*
*Medical University of South Carolina*
*Associate Chief of Staff for Research and*
*    Development*
*Ralph H. Johnson Veterans Administration*
*    Medical Center*
*Charleston, South Carolina*

**Kenrick J. Dennis, D.P.M.**
*Associate Clinical Professor*
*University of Texas Health Science Center*
  *at San Antonio*
*San Antonio, Texas*

**Michael Edmonds, M.D., F.R.C.P.**
*Senior Lecturer*
*Kings College School of Medicine*
*Consultant Physician*
*Kings College Hospital*
*London, England*

**Eva L. Feldman, M.D., Ph.D.**
*Assistant Professor of Neurology*
*University of Michigan*
*Assistant Professor of Neurology*
*University of Michigan Medical Center*
*Ann Arbor, Michigan*

**Vance Fiegel, B.S.**
*Scientist, Center for Wound Healing and*
  *Reparative Biology*
*Department of Surgery*
*University of Minnesota*
*Minneapolis, Minnesota*

**Althea V.M. Foster, B.A.(Hons),**
  **D.Pod.M., M.Ch.S.**
*Diabetic Department*
*Chief Hospital Podiatrist*
*Kings College Hospital*
*London, England*

**John J. Frank, J.D.**
*St. Louis University School of Law*
*St. Louis, Missouri*

**Joseph A. Frank, J.D.**
*St. Louis, Missouri*

**Robert G. Frykberg, D.P.M.**
*Attending Podiatrist*
*Department of Surgery*
*Division of Podiatry*
*Harvard Medical School*
*New England Deaconess Hospital*
*Boston, Massachusetts*

**Greta M. Gilson, R.N., B.H.S., M.S.A.**
*Fayetteville, Georgia*

**Louis A. Gilula, M.D.**
*Professor of Radiology*
*Washington University School of Medicine*
*Mallinckrodt Institute of Radiology*
*Consulting Radiologist*
*Barnes Hospital*
*St. Louis, Missouri*

**Dorothy M. Gohdes, M.D.**
*Director, Indian Health Service Diabetes*
  *Program*
*Albuquerque, New Mexico*

**Douglas A. Greene, M.D.**
*Professor of Internal Medicine*
*Division Chief*
*Endocrinology and Metabolism*
*Director, Michigan Diabetes Research and*
  *Training Center*
*University of Michigan*
*Ann Arbor, Michigan*

**David C. Hardy, M.D.**
*Attending Physician*
*LDS Hospital*
*University of Utah School of Medicine*
*Salt Lake City, Utah*

**Lawrence B. Harkless, D.P.M.**
*Clinical Professor*
*Department of Orthopaedics*
*University of Texas Health Science Center*
  *at San Antonio*
*San Antonio, Texas*

**Phala A. Helm, M.D.**
*Professor and Chairman*
*Department of Physical Medicine and*
  *Rehabilitation*
*The University of Texas Southwestern*
  *Medical Center at Dallas*
*Dallas, Texas*

**Falls B. Hershey, M.D.**
*Emeritus Director of Vascular Surgery*
*St. John's Mercy Medical Center*
*St. Louis, Missouri*

**Irl B. Hirsch, M.D.**
*Assistant Professor of Medicine*
*University of Washington Medical Center*
*Medical Director, Diabetes Care Center*
*Seattle, Washington*

**Thomas K. Hunt, M.D.**
*Professor of Surgery*
*University of California at San Francisco*
*San Francisco, California*

**Joseph J. Hurley, M.D.**
*Clinical Associate Professor*
*St. Louis University Medical School*
*Vascular Surgeon*
*St. John's Mercy Medical Center*
*St. Louis, Missouri*

**Dennis J. Janisse, C.Ped.**
*Chief Executive Officer*
*National Pedorthic Services, Inc.*
*Milwaukee, Wisconsin*

**J.E. Jelinek, M.D.**
*Clinical Professor of Dermatology*
*New York University Medical Center*
*Chief of Service, Skin and Cancer Unit*
*Tisch Hospital*
*New York, New York*

**Richard L. Klein, Ph.D.**
*Assistant Professor of Medicine*
*Medical University of South Carolina*
*Charleston, South Carolina*

**David R. Knighton, M.D.**
*Associate Professor of Surgery*
*University of Minnesota*
*Minneapolis, Minnesota*

**George S. Kobayashi, Ph.D.**
*Professor of Medicine and Molecular*
  *Microbiology*
*Washington University School of Medicine*
*Associate Director*
*Microbiology Laboratories*
*Barnes Hospital*
*St. Louis, Missouri*

**Karen J. Kowalske, M.D.**
*Assistant Professor*
*Department of Physical Medicine and*
  *Rehabilitation*
*The University of Texas Southwestern*
  *Medical Center at Dallas*
*Dallas, Texas*

**Marvin E. Levin, M.D.**
*Professor of Clinical Medicine*
*Washington University School of Medicine*
*Associate Director*
*Diabetes Metabolism Clinic*
*St. Louis, Missouri*

**J. Russell Little, M.D.**
*Professor of Medicine and Molecular*
  *Microbiology*
*Washington University School of Medicine*
*Chief, Infectious Diseases Division*
*Department of Medicine*
*The Jewish Hospital of St. Louis*
*St. Louis, Missouri*

**Maria F. Lopes-Virella, M.D., Ph.D.**
*Professor of Medicine*
*Medical University of South Carolina*
*Ralph H. Johnson Veterans Administration*
  *Medical Center*
*Charleston, South Carolina*

**Timothy J. Lyons, M.D., M.R.C.P.**
*Assistant Professor of Medicine*
*Medical University of South Carolina*
*Charleston, South Carolina*

**Kevin W. McEnery, M.D.**
*Instructor in Radiology*
*Washington University School of Medicine*
*Mallinckrodt Institute of Radiology*
*St. Louis, Missouri*

**Donald E. McMillan, M.D.**
*Professor of Internal Medicine*
*Professor of Physiology and Biophysics*
*Co-Director, Diabetes Center*
*University of South Florida College of*
  *Medicine*
*Tampa, Florida*

**Michael J. Mueller, M.H.S., P.T.**
*Instructor, Program in Physical Therapy*
*Washington University School of Medicine*
*Physical Therapist*
*Diabetic Foot Center*
*St. Louis, Missouri*

**Lawrence W. O'Neal, M.D.**
*Emeritus Professor of Clinical Surgery*
*St. Louis University School of Medicine*
*St. Louis, Missouri*

**Daniel Picus, M.D.**
*Associate Professor of Radiology*
*Washington University School of Medicine*
*Mallinckrodt Institute of Radiology*
*St. Louis, Missouri*

**Melvin Price, D.P.M., P.T.**
*Clinical Faculty*
*Department of Physical Medicine and*
  *Rehabilitation*
*Medical College of Wisconsin*
*Chief of Podiatry*
*Veterans Hospital*
*Milwaukee, Wisconsin*

**Gayle E. Reiber, M.P.H., Ph.D.**
*Assistant Professor of Health Services and*
*  Epidemiology*
*University of Washington*
*Research Health Science Specialist*
*Seattle Veterans Administration Medical*
*  Center*
*Seattle, Washington*

**Stephen J. Rith-Najarian, M.D.**
*Diabetes Control Officer*
*Indian Health Service*
*Bemidji, New Mexico*

**Lee J. Sanders, D.P.M.**
*Clinical Professor*
*College of Podiatric Medicine and Surgery*
*University of Osteopathic Medicine and*
*  Health Sciences*
*Des Moines, Iowa*
*Chief, Podiatry Section*
*Department of Veterans Affairs Medical*
*  Center*
*Lebanon, Pennsylvania*

**Gregorio A. Sicard, M.D.**
*Professor of Surgery*
*Washington University School of Medicine*
*Director, Vascular Service*
*Barnes Hospital*
*St. Louis, Missouri*

**David R. Sinacore, Ph.D., P.T.**
*Instructor, Program in Physical Therapy*
*Washington University School of Medicine*
*Physical Therapist*
*Diabetic Foot Center*
*St. Louis, Missouri*

**Tom W. Staple, M.D.**
*Adjunct Professor of Radiology*
*University of California at Irvine*
*Memorial Medical Center*
*Irvine, California*

**Martin Stevens, M.D.**
*Visiting Scientist*
*University of Michigan*
*Ann Arbor, Michigan*

**Jan S. Ulbrecht, M.D.**
*Adjunct Assistant Professor of Clinical*
*  Locomotion Studies*
*Pennsylvania State University*
*Clinical Assistant Professor of Medicine*
*Hershey Medical Center*
*University Park, Pennsylvania*

**Thomas M. Vesely, M.D.**
*Assistant Professor of Radiology*
*Washington University School of Medicine*
*Mallinckrodt Institute of Radiology*
*St. Louis, Missouri*

**Aristidis Veves, M.D., M.Sc.**
*Clinical Research Fellow*
*University of Manchester*
*Honorary Registrar*
*Manchester Royal Infirmary*
*Manchester, United Kingdom*

**Willard B. Walker, M.D.**
*Professor Emeritus*
*Washington University School of Medicine*
*St. Louis, Missouri*

**Paul F. White, Ph.D., M.D.**
*Professor and McDermott Chairman*
*Department of Anesthesiology and Pain*
*  Management*
*University of Texas Southwestern Medical*
*  School at Dallas*
*Dallas, Texas*

**John J. Woods, Jr., M.D.**
*Vascular Surgeon*
*St. John's Mercy Medical Center*
*St. Louis, Missouri*

**Matthew J. Young, M.B., M.R.C.P.**
*Clinical Research Fellow*
*University of Manchester*
*Honorary Registrar*
*Manchester Royal Infirmary*
*Manchester, United Kingdom*

# FOREWORD

Problems of the diabetic foot have been a lifelong passion for me, and my goal of decreasing amputations has gone from a dream to reality. To accomplish this nationally and internationally requires an ever increasing cadre of teachers and specialists. As I look at the names of contributors to this fifth edition of *The Diabetic Foot* I note that I know many of them personally. Some of them have come to the Hansen's Disease Center in Carville, Louisiana to study with me and to learn our techniques for saving the diabetic foot. Some of these physicians have told me that coming to Carville was a turning point in their understanding of the practical aspects of diabetic foot care. To see that these physicians are now carrying out our teachings by contributing to this text is a great pleasure to me. There is no greater satisfaction than seeing people who have studied with you go on to make important scientific contributions and teach others.

I am pleased to see that in this edition greater emphasis has been put on diabetic peripheral vascular disease. This is critically important because although it is the insensate foot that initiates most of the diabetic foot problems, proper healing depends on an adequate blood supply as well as on protection of the foot.

Of great importance in the pathogenesis of diabetic foot ulcers is the problem of abnormal foot pressures and shear stress areas, which I have studied for many years. Therefore I was pleased to see two chapters devoted to these problems, which continues our initial research. A chapter on the Charcot foot has been added. Proper footwear for these patients and the prevention and recurrence of foot ulcers has always been of special interest to me.

The addition of a third editor, John Bowker, an expert in orthopedics, rounds out this edition of *The Diabetic Foot*. The increased number of contributors to this text points out the multiple facets of management required for the complicated problems involving the diabetic foot. The text repeatedly emphasizes the importance of teamwork.

Again, I am pleased to see many of the physicians I have worked with over the years who have become teachers sharing their experiences and expertise.

**Paul W. Brand, M.D.**
Clinical Professor Emeritus
Department of Orthopaedic Surgery
University of Washington School of
Medicine
Seattle, Washington

# FOREWORD

New knowledge is meaningless unless presented effectively, such that it can be understood. The goal of the fifth edition of *The Diabetic Foot* is to assemble the most current or updated information relating to the diabetic foot from all specialities of medicine and to present it in a manner to guide all health care professionals in their approach to the patient with diabetes.

The increasing importance of ischemia complicating diabetic foot problems is recognized in this new edition. Revising and updating the chapters on hemorrheology and the pathogenesis of macrovascular disease provides understanding of the nature and pattern of diabetic atherosclerotic occlusive disease, especially recognizing the absence of occlusive microvascular disease of the diabetic foot. These concepts lay the foundation for the chapters dedicated to the diagnosis and treatment of ischemia. New approaches to radiologic imaging and interventional techniques are integrated with updated medical and surgical techniques to provide the reader options on how to best manage the patient with ischemia.

Our own team approach has changed to now evaluate all threatened limbs for ischemia. Aggressive revascularization even to the dorsalis pedis artery to achieve maximum perfusion of the foot can be justified only by outcome analysis. We have demonstrated long-term patency and a significant reduction in amputations at all levels, with no change in an already low mortality rate.

The challenge to the reader in any of the health care disciplines caring for the diabetic is to make it work. There can be no turf wars, recognizing instead strengths to achieve success using the knowledge illustrated in this new edition. Working together as a team can reduce not only the number of major amputations but also the physical and emotional costs to the patient and to society.

**Gary W. Gibbons, M.D.**
Associate Clinical Professor of Surgery
Harvard Medical School
Clinical Chief
Division of Vascular Surgery
New England Deaconess Hospital
Boston, Massachusetts

# FOREWORD

As an editor of four editions of the text *Diabetes Mellitus: Theory and Practice*, I fully understand the manifold problems of a multiauthored text. Therefore I am much impressed with this text, which interweaves 28 multiple disciplines and whose message, it is hoped, if followed will reduce the number of diabetic amputees.

As an internist and diabetologist with 45 years of experience in taking care of literally thousands of diabetic patients, I have seen too many amputations. Today a prime goal of every physician caring for the diabetic is to prevent amputation. This cannot be accomplished in every case; however, with a combination of medical, surgical, radiologic, and podiatric approaches described in detail in this text the amputation rate certainly can be decreased significantly.

I am pleased to see contributions by internationally known experts in diabetic foot care incorporated into this new edition. New chapters on dermatology, Charcot foot, wound healing factors, special wound dressings, and hyperbaric oxygen therapy have increased the depth of this work. Especially helpful and important is a new chapter on foot care in minorities, a group in which foot problems and amputations are especially high. The addition of a third editor, Dr. John Bowker, and his chapter on amputation have increased significantly the scope of this edition.

Amputations can and do lead to legal issues. The new chapter on legal issues stresses the need for consultation, the importance of avoiding substandard care, and pertinent information on how to avoid a legal suit in cases involving the diabetic foot.

*The Diabetic Foot* since its inception and first edition in 1973 has set the standard for diabetic foot management. Each edition has been updated with new topics, new authors, and new references; this fifth edition is no exception. The text is not just for surgeons, orthopedists, podiatrists, and shoe specialists, but for internists, diabetologists, primary care physicians, diabetes educators, and nurses. This edition is a landmark book and should be in the library of every medical school, hospital, and nursing facility. It deserves a prominent place in the personal library shelf of all physicians who treat the diabetic patient.

**Harold Rifkin, M.D.**
Professor of Clinical Medicine
New York University School of Medicine
Clinical Professor of Medicine
Albert Einstein College of Medicine
Principal Consultant
Diabetes Research and Training Center
Montefiore Medical Center–Albert Einstein College of Medicine
New York, New York

# PREFACE TO FIRST EDITION

Patients affected with diabetes mellitus, no longer dying of coma or starvation, have acquired an increased life span. These added years have brought into focus the diabetic complications of retinopathy, nephropathy, neuropathy, and vascular disease. Perhaps nowhere in the body do we see so plainly the ravages of the diabetic complications of vascular disease and neuropathy as in the foot. These common and often disabling foot problems lead to suffering, disability, time lost from work, hospitalization, and great expense, to both the patient and the community. To prevent and treat these complex diabetic foot problems the talents of multiple medical disciplines are required; therefore the goal of this monograph is to bring together in a single volume an in-depth discussion of the varied factors affecting the diabetic foot, including their pathogenesis, and to stress the need for a team effort in their management.

The primary approach to the problem must begin with an understanding of the basic metabolic abnormalities of diabetes. These deal not only with insulin, carbohydrate, and lipid abnormalities, but also with the pathologic processes that develop in the blood vessels and nerves. Currently we do not know the basis for the development of the angiopathy and neuropathy in diabetes. It does not appear to be directly related to the elevated body sugars, as blood vessel disease and abnormal nerve conduction can be found in some patients prior to the occurrence of hyperglycemia. Furthermore good control of the blood sugar by our present criteria does not always prevent diabetic complications. For these reasons it is apparent that with our current therapy we cannot prevent vascular and nerve disease in the diabetic and can therefore expect to see a continuing high frequency of diabetic foot problems.

The physician who is to treat the diabetic foot successfully must be knowledgeable in the anatomy of the foot. He must also be aware of the pathophysiology and the signs and symptoms of the neuropathies and angiopathies so that when these problems arise he can institute early and proper therapy. Since early recognition and proper therapy of ischemic and neuropathic problems may save the diabetic's foot and leg, a detailed discussion of these factors is presented. Because of the frequency of surgery involving the diabetic foot, a discussion is also included on the management of the diabetic and his insulin requirement during surgery.

The vascular problems can be divided into two major groups: the large vessels—macrovascular disease—and the small blood vessels comprising the small arteries, arterioles, and the capillaries and venules—microvascular disease. Because large vessel disease in the diabetic often is associated with atherosclerosis and thrombosis, reconstructive arterial surgery is a frequent event in these patients and can be a foot-and-limb–saving procedure. However, before vascular surgery can be recommended, the site and degree of the arterial block and the degree of patency of the adjacent vascular tree must be established by angiography. At this point the radiologist becomes a vitally important member of the team. Roentgenography is also of great importance in establishing the presence or absence of osteomyelitis and the degree of neuropathic bone involvement. Small blood vessel disease consists of the narrowing or occlusion of the small arteries and the arterioles as well as thickening of the basement membrane of the microvascular capillaries. The latter may be the most important and specific vascular lesion in the diabetic. Hopefully the identification of the pathogenesis of this lesion and its effect on tissue metabolism may lead to a major breakthrough in the total understanding of diabetic vascular disease. Because of the importance of this lesion and other vascular lesions in the diabetic, the pathology of blood vessel disease is presented in detail, with particular emphasis on the microvascular lesions.

Diabetic neuropathy, although frequently accompanied by pain and paresthesias, causes its greatest problem by the opposite effect, the loss of pain sensation. The patient without pain perception unwittingly allows his foot to endure repeated trauma until trophic changes and, frequently, secondary infection develop. With the appearance of infection, he now has the classic pathologic triad of the diabetic foot: vascular disease, neuropathy, and infection. The development of significant infection may be the harbinger of the final cataclysmic events: gangrene and amputation. The expert in infectious disease therefore plays a vital role in the care of the diabetic foot. His knowledge of the effect of diabetes on infectious processes and his expertise in the use of sensitivity studies, the choice of antibiotics, and the route of administration may result in the control of infection and the ultimate saving of the foot and lower extremity.

Not too many years ago, when amputation was required, there was a tendency to do a rather extensive procedure based on the philosophy that patients with progressive vascular disease would eventually require surgery and therefore the first amputation should be the last. Today the approach is quite different. Surgical techniques are conservative. Debridement and minor amputations are used to preserve as much of the foot as possible and to keep the patient ambulatory. It has been possible to salvage a functional foot for many diabetics, even those with severe vascular and neurotrophic disease.

Despite advancement in diabetic foot care, however, amputation requiring a prosthesis is still a major problem. Over 80% of lower-extremity amputations in the civilian population are the result of vascular disease.* Based on several series it can be estimated that 50%† to 70%* of these amputations are in diabetics; therefore anyone who sees even a small number of diabetics will eventually be faced with the problem of amputation and subsequent rehabilitation. For this reason a thorough discussion of amputation techniques and orthopedic and rehabilitation management has been included in this book.

Perhaps the most important facet in the care of the diabetic foot is the education of the patient in the proper care of his very vulnerable foot. A foot can be lost from complications following a patient's careless home surgical attempts. Proper care of nails, calluses, corns, and other local foot problems can be accomplished only after the patient has been carefully instructed. At other times these tasks should be performed by the patient's physician, surgeon, or podiatrist. Today the podiatrist plays such a vital role in the care of the diabetic foot that every diabetes clinic should have one as a member of its staff.

Currently diabetes mellitus cannot be prevented, nor is there any significant means to prevent or control the development of its complications. When these complica-

---

*Mooney V, Harvey MP, McBride E, et al: Comparison of postoperative stump management: plaster versus soft dressings, *J Bone Joint Surg [Am]* 53:241, 1971.

†Warren R, Kihn RB: A survey of lower extremity amputations for ischemia, *Surgery* 63:107, 1968.

tions involve the diabetic's foot, they are frequently multiple and complex, requiring many medical skills for their management. The chapters in this monograph have been written by authorities in the fields of diabetes, vascular disease, neurology, vascular surgery, bacteriology, radiology, amputation techniques, orthopedics, rehabilitation, and podiatry. The book provides not only a fundamental background for understanding the pathogenesis of diabetic foot lesions but also includes a practical clinical approach to therapy for those involved in the care of the diabetic and his foot.

**Marvin E. Levin, M.D.**
**Lawrence W. O'Neal, M.D.**

# PREFACE TO FIFTH EDITION

The goal of this text has always been to decrease the incidence of foot ulcers and amputations. In the late 1960s and early 1970s the editors realized that the pathogenesis and management of diabetic foot problems were very complex and required multiple approaches. There was no single text devoted to this topic; those who wanted to learn about the diabetic foot had to consult several books. For this reason the first edition of *The Diabetic Foot* was created, comprising 10 chapters, with twelve contributors, and 262 pages. Over the past 20 years subsequent editions have addressed the complexities of the pathogenesis and management of the diabetic lower limb. Because of the many advances in the care of the foot of the diabetic, the fifth edition has become necessary to bring readers up to date. This fifth edition has 28 chapters, with 57 contributors, and more than 600 pages. The number of color plates has been increased to 31.

Included in this text are new chapters on epidemiology and dermatology. The increasing understanding of foot biomechanics and abnormal foot pressures has necessitated two new chapters. New approaches to wound healing are also addressed in this edition, including special dressings, hyperbaric oxygen therapy, and topically applied wound healing growth factors. Because there is a higher incidence and prevalence of foot problems in minorities, a chapter on this topic is included. Appropriate footwear for the diabetic has always been a problem, and a chapter on the role of the pedorthist rounds out this area. Because the orthopedist plays such an important role in the management of the diabetic foot, John H. Bowker, a specialist in this area and the newest editor, has added an important chapter to this text.

Frequently in the front line of caring for the foot of the diabetic is the podiatrist. Podiatrists frequently make the diagnosis, educate the patient in proper foot care, and perform prophylactic and surgical procedures. Podiatrists have made significant contributions to past editions of this text. The number of contributing podiatrists to this edition has increased to seven.

The diabetic population is becoming more sophisticated and knowledgeable about the disease and their care. Therefore, when a foot lesion does not heal or becomes larger, infection is not controlled, or amputation, becomes necessary, diabetic patients frequently question whether they have received proper care. Because of this, an increasing number of malpractice cases have resulted. A chapter on how to address legal issues related to the diabetic foot has been added.

Because the diabetic population is growing and aging, the magnitude of diabetic foot problems is increasing. Approximately

60,000 major amputations related to diabetes are performed in the United States every year. The annual cost of these amputations is more than $1 billion, not including surgeons' fees, rehabilitation costs, prostheses, time lost from work, and disability payments. Nevertheless, our original goal of reducing the number of amputations is being achieved in the hospitals, clinics, and offices where the care of the diabetic foot is comprehensively approached. This includes aggressive treatment of foot ulcers, use of special shoes, appropriate consultation, regular examination of the patient's feet, and education of the patient in foot care. These approaches, discussed in detail in this edition, have reduced amputation rates by 50% and more. This is an achievable goal. We hope our updated text will help physicians and other health care professionals to continue to decrease the number of foot ulcers and amputations.

**Marvin E. Levin, M.D.**
**Lawrence W. O'Neal, M.D.**
**John H. Bowker, M.D.**

# CONTENTS

# CHAPTER 1

# Epidemiology of the Diabetic Foot

**Gayle E. Reiber, M.P.H., Ph.D.**

Many of the estimated 14 million persons in the United States with diagnosed or undiagnosed diabetes will experience pathologic changes in their lower extremities, which when combined with minor trauma and infection may lead to serious foot problems. In this chapter the epidemiology of the diabetic foot is presented focusing on the major outcomes, lower extremity ulcers, and amputations. The chapter begins with general epidemiologic considerations for evaluating diabetic foot data. Next, select population-based analytic and experimental data are presented that describe the epidemiology and risk factors for lower extremity ulcers and amputations. Analytic and experimental diabetic foot studies provide more robust information and allow findings to be generalized to similar populations, a feature not possible with case-series studies; thus they are emphasized in this chapter. Information on subsequent amputation and mortality experience is briefly reviewed, and the chapter concludes with economic considerations.

## GENERAL EPIDEMIOLOGY

The full extent of the U.S. diabetic foot problem is unknown, because these heterogeneous pathologic conditions are not uniformly classified or reported. The most commonly described diabetic foot conditions include neuropathy, structural deformities, calluses, skin and nail changes, foot ulcers, infection, and vascular disease.[1, 21, 37] Al-

though several foot pathology classification systems have been published,[18, 33, 53, 63] a systematic and widely accepted diabetic foot classification with the ability to grade structural and select physiologic characteristics is needed for clinical, research, and surveillance purposes.[52]

The extent of the diabetic foot problem as described in U.S. hospital discharge data includes annual estimates of civilian, noninstitutionalized, hospitalized individuals. However, the ability to track an individual from year to year is limited by the population sampling strategies used.[48] Absent from this source are data from the 172 Veterans Affairs (VA) hospitals and numerous military hospitals. Further limitations of diabetic foot surveillance data include underreporting of diabetes status on hospital discharge abstracts, absence of uniform outpatient data describing major foot problems, and the growing number of minor outpatient surgical procedures.

Lower extremity diabetic ulcers are identified by ICD (*International Classification of Diseases*, rev 9) code 250 for diabetes and code 707 for ulcer.[30] Other codes may be used in the presence of infection, peripheral vascular disease, or other conditions. The unequivocal end point amputation includes surgical procedures performed to remove a nonviable portion of a lower extremity (ICD codes 84.10 to 84.18, including toe, ray, transmetatarsal, Syme, below knee, above knee, and hip disarticulation amputations).[30] These surgical procedures are performed for multiple indications, including gangrene, peripheral arterial occlusion, nonhealing ulcers, severe soft tissue infections, and osteomylitis.

A variety of numerators and denominators have been used in published international reports on diabetic amputation, making summary and comparison of data difficult. Amputation numerator data are reported alternatively as number of patients or number of procedures. Data sources do not uniformly indicate whether an amputation represents the first amputation, first amputation to an extremity, revision of an amputation, or higher level amputation. Some reported amputation data include only major amputations (usually BK and above); others include all amputations. Published "diabetes amputation rates" use as denominators all persons with diabetes, those with diabetes in "at risk" age groups, or all persons regardless of diabetes status. If the indication for amputation is major trauma or malignancy, those patients should be excluded from diabetic amputation studies.

Awareness of these considerations may help the reader assess the strengths of available data.

## EPIDEMIOLOGY OF FOOT ULCERS

Foot disease is the most common complication of diabetes leading to hospitalization.[21, 34] In a controlled trial of 854 diabetic outpatients observed in the general medicine clinic of a large community hospital, the indications for hospitalization suggested that 16% of admissions over a 2-year period, and 23% of total hospital days were because of diabetic foot problems.[59] It is estimated that 15% of diabetic patients will develop an ulcer on the feet or ankles at some time during the disease course.[51] Outpatient studies have reported that diabetic ulcer healing rates, depending on ulcer classification, range from 57% to 94%.[2, 11, 15, 24] A majority of patients with wound healing failure will require subsequent surgery or amputation.

**TABLE 1–1.**

Population-Based Foot and Ulcer Findings From Selected Studies of Patients With Diabetes Mellitus

| Author | Population Studied | Clinical Assessment | Diabetes Type | | | Foot Ulcers | | | Neuropathy (%) |
| | | | IDDM | NIDDM | NS | History (%) | Current (%) | Annual Incidence per 100 | |
|---|---|---|---|---|---|---|---|---|---|
| Borssen et al.[6] | 375 patients from Umea County Sweden; age 15–50 yr | Yes | 298 | 77 | | 10 | 2 | | |
| Boulton et al.[8] | 811 patients from three cities in UK | Yes | 811 | | | 5 | 1 | | 42 |
| Moss et al.[46] | Cohort of 2,990 patients with late- and early-onset diabetes | Partial | 1,210 | 1,780 | | | | 2.5 | |
| Rosenqvist[57] | 617 patients from Stockholm County, Sweden | No | | | X | 4 | | | |

*IDDM = insulin-dependent diabetes mellitus, NIDDM = non-insulin-dependent diabetes mellitus, NS = not stated.*

**TABLE 1–2.**

Risk Factors for Development of Foot Ulcers in Patients With Diabetes Mellitus From Select Analytic and Experimental Studies

| Author | Population Studied | Diabetes Type | Long DM Duration | Neuropathy (vibration or pressure) | Low Ankle/Arm Index | Smoking History | High Hb A$_{1c}$ | Outpatient Education | Poorly Fitting Shoes |
|---|---|---|---|---|---|---|---|---|---|
| Boulton[7] | 135 clinic/ER patients | NS | + | + | 0 | | | | |
| Bakker and Drent[4] | 60 clinic patients | NS | | + | | | 0 | | |
| Delbridge et al.[12] | 80 clinic patients | NS | 0 | 0 | + | + | 0 | | |
| Litzelman et al.[39] | 306 clinic patients | NIDDM | | | | | | | + |
| Litzelman et al.[40, 41] | 396 clinic patients | NIDDM | | + | | + | + | | |
| Malone et al.[44] | 203 clinic patients | NS | | | | | | + | |
| Moss et al.[46] | Cohort of 2,990 patients with late- and early-onset diabetes | IDDM NIDDM | + | | | + in young | + | | |
| Sosenko et al.[61] | 314 clinic patients | NIDDM | + | + | | | 0 | | |

*IDDM = Insulin-dependent diabetes mellitus, NIDDM = non-insulin-dependent diabetes mellitus, NS = not stated, + = statistically significant association, 0 = no statistically significant association.*

A cross-sectional San Francisco VA study comparing diabetic individuals with and without prior ulcer or amputation reported a significantly increased frequency of hammertoe deformity, abnormal cutaneous pressure sensation, intermittent claudication, and low ankle brachial index.[26] A population-based Swedish study[6] of individuals with insulin-dependent (IDDM), non-insulin-dependent (NIDDM) diabetes mellitus, and without diabetes reported important differences among individuals by diabetes type, including hammertoes, callosities, and dry feet. In this study the prevalence of current and prior foot ulcers was 2% and 10%, respectively. A Wisconsin cohort study[46] reported the 4-year ulcer incidence for individuals diagnosed with early- and late-onset diabetes was 9.5% and 10.5%, respectively. Table 1–1 summarizes data from selected population-based diabetic foot studies on the history, prevalence, and incidence rates for diabetic foot ulcers. Risk factor data in Table 1–2 indicate pathophysiologic, behavioral, and education variables have been associated with development of foot ulcers.

## EPIDEMIOLOGY OF LOWER EXTREMITY AMPUTATIONS

Only a small fraction of foot lesions progress to the most severe diabetic foot complication, lower extremity amputation. The importance of amputation among diabetic patients has been described.[37] Provider, patient care, and educational strategies have been developed to assist agencies and practitioners realize the proposed 40% diabetic amputation reduction.[25]

Table 1–3 displays available population-based data on nontraumatic amputation for selected states and populations. Annual amputation incidence rates are considerably higher among patients with diabetes mellitus. The percentage of patients with diabetes among all individuals undergoing nontraumatic lower extremity amputations approximates 50% in VA and U.S. populations.[13, 62] State-specific age-adjusted risk for lower extremity amputation has been reported to be 15 to 40 times higher in diabetic compared with nondiabetic persons.[42, 47] Excluding military and VA hospitals, national hospital

**TABLE 1–3.**
Population-Based Nontraumatic Lower Lower Extremity Amputation Findings From Selected Studies of Patients With Diabetes Mellitus

| Investigation | | | Amputation Rates and % Amputations in Diabetics | | | Diabetes Specific Findings | |
|---|---|---|---|---|---|---|---|
| Author | Lower Extremity Amputation | Group Studied | Incidence of LEA in Nondiabetics (LEA/10,000 person-years) | Incidence of LEA in Diabetics LEA/10,000 person-years) | Percent Diabetes Among Patients with LEA | Percent Below-Knee and Above-Knee of Total LEA | Mean Duration of Hospital Stay (days) |
| U.S. Hospital discharge data[13] | Any | United States | | 57 | 50 | | |
| Goldman and Ellis[22] | Any | Rhode Island | 2.5 | 88 | 53 | 57 | 33 |
| Humphrey et al.[28] | First | Rochester, Minn. | | 35 | 50 | | |
| Lindegard et al.[38] | Major | Gotland and Umea, Sweden | | | 54 | | |
| Washington State diabetes program[42] | Any | Washington | 1.0 | 52 | 53 | | |
| Miller et al.[45] | Any | New Jersey | | 77 | 63 | 56 | 40 |
| Most and Sinnock[47] | Any | United States; 6 million | 2.0 | 58 | 45 | 65 | 30 |
| Nelson et al.[49] | First | Pima Indians | 1.3 | 137 | 95 | 16 | |
| Wright and Kaplan[65] | Any | California | 1.2 | 47 | 55 | 62 | 21 |
| VA Hospital discharge data[62] | Any | Veterans Administration | | | 50 | 55 | |

LEA = Lower extremity amputation.

**TABLE 1–4.**

Nontraumatic Lower Extremity Amputations, VA Hospitals, Fiscal Years 1986–1990*

| Fiscal yr | Procedures in Patients With DM | | Procedures in Patients Without DM | |
|---|---|---|---|---|
| | Amputation ICD 84.10–84.18 | Revision ICD 843 | Amputation ICD 84.10–84.18 | Revision ICD 843 |
| 1986 | 9,944 | 1,384 | 8,516 | 1,322 |
| 1987 | 8,942 | 1,367 | 8,407 | 1,354 |
| 1988 | 8,910 | 1,323 | 8,296 | 1,288 |
| 1989 | 8,638 | 1,229 | 7,997 | 1,190 |
| 1990 | 8,551 | 1,159 | 7,899 | 1,128 |
| Total | 44,985 | 6,462 | 41,115 | 6,282 |
| Average | 8,997 | 1,292 | 8,223 | 1,256 |

*J. Taylor, Department of Veterans Affairs, personal communication, 1992.
DM = Diabetes mellitus, ICD = International Classification of Disease codes[30]

discharge data in 1990[13] indicated that 54,000 diabetic patients had at least one amputation. Although the actual number of patients in the United States undergoing at least one nontraumatic diabetic amputation per year increased 70%, from 31,700 in 1979 to 54,000 in 1990, the age-adjusted rates fluctuated between 5.1 and 8.6 per 1,000 persons with diabetes,[13] and overall the trend in age-adjusted amputation rates

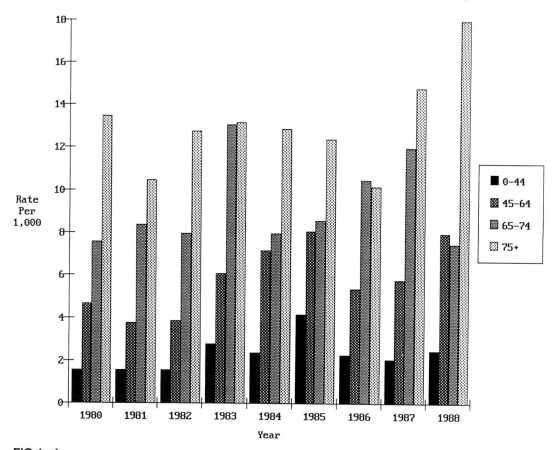

**FIG 1–1.**
Civilian hospital discharge rates for nontraumatic lower extremity amputation per 1,000 diabetic patients, by age, 1980 to 1988. (*From* Diabetes surveillance: Annual report. *Atlanta, 1991, Centers for Disease Control, Division of Diabetes Translation.*)

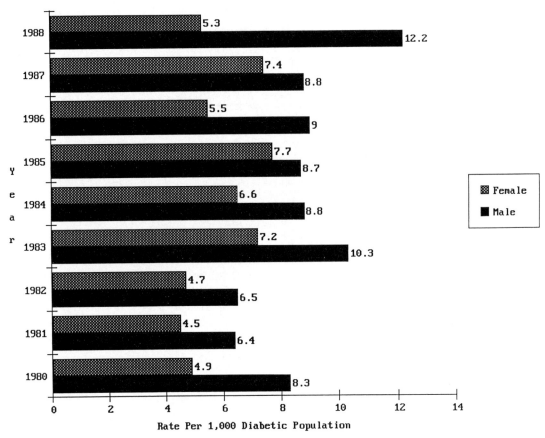

**FIG 1–2.**
Civilian age-adjusted hospital discharge rates for nontraumatic lower extremity amputation per 1,000 diabetic patients, by sex, 1980 to 1988. (*From* Diabetes surveillance: Annual report. *Atlanta, 1991, Centers for Disease Control, Division of Diabetes Translation.*)

showed no striking increase or decrease.

VA hospitals averaged 8,997 amputation procedures per year among persons with diabetes, and 8,223 amputation procedures among persons without diabetes during fiscal years 1986 to 1990.[62] In both groups the average number of amputation revisions per year approximated 1,300. Table 1–4 shows a modest reduction in the number of amputations and revisions across these surgical procedures by diabetes status for VA hospitals. These data are limited in that they reflect procedures rather than patients. They do, however, suggest that as many as 15% of amputations in the United States may be performed in VA hospitals.

## Demographic Findings

### Age

Diabetic amputation rates are reported to increase with advancing age.[13, 22, 28, 42] To quantify the risk of age on lower extremity amputations using 1988 U.S. hospital discharge data, diabetic patients aged from birth to 44 years were used as the baseline, and the increased amputation risk for ages 45 to 64 years and ages 65 to 74 years was threefold, whereas for individuals age 75 years or older the risk increased more than seven times.[13] Figure 1–1 shows the U.S. hospital discharge summary rates for amputation from 1980 to 1988 by age. Proportional hazards analysis of population-based amputation data for Rochester, Minnesota, indicated that after adjusting for sex and year of diabetes diagnosis, each 10-year increase in age at diagnosis imparted a hazard ratio of 1.5 (95%, confidence interval [CI] 1.2–1.9).[28]

### Sex

Specific studies have reported elevated risk for amputation among males, ranging from 1.4 to 2.7.[22, 45, 47] As can be seen in Figure 1–2, after adjusting for age the 1980–1988 U.S. hospital discharge amputation rates are noticeably higher in males than in female patients. These data in 1988 indicated a 2.3-fold higher amputation risk in males compared with females. This higher risk was more pronounced in younger male patients.[13]

### Race

After adjusting for age, the U.S. hospital discharge rates for 1980 to 1988 (Fig 1–3) show that despite the annual variation, a higher rate exists among blacks than in whites.[13] In American Indians on the Gila River Reservation the overall amputation rate was 24.1 per 1,000 person-years, compared with 6.5/1,000 person-years for the general U.S. diabetic population.[49] Although nonwhite race has been associated with amputation more often than white

race, population-based findings have not been able to control for the potentially confounding effects of socioeconomic and health care factors.

### Geographic Region

Figure 1–4 shows the age-adjusted amputation rates by U.S. geographic region. Despite year-to-year variation, amputation rates tend to be lower in the West, and generally are higher in the Northeast.

### Amputation Risk Factors Identified in Analytic and Experimental Studies

Several recent studies provide solid information on amputation risk factors. These are summarized in Table 1–5 for selected pathophysiologic, diabetes-specific, health care and health history, and social and behavioral factors.

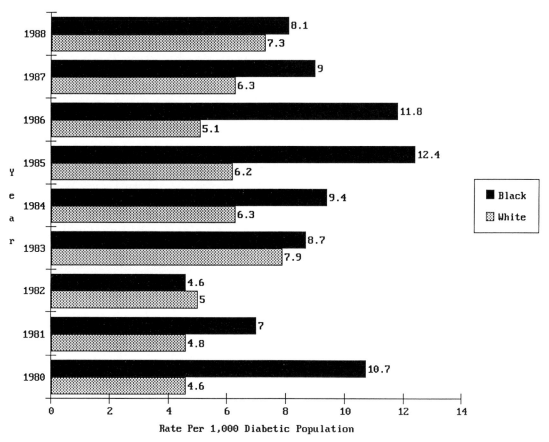

**FIG 1–3.**
Civilian age-adjusted hospital discharge rates for nontraumatic lower extremity amputation per 1,000 diabetic patients, white and black populations, 1980 to 1988. (*From* Diabetes surveillance: Annual report. *Atlanta, 1991, Centers for Disease Control, Division of Diabetes Translation.)*

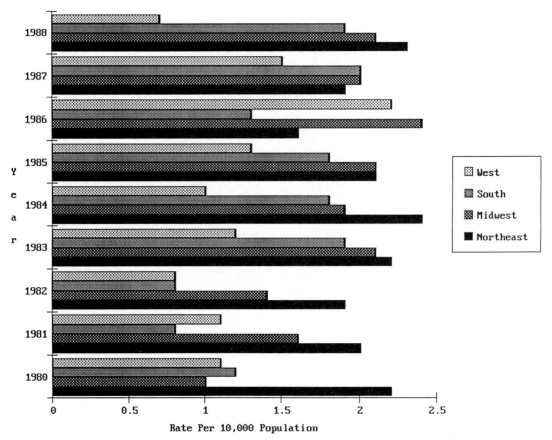

**FIG 1–4.**
Civilian age- and race-adjusted hospital discharge rate per 10,000 population, by U.S. region, 1980 to 1988. (*From* Diabetes surveillance: Annual report. *Atlanta, 1991, Centers for Disease Control, Division of Diabetes Translation.)*

## Pathophysiologic Risk Factors for Amputation

### *Peripheral Neuropathy*

Evidence for an association between neuropathy and lower extremity amputation was provided in two analytic studies. Impaired vibratory perception was a statistically significant risk factor for amputation after controlling for age, sex, and diabetes duration in the cohort study of Pima Indians[49] and the Seattle VA case-control study.[55] In the latter study the significance of this predisposing condition in terms of population-attributable risk was high because of the high prevalence of hypoesthesia among cases (78%) and controls (18%). Absence of patellar tendon reflexes also was associated with subsequent risk for amputations.[49] Although some vascular factors may

have higher estimated relative risk for amputation, they affect relatively fewer diabetic patients from the total at-risk population.

### *Impaired Cutaneous Circulation*

Circulatory insufficiency has been considered among the most important reasons for amputation for patients with or without diabetes who have severe peripheral vascular disease. However, until recently, clinicians have made little distinction between the relative adequacy of cutaneous circulation and its relationship to major arterial circulation. The literature regarding healing of surgical amputation sites strongly suggests that parameters that reflect principally arterial perfusion provide different clinical information regarding cutaneous circulation than do more direct techniques for

**TABLE 1–5.**
Risk Factors for Nontraumatic Lower Extremity Amputation in Individuals With Diabetes Mellitus Identified Through Analytic and Experimental Studies

| Author | Study Type; Group | Diabetes Type | Neuropathy | Cutaneous Circulation | Peripheral Vascular Neuropathy | History of Smoking | Hypertension | Total Cholesterol | High Hb $A_{1c}$ or Glucose | Outpatient Education | Self-Care | History of Ulcer | History of Retinopathy |
|---|---|---|---|---|---|---|---|---|---|---|---|---|---|
| Litzelman et al.[41] | Experimental; 398 clinic patients | NIDDM | | | | | | | | | + | | |
| Malone et al.[44] | Experimental; 203 clinic patients | NS | | | | | | | | + | | | |
| Moss et al.[46] | Cohort, 2,990 late and early onset | IDDM NIDDM | | | | + | + DBP Young | | + | | | + | + |
| Nelson et al.[49] | Cohort, 4,399 Pima Indians | NIDDM | + | + | | 0 | 0 | 0 | + | | | | + |
| Reiber et al.[55] | Case-control, Seattle VA hospital | IDDM NIDDM | + | + | + | 0 | 0 | 0 | + | | | + | + |

DPB = diastolic blood pressure, IDDM = Insulin-dependent diabetes mellitus, NIDDM = non-insulin-dependent diabetes mellitus, + = statistically significant association, 0 = no statistically significant association assessing this compartment.[9, 10, 50, 51] Furthermore, there is evidence that adequate cutaneous perfusion not only depends on the underlying arterial circulation but may be critically influenced by other factors, including skin integrity, mechanical effects of repetitive pressure, and presence of tissue edema.

Cutaneous circulation (measured using transcutaneous oxygen tension, $TcPo_2$), reflects oxygen diffusion across the skin barrier resulting from tissue equilibration after capillary delivery and tissue utilization at the dermis.[17] $TcPo_2$ values associated with below-knee amputation healing potential suggest that values less than 20 mm Hg are associated with poor healing, 20 to 40 mm Hg with intermediate healing potential, and greater than 40 mm Hg with high likelihood of healing.[66] Findings reported from the Seattle VA study showed that average below-knee and dorsal foot values less than 20 mm Hg when compared with the 40 mm Hg reference group yielded an odds ratio of 161 (95%, CI 55–469), whereas for those between 20 and 40 mm Hg the odds ratio was 7.5 (CI 4.0–14.1).[55] This association persisted after controlling for the potentially confounding effects of age, race, duration, diabetes type, socioeconomic status, and diabetes severity.

### Impaired Major Peripheral Arterial Circulation

Atherosclerosis obliterans defined by the presence of intermittent claudication was reported in the Framingham Study to be 3.8 and 6.5 times more common in diabetic than in nondiabetic males and females, respectively.[32] Mayo Clinic data indicated that arteriosclerosis obliterans, defined as peripheral pulse deficit, was present in 8% of subjects at diabetes diagnosis, 15% after 10 years, and 45% after 20 years of clinical diabetes.[51] In subjects in the University Group Diabetes Study, although the predicted 13-year cumulative risk for intermittent claudication was 38% and 24%, respectively, for male and females subjects, intermittent claudication seldom led to amputation.[35] Doppler ankle arm index (normal range ≥0.90) measured in the

Seattle VA study compared patients with values less than 0.45 with those greater than 0.70 and found the amputation odds ratio for amputation to be 55.8 (95%, CI 15–209).[55]

Cigarette smoking, lipoprotein abnormalities, and hypertension are major alterable risk factors that have been implicated in development of atherosclerosis in nondiabetic subjects,[23] and are assumed to be similarly atherogenic in diabetic populations.[17, 31] The prevalence of smoking in the United States is well described in numerous publications, although separate prevalence figures for patients with diabetes are not provided.[58, 60] Several authors have reported no consistent relationship, either positive or negative, between smoking and diabetes itself.[31] Although many studies, including the Framingham Study, show a relationship between smoking and coronary heart disease, intermittent claudication, and arteriosclerosis obliterans, direct evidence is more limited for the effect of smoking on lower leg lesions and amputation in diabetes.[20, 32, 42]

Smoking was a statistically significant risk factor for amputation in the Indianapolis study,[41] of borderline significance in the Wisconsin study,[46] but not significant in two other analytic studies measuring this association,[49, 55] although a low smoking prevalence was reported among Pima Indians.[49]

Some researchers have questioned the role of hypertension in amputation, stating that lesions related to arteriosclerotic changes more likely were a result of increased weight and age and further postulating that hypertension may be an isolated or independent risk factor,[31] an association not confirmed by others.[49, 55]

Lipoprotein abnormalities may be more prevalent among diabetic individuals, including elevated plasma triglyceride levels, and decreased very low-density, low-density lipoprotein levels, and high-density lipoprotein levels. Although lipoprotein abnormalities have been associated with macrovascular disease in diabetics, there are scant data to evaluate direct effects on risk for amputation. Two analytic studies examined the possible effect of serum cholesterol level on amputation risk and reported no statistically significant association between increasing levels of total cholesterol and amputation.[49, 55] However low levels of high-density lipoprotein subfraction 3 have been reported as statistically significant risk factors for amputation.[55] In general, the risk factors for peripheral arterial disease established in nondiabetic subjects need to be further examined together with metabolic and diabetes-specific factors for accurate amputation risk assessment in diabetic patients.

## Diabetes-Specific Factors

### Diabetes Type

Diabetes is a heterogeneous disorder with differing causes, requirements for treatment, and manifestations of IDDM and NIDDM.[16] For clinical and research purposes, characterizing diabetes by type is important,[35] although precise classification may be problematic because of lack of an unequivocal marker. Four-year amputation incidence for both early- and late-onset diabetes was 2.2% in the Wisconsin cohort study.[46] In the population-based Rochester study, amputation risk was higher for NIDDM than for IDDM (35.6 vs. 28.3 per 10,000 patients).[28] The Seattle VA study indicated that the odds ratio comparing IDDM with NIDDM was 1.7; however, the confidence interval included 1. Other analytic or experimental studies with information on diabetes type used exclusively patients with NIDDM.[35, 44, 49]

### Glycemic Control

Many investigators have postulated that the presence of chronic hyperglycemia accelerates development of chronic complications of diabetes.[36, 56] The glycemic control-amputation relationship was addressed by West,[64] who found among patients with diabetes and higher blood glucose levels a two-fold increased risk for leg lesions, including gangrene, than in those with lower blood glucose concentrations. Findings in three analytic studies demonstrated statistically significant increased amputation

risk with elevated plasma glucose levels, 2-hour postload findings, or glycated hemoglobin.[46, 49, 55] The availability of health care should be evaluated as a potential confounding factor when the relationship between glycemic control and amputation relationship is assessed.

### Clinical Duration of Diabetes

Clinical duration of diabetes represents the time from diabetes diagnosis to the time of study. Although diabetes diagnosis usually marks the onset of "clinical duration," disease processes could have been ongoing prior to diagnosis, particularly in NIDDM. After adjustment for age and sex, clinical duration of diabetes remained a statistically significant risk for lower extremity amputation in two analytic studies.[46, 49]

## Health Care Factors and Health History

Measures reflecting availability and parameters of health care have been addressed directly and found to be significant factors in experimental and analytic amputation studies.[41, 44, 55] Prior history of lower extremity ulcers was a strong risk factor in several studies.[46, 55] A positive history of retinopathy also was strongly associated with amputation in three of these studies.[46, 49, 55]

### Outpatient Diabetes Education

Major international diabetes patient education efforts have been mounted over the last 10 years to provide patients with information and skills to better manage their diabetes.[3] Strong associations have emerged in an experimental and case-control study showing a threefold increased risk in subjects who did not receive targeted foot or general outpatient diabetes education.[44, 55] Patient education provided at the time of diabetes diagnosis and in hospital settings did not show the same effectiveness as formal outpatient diabetes education closer to the time of actual risk for amputation.[55] In the Indianapolis experimental study the educated intervention group was significantly more likely to report appropriate foot care behaviors than the control group.[41]

## Social Connectedness

Social ties have been suggested to increase a person's resistance to physical illness. Adequate support by the family or community may enhance the attention to health problems. Conversely, lack of social and community support has been associated with increased overall mortality.[27] One study quantified an increased amputation risk in the absence of family support, social networks, or other social support.[55]

## REAMPUTATION, CONTRALATERAL AMPUTATION, AND SUBSEQUENT MORTALITY

Statewide hospital discharge data for California and New Jersey, excluding patients who may have had multiple amputation during their index hospitalization, indicated that, respectively, 13% and 9% of patients required a subsequent amputation in separate hospitalizations within the year.[45, 65] The ability to track a patient's ulcer and amputation history over many years is a limitation of current U.S. hospital discharge data. Additional population-based research is needed to quantify "events" during the time interval that spans lower extremity disease.

Descriptive studies have reported that approximately 30% to 50% of amputees will undergo contralateral limb amputation within 1 to 3 years of the initial amputation.[5, 37] There has been little improvement over the last two decades in preventing this morbidity.[37] Even in those patients who have undergone an initial amputation, the obvious increased risk for subsequent amputation is not uniformly translated into preventive patient and provider care actions. More programs like the Department of Veterans Affairs Special Team for Amputation, Mobility and Prosthetics/Orthotics (STAMP) program, instituted in eight regional medical centers, are needed to diminish postamputation morbidity and mortality in these high-risk patients.

In-hospital mortality was reported at 10% in the 3-year statewide New Jersey amputation study.[45] Reported in-hospital mortality has declined in case-series reports, from as high as 50% in the mid-1930s to 1.5% in the mid-1980s.[37] Higher overall mortality has been reported for diabetic amputees than for other patients with diabetes.[49] Factors such as comorbidity, disease severity, and age should be considered in future population-based studies of postamputation survival.

## ECONOMIC CONSIDERATIONS

Although the actual cost of diabetic foot problems in the United States is not known, various studies provide helpful information on utilization and cost, particularly for ulcers and amputations. The U.S. economic costs of NIDDM estimated that in 1986 "chronic skin ulcers" alone accounted for $150 million of the $11.6 billion direct costs related to this disease.[29] Costs were not reported similarly for peripheral neuropathy, peripheral vascular disease, or amputation. A Southern California referral hospital computed costs for 94 patients undergoing lower extremity bypass graft procedures (35% with diabetes) and 53 undergoing primary below the knee amputation (56% with diabetes). The average cost (in 1985 dollars) was $23,500 for each patient having bypass surgery, compared with $24,700 for those undergoing primary amputation; and the duration of hospital stay averaged 17.6 and 21.0 days, respectively.[54]

Statewide California hospital discharge data, excluding military and VA data, indicated the average cost and duration of stay for a nontraumatic diabetic amputation in 1987 to be $20,085 and 19.3 days, respectively.[65] The Medstat System[14] reported in fiscal year 1989 on health care claims for 3.1 million patients whose health benefits were provided by large employers. Their average cost for diagnosis-related group (DRG) 113 (lower extremity amputation) was $33,771, with the average duration of hospitalization 26 days. The fiscal year 1989 Health Care Finance Administration report on Medicare data indicated that there were 32,597 bills for DRG 113, averaging 18.3 days duration of stay. The average charge per bill was $15,684, whereas the average reimbursement was only 54% of that total, or $8,457; however, all costs of care, including rehabilitation, prosthetics, and orthotics, may not be reflected in these figures.

Costs were reported in a follow-up study of 106 patients (diabetes status unreported), with limb-threatening ischemia treated at a New England medical center.[43] The average cumulative cost of care was $40,769 for a lower extremity bypass procedure with an average follow-up of 2.2 years, compared with $40,563 for an amputation with follow-up averaging 1.8 years, although severity of lower extremity ischemia differed among patients undergoing these procedures. After presenting information on charges and costs, the authors concluded that DRG reimbursement closely approximated current cost (73.6% times charge), or $19,932 for reconstruction and $19,241 for amputation.[43]

## SUMMARY

The epidemiologic data presented in this review of diabetic foot problems suggests a heterogeneous, multifactorial problem of considerable magnitude. Available analytic and experimental studies provide valuable information, although other possible foot ulcer and amputation risk factors have not received adequate study.

This review suggests that clear numerator and denominator definitions must be stated for future foot ulcer and amputation ascertainment, surveillance, and research. Measuring and stratifying by socioeconomic status will be important to better understand the race-amputation relationship. A variety of studies suggest that pathophysiologic risk factors for diabetic ulcers and amputation extend beyond neuropathy, vascular disease, and infection. Although impaired cutaneous circulation and failed wound healing have not been studied adequately, available evidence indicates that they confer major risk for amputation in diabetes. Additional research is needed to assess concurrently the underlying pathophysiologic factors and

their interactions with other important exposures.

Interrelationships between diabetes-specific factors, such as diabetes type, duration, and disease severity, and other biomedical factors, such as age and weight, and their position in the chain of causation leading to ulcer and amputation, need investigation. Risk factors from health care and history and from social and behavioral categories suggest there may be multiple nonphysiologic exposures that may lend themselves to modification and ulcer or amputation prevention. Evidence supporting the reduction in risk with patient education and self-care is encouraging. This type of information provides a scientific basis for productive interventions by both care providers and patients with diabetes to prevent or delay limb ulcers and amputations.

## REFERENCES

1. American Diabetes Association: Foot care in patients with diabetes mellitus, *Diabetes Care* 14(suppl 2):18–19, 1991.

2. Apelqvist J, et al: Wound classification is more important that site of ulceration in the outcome of diabetic foot ulcers, *Diabetic Med* 6:526–530, 1989.

3. Assal JP, et al: Patient education as the basis for diabetes care in clinical practice and research, *Diabetologia* 28:602–613, 1985.

4. Bakker K, Drent ML: Foot ulceration in relation to risk factors and complications in type II diabetes mellitus, *Diabetes* 40(suppl 1):3555A, 1991.

5. Bodily KC, Burgess EM: Contralateral limb and patient survival after leg amputation, *Am J Surg* 146:280–282, 1983.

6. Borssen B, Bergenheim T, Lithner: The epidemiology of foot lesions in diabetic patients aged 15–50 years, *Diabetic Med* 7:438–444, 1991.

7. Boulton AJM: Impaired vibratory perception and diabetic foot ulceration, *Diabetic Med* 3:335–337, 1986.

8. Boulton AJM, et al: High prevalence of risk factors for ulceration in type 2 diabetic patients: a population based study, *Diabetologia* (in press).

9. Christensen KS, et al: Results of amputation for gangrene in diabetic and nondiabetic patients, *J Bone Joint Surg* 70A:1514–1519, 1988.

10. Cina C, et al: Utility of transcutaneous oxygen tension measurements in peripheral arterial occlusive disease, *J Vasc Surg* 1:362–371, 1984.

11. Crausaz S, et al: Additional factors associated

with plantar ulcers in diabetic neuropathy, *Diabetic Med* 5:771–775, 1988.

12. Delbridge L, et al: Factors associated with development of foot lesions in the diabetic, *Surgery* 93:78–82, 1983.

13. *Diabetes surveillance.* Atlanta, 1991, Centers for Disease Control, Division of Diabetes Translation.

14. *DRG Guide.* Ann Arbor, Mich, Medstat Systems.

15. Edmonds ME, et al: Improved survival of the diabetic foot: the role of a specialized foot clinic, *Q J Med* 60:763–771, 1986.

16. Fajans SS, Cloutier MC, Crowther RL: Clinical and etiologic heterogeneity of idiopathic diabetes mellitus, *Diabetes* 27:1112–1125, 1978.

17. Faris I, Duncan H: Vascular disease and vascular function in the lower limb in diabetes, *Diabetes Res* 1:171–177, 1984.

18. Forrest RD, Gamborg-Nielsen P: Wound assessment in clinical practice—a critical review of methods and their application, *Acta Med Scand* 687:69–74, 1984.

19. Franzeck UK, et al: Transcutaneous $PO_2$ measurements in health and peripheral arterial occlusive disease, *Surgery* 91:156–163, 1982.

20. Garcia MJ, et al: Morbidity and mortality in diabetics in the Framingham population—sixteen year follow-up study, *Diabetes* 23:105–111, 1974.

21. Gibbons G, Eliopolos G: Infection of the diabetic foot, in Kozak G, et al, editors: *Management of diabetic foot problems*, Philadelphia, 1984, WB Saunders, pp 97–102.

22. Goldman D, Ellis S: Centers for Disease Control cooperative agreement No U32/CCU100351-08, Providence, Rhode Island Department of Health, 1988, p 76.

23. Gordon T, Kannel WB: The Framingham study: predisposition to atherosclerosis in the head, heart and legs, *JAMA* 221:661–666, 1972.

24. Hawkins ES, Birke JA: Diabetic foot ulcer healing rates, personal communication, Hansen's Disease Center, 1992.

25. *Healthy people 2000: National health promotion and disease prevention objectives.* (DHHS publ no (PHS)91-50213.) Rockville, Md, 1991, US Government Printing Office, pp 73, 117.

26. Holewski J, et al: Prevalence of foot pathology and lower extremity complications in a diabetic outpatient clinic, *J Rehabil Res Dev* 26(3):35–44, 1989.

27. House JS, Robbins C, Metzner H: The association of social relationships and activities with mortality: prospective evidence from the Tecumseh Community Health Study, *Am J Epidemiol* 116:123–140, 1982.

28. Humphrey LL, et al: The epidemiology of lower extremity amputation in diabetics: a population-based study in Rochester, Minnesota, *Diabetes* 2(suppl):33A, 1989.

29. Huse DM, et al: The economic cost of non-insulin dependent diabetes mellitus, *JAMA* 262:2708–2713, 1989

30. *International Classification of Diseases, Ninth Revision: Clinical Modifications* (ICD 9 CM), vol 3, ed 2 (DHHS publ no (PHS)80-1260). Rockville, Md, 1980, US Government Printing Office, p 235.

31. Jarrett RJ, Keen H: Diabetes and atherosclerosis, in Keen H, Jarrett RJ, editors: *Complications of diabetes*, London, 1975, Edward Arnold Publishing, pp 179–204.

32. Kannel WB, McGee DL: Diabetes and cardiovascular disease: the Framingham study, *JAMA* 241:2035–2038, 1979.

33. Knighton DR, et al: Classification and treatment of chronic nonhealing wounds: successful treatment with autologous platelet-derived wound healing factors (PDWHF), *Ann Surg* 204:322–329, 1986.

34. Kozak GP: Diabetic foot disease: a major problem, in *Management of diabetic foot problems*, Philadelphia, 1984, WB Saunders, pp 1–8.

35. Kreines K, et al: The course of peripheral vascular disease in non-insulin dependent diabetes, *Diabetes Care* 8:235–243, 1985.

36. Kroc Collaborative Study Group: Blood glucose control and the evolution of diabetic retinopathy and albuminuria: a preliminary multicenter trial, *N Engl J Med* 311:365–372, 1984.

37. Levin ME: The diabetic foot: pathophysiology, evaluation and treatment, in Levin ME, O'Neal LW, editors: *The diabetic foot*, 4 ed, St Louis, 1988, Mosby–Year Book, pp 1–50.

38. Lindegard P, Jonsson B, Lithner F: Amputations in diabetic patients in Gotland and Umea Counties, 1971–1980, *Acta Med Scand* 687(suppl):89–93, 1984.

39. Litzelman DK, et al: Prevention of diabetic foot complications, *Clin Res* 38:7228A, 1990.

40. Litzelman DK, et al: Risk factors for foot lesions in persons with diabetes, *Clin Res* 39:746A, 1991.

41. Litzelman DK, Slemenda CW, Langefeld CD: Lower extremity amputation risk reduction in persons with diabetes, *Clin Res* 39:581A, 1991.

42. *Lower extremity amputations among people with diabetes, Washington State 1985–1988.* Olympia, Washington State Department of Health Diabetes Control Program, 1991.

43. Mackey WC, et al: The costs of surgery for limb-threatening ischemia, *Surgery* 99:26–35, 1986.

44. Malone JM, et al: Prevention of amputation by diabetic education, *Am J Surg*, 158:520–524, 1989.

45. Miller AD, et al: Diabetes-related lower extremity amputations in New Jersey, 1979 to 1981, *J Med Soc NJ* 82:723–726, 1985.

46. Moss SE, Klein R, Klein B: The prevalence and incidence of lower extremity amputation in a dia-

betic population, *Arch Intern Med* 152:610–615, 1992.

47. Most RS, Sinnock P: The epidemiology of lower extremity amputations in diabetic individuals, *Diabetes Care* 6:87–91, 1983.

48. National Center for Health Statistics, Hospital Care Statistics Branch: 1987 Summary: National Hospital Discharge Survey. *Advance Data. Vital Health Stat* 1988; 159(rev):12. (DHHS publ no (PHS)88–1250).

49. Nelson RG, et al: Lower-extremity amputations in NIDDM: 12-yr follow-up study in Pima Indians, *Diabetes Care* 11:8–16, 1988.

50. Oishi CS, Fronek A, Golbranson FL: The role of non-invasive vascular studies in determining levels of amputation, *J Bone Joint Surg* 70A:1520–1530, 1988.

51. Palumbo, PJ, Melton, LJ: Peripheral vascular disease and diabetes, in MI Harris, RF Hamman, editors: *Diabetes in America.* NIH pub no 85-1468. Bethesda, Md, 1985, National Institutes of Health, p XV 1–21.

52. Pecoraro RE: Diabetic skin ulcer classification for clinical investigations, *Clin Materials* 8:257–262, 1991.

53. Pecoraro RE, Reiber GE: Classification of wounds in diabetic amputees, *Wounds* 2:65–73, 1990.

54. Raviola CA, et al: Cost of treating advanced leg ischemia—bypass graft vs primary amputation, *Arch Surg* 123:495–496, 1988.

55. Reiber GE, Pecoraro RE, Koepsell TD: Risk factors for amputation in patients with diabetes mellitus: a case-control study, *Ann Intern Med* 117:97–105, 1992.

56. Riechard P, et al: The Stockholm Diabetes Intervention Study (SDIS): 18 months' results, *Acta Medica Scand* 224:115–22, 1988.

57. Rosenqvist U: An epidemiological survey of diabetic foot problems in the Stockholm County 1982, *Acta Med* 687(suppl):55–60, 1984.

58. Shopland DR, Brown C: Toward the 1990 objectives for smoking: measuring the progress with 1985 NHIS Data, *Public Health Rep* 102:68–73, 1987.

59. Smith D, Weinberger M, Katz B: A controlled trial to increase office visits and reduce hospitalizations of diabetic patients, *J Gen Intern Med* 2:232–238, 1987.

60. *Smoking and health: A report of the Surgeon General.* Department of Health Education and Welfare DHEW (DHEW publ no (PHS)79-50066 1979.

61. Sosenko J, et al: Comparison of quantitative sensory threshold measures for their association with foot ulceration in diabetic patients, *Diabetes Care* 13:1057–1061, 1990.

62. Taylor J, Department of Veterans Affairs, personal communication, 1992.

63. Wagner FW: A classification and treatment program for diabetic, neuropathic, and dysvascular foot problems, in *The American Academy of Orthopaedic Surgeons instructional course lectures,* St Louis, 1979, Mosby–Year Book, pp 143–165.

64. West KM: *Epidemiology of diabetes and its vascular lesions,* New York, 1978, Elsevier.

65. Wright, WE, Kaplan, GA: Trends in lower extremity amputations California, 1983–1987, in *California chronic and sentinel diseases surveillance program resource document,* Sacramento, 1989, California Department of Health Services.

66. Wyss CR, et al: Transcutaneous oxygen tension as a predictor of success after an amputation, *J Bone Joint Surg* 70A:1514–1519, 1988.

67. Wyss CR, et al: Transcutaneous oxygen tension measurements on limbs of diabetic and nondiabetic patients with peripheral vascular disease, *Surgery* 95:339–346, 1984.

# CHAPTER 2

# Pathogenesis and Management of Diabetic Foot Lesions

**Marvin E. Levin, M.D.**

Diabetes is one of the oldest diseases known to mankind. The Ebers Papyrus of 1500 BC mentions its symptoms and suggests treatment. Moreover, the history of gangrene of the foot was known in Biblical times, when the first case, perhaps due to diabetes, was described:

In the 39th year of his reign, King Asa became affected with gangrene of his feet; he did not seek guidance from the Lord but resorted to physicians. He rested with his forefathers in the 41st year of his reign. (*Chronicles XVI:12–14*)

Whether King Asa had diabetic gangrene is a moot point. Certainly in Biblical times there was not much one could do for a foot lesion but pray. By the 1500s healing continued to depend on prayer alone. The famous surgeon Ambroise Paré (1510–1590) said, "I dressed [the wound] and God healed him." Today the skills of multiple medical disciplines are significantly reducing amputation rates. With increasing awareness of diabetic foot problems and improved treatment, amputation rates will continue to decrease.

The human foot is a mechanical marvel. It consists of 26 bones, 29 joints, 42 muscles, and a multitude of tendons and ligaments. In a lifetime this phenomenal machine with its multiple moveable parts walks between 75,000 and 100,000 miles, three to four times around the world, and is exposed to significant pressures with each step. In the diabetic patient, particularly those with ulceration, the foot is exposed to unusually high pressures (see Chapter 10). Foot problems are common in the population at large. However, the diabetic patient is especially vulnerable because of the frequent complications of peripheral neuropathy, infection, and peripheral vascular disease (PVD). This triad leads to the final cataclysmic events, gangrene and amputation. More than 56,000 major amputations were reported in 1987 in the United States.[76] Fifty percent of all nontraumatic amputations are performed because of diabetes. Multiple epidemiologic factors are associated with diabetic foot problems and amputation (see Chapter 1). Suffice it to say that of all complications of diabetes, those involving the foot are the most common. Bild et al.[12] reported the annual incidence of leg and foot ulcers to be 200,000, diabetic coronary artery disease 101,000, stroke 27,000, blindness 6,900, and kidney failure 5,900. The diabetic patient most likely to develop a foot lesion is older than 40 years. Today 90% of diabetic patients in the United States are in this age group.[36] Fifteen percent of all diabetics will develop a foot ulcer during their lifetime.[96] Most of these ulcers are the result of peripheral neuropathy leading to an insensate foot, which is then vulnerable to painless trauma and ulceration. Peripheral neuropathy is extremely common in the type I diabetes, with the incidence gradually increasing with age and duration. After 20 years duration of diabetes, 42% of patients have clinical evidence of peripheral neuropathy.[94]

PVD is present at diagnosis in 8% of diabetic patients, in 15% after 10 years, and in 42% after 20 years.[85] Kreines et al.[63] have reviewed the natural history of PVD in type II non-insulin-dependent diabetes mellitus (NIDDM) and found similar results. Twenty percent of diabetics who enter the hospital do so because of foot problems.[14] Thirty percent have symptomatic PVD, and 7% require vascular surgery and/or amputation.[14]

The long- and short-term prognosis for the diabetic undergoing amputation has always been poor. In the preantibiotic era the principal cause of in-hospital mortality in patients with diabetic gangrene was toxemia and infection.[78] With the availability of antibiotics and newer management techniques a mortality rate of 50% in the 1930s[68] is now in the range of 1.5% to 3%.[15, 43] McDermott and Rogers[82] stated that curing all cancers would add just 2 years to the life expectancy for Americans, but the introduction of antibiotics has added 10 years.

Postoperative morbidity is a frequent occurrence in these patients. Fearon et al.[43] found local complication rates of 18% and systemic complication rates of 36%, including gastrointestinal hemorrhage, myocardial infarction, congestive heart failure, and cerebral vascular accident. In the diabetic the major postoperative concern is not the operative site but control of blood glucose and management of medical problems, such as cardiac and renal complications. These require the constant attention of trained medical personnel. It is my strong opinion that any diabetic patient undergoing surgery should be returned to the medical division for systemic and metabolic postoperative care.

The long-term outlook for the diabetic amputee has not improved significantly since Silbert's[115] report in 1952. In a follow-up of 294 cases he found a 65% survival rate for 3 years but only a 41% rate at the end of 5 years. Eighteen years later Ecker and Jacobs[39] found data similar to those of Silbert. In their series of 103 patients they found a survival rate of only 61% 3 years after the first amputation.[39] Because of the high mortality, primarily from heart attack and stroke, in this group of diabetics, many do not live long enough to undergo a second

amputation. For those who do, the long-term outlook for the remaining leg is poor. This poor prognosis is not new. Marchal de Calvi[80] in 1864 stated that "often the opposite leg is affected, gangrene sets in and soon the patient succumbs to horrible suffering. Having relieved him only of his local affliction [by amputation], I have done nothing but mutilate him." This problem still exists. On average, 40% of these patients will have amputation of the remaining leg in 1 to 3 years, and 55% in 3 to 5 years.

## PATHOGENESIS OF DIABETIC FOOT LESIONS

The diabetic foot is especially prone to vascular disease and neuropathy. The signs and symptoms of either ischemia or neuropathy may predominate; however, neither is present to the exclusion of the other. The clinical picture therefore is the result of complications stemming from a combination of both. Peripheral neuropathy is the leading cause of most diabetic foot lesions. A majority of patients who enter the hospital because of diabetic foot lesions do so because of ulceration secondary to painless trauma. Very few diabetic patients are admitted for ischemic pain alone. Impaired blood flow to the injured or ulcerated areas prevents healing, and in the presence of infection limits the delivery of oxygen and antibiotics. The most important effect of peripheral neuropathy on the diabetic foot is the loss of sensation, making the foot vulnerable even to trivial trauma. A break in the skin, even though inconspicuous and miniscule, can become a portal of entry for bacteria. Unsuccessfully treated infection leads to gangrene and amputation. Figure 2–1 outlines the pathogenesis of diabetic foot lesions leading to amputation.

## PERIPHERAL VASCULAR DISEASE

The deposits of lipids, cholesterol, calcium, smooth muscle cells, and platelets in the plaques are qualitatively the same in the diabetic and nondiabetic, although acceler-

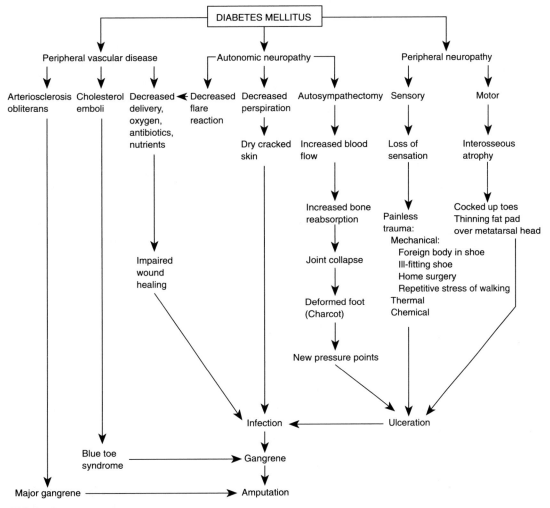

**FIG 2–1.**
Pathogenesis of diabetic foot lesions.

ated in the diabetic. There are, however, important differences, as shown in Table 2–1. In the diabetic the vessels involved are primarily those below the knee, the tibial and peroneal arteries. In the series of Janka et al.[54] the overall prevalence of isolated proximal vascular disease involving femoral and iliac vessels was 5.8% in the diabetic, the same percentage as in the general population. They concluded that proximal vascu-

**TABLE 2–1.**

Differences in Diabetic and Nondiabetic Periperal Vascular Disease

|  | Diabetic | Nondiabetic |
|---|---|---|
| Clinical | More common | Less common |
|  | Younger patient | Older patient |
|  | More rapid | Less rapid |
| Male/female | M > F | M ≫ F |
| Occlusion | Multisegmental | Single segment |
| Vessels adjacent to occlusion | Involved | Not involved |
| Collateral vessels | Involved | Usually normal |
| Lower extremities | Both | Unilateral |
| Vessels involved | Tibial | Aortic |
|  | Peroneal | Iliac |
|  |  | Femoral |

lar disease in the diabetic may represent the atherosclerotic process with coexisting diabetes but did not necessarily represent diabetogenic macroangiopathy.[54] Atherosclerotic involvement of the larger proximal vessels, the aorta and the iliac and femoral arteries, is accelerated by smoking. For example, we saw a 27-year-old patient with type I insulin-dependent diabetes mellitus (IDDM) since age 5 years who had been a heavy smoker since age 13 years. At age 27 years severe intermittent claudication developed in his right leg. Vascular laboratory studies demonstrated a right superficial femoral artery obstruction (Fig 2–2). It was believed that his prolonged heavy smoking had contributed significantly to the proximal ar-

tery atherosclerotic process. He required vascular surgery. Despite warnings to stop smoking, he continued. Two years later severe PVD developed in the left lower extremity. This time vascular surgery was unsuccessful, and the left leg was amputated. He continued to smoke. Angina developed, and the patient died of a massive myocardial infarction 2 years later at age 31 years.

This young patient's inability to stop smoking is not unique. Ardron et al.[4] found conventional antismoking strategies to be completely ineffective in young diabetic subjects.

Further evidence of which vessels are involved is demonstrated by the type of vascular surgery that is performed in these pa-

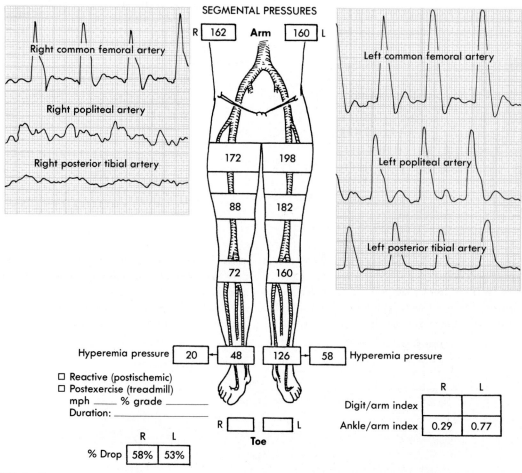

**FIG 2–2.**
Severe PVD in 27-year-old man. Doppler pressures reveal evidence of right superficial femoral artery obstruction. Note blunted waveforms in right popliteal and right posterior tibial arteries, with ankle-arm index of only 0.29. Patient had been diabetic since age 5 years, and a heavy smoker since his early teens. He required right femoral-popliteal Gore-Tex bypass graft. *(Courtesy of Dr. Charles B. Anderson, St. Louis.)*

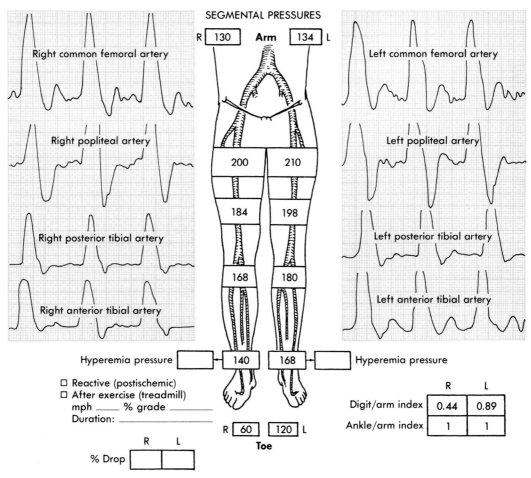

**FIG 2–3.**
Doppler waveforms in lower extremity of 62-year-old woman with type II diabetes who had ischemic changes in right great toe. Low toe pressure and normal ankle pressure confirm small-vessel disease of the great toe.

tients. Although vascular surgery of all types is more common in the diabetic than in the nondiabetic, the procedure most frequently performed in the diabetic is tibioperoneal bypass surgery, involving the vessels below the knee.[69] Large and smaller vessel diseases do not always progress at the same rate. It is not uncommon, for example, for small vessels in the toes to have evidence of ischemia, whereas the dorsalis pedis or posterior tibial pulses may be present and adequate. Figure 2–3 illustrates a significant decrease in toe pressure in a patient with normal ankle pressure. It is also common in the diabetic to have very high ankle Doppler pressure compared with brachial pressure. This occurs in about 15% of diabetics, because of deposits of calcium in the arteries, making them noncompressable.

Microangiopathy is not a significant factor in the pathogenesis of diabetic foot lesions. Although there may be capillary basement membrane thickening, there is no evidence that this contributes to the foot lesions. This has been noted by LoGerfo and Coffman.[75] They stressed that in many instances there are enough patent vessels at the ankle to allow vascular surgery, usually a tibioperoneal bypass procedure, from the femoral arteries in the thigh to the tibial vessels at the ankle. (Vascular surgery techniques are discussed in Chapter 18.)

## Gangrene of Toes

Ischemia or gangrene of the toes can result from (1) atherosclerosis with thrombosis, (2) microthrombi formation resulting from infection (microthrombi secondary to infection can convert the small vessels in the toes to end-arteries with resultant gangrene), (3) cholesterol emboli, and (4) drugs that decrease blood flow.

The classic blue toe syndrome is caused by cholesterol emboli that break off from ulcerated atheromatous plaques in the proximal larger vessels. The toe takes on a deep purplish color, and gangrene can develop. Cholesterol emboli to the foot result in painful petechia and occasionally a livedo reticularis pattern of the skin due to embolization of the arterioles in the skin. The atheromatous plaques may be present in the aorta, iliac artery, or more distant vessels. The syndrome is characterized by the sudden onset of pain in the toe. Leg and thigh myalgia may be present if muscular arteries are involved. When digital artery blood flow becomes sluggish, the toe becomes bluish purple. A sharp demarcation frequently occurs

between normally perfused skin and ischemic areas. Some patients have received anticoagulation therapy with warfarin.[89] It is therefore extremely important to periodically check the toes and feet of patients receiving anticoagulants. Repeated attacks of acute ischemic changes in the toes occurring bilaterally suggests ulcerated atherosclerotic plaque in the aorta.

The development of painful cyanotic toes, myalgias, painful petechia, and a livedo reticular pattern of the skin strongly suggests microemboli. Plate 1 shows purplish discoloration of the right fifth toe and a livedo reticularis pattern on the sole of the foot in a 60-year-old man with a painful, cyanotic fifth toe on his right foot and painful petechial lesions on both feet. These did not blanch on compression. He also complained of myalgias of the lower extremities. An arteriogram (Figure 2–4) showed a large atheromatous plaque in the left lateral wall

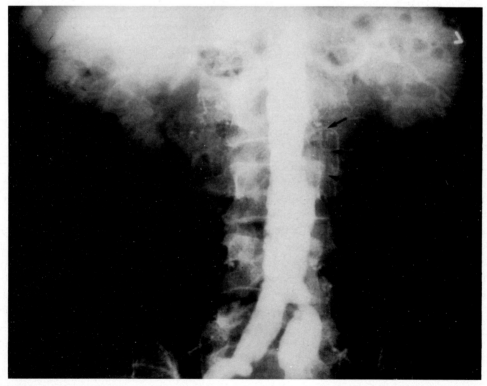

**FIG 2–4.**
Arteriogram shows large filling defect caused by an atheroscleromatous plaque of the aorta just inferior to the renal artery in a patient with evidence of cholesterol emboli to the foot (see Plate 1). *(Courtesy of Georgio Sicard, M.D., St. Louis.)*

of the infrarenal portion of the aorta with ulceration; the ulcerated plaque was removed successfully. The treatment in such cases is vascular surgery with removal of the plaque, thereby preventing further embolization.

Virtually all of the earliest reports suggest that atheromatous embolization occurred in the aortic and iliac segments. Mehigan and Stoney[84] were the first investigators to identify femoropopliteal disease as causing distal embolization. However, a dilemma exists in establishing the exact location of the lesions, because the current treatment of choice is vascular surgery to remove the atherosclerotic plaque and prevent further embolization. In the study by Fisher et al.[44] in patients with multilevel atherosclerotic occlusive disease the peripheral lesions were treated first. In their small series the authors reported no morbidity or mortality. Recurrent embolization did not occur during follow-up of 8 to 24 months.

Recently Vannini et al.[121] found that the local intra-arterial thrombolysis by urokinase in eight patients with NIDDM with angiographic evidence of infrapopliteal occlusive disease and rapidly progressive foot lesions had improved clinical symptoms. Six patients showed immediate improvement of symptoms. Angiography revealed reestablishment of blood flow in the collateral vessels of the leg and foot in the dorsal pedal artery in three patients, and in the plantar arch in two. It was their conclusion that intra-arterial urokinase, which opens collateral and smaller vessels of the leg and foot in patients with diabetes, may be effective in improving blood flow in the lower extremity, making the patient a better candidate for vascular surgery.[121] They did not specifically suggest vascular surgery for patients with blue toe syndrome; however, this form of therapy might be considered. The diagnosis of ulcerated atheromatous plaques can be made by angiography. Protruding atheromas in the thoracic aorta also can be detected by transesophageal echocardiography.[119] It was of interest in this report that diabetes was not considered an increased risk factor. However, hypertension was a major risk factor, and hypertension is extremely common in diabetes.

Certain drugs can cause gangrenous changes in the toes. Vasopressors such as dopamine (Intropin) frequently are used to treat shock. Because of the norepinephrine-like and vasoconstriction effects of these agents, ischemic gangrene can develop in the toes and feet, particularly in diabetics who already have PVD. Dopamine exerts positive inotropic effects by direct action on the adrenergic receptors. When sufficiently large doses of these inotropic drugs are administered, the predominant effect is vasoconstriction in all vascular beds.[49] Dopamine should be used with caution, in as low a dose as possible. If a patient is in shock, the risk-benefit ratio will dictate the use of this family of drugs despite the peripheral vascular risks. However, the feet of these patients must be observed daily.

Peripheral circulation also can be impaired by β-blockers, which are commonly used for treatment of angina and hypertension and after myocardial infarction. Zacharias et al.[131] found peripheral vascular complications to be a side effect in 22 of 305 patients given a β-blocker. This mechanism appears to result from unopposed α-vasoconstriction subsequent to β-blockade.

Diabetes is a hypercoagulable state resulting in increased blood viscosity[105] and impaired flow in the microvascular vessels. The increase in hypercoagulability or blood viscosity is the result of several factors. Increased platelet hyperactivity has been well documented. Elevated levels of fibrinogen have been reported, and a decrease in fibrinolysis has been documented in diabetes mellitus and may play a role in the increased fibrinogen levels.[48] von Willebrand factor is elevated.[17] Increase in red blood cell rigidity also has been demonstrated.[83] An increased tendency for hypercoagulability has been demonstrated in smokers compared with controls.[10] All of these factors can lead to an increase in blood viscosity and a decrease in blood flow. A detailed discussion of the pathogenesis of diabetic PVD is found in Chapter 4.

## Risk Factors

Risk factors for the development of diabetic macrovascular disease include (1) genetic predisposition, (2) age, (3) duration of diabetes, (4) smoking, (5) hypertension (systolic or diastolic), (6) hypercholesterolemia, (7) hypertriglyceridemia, (8) hyperglycemia, (9) truncal obesity, (10) hyperinsulinemia, (11) proteinuria, (12) dialysis, and (13) drugs (e.g., inotropic agents, β-blockers). Age, duration of diabetes, diabetes itself, and genetic factors may be the most important factors, but these cannot be corrected; other risk factors can be treated. Of the correctable risk factors, smoking tops the list. The evils of smoking were noted many years ago by King James I of England (1566–1625):

A custom loathsome to the eye, hateful to the nose, harmful to the braine, dangerous to the lungs, and the black stinking fume thereof, nearest resembling the horrible stigian smoke of the pit that is bottomless.

An excellent review on the consequences of smoking has been written by Couch.[27] Pollin[103] has estimated that cigarette smoking causes an estimated 325,000 to 355,0000 deaths annually in the United States. This is more than all other drug and alcohol abuse deaths combined, 7 times more than all automobile fatalities per year, more than 11 times all reported deaths caused by acquired immune deficiency syndrome, and more than all American military fatalities in World War I, World War II, and Viet Nam combined.[103] A clinical series from New Zealand found that cigarette smoking was noted two and one-half times more frequently in diabetic patients with ischemia and gangrene as in a control series of persons without diabetes.[33] Kannel,[57] in a 26-year follow-up of the Framingham Study of 5,209 subjects, found that cigarette smoking together with impaired glucose tolerance and hypertension were powerful predisposing factors for PVD. The series of Beach and Strandness[9] on arteriosclerosis obliterans and associated risk factors in diabetics showed a high correlation between smoking and atherosclerosis. They found this to be one of the most important risk factors, and presented evidence to show that the cessation of smoking was associated with a decrease in the progression of atherosclerosis. Cigarette smoking approximately doubled the risk in both sexes. The impact was discernible into advanced age and was dose related.[9] Smoking is atherogenic, decreases blood flow through vasospasm, and increases blood viscosity and clotting factors (Table 2–2).

The mechanisms by which smoking is atherogenic is unknown, but may be related to intimal injury from increased levels of carboxyhemoglobin and carbon monoxide.[123] Another effect of smoking is its possible influence on prostacyclin ($PGI_2$), an important prostaglandin that prevents platelet aggregation and promotes vasodilation. Nadler et al.[91] have shown that cigarette smoking inhibits $PGI_2$ formation. In their study, smoking tobacco with nicotine abolished $PGI_2$ production. This may be a factor in developing accelerated cardiovascular disease.

Although the nicotine and carbon monoxide content of cigarette smoke has been be-

**TABLE 2–2.**

Vascular Complications of Smoking

| Atherosclerosis | |
|---|---|
| ↑ | Carboxyhemoglobin |
| ↑ | Carbon monoxide |
| ↑ | Cholesterol |
| ↑ | Triglycerides |
| ↑ | Very low-density lipoproteins |
| ↓ | High-density lipoproteins |
| ↓ | Prostacyclin |
| ↑ | Truncal obesity |
| ↑ | Hypertension |
| ↑ | Albuminuria |
| Decreased blood flow | |
| ↑ | Vasospasm |
| ↑ | Hypercoagulability |
| ↑ | Viscosity |
| ↓ | Red blood cell deformability |
| Increased clotting | |
| ↑ | Thrombus formation |
| ↑ | Platelet aggregation |
| ↑ | Fibrinogen |
| ↑ | von Willebrand factor |
| ↓ | Plasminogen |
| ↓ | Plasminogen activator |

lieved to be the major risk, a recent article by Kaufman et al.[59] has shown that patients who smoked cigarettes with a reduced amount of nicotine and carbon monoxide did not have any lower risk factor for myocardial infarction than did those who smoked cigarettes containing a larger amount of nicotine. This was confirmed by Palmer et al.,[95] who found that smoking "low yield" cigarettes did not lower the risk of a first nonfatal myocardial infarction.

Cigarette smoking also may contribute to the pathogenesis of atherosclerosis through its effect on lipid metabolism. Brischetto et al.[20] showed the plasma lipid and lipoprotein profiles of cigarette smokers from randomly selected families to be abnormal. The study demonstrated that those who smoked had higher plasma cholesterol, triglyceride, and very low-density lipoprotein (VLDL) levels and a lower high-density lipoprotein (HDL) cholesterol concentration.[20] Smoking causes a greater reduction in HDL concentration in women than in men.[35]

One proposed mechanism by which smoking can cause an abnormal atherogenic lipoprotein profile has been proposed by Dullaart et al.[37] They found that smoking in type I diabetic men resulted in an elevation of cholesteryl ester transfer protein activity. Cholesteryl ester transfer protein activity elevations have been associated with an unfavorable lipoprotein profile.

Obesity, especially abdominal or truncal, with an increase in waist-hip ratio has been associated with atherosclerosis.

Smoking also may have a tendency to increase abdominal obesity. Shimokata et al.[114] found the waist-hip ratio in smokers to be significantly higher than in nonsmokers, and that waist-hip ratio in patients who started smoking actually increased despite weight loss. Barrett-Connor and Khaw[8] also have demonstrated that cigarette smokers have more central obesity than do nonsmokers. The explanation for this effect of cigarette smoking is not known. However, cigarette smoking is associated with increased adrenal androgens in both men and women, and androgens contribute to truncal obesity.[30, 42, 46, 60]

Hypertension is an atherosclerotic risk factor that may be influenced by smoking. Mann et al.[79] found that hypertensive patients older than 50 years who were smokers maintained a higher daytime ambulatory systolic pressure than did nonsmokers, even though the blood pressure measured in the office was not different between the smokers and nonsmokers.

Cigarette smoking also increases the rate of albuminuria among subjects with type I diabetes, and albuminuria is related to hypertension and atherosclerosis.[24] Muhlehuser et al.[90] also found cigarette smoking to be a risk factor for macroproteinuria. This may be another factor in the development of atherosclerosis. A cooperative study by a group of pathologists indicated strong evidence for the effect of smoking on atherosclerosis in the young.[108]

Smoking also impedes blood flow by increasing vasospasm; one cigarette can cause vasoconstriction for more than 1 hour. Smoking increases blood viscosity and hypercoagulability and decreases erythrocyte deformability, which also contributes to increased blood viscosity. Increased hypercoagulability has been found in chronic smokers compared with nonsmokers.[10] It became pronounced immediately after smoking three cigarettes. Cigarette smoking also can cause increased clotting. Smoking causes an increase in platelet aggregation and von Willebrand factor and a decrease in red blood cell deformability.[10] The group who smoked had higher plasma fibrinogen levels, lower plasminogen levels, lower plasminogen activator levels, and higher plasma viscosity.[10] These factors contribute not only to increased coagulability but to increased in clotting as well. Smoking affects platelet function and increases the tendency for thrombus formation.[71]

Despite the deleterious effects of smoking on atherosclerosis, the percentage of diabetics who smoke is high. Ford and Newman,[45] in a study of 3,000 persons older than 30 years with diabetes and 5,300 older than age 30 years without diabetes, found that 26% of the diabetic population were smokers, 26% were former smokers, and 48% had never smoked; the figures were similar for the nondiabetic population. They found that the prevalence of smoking was higher among diabetics between the ages of 18 and 34 years, among diabetics who had not graduated from high school, and in black men. Despite the risk, the overall prevalence of smoking in the diabetic population is comparable to that of the general population. This only emphasizes the increasing need for education of this group about the dangers of smoking, particularly from a vascular point of view.[45]

Smoking also may have an effect on neuropathy. Mitchell et al.[87] investigated lifetime cigarette smoking and its association with the presence of diabetic neuropathy in patients with IDDM. Current or former smokers were significantly more likely to have neuropathy than persons who never had smoked. The prevalence of neuropathy increased with the number of pack-years. The theoretical explanation for this finding was that cigarette smoking may contribute to tissue hypoxia and subsequent injury to the neural microvasculature. That this finding was restricted to patients with IDDM might be because of the much lower overall incidence of smoking in the NIDDM patients in their sample.[87]

A final comment to our patients regarding smoking comes from the cigar-smoking Mark Twain's Aunt Mary, who said to him, "I beg you. I beseech you. I implore you, crush out that fatal habit."

Hypertension is a well-known risk factor for atherosclerosis. Approximately 2.5 million Americans have both diabetes and hypertension.[129] Hypertension, both systolic and diastolic, is a risk factor for PVD. The initial treatment of hypertension is a low-salt diet, weight reduction, and exercise. When these approaches are unsatisfactory, pharmacologic treatment is indicated. The older antihypertensive drugs, β-blockers, and diuretics, especially thiazides, may have an adverse effect on atherosclerosis. β-Blockers increase fasting blood glucose levels, hemoglobin $A_{1C}$ levels, insulin levels, VLDL levels, and triglyceride levels, and lower HDL levels. Thiazides increase blood glucose,

cholesterol, LDL cholesterol, and triglyceride levels and insulin resistance. A recent report by Warram et al.[125] showed that the use of diuretics was associated with a higher degree of mortality than in patients receiving no antihypertensive treatment or antihypertensive drugs other than diuretics. Diuretics were associated with a fourfold risk for cardiovascular mortality in patients without proteinuria and a tenfold risk in those with proteinuria. Multivariate analysis revealed that diuretic therapy alone as treatment of hypertension was associated with increased risk for cardiovascular mortality in both the proteinuric and nonproteinuric groups, and especially those with proteinuria. Thiazides sometimes are indicated as an adjunct in the treatment of hypertension, but in these cases the dose should be low, not exceeding 12.5 to 25 mg/day. There is some evidence that thiazide therapy in low doses may be more effective in black patients. The antihypertensive drugs of choice for diabetes today are calcium channel blockers and angiotensin converting enzyme inhibitors.

There is no question that a strong correlation exists between hypercholesterolemia and cardiovascular disease. However, not all authorities have found a correlation between PVD and hypercholesterolemia.[54, 92] In most of these studies triglyceride, LDL, and HDL levels were not reported. Laakso and Pyorala[64] confirm a strong relationship between total cholesterol and lipid abnormalities and PVD, as demonstrated by intermittent claudication in both type I and II diabetes. They found that the total LDL cholesterol, VLDL, and triglyceride levels tended to be higher and HDL and $HDL_2$ cholesterol levels to be lower in those patients with claudication. Therefore, control of cholesterol and lipid abnormalities should be as vigorous in patients with PVD as in those with coronary artery disease.

The role of hyperglycemia in the pathogenesis of atherosclerosis is debatable. Nelson et al.[92] found a correlation between hyperglycemia and PVD; others, however, have not.[9, 54, 102, 120]

Hyperinsulinemia itself may be atherogenic by contributing to hypertension and dyslipidemia and by indirectly causing atherosclerotic changes in the arteries. Current data suggest a possible direct relationship between fasting insulin levels and blood pressure, especially in the obese patient and those with impaired glucose tolerance levels,[81] and in fact hypertensive patients have exhibited a decrease in systolic and diastolic blood pressures after insulin reduction. Hyperinsulinemia can contribute to hypertension by stimulating the sympathetic nervous system.[88] Insulin also stimulates the reabsorption of sodium and water in the kidney, which may lead to increase in the blood volume and hypertension.[126]

Insulin is a growth hormone—like factor, and has been found by several investigators to stimulate the duplication of smooth muscle cells and their migration into the arterial lumen.[22, 113] This process plays a major role in the formation of atherosclerotic plaque. Evidence of atherosclerosis caused by hyperinsulinemia has been reported to occur in the presence of normal glucose tolerance. Zavaroni et al.[132] found that a group of "healthy individuals" with hyperinsulinemia and normal glucose tolerance had an increase in vascular risk factors and triglycerides levels and lower HDL concentrations. In the experimental diabetic BB rat, Larson and Haudenschild[66] found a genetic predilection, sensitivity of the vascular smooth muscle cells to insulin, and a dissociation of this effect from hyperglycemia.

As noted, adiposity, especially fat distribution, is a vascular risk factor. Distribution of body fat has been found to be an independent predictor of metabolic aberrations, including cardiovascular morbidity and mortality.[65] Abdominal or truncal obesity has been associated with hyperinsulinemia, hypertriglyceridemia, hypertension, and decreased HDL levels.[2, 52] An excellent review of the reasons why abdominal fat may relate to insulin resistance has been reported by Bjorntorp.[13] Peiris et al.[100] measured intra-abdominal fat using computed tomography. They found that intra-abdominal fat deposition constitutes greater cardiovascular risk than obesity alone. They also reached the conclusion that hyperinsulinemia is associated with abdominal obesity and is an important component of increased vascular risk associated with abdominal obesity. Kaplan[58] has aptly termed the deadly quartet as upper body obesity, glucose intolerance, hypertriglyceridemia, and hypertension.

A cluster of variables, resistance to insulin-stimulated glucose uptake, glucose intolerance, hyperinsulinemia, increased VLDL triglyceride levels, decreased HDL cholesterol levels, and hypertension, have been termed syndrome X by Reaven.[107] These factors may be of enormous importance in the pathogenesis of macrovascular disease. Proteinuria is an established macrovascular risk factor.

Patients with IDDM have a significantly increased risk for macrovascular disease, particularly if they have persistent proteinuria. Apolipoprotein A (apo A) contributes to the increased risk for atherosclerosis. Jenkins et al.[55] found elevated levels of apo A in diabetic patients with both microalbuminuria and albuminuria than in patients without these. They believed that elevated apo A levels in patients with IDDM and increased urinary albumin loss may contribute to the heightened risk for macrovascular disease.[55] Cardiovascular mortality in patients with proteinuria is 10 times that of those without it.[16] (See Chapter 4 for a detailed discussion of the pathogenesis of diabetic atherosclerosis.)

## Signs and Symptoms

The signs and symptoms of PVD include the following:

1. Intermittent claudication
2. Cold feet
3. Nocturnal pain
4. Rest pain
5. Nocturnal and rest pain relieved with dependency
6. Absent pulses
7. Blanching on elevation
8. Delayed venous filling after elevation

9. Dependent rubor
10. Atrophy of subcutaneous fatty tissues
11. Shiny appearance of skin
12. Loss of hair on foot and toes
13. Thickened nails, often with fungal infection
14. Gangrene
15. Miscellaneous: blue toe syndrome, acute vascular occlusion

Intermittent claudication is a common symptom of PVD. It was originally described by veterinary surgeons as a disease of horses. The first case of intermittent claudication in humans was described by Charcot in 1858.[23] The word claudication comes from the Latin word meaning "to limp," but patients with claudication do not limp; they stop to rest. The pain associated with intermittent claudication is characterized by cramping or aching, most often in the calf. The pain occurs with walking, and is relieved when the person stops walking, without the need to sit down. The pain of intermittent claudication must be differentiated from similar pain that also may be induced by walking, such as arthritis, muscle pain, radicular pain, spinal cord compression, thrombophlebitis, anemia, and myxedema.

This nonischemic pain, called pseudoclaudication, also can be relieved by rest. However, the pain associated with these problems usually takes longer to disappear and these patients usually need to sit down and/or change position. Thus, nonischemic causes of intermittent claudication must be considered in the differential diagnosis of leg pain associated with walking. Intermittent claudication most commonly occurs as calf pain, but higher vascular obstruction (e.g., in the aorta) will cause pain in the buttocks and upper thighs and frequently is accompanied by impotence. This is known as Leriche's syndrome. Obstruction of the iliac arteries will cause pain in the lower thigh.

The symptoms of intermittent claudication depend on ischemia in the muscle. Thus, despite extensive involvement of the small vessels in the diabetic foot, symptoms of claudication in the foot may be infrequent because of the small muscle mass. Some investigators believe that claudication does not occur in the foot. The distance a person can walk will vary from patient to patient. Pain occurs after a shorter distance if a person is walking uphill, on a hard surface, or is walking fast. Persons with progressive intermittent claudication note that over time they are able to walk a shorter distance before the discomfort develops.

Examination of the patient with intermittent claudication involving the calf muscle may reveal both femoral and pedal pulses but no popliteal pulse. The pedal pulses are present because of the collateral arteries. After the patient takes a brisk walk the foot will become pale and pulseless because the blood bypasses the skin of the foot and flows to the skeletal muscles of the calf instead. Intermittent claudication usually results from a single arterial block. However, because of multiple-vessel involvement in the diabetic, several blocks may be present.

Among the several approaches to the treatment of intermittent claudication, the most important is cessation of smoking, and the next is walking. Jonason et al.[56] demonstrated the beneficial effects of a supervised training and exercise program in patients with intermittent claudication. Patients with angina were limited in their ability to participate in the program. A minimum of 3 months training was required to achieve maximum improvement. Some of this improvement may be attributed to the effect of exercise on platelets. Peterson[101] demonstrated that the percentage of platelet adhesiveness in diabetic subjects decreased from 74% before exercise to 53% after exercise. However, other studies have not confirmed this effect of exercise on platelet function, and most of these studies have not confirmed a decrease in platelet aggregation with exercise.[26]

Exercise is the cornerstone of conservative management. A regular walking program will improve distance in 80% of the patients. Although leg exercises may be helpful, walking is the best exercise. Bicycling is probably less beneficial, because it exercises the thigh muscles more than the calf muscles. A good walking program consists of a definite daily walking routine over and above normal activities. The exercise can be divided to suit the patient's daily schedule, but the program should be supervised by a physician.

Recently the Food and Drug Administration (FDA) released a drug called pentoxifylline (Trental) for the treatment of intermittent claudication. This new drug does not dilate blood vessels; rather, its major effect appears to be on the red blood cells. This drug makes the red blood cells more flexible or deformable, so that they can pass through a narrowed blood vessel. A red blood cell measures approximately 7.4 μm, a capillary 3 to 5 μm. Therefore a red blood cell must be flexible to easily pass through a capillary. White blood cell flexibility also may be improved with pentoxifylline. Although pentoxifylline does not improve intermittent claudication in every patient, it does so in a significant number, and certainly is worth a trial. The drug does not work instantly, and it may be several months before its effect is noted. A detailed discussion of the mechanism of action of pentoxifylline on red blood cell deformability is found in Chapter 5.

Although the FDA has approved pentoxifylline only for treatment of intermittent claudication, the Canadian equivalent of the FDA has approved it for the treatment of ischemic trophic ulcers. Others, as well as myself, have found it helpful in treating painful ischemic ulcers on the tips of the toes in patients who are not candidates for vascular surgery.

Vasodilators have been ineffective in the treatment of intermittent claudication.[25] The arteries in the diabetic are sclerosed and have very little vasospastic disease. In many cases dilation already has been achieved by "autosympathectomy" because of involvement of the autonomic nervous system.

In fact, vasodilators can theoretically worsen an ischemic area by causing the "steal effect," in which dilation of the healthy vessels steals blood away from the sclerosed vessels and the tissues they supply.

The ultimate treatment for intermittent claudication is vascular surgery to bypass narrowed areas or endarterectomy. Transcutaneous angioplasty (see Chapter 17) seldom is useful in diabetes, because its greatest applicability is in the larger vessels, and PVD in the diabetic occurs most often in the smaller vessels. Surgery is rarely indicated as therapy for intermittent claudication, and then only if the patient is severely disabled. The strongest indication would be for persons whose livelihood depends on walking (e.g., mail carrier).

The long-term outlook for patients with intermittent claudication is relatively good with conservative management. Long-term follow-up has shown that in most patients the condition will stay the same or actually improve.

The effectiveness of vasodilator drugs and hemorheologic agents in the treatment of claudication has recently been reviewed by Taylor and Porter.[117] The use of prostaglandins in peripheral arterial ischemia has been reviewed by Cronenwett.[28] Weismann[127] recently discussed the role of platelets and treatment with pharmacologic agents used to alter platelet function.

Cold feet are a common complaint in patients with peripheral vascular insufficiency, prompting them to use hot water bottles, heating pads, and hot water soaks. These practices can result in severe burns to a foot that has become insensitive to heat because of peripheral neuropathy.

Rest pain usually indicates at least two hemodynamically significant arterial blocks in a series. Rest pain is persistent pain caused by nerve ischemia. It has peaks of intensity, is worse at night, and may require the use of narcotics for relief. Rest pain decreases with dependency of the lower extremities and is aggravated by heat, elevation, and exercise. The studies of Rayman et al.[106] suggest that postural control of blood flow to the foot is disturbed in patients with diabetic neuropathy. This disturbance relates to loss of sympathetic vascular tone. The result is hyperperfusion on dependency, which may account for some of the edema and ischemic pain relief seen in these patients after dependency of the legs. Consequently these patients often sleep in a chair, and leg edema secondary to prolonged dependency is common. Laboratory proof of improved peripheral circulation with the foot in a dependent position is seen from the early studies of Dahn et al.[29] and Gaskell and Becker.[47] They demonstrated an increase in the clearance rate of xenon 133 from the anterior tibial muscles[29] and from the dermal tissues of the forefoot when patients with occluded arteries of the lower limbs moved from a supine to a sitting position.[47]

Nocturnal ischemic pain is a form of ischemic neuritis that usually precedes rest pain. It occurs at night because during sleep the circulation is essentially of the core variety, with little perfusion of the lower extremity. The resulting ischemic neuritis becomes intense and disrupts sleep. The patient invariably gains relief by standing up or dangling the feet over the edge of the bed, and on occasion by walking a few steps. This increases cardiac output, leading to improved perfusion of the lower extremities and relief of ischemic neuritis. If the lesions that produce nocturnal and rest pain are not corrected by vascular surgery, tissue necrosis and gangrene almost always develop, necessitating amputation. Rest pain and nocturnal pain therefore are indications for vascular surgery to relieve arterial occlusions. In the diabetic, rest and nocturnal pain may be absent despite severe ischemia because diabetic neuropathy has destroyed the sensory perception of pain.

Severe pain in the legs at night may be caused by diabetic neuropathy or vascular insufficiency. To differentiate the two, keep in mind that the diabetic with vascular disease gets relief by sitting up and dangling the legs. Walking more than a few feet makes the pain worse. The patient with neuropathic pain tends to get relief by walking.

Cold sensation in the feet can be caused by neuropathy and vascular disease. To determine the cause, feel the foot and leg to evaluate skin temperature.

If the popliteal area is obstructed, there may be a difference in skin temperature in the two patellar areas. The skin around the knee on the ischemic side often is warmer, due to collateral vessels that form around the obstructed popliteal artery.[32]

Pallor of the foot on elevation and delayed capillary filling are other signs of ischemia. With the patient in the supine position

**TABLE 2–3.**

Capillary Filling Time on Dependency

Normal: 10–15 sec
Moderate ischemia: 15–25 sec
Severe ischemia: 25–40 sec
Very severe ischemia: ≥40 sec

the feet are elevated to a 45-degree angle and held in this position until one or both feet blanch. The patient is then instructed to sit upright with the feet in a dependent position. Normally the venous and capillary filling time is less than 15 seconds; it can be prolonged to minutes in the severely ischemic extremity. A capillary filling time more than 40 seconds indicates very severe ischemia (Table 2–3).

The extremity with severe PVD will develop rubor after dependency. Patients with varicose veins also may have dependent rubor because of venous stasis. Pallor on elevation, prolonged filling time, and dependent rubor are the hallmarks of significant lower extremity vascular insufficiency.

Ischemic skin changes are characterized by shiny atrophic cool skin, loss of hair on the dorsum of the foot and toes, thickening of the nails, and frequently fungal infections. The nails tend to grow more slowly when the blood supply is decreased. As further ischemia develops the subcutaneous tissue atrophies. The skin appears shiny and tightly drawn over the foot. Ulcerations in these vulnerable feet may occur from minor trauma (Fig 2–5). The ulcerations heal slowly and frequently become infected.

Treatment of infection is difficult in these patients because of poor blood supply. It has been known for many years that peripheral vascular insufficiency is one of the major factors contributing to the increased incidence of infection of the lower extremity.[130]

PVD contributes to amputation by impeding the delivery of antibiotics, oxygen, and nutrients and by delaying wound healing and the ability to fight infection. Taylor and Porter[118] reported that aggressive therapy with debridement, antibiotic therapy, and, when indicated, revascularization resulted in long-term salvage of 73% of threat-

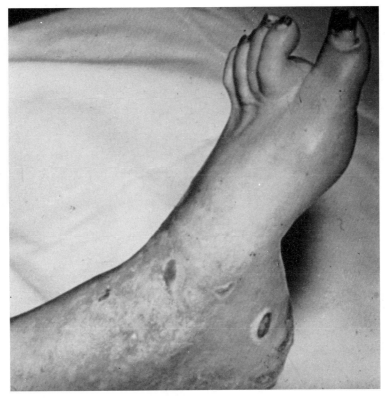

**FIG 2–5.**
Classic diabetic foot with ischemic skin changes: atrophy of subcutaneous tissues, hair loss on dorsum of foot, thickening of nails, atrophy of interosseus muscles resulting in cocked-up toes, and commonly seen superficial ulcerations. *(Courtesy of John F. Fiarbairn II, M.D., Rochester, Minn., and The Upjohn Company, Kalamazoo, Mich.)*

ened limbs even in high-risk patients. Clearing of infection and wound healing is unlikely if the ankle brachial index is less than 0.45 or the transcutaneous oxygen pressure ($tcPo_2$) is less than 30 mm Hg. If $tcPo_2$ is less than 20 mm Hg, healing is very unlikely.

### Acute Occlusion

In the diabetic patient most ischemic changes occur slowly, although sudden occlusion from emboli or acute complete thrombosis can occur. Most emboli (>70%) originate in the heart. The most common underlying cardiac pathologic condition is atrial fibrillation. Myocardial infarction with mural thrombi is the second most common cause. Acute thrombosis has atherosclerosis as the underlying cause. The signs and symptoms of acute arterial occlusion usually are referred to as "the five Ps" (Table 2–4). Pale leg develops, which may appear waxy. Paresthesias and numbness are common.

The patient may have sudden weakness in the leg, and on physical examination, pallor, paralysis, and pulselessness below the block are noted. Most sudden occlusions are the result of emboli. The extent of ischemia and final outcome depend on collateral circulation, size, clot location, and the time between onset of acute occlusion and treatment. These occlusions must be treated as soon as possible, because peripheral nerve and skeletal muscles have less resistance to ischemia than skin and bone do. Irreversible changes of skeletal muscle and peripheral

**TABLE 2–4.**

"Five Ps" of Acute Arterial Occlusion in Lower Extremity

| |
|---|
| Pain: sudden onset |
| Pallor: waxy |
| Paresthesias: numbness |
| Pulselessness: no pulse below block |
| Paralysis: sudden weakness |

nerves may occur after 4 to 6 hours of severe ischemia. The skin may tolerate severe ischemia for 10 hours. Pallor is usually more severe with embolism than with thrombosis. With embolism the effected extremity is waxlike and lemon yellow. With thrombosis, the extremity appears less cadaverous and tends to be somewhat cyanotic. Paresthesias are caused by peripheral nerve ischemia. Treatment of sudden arterial occlusion requires surgical intervention or thrombolytic therapy.

## PERIPHERAL NEUROPATHY

The first description of the manifestations of diabetic neuropathy was made by Marchal de Calvi[80] in 1864. More than 100 years later, despite much research and many publications, the exact cause of diabetic neuropathy remains unexplained. The pathogenesis no doubt is multifactorial. Decreased blood flow in the vasonervorum caused by vascular narrowing of the vessel or increased blood viscosity is a factor. Another possible factor under investigation is the trapping of immunoglobulins on peripheral nerve myelin.[21] This does not occur in the brain, and may account for the fact that rarely is there central nervous system neuropathy.[21] Metabolic change probably is the most significant factor.[50, 53] (A detailed discussion of the pathogenesis and treatment of diabetic peripheral neuropathy is found in Chapter 6.)

A number of syndromes are associated with diabetic neuropathy. The most common of these involving the foot are distal symmetric sensorimotor polyneuropathies, resulting in pain; paresthesias; muscle atrophy; loss of sensation; autonomic neuropathy with dry, scaly feet; radiculopathy; and entrapment syndromes. An important entrapment syndrome affecting the foot is the tarsal tunnel syndrome. This syndrome results from compression of the posterior tibial nerve at the tarsal tunnel or of the plantar nerves, causing sensory impairment in the sole of the foot and weakness of the intrinsic pedal musculature. Tarsal tunnel syndrome usually occurs unilaterally, which differentiates

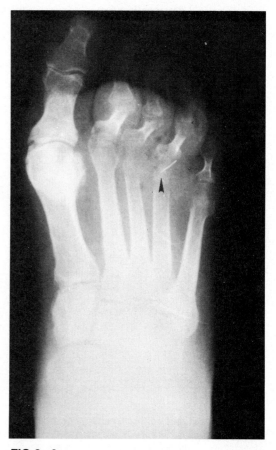

**FIG 2–6.**
Carpenter's nail present for approximately 1 month in tissues of foot of an insulin-requiring diabetic patient. He had no knowledge of having stepped on this nail, nor did he have any pain or discomfort. *(Courtesy of Dr. Joseph Marr, Senior Vice-president, Discovery Research, Searle, Skokie, Ill.)*

it from metabolic bilateral symmetric polyneuropathy. Symptoms include burning pain and paresthesias at the ankle and plantar surface of the foot.[1]

Peripheral neuropathy in diabetic patients is not always due to the diabetes; other causes include alcoholism, herniated nucleus pulposus, heavy metals, vitamin deficiencies, collagen disease, pernicious anemia, malignancy, pressure neuropathy, uremia, porphyria, Hansen disease (leprosy), and drugs.

Malignancies may cause peripheral neuropathy by humoral effect or by nerve compression. Recently we saw a woman with diabetes and peripheral neuropathy. The neuropathy was unilateral, which was atypical. Further evaluation revealed a meningioma of the spinal cord. Treatment for diabetic peripheral neuropathy in this patient would have resulted in a missed diagnosis.

As noted in Figure 2–1, neuropathy ultimately can result in amputation through various pathways, including loss of autonomic, sensory, or motor nerve function. Autonomic involvement results in decreased perspiration. This leads to dryness, cracking, and fissures of the skin, which can be portals of entry for bacteria. Autonomic dysfunction also can lead to loss of the flare reaction.[97] Any noxious stimuli to the skin results in increased blood flow. In the diabetic with significant foot lesions this autonomic effect is blunted, thereby impeding wound healing. Orthostatic hypotension, a complication of autonomic involvement, may lead to a decrease in pressure and arterial perfusion with standing.

The most important neuropathic factor is the loss of pain and temperature sensation. The patient with nerve impairment develops an insensate foot that endures painless trauma from mechanical, chemical, or thermal sources, frequently resulting in ulceration and infection (see Fig 2–1).

Painless mechanical trauma can occur from a variety of causes. The most common

is walking. The repetitive stress of walking results in callus buildup and hot spots. Because there is no pain, the patient continues to walk. The callus builds up, and pressure necrosis and ulceration result (Plate 2). Abnormally high pressures, especially under the forefoot, have been found in such feet.[18]

Trauma from painless puncture wounds is not rare. Figure 2–6 shows a carpenter's nail deep in the tissues of the foot of a 45-year-old who had required insulin for 10 years. He had a small, painless draining area on his foot for approximately 1 month, and sought medical attention only because the area had failed to heal. The dorsalis pedis and posterior tibial pulses were of good quality; however, vibratory sense and pain and touch sensation were markedly diminished. Radiographs of the foot revealed the carpenter's nail, which must have been present for at least a month without any discomfort to the patient. The area involved had caused severe osteomyelitis, and the foot ultimately was amputated.

I agree with Dr. Paul Brand, who stated that "the diabetic who claims his shoes are killing him may well be right." Painless ulceration from ill-fitting shoes may become

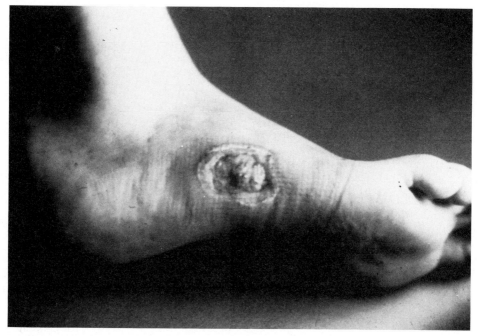

**FIG 2–7.**
Ulceration on the side of the foot, suggestive of ill-fitting shoe. *(From Levin ME: Diabetic foot lesions, in Young JR, Graor RA, Olin JW, et al, editors:* Peripheral vascular diseases, *St Louis, 1991, Mosby–Year Book.)*

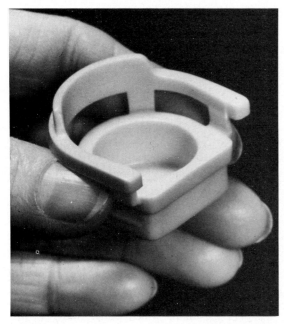

**FIG 2–8.**
Doll's chair measuring 2.5 by 3.8 cm found in patient's shoe. He had worn the shoe all day without being aware of the chair's presence because of almost total absence of sensory perception produced by severe diabetic neuropathy.

infected; gangrene may follow, and amputation may be necessary. Ulcers caused by ill-fitting shoes occur most often on the side of the foot (Fig 2–7). The number of foreign objects found in patients' shoes that they have walked on without pain or awareness is legion, and includes pebbles, coins, and unbelievably large objects such as doll chairs (Fig 2–8) and shoehorns (Fig 2–9), to mention only a few.

Another extreme example of painless trauma is noted in Figure 2–10,A, which shows ulceration over the Achilles tendon of a patient who kept the back of his heel against a chair while on jury duty. Blisters developed, which ulcerated and penetrated to the Achilles tendon. The patient's physician advised using a bandage and returning to work. Fortunately the patient sought a second opinion. A skin graft flap procedure was done (Fig 2–10,B), and the ulceration healed (Fig 2–10,C).

Another common cause of painless injury results from "home surgery." Because persons with diabetic neuropathy feel no pain, they frequently cut their calluses too deep and their nails too short, resulting in ulceration and infection. Figure 2–11 shows an infected and gangrenous great toe that resulted when a patient practiced home surgery. Even though she was partially blind, she attempted to cut the nail, and in doing so, cut into the tissue. This resulted in infection and gangrene, which necessitated partial amputation.

Chemical trauma results from the use of callus and corn removers, and also has occurred from soaking the feet in chemical solutions and strong antiseptics.

Thermal injuries are common in the insensitive diabetic foot. Figure 2–12 shows gangrene of the toes of a diabetic who had soaked his cold foot in a bucket of hot water. The patient had good dorsalis pedis and posterior tibial pulses, and midtarsal amputation was successful. Severe burns have occurred in patients with insensitive feet who have walked on hot sandy beaches or other hot surfaces. We have seen a number of these patients ultimately require amputation

**FIG 2–9.**
Shoehorn in shoe worn by patient who, because of insensitive foot resulting from diabetic neuropathy, was unaware of its presence until removing the shoe at end of day.

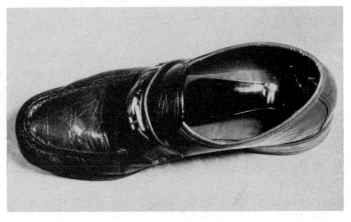

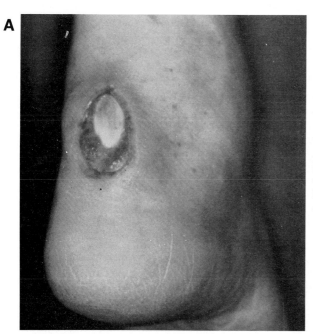

**FIG 2–10.**
**A,** ulceration resulting from breakdown of painless blisters that penetrated to the Achilles tendon. **B,** outline of skin flap for treatment of ulceration. **C,** healed skin flap graft. *(Courtesy of Leroy Young, M.D., St. Louis.)*

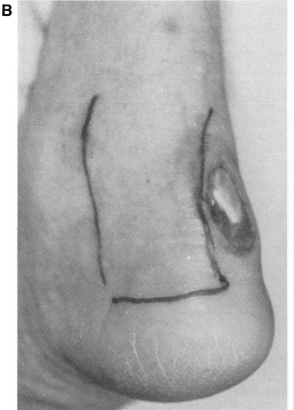

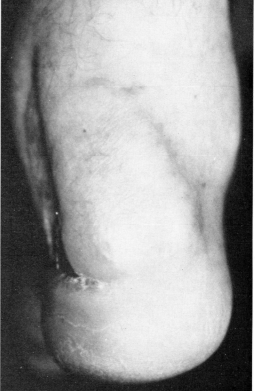

of the feet. Diabetic patients going to the beach or to swimming pools should wear protective footwear. Not uncommonly, patients who have placed their feet in front of the fireplace to warm them have sustained

severe burns. Perhaps the most dramatic case of painless thermal injury that I have seen was in a diabetic patient who had had a previous below-knee amputation. He had purchased a riding lawn mower, and in posi-

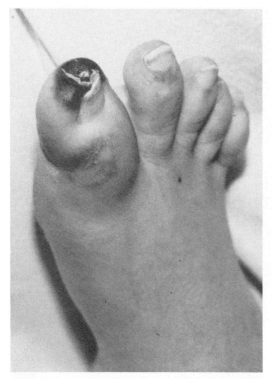

**FIG 2–11.**
Gangrenous toe resulting from patient's attempt at home surgery. Toenail was cut too short and became infected, and gangrene developed.

tioning the good leg, inadvertently placed it on the manifold, which became extremely hot. Only when he "smelled something burning" did he look down to discover that his shoe and foot were on fire. Subsequent amputation of his remaining foot was necessary.

## FOOT DEFORMITIES

Muscle atrophy caused by involvement of the motor nerves leads to an imbalance of the interosseous muscles in the foot. This frequently leads to cocked-up toes. Ulceration may occur on the tips and tops of the toes. I refer to this as tip-top-toe ulcer syndrome. Because of thinning of the fat pad underneath the first metatarsophalangeal joint, ulceration may occur in this area (Fig 2–13). Prevention of ulceration in these areas requires straightening of these cocked-up, claw, or hammer toes at a time when circulation is good. However, if this cannot be

done, it is important to make sure the toe box of the shoe is large enough to accommodate the top of these deformed toes. Cushioned insoles should be worn to protect the tips of the toes.

The most extreme example of diabetic foot deformity is the Charcot foot, or neuroarthropathy.

Classically, the Charcot foot at its acute onset is hot, erythematous, and swollen, with bounding pulses and prominent veins. Despite what is written in some textbooks, patients with Charcot foot frequently have moderate pain and discomfort. It may be difficult to differentiate the warm, red Charcot foot from cellulitis. However, the patient with Charcot foot is afebrile, and the white blood cell count is normal; sedimentation rate may be slightly elevated. The neuropathic component of Charcot foot probably stems from involvement of the autonomic nervous system. The result is the equivalent of sympathectomy to the arteries in the foot. The arteries dilate, and arteriovenous (AV) shunts have been demonstrated in these feet.[19] X-ray examination in the acute state usually reveals no bony abnormality (Fig 2–14,A). If the patient continues to walk, there can be gradual dissolution and fragmentation of the distal ends of the metatarsals (Fig 2–14,B) and the ankle bones. The distal ends of the metatarsals become pointed, the "peppermint stick sign," as if the ends of the bone were licked away.[110] X-ray films also show the absence of calcification in the interosseous arteries, further evidence that there is no significant vascular insufficiency. It is believed that the increased circulation causes resorption of the bone. Evidence that increased circulation contributes to Charcot foot has been suggested by the report of Edelman et al.[40] These authors reported three cases of Charcot foot that developed after successful peripheral vascular surgery. These cases demonstrate the important role of increased blood flow in the absorption of calcium from the bones in the foot, their collapse, and the development of Charcot foot. Because there is relative insensitivity in these feet, patients continue to walk, subsequently developing so-called stress fractures and further bone

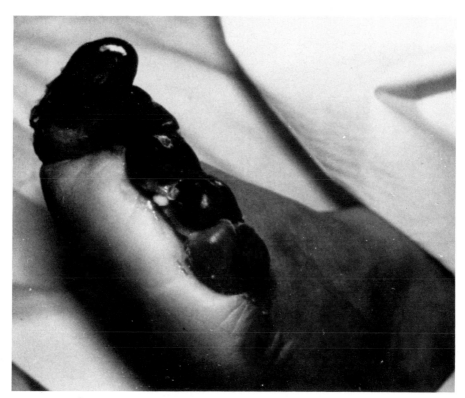

**FIG 2–12.**
Gangrene in toes of patient who had soaked his cold foot in hot water.

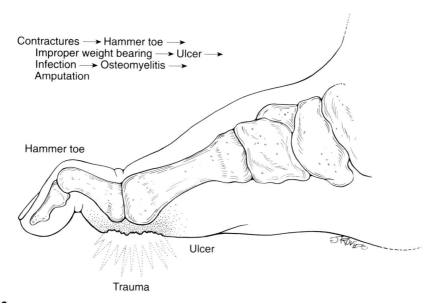

Contractures ⟶ Hammer toe ⟶
Improper weight bearing ⟶ Ulcer ⟶
Infection ⟶ Osteomyelitis ⟶
Amputation

Hammer toe

Ulcer

Trauma

**FIG 2–13.**
Progression of contractures leading to hammer toes, improper weight bearing, ulceration, infection, and osteomyelitis. Because ulcerations can occur at tip and on top of toe, I refer to this as tip-top-toe ulcer syndrome. *(From the Michigan Diabetes Research and Training Center, University of Michigan, Ann Arbor, 1983.)*

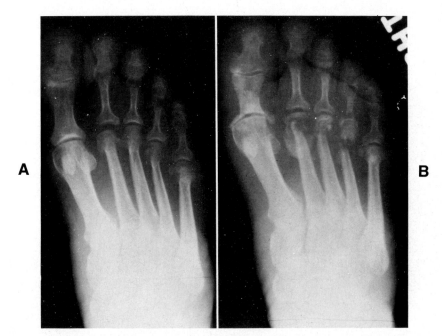

**FIG 2–14.**
**A,** radiograph of the foot of a 60-year-old man with known diabetes of 4 years duration. **B,** same foot 3 months later shows classic osteolytic bone changes of diabetic neuropathy involving the distal segment of the metatarsals. *(Courtesy of Robert Karsh, M.D., St. Louis.)*

destruction. Treatment in the acute stage is non–weight bearing, frequently with the aid of a contact cast. If the process is allowed to progress the arch collapses, and the foot becomes everted and shortened and takes on a clubfoot shape. The arch is lost, and the foot takes on a rocker bottom configuration (Fig 2–15,A). Maximum pressure now occurs at the plantar surface of the arch. This area breaks down and becomes ulcerated (Fig 2–15,B). The plantar surface of the arch is the classic site of ulceration in the Charcot foot. (Discussion of the pathogenesis and management of the Charcot foot is found in Chapter 7.)

## INFECTION

Infection is the third major factor in the pathogenesis of diabetic foot lesions, and when associated with ischemia frequently leads to amputation.[61] Breaks in the skin, which may be almost imperceptible (e.g., cracks, fissures in calluses), and major wounds (e.g., neurotrophic foot ulcers) act as portals of entry for bacteria. A variety of factors contribute to the diabetic's difficulty in handling infection. In the nondiabetic, infection leads to increased blood flow. In the diabetic, however, infection frequently leads to microthrombi formation in the small arterioles, which further impair circulation. When this occurs in the small arteries of the toes, the vessels can convert to end-arteries, resulting in gangrene of the toes. Vascular disease impairs the delivery of antibiotics and oxygen to the affected areas. Autonomic neurogenic vascular responses are impaired. Leukocyte function frequently is impaired, with defective adherence, diapedesis, chemotaxis, phagocytosis, and microbicidal activity, particularly in patients with uncontrolled diabetes and ketosis. (The pathogenesis and management of the diabetic foot infection are found in Chapter 8.)

## SPECIAL DIABETIC FOOT PROBLEMS IN THE HEEL

The heel of the diabetic foot is particularly vulnerable to trauma. The heel is exposed to a great deal of pressure, resulting in callus buildup. As the callus becomes

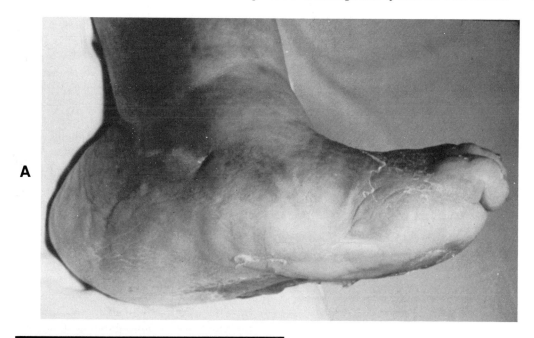

A

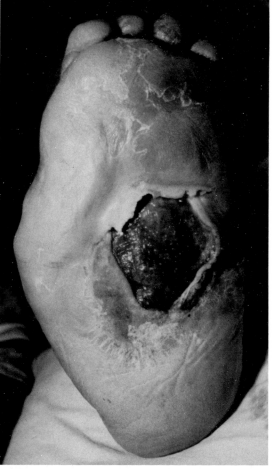

B

**FIG 2–15.**
Charcot foot. **A,** note clubfoot appearance, with collapse of tarsal metatarsal joints. **B,** massive ulcer on plantar surface of arch. *(From Levin ME: Pathophysiology of diabetic foot lesions, in Davidson J: Clinical diabetes mellitus: a problem-oriented approach, New York, 1986, Thieme Medical Publishers. Used by permission.)*

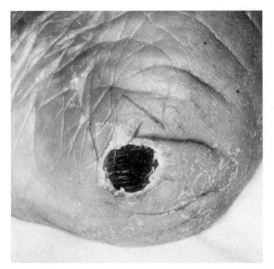

**FIG 2–16.**
Small painless gangrenous area on heel of the foot caused by pressure necrosis in a diabetic neuropathic foot.

thicker it tends to crack, and becomes a site of infection. When the heel is infected, the infection tends to penetrate deeply. The skin of the heel is tightly bound by numerous vertical septa extending through the subcutaneous tissue to the surface of the calcaneous. These septa result in formation of

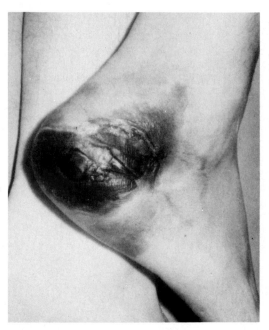

**FIG 2–17.**
Gangrene of heel of bedridden diabetic patient caused by weight of immobile neuropathic foot on mattress.

small cylinders packed with fatty tissue. These small fat-containing tubes act like shock absorbers on heel impact. With ischemic changes there is atrophy of the subcutaneous fatty tissue, thus decreasing the effectiveness of the "shock absorber" effect. When the skin covering the heel is destroyed much of the subcutaneous fat colliquates and the septa are disrupted. If healing does occur, a tight scar will result, which makes the heel susceptible to further trauma.

When the diabetic patient requires bed rest for any length of time, as when hospitalized, particular attention must be paid to the heel. Because of loss of sensation the patient tends to keep the heels in the same position, which results in pressure necrosis (Figs 2–16 and 2–17). The skin breaks down, and infection and gangrene can develop. The heels of these patients should be inspected at least once, and preferably twice, daily. If erythema is present, aggressive protective intervention must be instituted.

Prevention is critically important. Turning the patient and use of heel protectors or foam rubber or egg crate–type sponge-rubber mattresses is essential. The heel protectors may not stay in place; therefore daily checks of the heel are necessary.

## EXAMINATION OF DIABETIC FOOT

One of the most important aspects of the office or clinic visit is examination of the diabetic patient's foot and leg. Despite the problems associated with the diabetic foot, it is frequently the most neglected part of the examination. The low rate of foot inspection in a clinic setting has been documented by Cohen,[25] who found that only 15% to 19% of patients who entered the examining room had their feet inspected, and by Bailey et al.,[6] who reported that only 12.3% of diabetic patients' feet were examined. The foot and lower extremity of the diabetic should be examined at every routine office visit at least three or four times each year, and more often when indicated. This examination should include not only the removal of shoes and stockings but also of trousers or

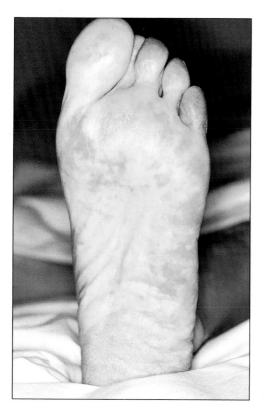

**PLATE 1.**
Cyanotic changes in the fifth toe and livedo reticularis pattern on the foot secondary to cholesterol emboli from atheroscleromatous plaque (see Fig 2–4). *(Courtesy of Gregorio Sicard, M.D., St. Louis.)*

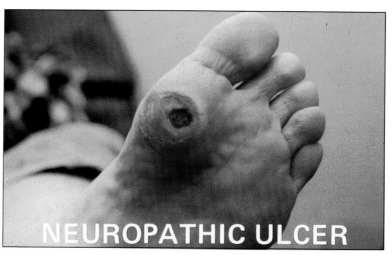

NEUROPATHIC ULCER

**PLATE 2.**
Classic neuropathic diabetic foot ulcer. Note ulceration in callus is well-circumscribed. Lesion is painless. *(From the Michigan Diabetes Research and Training Center, University of Michigan, Ann Arbor, 1983. Used by permission.)*

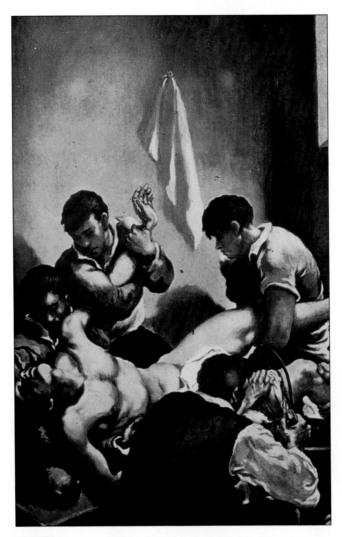

**PLATE 3.**
Painting depicts agonies of patient undergoing amputation in ancient times. Amputations were performed with only alcohol as anesthetic. Many patients died during this guillotine operation; some even died of shock and terror before the operation began! Teamwork today should be geared to saving, not removing, the leg. *(Painting by Italian Count Gregorio Calvi de Bergolo in 1953. From the International Museum of Surgical Sciences and Hall of Fame, International College of Surgeons, Chicago.)*

pantyhose as well. Only then can the lower extremity be examined properly. Patients are reluctant to remove their shoes and stockings because they seldom feel pain or discomfort and therefore assume that all is well. Second, it is embarrassing to many of these patients to remove their shoes and stockings. However, if the feet are not examined on a routine basis, lesions will be missed and treatment delayed, and amputation may be the result. Examination of the foot and lower extremity should include inspection and palpation, and neurologic and vascular tests.

## Inspection

Simply inspecting the legs and feet will give many clues to vascular status. Evidence of significant ischemia in the foot includes the loss of hair on the dorsum of the foot and toes, skin that is shiny and atrophic and appears to be drawn tightly around the foot because of loss of the subcutaneous fat layers, and dependent rubor (see Fig 2–5). All of these findings are indicative of severe PVD. One of the simplest evaluations for vascular insufficiency is to measure delayed capillary filling time. The extremity with severe PVD will develop dependent rubor. Patients with varicose veins also may have dependent rubor. Shiny atrophic skin, pallor

on elevation, delayed filling time, and dependent rubor are the hallmarks of significant lower extremity vascular insufficiency.

Inspection between the toes is of the utmost importance. Figure 2–18 shows an example of a painless interdigital ulcer in an elderly woman. When this patient came into the office and was asked to remove her shoes and socks, she refused, saying that her feet felt fine and that she had no problems with them. After much insistence she removed her shoes and stockings, and the ulcer was identified. When asked how long the ulcer had been present, the patient looked down and with great surprise stated that she did not know that she had an ulcer because she had felt no pain. Foot inspection frequently reveals interosseous muscle atrophy with resulting contractions and hammer and cocked-up toes.

## Palpation

Touching the skin is a simple and important part of the examination. The experienced hand and eye (see Inspection) are extremely important in the evaluation of PVD. Palpation consists of evaluating the femoral, popliteal, dorsalis pedis, and posterior tibial pulses. Auscultation for bruits will help identify the presence of atheromatous plaques and narrowing of the arterial lu-

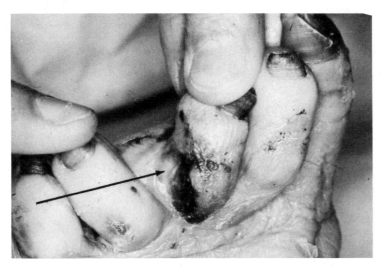

**FIG 2–18.**
Nonpainful interdigital ulcer in elderly diabetic woman. *Arrow* points to exposed tendon, indicating depth of ulceration. The painless ulcer was found on routine foot examination.

men. One of the most important aspects of palpation is detecting whether the skin is warm or cool. Sophisticated instruments are available for quantitative measurements of skin temperature, for example, the Mikron digital infrared thermometer, (Mikron Instrument Co., Ridgeway, N.J.; Biomedical Instruments, Newburg, Ohio). The approximate cost is $1,800. This instrument is useful for research, but is not necessary for routine examination of the foot. Palpation with the palm or back of the hand is sufficient. In the office a hand-held Doppler, relatively inexpensive and easy to use, can be used to evaluate the peripheral vascular status. The use of Doppler and other laboratory techniques for evaluating PVD are found in Chapter 15.

## Sensory Examination

Although a variety of sophisticated techniques are available for measurement of vibratory sense (large nerve fibers), such as the Biothesiometer, a simple tuning fork with a 128 cycle is sufficient. This examination should include vibratory sense, not only at the ankle but also at the tips of the toes. Once the patient can no longer feel the vibration the examiner can apply the tuning fork to the same area of his or her own foot to see whether further vibrations can be detected.

The examination to assess the ability to perceive temperature, a small nerve fiber modality, also can be carried out. Guy et al.[51] found the lateral aspect of the foot to be the most sensitive location for the measurement of thermal sensation. These authors noted loss of thermal sensation in all feet with neuropathic ulcerations and in feet with Charcot joint. When thermal sensitivity was compared with vibratory perception threshold, it was found that thermal sensitivity sometimes was selectively affected, especially in those patients with painful neuropathy, suggesting that the small fibers are more vulnerable in the diabetic.[51] Quantitative measurements of thermal sensation can be made with sophisticated instruments.

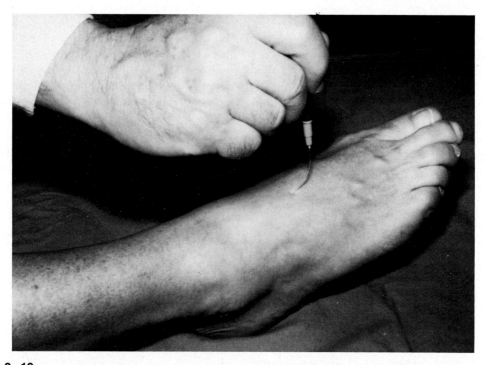

**FIG 2–19.**
Semmes-Weinstein monofilament being used to evaluate sensory perception. Patient should be able to detect sensation at the time the monofilament buckles. The 5.07 filament equals 10 g of linear strength to buckle and represents the threshold for loss of touch sensation. *(From Levin ME: J Diabetic Complications 3:211, 1989. Used by permission.)*

However, using test tubes of cold and warm water is a simple and reasonable means of detecting thermal sensation.

Sensory evaluation to perceive protective sensation is frequently carried out by using a pin. This is an inadequate way to evaluate sensation because it varies with each investigator, depending on how forcefully the pin is used. Today state-of-the-art evaluation for the ability to perceive touch is done using the Semmes Weinstein monofilaments. These filaments come in three thicknesses, 4.17, 5.07, and 6.10. The monofilament is placed against the skin and pressure applied until the filament buckles (Fig 2–19). The monofilament usually is applied to the bottom of the foot and to different areas; the patient should be able to identify the area being touched. The patient should also be able to detect the presence of the monofilament at the time it buckles. A thickness of 5.07 is equal to 10 g of linear pressure and is the limit used to determine protective sensations.

Although there is variability from patient to patient, the loss of peripheral nerve function progresses as follows: first the vibratory sense is lost, followed by loss of reflexes (Achilles reflex is usually the first to go), and finally loss of sensations of pain and touch.

## TREATMENT OF DIABETIC FOOT ULCERS

### Primary Treatment

Ulcers occur in the diabetic foot because of repetitive stress on insensitive feet. When repetitive stress continues the foot develops hot spots, callus buildup, pressure necrosis, and ultimately ulceration. This occurs most often at the site of the most pressure and excessive callus buildup, usually over the metatarsal heads, especially the first, and on the plantar surface of the hallux. Patients who develop ulcers have increased foot pressures.[18] Plate 2 illustrates the classic diabetic foot ulcer, sometimes referred to as a malperforans ulcer. Note the marked callus buildup surrounding the ulcer. Ulceration on the dorsum of the foot is caused by trauma. When on the side of the foot (see

**TABLE 2–5.**

Primary Treatment of Diabetic Foot Ulcers

1. Evaluation
   a. Clinical appearance
   b. Depth of penetration
   c. X-rays to detect
      (1) Foreign body
      (2) Osteomyelitis
      (3) Subcutaneous gas
   d. Location
   e. Biopsy
   f. Blood supply (noninvasive vascular studies)
2. Debridement, radical
3. Bacterial cultures (aerobic and anaerobic)
4. Metabolic control
5. Antibiotics
   a. Oral
   b. Parenteral
6. Do not soak feet
7. Decrease of edema
8. Non–weight bearing
   a. Bed rest
   b. Crutches
   c. Wheelchair
   d. Special sandals
   e. Contact casting
9. Improvement of circulation (vascular surgery)

Fig 2–7), ulceration most likely is caused by an ill-fitting shoe. Persistent ulceration in the diabetic foot leads to lower limb amputation in 84% of cases.[99]

Table 2–5 lists the management of diabetic foot ulcers. X-ray films are necessary to rule out osteomyelitis, gas formation, and the possibility of the presence of foreign objects (see Fig 2–6). I believe a radiograph should be taken of any foot with a diabetic foot ulcer or infection.

Treatment of diabetic foot ulcers requires the establishment of depth and degree of ulceration. What may appear to be a superficial ulceration may in fact penetrate deep into the tissues. Figure 2–20,A shows what appears to be a relatively small ulcer on the plantar surface of the foot in a 60-year-old woman. She had been diabetic for 20 years and had severe peripheral neuropathy with an insensate foot. While walking barefoot she stepped on a nail and developed a painless ulceration on her instep, which she treated with a variety of "home remedies." When the wound failed to heal after several weeks she sought medical attention. The wound appeared to be a small superficial ul-

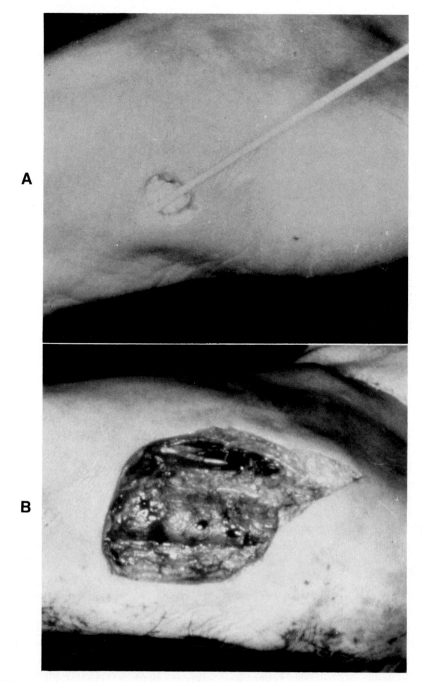

**FIG 2–20.**
**A,** ulcer appears to be small and superficial on plantar surface of foot. **B,** exploration of ulcer reveals infection to penetrated tissues and interfascial plane. **C,** successful skin graft of lesion. *(Courtesy of Dr. David Caplan, St. Louis.)*                                                                  (Continued.)

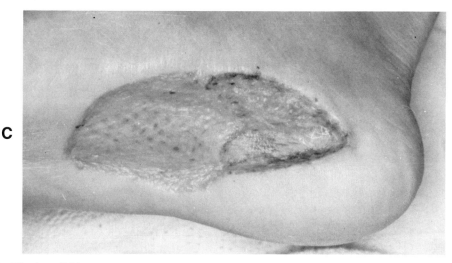

**C**

**FIG 2–20 (cont'd).**

cer with minimal infection. However, extensive debridement revealed the infection to have penetrated deep into the interfascial spaces (Fig 2–20,B). Because this patient's circulation was good, she responded to parenteral antibiotic therapy, and a skin graft was successful (Fig 2–20,C). Multiple lessons can be learned from this case. First, patients should not go barefoot. Second, the physician should not assume that what appears to be a superficial ulceration is simply that, and treat it only with topical agents. Finally, vigorous debridement of the ulcer must be done to establish the degree of penetration and to remove all necrotic material. It is currently believed that debridement should be taken down to healthy tissue. The ulcer after debridement in all probability will be larger than it was at manifestation. Eschars should be completely removed. Whirlpool is not the method of choice for debridement. When the foot is insensitive, minor debridement can be carried out at the bedside; however, frequently the patient must be taken to the operating room for adequate debridement under anesthesia.

Biopsy should be considered when the ulcer appears at the atypical location (e.g., not over the metatarsal heads or the plantar surface of the hallux), when it cannot be explained by trauma, and when it is unresponsive to aggressive therapy. On numerous occasions biopsies of atypical ulcers have revealed malignancies.

Evaluation should include testing for peripheral neuropathy and status of the blood supply by noninvasive vascular studies. Cultures should be taken aerobically and anaerobically. However, Wheat,[128] commenting on the report of Lipsky et al.,[74] believed that baseline cultures were not always required when the lesions were not septic and there was no extensive infection, cellulitis, lymphangitis, soft tissue necrosis, gangrene, crepitus, or gas in the tissues and when baseline x-ray films did not show focal erosive changes suggestive of osteomyelitis. Other criteria for not culturing were patient compliance and ability to return at least weekly. The patient should have adequate local care, including debridement, toenail removal if indicated, and incision and drainage of abscesses. The patient must keep the legs elevated, minimize ambulation, and use protective shoes. The patient and or family member must be able to assist in home management. Wheat[128] believed that if these criteria were met the following approaches were reasonable: (1) Obtain x-ray films, and (2) initiate oral treatment with an antibiotic with good activity against gram-positive organisms. If the lesion does not improve, appropriate curettage cultures should be obtained on which to base proper antibiotic therapy and the patient should be hospitalized for additional workup and treatment. Parenteral antibiotics are necessary when significant infection is present.

It should be kept in mind that many of these diabetic foot infections contain gram-negative organisms. Consideration therefore should be given to choosing an oral antibiotic effective against both gram-positive and gram-negative organisms.

The selection of an oral antibiotic or parenteral antibiotic for the treatment of a diabetic foot infection is based on medical judgment. However, certain criteria strongly suggest the need for hospitalization and the use of parenteral antibiotics. These include patients who are septic or febrile or have luekocytosis, cellulitis, or deep infection. Patients with what appears to be a minor infection on the plantar surface of the foot but with evidence of infection on the dorsum of the foot suggested by erythema should be hospitalized. Although sepsis may not be present, there is a high probability of severe infection deep in the tissues. Patients with severe PVD should be hospitalized and given parenteral antibiotics to achieve higher concentration of antibiotics in the peripheral tissues than frequently can be achieved by oral therapy alone. Furthermore, the antibiotic of choice can be given only parenterally.

Infection in the diabetic foot can deteriorate within 24 hours. If an oral antibiotic is selected, I believe the patient should be seen every 2 to 3 days until the infection is under control. The patient must be carefully instructed to notify the physician at once should there be increased redness, drainage, and pain or evidence of lymphangitis. Although many of these patients have insensate feet, the development of pain is indicative of deep infection and requires immediate attention. The development of odor also indicates worsening infection and frequently the presence of anaerobes. It is important that patients with infection monitor their blood glucose levels closely. A rising blood glucose level strongly suggests worsening infection. These instructions should be documented in the patient's chart.

When infection does not respond to aggressive debridement and antibiotic therapy, the wound should be debrided again and another culture done, because the flora may have changed. Chronic recurrent or resistant infection suggests the presence of

**TABLE 2–6.**

Indications of Worsening Infection

1. Signs and symptoms
   a. ↑ Drainage,
   b. ↑ Erythema,
   c. ↑ Pain
   d. ↑ Temperature
   e. Foul odor
   f. Lymphangitis
   g. Lymphadenopathy
   h. Gangrene
2. Laboratory results
   a. ↑ Blood glucose level
   b. ↑ WBC level
   c. ↑ Sedimentation rate

osteomyelitis. Vascular status should be evaluated carefully, and vascular surgery considered when indicated. Impending or developing gangrene also suggests possible progression of infection. Indications of worsening infection are noted in Table 2–6.

Edema frequently is present. Elevation of the feet, no more than the thickness of one pillow, can be beneficial. Higher elevation may impede circulation.

Soaking the feet has no benefit, although it has been a traditional approach.[70] Soaking can lead to maceration and further infection. Because of the insensitivity of the foot, the patient may soak it in water that is too hot (see Fig 2–12), resulting in severe burns. Chemical soaks can result in chemical burns.

No weight bearing is essential. Because the feet are insensitive and the ulcer does not hurt, patients continue to walk. The result is increased pressure necrosis, forcing bacteria deeper into the tissues, and failure to heal. The use of crutches and wheelchairs is seldom successful in achieving total and consistent non–weight bearing. Many patients with neuropathy have ataxia, making the use of crutches potentially dangerous. The best method for non–weight bearing in appropriately selected patients is the use of a contact cast. This cast allows the patient to be ambulatory by redistributing the weight, thereby decreasing the pressure on the ulcer area. (Use of the contact cast is discussed in Chapter 13.)

When an ulcer does not heal despite good metabolic control, adequate debridement,

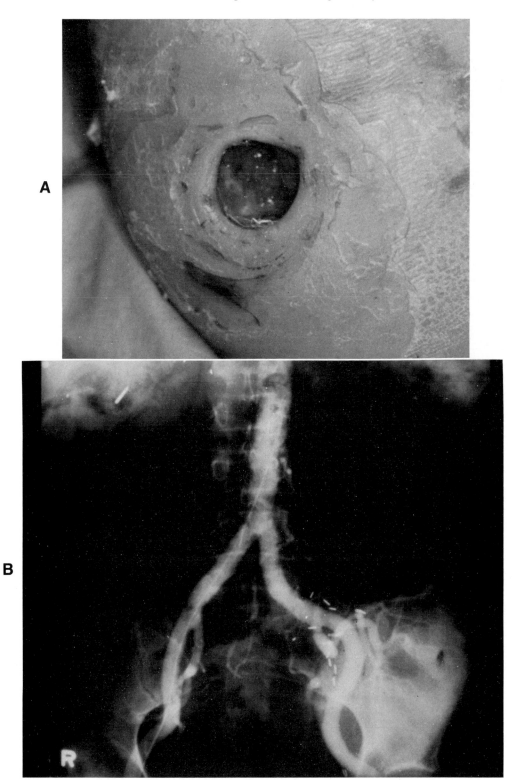

**FIG 2–21.**
**A,** ulceration of plantar surface of heel, which was debrided to the periosteum of the calcaneus. **B,** arteriogram revealed normal aorta and iliac arteries. Previously transplanted kidney is noted on left side of the pelvis. **C,** arteriogram shows occlusion of both left and right tibial and peroneal vessels at their origin. **D,** extent of surgery for popliteal posterior tibial bypass. **E,** healed ulcer 3 weeks after vascular surgery. *(Courtesy of Dr. Gregorio Sicard, St. Louis.)*                                                                          (Continued.)

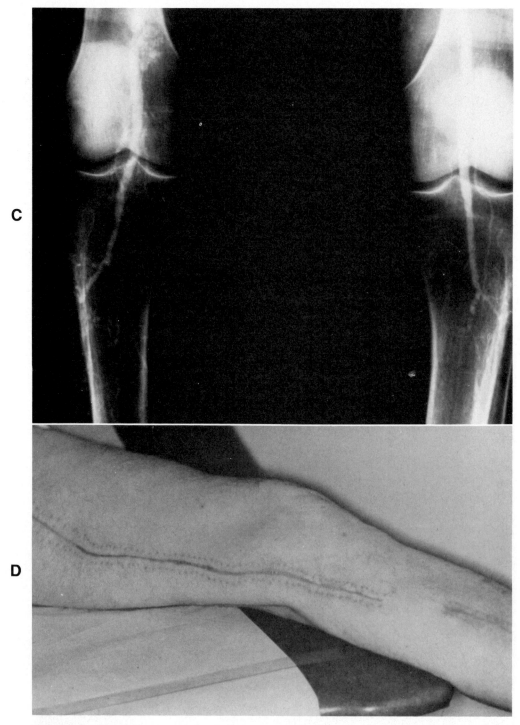

**C**

**D**

FIG 2–21   (cont'd.).

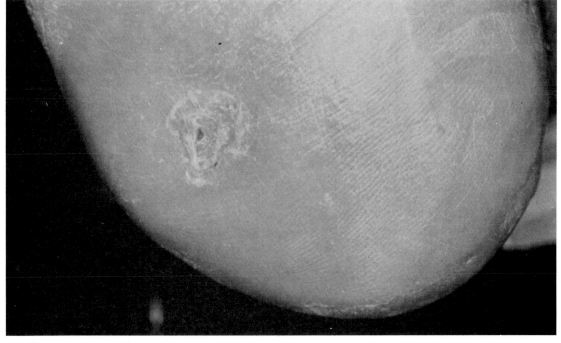

E

**FIG 2–21  (cont'd.).**

parenteral antibiotic therapy, and non–weight bearing, underlying osteomyelitis, changes in bacterial flora, and inadequate blood supply should be considered. In the presence of ischemia in cases of impaired healing, vascular surgery should be considered. Ankle brachial indexes of less than 0.45 or $tCPo_2$ less than 30 mm Hg, and certainly less than 20 mm Hg, is highly predictive that the infection will not resolve and that the ulcer will not heal. For example, Pecoraro et al.[98] found a 39-fold increased risk of early wound failure if the average periwound $tcPo_2$ was less than 22 mm Hg.

Figure 2–21,A shows an ulceration on the plantar surface of the heel. The patient had an insensitive foot and had worn a shoe with a rough area in the heel. He was hospitalized, and aggressive therapy was carried out. Debridement was continued to the periosteum of the calcaneous, but 4 weeks later there had been no progress in healing. Vascular surgery was considered. Arteriograms revealed a previously transplanted kidney in the left iliac fossa, and good aorta and iliac vessels (Fig 2–21,B); and slight atherosclerosis in both superficial femoral arteries but

occlusion of both left and right tibial and peroneal vessels at their origins (Fig 2–21,C). The patient underwent a left posterior tibial bypass (Fig 2–21,D). The initial left ankle Doppler index, 0.66 preoperatively, probably an erroneously high reading because of noncompressible vessels, had now risen to 0.95. Within 3 weeks the plantar ulcer had completely healed (Fig 2–21,E). The importance of treating diabetic foot ulcers by improving circulation has been noted by Sage and Doyle.[112] They believe, and I agree, that the degree of ischemia and not necessarily the extent of the ulcer is the most significant factor in predicting the potential outcome of treatment. Their success rate in the ischemic group was 25%, and in the nonischemic group 83%. Impediments to wound healing are noted in Table 2–7 and have been reviewed by Rosenberg.[111] One of the most overlooked factors is poor nutrition. A serum albumin level of less than 3.0 g or a lymphocyte count of less than 1,500 $mm^3$ is evidence of preexisting malnutrition.[34] Duncan and Faris[38] have shown that the presence of diabetes, hypertension, and advanced age also are factors that reduce

**TABLE 2–7.**

Impediments to Wound Healing

1. Vascular
   a. Atherosclerosis
   b. Increased viscosity
2. Neurologic
   a. Insensate foot
   b. Decreased flare reaction
3. Infection
   a. Inadequate debridement
   b. Poor blood supply
   c. Microthrombi
   d. Hyperglycemia
   e. Decreased polymorphonuclear neutrophil
      function
   f. Polymicrobial infection
   g. Changing bacterial flora
   h. Osteomyelitis
4. Mechanical
   a. Edema
   b. Weight bearing
5. Poor nutrition
   a. Low serum albumin level
6. Decreased growth factors
7. Poor patient compliance

the likelihood of wound healing. Other investigators have attributed delay in wound healing to a variety of factors, as noted earlier. Pecoraro et al.,[98] in a study of 46 diabetic patients with lower extremity ulcers, found that age, type of diabetes, duration, or treatment, the level of glycosylated hemoglobin, current smoking, presence of sensory neuropathy, ulcer location, initial infection, frequency, and recurrent infections were not factors. However, the absence of these factors in wound healing should not deter from the fact that many of these ulcers were initiated or contributed to by some of the previously mentioned factors. Their most important finding was one that has been repeated throughout this chapter, namely, that local cutaneous perfusion estimated by periwound measurements of $tcPo_2$ were significantly associated with the initial rate of tissue repair. Pecoraro et al.[98] concluded that periwound cutaneous perfusion is the critical physiologic determinant of diabetic ulcer healing. They found a 39-fold increased risk of early healing failure when the average periwound $tcPo_2$ was less than 20 mm Hg. They found that the prediction of early healing of local skin perfusion was independent of segmental Doppler arterial

pressure at the dorsalis pedis, although eventual ulcer reepithelization was significantly related to foot blood pressure and periwound $tcPo_2$. A variety of theoretical possibilities that might contribute to decreased skin oxygenation and wound healing include inadequacy of capillary filling,[109] tissue edema,[3] AV shunting,[41] and atypical microvascular response to physiologic stimuli because of autonomic neuropathy.[124]

The efficacy of hyperbaric oxygen in treating diabetic foot ulcers continues to be investigated. The use of topical hyperbaric oxygen is of no benefit. Leslie et al.[67] conducted a prospective and randomized study of 28 diabetic patients treated with topical hyperbaric oxygen. These patients were followed for 14 days. At 7 days and 14 days there were no differences in the type of microorganisms isolated by curettage. Changes in ulcer size did not differ between the control and the topical hyperbaric oxygen group. It was their conclusion that the healing of diabetic foot ulcers was not accelerated by topical hyperbaric oxygen.[67] Results obtained from the use of the hyperbaric oxygen chamber are more encouraging. Baroni et al.[7] treated 18 hospitalized adult diabetic patients with gangrenous lesions of the foot. These patients wee compared with a group of ten diabetic patients with comparable foot lesions who were not treated in the chamber.[7] They found that hyperbaric oxygen treatment greatly reduced leg amputations. However, confirmation that the hyperbaric oxygen chamber for treatment of diabetic foot ulcers is a beneficial modality will require a study that has a larger patient population and is better controlled. The use of hyperbaric oxygen is covered in Chapter 14.

## Topical Treatment

The use of topical therapy goes back to ancient times, when an unbelievable number of substances, ranging from wine to human excreta, were used to treat wounds (Table-Talk, XCII "Of God's Works," Martin Luther [1483–1546]). Today the list of topically applied agents remains long, and is growing. Like various weight-loss diets, if one of these treatments was specifically effective, we would not see a continuing stream of new diets or topical preparations being advocated. Currently the use of resins and enzyme therapy to help debride are advocated by some. Although these are of some benefit, they represent adjunct therapy and should not be substituted for total aggressive surgical debridement. It remains traditional to use povidone-iodine (Betadine), acetic acid, hydrogen peroxide, and sodium hypochlorite (Dakin's solution). Although these substances will destroy surface bacteria, they are cytotoxic to granulation tissue.[72] Oberg and Lindsey[93] also have cautioned against the use of hydrogen peroxide and povidone-iodine in wounds. Henri de Mondeville (1260–1320) said, "Many more surgeons know how to cause suppuration than to heal a wound." I think many surgeons, but not all, are learning how to manage wounds and are now doing more good than harm. Current therapy does not recommend the use of these topical agents. Other topical antibiotics such as silver sulfadiazine (Silvadene) or topical triple antibiotic therapy can be used but are only beneficial for removing surface bacteria. The use of topical preparations and allowing these patients to bear weight puts them at great jeopardy for amputation (see Chapter 12).

The latest addition to topical therapy is topically applied wound healing growth factors. Current investigation suggests that the use of platelet-derived growth factors is an important adjunct to wound healing.[62, 104] A wound-healing formula derived from platelets consists of a variety of factors. The most important function of the growth factors is chemoattractive, which attracts the neutrophils and monocytes; fibroblast growth factor, which promotes matrix formation by stimulating fibroblasts; angiogenesis factor, which stimulates endothelial cells to form granulation tissue; and epidermal growth factor to promote skin growth. As many as 19 growth factors are currently being developed by more than 60 companies focusing on a broad range of indications in addition to wound healing. See Chapter 11 for a discussion of wound healing factors and wound healing formula. It is obvious that there are many impediments to diabetic wound heal-

ing (see Table 2–7). To achieve success in healing the wound, one must address all of these.

## Posttreatment of Healed Diabetic Foot Ulcers

Even though the diabetic foot ulcer has healed, the job is not complete. The underlying etiologies such as foot deformities, calluses, and increased pressure responsible for the ulceration are still present. In addition, scar tissue from previously healed ulcers is not strong tissue and is very vulnerable to the shearing forces of walking. Therefore special measures are necessary to protect the vulnerable sites of previous breakdown. This requires reeducation of the patient in walking, teaching him or her to take shorter steps, and frequently a change in jobs is necessary. Internal pressure from metatarsal heads or sesmoid bones may cause recurrence of ulceration. In selected cases, removal of these may be necessary. Special shoes are very important.

## SPECIAL SHOES

Patients who have cocked-up toes require a shoe with a bigger toe box. The patient with a markedly deformed foot such as the Charcot foot needs a specially molded shoe. The use of special therapeutic shoes is critically important in preventing ulcerations or recurrence of ulcers. This frequently requires an extra-depth shoe with a plasticlike material, frequently a Plastazote insole to redistribute the weight and to prevent recurrence of ulceration. This was clearly demonstrated at a study at King's College in London, which showed an 83% recurrence of ulcers when patients returned to wearing regular shoes. However, with the use of special shoes, there was only a 17% recurrence of ulceration.[41] The importance of therapeutic shoes and proper fitting is being recognized with increasing frequency. Figure 2–22 shows an x-ray film of an unusual case, a patient, who was not diabetic, with eight toes and fully developed metatarsal bones. This patient's major problem was

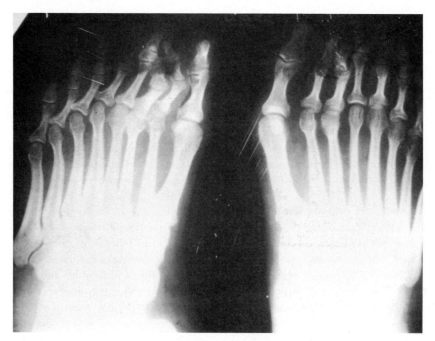

**FIG 2–22.**
This patient has difficulty finding shoes that fit because he has eight toes and eight metatarsal bones on each foot. *(Courtesy of Cheryl Strickland Allen, P.T., Oklahoma City.)*

finding a shoe that fit. He obviously required very special shoes (see Chapters 24 and 25). As previously noted, abnormally high pressures contribute to callus buildup and ulceration. A recently developed stocking has been shown to significantly decrease forefoot pressure by 27% compared with barefoot pressures.[122] The use of such a stocking may prove beneficial in preventing callus buildup and ulceration and in postulcer management.

## TEAMWORK

The team needed for the care of the diabetic is not the one depicted in Plate 3. It is a team that will save the foot, not amputate it. I believe the 11th commandment should be "Thou shalt not amputate."

It becomes quite obvious that the management of the diabetic foot requires many medical disciplines, including the primary physician, endocrinologist, diabetologist, podiatrist, nurse educator, physician assistant, enterstomal nurse, infectious disease specialist, neurologist, vascular surgeon, orthopedist, physiatrist, pedorthist, orthotist, phys-

ical therapist, prosthetist, occupational therapist, social worker, and home care nurse. The primary physician's most important role is examining the foot at every visit and educating the patient in foot care. The physician who does not carry out these tasks loses the advantage of the old adage, "an ounce of prevention is worth a pound of cure." The nurse educator or trained assistant is an important member of the team. The nurse educator not only educates the patient about the various aspects of diabetes but also examines the feet. The expert in infectious disease has a very important role in the care of the diabetic. The vascular surgeon, because of expertise in revascularization, has saved many patients from amputation. Many enterostomal nurses have developed an expertise in wound management and have assumed a significant role in diabetic foot management, including debridement and wound dressings (see Chapter 12). The podiatrist frequently is the first to detect a diabetic foot lesion and occasionally the first to diagnose the patient's diabetes. The podiatrist can surgically correct foot problems such as cocked-up toes and bunions and can treat chronic nail problems. The podiatrist's role in patient education in foot care is paramount (see Chapter 23). The frequency of neuropathic syndromes and their differential diagnoses may require a neurologist. The orthopedist frequently sees the patient because of foot deformities. The expertise of the orthopedist in prophylactic or other corrective surgery is of the upmost importance. Other important members of the team managing diabetic foot deformities consist of the certified pedorthist and orthotist. These specialists in fitting therapeutic shoes and braces are critically important. The physical therapist may have two roles. In medical centers where contact casting is practiced, it is frequently the physical therapist who is trained to apply these special casts. When amputation occurs, the physiatrist's skills, along with the physical therapist and the prosthetist, are required for rehabilitation. Treatment of diabetic foot lesions can be prolonged, and because hospital stays must be shortened, many patients require home nursing care services. The home care nurse may be needed to carry out prolonged parenteral antibiotic therapy, change dressings, debride, and observe the clinical course. Financial problems resulting from loss of a job can be monumental. The social worker becomes an important team member in these cases.

From the foregoing, it is clear that the management of diabetic foot problems can be complicated. It should not be left to the neophyte or the uninterested. Success in saving the diabetic foot is achieved only from the expertise requiring multiple disciplines.

## PATIENT EDUCATION

Of all the approaches to saving the diabetic foot, the most important is patient education. Despite our current knowledge and good diabetic control, physicians cannot totally prevent PVD and peripheral neuropathy. However, the patient can be educated in proper foot care, teaching him or her how to prevent injury to insensitive feet and de-

tect foot lesions as early as possible. At the time of the office visit and while the shoes and socks are off, the nurse or physician should review the do's and don'ts of foot care with the patient (Table 2–8). This cannot be adequately accomplished by simply handing the patient a list of instructions. The instructions should be explained and questions encouraged and answered. If this is done, the patient will have a better understanding of the importance of foot care. The patient should be instructed to not only look at the feet but to also inspect the areas between the toes (see Fig 2–18). Patients with impaired vision, extreme obesity, or arthritis who cannot inspect their feet adequately can have this performed by a family member. If a family member is not available to do this, the patient can place a mirror on the floor, allowing him or her to inspect the bottom of the foot. The feet should be kept clean, and the patient should be cautioned to dry them carefully, making sure that the areas between the toes are dried thoroughly. Moisture left in these areas can lead to maceration and infection.

Because autonomic neuropathy leads to the inability of the foot to perspire, the skin becomes dry, flaky, and cracked. The application of a very thin coat of lubricating material to the foot after bathing helps to seal in the moisture. It is moisture rather than the oil alone that keeps the skin pliable and decreases the dryness. Any type of cream can be used. Each practitioner has his or her favorite. Even vegetable oils can be used. Exotic oils such as mink oil have been suggested.[11] It is important that lubricants not be placed between the toes, because this can cause moisture to accumulate and lead to maceration and infection (see Chapter 12).

Extremes of temperature should be avoided. Many patients with cold insensitive feet because of neuropathy and PVD have incurred severe burns by using a heating pad or hot water bottle or by soaking them in water that is too hot (see Fig 2–12). The temperature of the water should be tested before bathing. This should be done with the elbow or a thermometer, not with the hand, which may be insensitive because of periph-

**TABLE 2–8.**

Patient Instructions for the Care of the Diabetic Foot

1.  Do not smoke.
2.  Inspect the feet daily for blisters, cuts, and scratches. The use of a mirror can aid in seeing the bottom of the feet. Always check between the toes.
3.  Wash feet daily. Dry carefully, especially between the toes.
4.  Avoid extremes of temperatures. Test water with hand, elbow, or thermometer before bathing.
5.  If feet feel cold at night, wear socks. Do not apply hot water bottles or heating pads. Do not use an electric blanket. Do not soak feet in hot water.
6.  Do not walk on hot surfaces such as sandy beaches or on cement around swimming pools.
7.  Do not walk barefoot.
8.  Do not use chemical agents for removal of corns and calluses, corn plasters, or strong antiseptic solutions.
9.  Do not use adhesive tape on the feet.
10. Inspect the inside of shoes daily for foreign objects, nail points, torn linings, and rough areas.
11. If your vision is impaired, have a family member inspect feet daily, trim nails, and buff calluses.
12. Do not soak feet.
13. For dry feet, use a very thin coat of a lubricating oil or cream. Apply this after bathing and drying the feet. Do not put the oil or cream between the toes. Consult your physician for detailed instructions.
14. Stockings: Wear properly fitting stockings. Do not wear mended stockings or stockings with seams. Change stockings daily.
15. Do not wear garters.
16. Shoes should be comfortable at time of purchase. Do not depend on them to stretch out. Shoes should be made of leather. Purchase shoes late in the afternoon when feet are the largest. Running or special walking shoes may be worn after checking with your physician. Purchase shoes from shoe salesman who understands diabetic foot problems.
17. Do not wear shoes without stockings.
18. Do not wear sandals with thongs between the toes.
19. In winter time, take special precautions. Wear wool socks and protective foot gear such as fleece-lined boots.
20. Cut nails straight across.
21. Do not cut corns and calluses: follow instructions from your physician or podiatrist.
22. Avoid crossing your legs; this can cause pressure on the nerves.
23. See your physician regularly and be sure that your feet are examined at each visit.
24. Notify your physician or podiatrist at once should you develop a blister or sore on your feet.
25. Be sure to inform your podiatrist that you are a diabetic.

eral neuropathy. Hot cement around swimming pools and hot sandy beaches are potentially disastrous for the diabetic foot. Many diabetic patients with insensitive feet have suffered severe burns secondary to walking on these surfaces. Patients should be advised to wear protective footwear at the beach and around the pool.

Chemical burns can occur from agents used to remove corns and calluses. The use of these substances should be avoided. The diabetic should inspect the inside of the

shoes daily for foreign objects, nail points, and torn linings.

A critically important part of the diabetic's educational program is instruction in proper footwear. The shoes should be comfortable at the time of purchase, and the patient should not depend on them to "stretch out." Shoes should be purchased late in the day when the feet are at their largest. Shoes that feel comfortable at the time of purchase may actually be too small, because the patient with an insensitive foot cannot detect

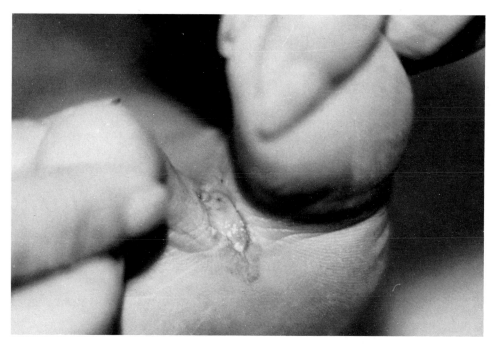

**FIG 2–23.**
Ulceration between toes from wearing thongs.

discomfort. New shoes should be worn only a few hours each day. The shoes should be made of leather, not manmade materials. However, walking or running shoes may reduce the rate of callus buildup.[116] Patients with foot deformities should wear special therapeutic or molded shoes. The patient should be instructed not to wear thongs. Figure 2–23 shows an ulceration between the first and second toes of a patient who had worn thonged sandals.

The patient should be taught the proper method of cutting nails straight across or following the curve of the nails but never to cut deep into the corners. Improper trimming can result in an ingrown toenail. Recurring ingrown toenails can be treated conservatively but are always a potential source of infection and, when indicated, should receive definitive therapy. Patients must be instructed repeatedly not to do home surgery. Serious complications can result when the patient "operates" on insensitive feet (see Fig 2–11).

Calluses should not be cut by the patient. They can be planed down with pumice stones, emery boards, and callus files; used cautiously, they can be helpful. Patients with insensitive feet should be cautioned on the use of the callus file, because there is a tendency to file too deeply. If the callus is particularly thick, it should be trimmed by a physician, surgeon, or podiatrist. Patients should be reminded to inform any physician working with their feet that they are diabetic so that the necessary precautions can be taken. See Table 2–8 for a list of patient instructions.

The effectiveness of education and total foot care programs in reducing amputation has been noted by Malone et al.[77] In many instances the amputation rate has been reduced by 50% or more.[5, 31, 41] Lippman[73] has reduced the amputation rate of 8 to 15 cases a year to zero with a special foot care program in nursing homes.

## PATIENT ADHERENCE

Despite the most detailed and repeated instructions, many patients will not adhere to a foot care program. For instance, it is very difficult to convince some women to forego wearing high-fashion, high-heeled shoes despite their lament that "these shoes are killing me." As previously noted, despite warnings, many patients succumb to that irresistible urge to do "home surgery." For many patients, going barefooted "feels too good to give up," or they are simply not motivated enough to put on their shoes for their own protection. Cessation of smoking is almost impossible for many patients. It is not a rare experience for a physician to visit his postamputation patient and find him or her lying in bed, smoking. When the danger and risk to the remaining limb are explained for the "hundredth time," the response is usually, "You are right, Doc. I know that smoking can cause the loss of my other leg. I am going to quite smoking—some day." For all of these reasons and despite the constant effort of health care professionals, patient adherence is difficult to accomplish. The problem is compounded even further by patients who do not keep their clinic appointments. Miller[86] many years ago documented that an intensified foot care program resulted in approximately two thirds fewer hospital admissions of those patients with foot problems who faithfully participated in the program compared with those who did not attend the clinic on a regular basis.

## REHABILITATION AFTER LOWER LIMB AMPUTATION IN THE DIABETIC

Unfortunately, not all amputations can be prevented. Therefore, rehabilitation becomes an important facet in the overall management of the diabetic amputee. If we achieve our goal of reducing the amputation rate by 50%, we will still have more than 25,000 to 30,000 amputations each year. A significant number of these patients can benefit from a prosthetic rehabilitation program. (see Chapter 22).

## SUMMARY

The pathogenesis of diabetic foot lesions is multifactorial. Physicians involved in the management of the diabetic foot must understand the pathogenesis and risk factors involved so that whenever possible the development of foot problems can be prevented or delayed. Management is complicated, and consultation can help save the foot. The physician who does not seek help is not being fair to himself or herself or to the patient. Aggressive treatment of foot ulcers, the use of special shoes, and patient education have been stressed. Taking all of these factors into consideration, the goal of all physicians and clinics managing the diabetic foot should be to reduce their amputation rate by at least 50%. This goal is a realistic one and can be achieved.

## Acknowledgment

I wish to thank Barbara Levin for her excellent assistance in the preparation of this chapter.

## REFERENCES

1. Aguayo AJ: Neuropathy due to compression and entrapment, in Dyck PJ, Thomas PK, Lambert EH, editors: *Peripheral neuropathy*, Philadelphia, 1975, WB Saunders.

2. Anderson AJ, Sobocinski KA, Freedman DS, et al: Body fat distribution, plasma lipids, and lipoproteins, *Arteriosclerosis* 8:88, 1988.

3. Apelqvist J, Larsson J, Agardh C-D: The importance of peripheral pulses, peripheral oedema and local pain for the outcome of diabetic foot ulcers, *Diabetic Med* 7:590, 1990.

4. Ardron M, MacFarlane IA, Robinson C, et al: Anti-smoking advice for young diabetic smokers: is it a waste of breath? *Diabetic Med* 5:677, 1988.

5. Assal JP, Muhlhauser I, Pernat A, et al: Patient education as the basis for diabetes care in clinical practices, *Diabetologia* 28:602, 1985.

6. Bailey TS, Yu HM, Rayfield EJ: Patterns of foot inspection in a diabetes clinic, *Am J Med* 78:371, 1985.

7. Baroni G, Porro T, Faglia E, et al: Hyperbaric oxygen in diabetic gangrene treatment, *Diabetes Care* 10:81, 1987.

8. Barrett-Connor E, Khaw KT: Cigarette smoking and increased central adiposity, *Am Coll Phys* 111:783, 1989.

9. Beach KW, Strandness DE Jr: Arteriosclerosis obliterans and associated risk factors in insulin dependent and noninsulin dependent diabetics, *Diabetes* 29:882, 1980.

10. Belch JJF, McArdle BM, Burns P, et al: Effects of acute smoking on platelet behaviour, fibrinolysis and haemorheology in habitual smokers, *Thomb Haemostas (Stuttgart)* 51:6, 1984.

11. Bernstein RK: Two tips for care of diabetic feet, *Diabetes Care* 8:525, 1985.

12. Bild D, Teutsch SM: The control of hypertension in persons with diabetes: a public health approach, *Public Health Rep* 102:522, 1987.

13. Bjorntorp P: Abdominal obesity and the development of noninsulin-dependent diabetes mellitus, *Diabetes Metab Rev* 4:615, 1988.

14. Block P: The diabetic foot ulcer: a complex problem with a simple treatment approach, *Milit Med* 146:644, 1981.

15. Bodily KC, Burgess EM: Contralateral limb and patient survival after leg amputation, *Am J Surg* 146:280, 1983.

16. Borch-Johnsen K, Kreiner S: Proteinuria value as predictor of cardiovascular mortality in insulin-dependent diabetes mellitus, *Br Med J* 294:1651, 1987.

17. Borkenstein MH, Muntean WE: Elevated factor VIII activity and factor VIII-related antigen in diabetic children without vascular disease, *Diabetes* 31:1006, 1982.

18. Boulton AJM, Hardisty CA, Betts RP, et al: Dynamic foot pressure and other studies as diagnostic and management aids in diabetic neuropathy, *Diabetes Care* 6:26, 1983.

19. Boulton AJM, Scarpello JHB, Ward JD: Venous oxygenation in the diabetic neuropathic foot: evidence of arterial venous shunting, *Diabetologia* 22:6, 1981.

20. Brischetto CS, Connor WE, Connor SL; et al: Plasma lipid and lipoprotein profiles of cigarette smokers from randomly selected families: enhancement of hyperlipidemia and depression of high-density lipoprotein, *Am J Cardiol* 52:675, 1983.

21. Brownlee M, Vlassara H, Cerami A: Trapped immunoglobulins on peripheral nerve myelin from patients with diabetes mellitus. *Diabetes* 35:999, 1986.

22. Capron L, Jarnet J, Kazandjian S, et al: Growth-promoting effects of diabetes and insulin on arteries: an in-vivo study of rat aorta, *Diabetes* 35:973, 1986.

23. Charcot JM: Sur la claudication intermittente, observee dans un cas d'obliteration complete de l'une des arteres iliaque primitive, *C R Soc Biol* 10:225, 1858.

24. Chase HP, Garg SK, Marshall G, et al: Cigarette smoking increases the risk of albuminuria among subjects with type I diabetes, *JAMA* 265:614, 1991.

25. Cohen SJ: Potential barriers to diabetes care, *Diabetes Care* 6:499, 1983.

26. Colwell JA: Effects of exercise on platelet function, coagulation, and fibrinolysis, *Diabetes Metab Rev* 1:501, 1986.

27. Couch NP: On the arterial consequences of smoking, *J Vasc Surg* 3:807, 1986.

28. Cronenwett JL: The use of prostaglandins PGE1 and PGE2 in peripheral arterial ischemia. Symposium: use of drugs in peripheral vascular disease, *J Vasc Surg* 3:370, 1986.

29. Dahn I, Eckman CA, Lassen NA, et al: Conservative treatment of severe ischemia of the leg, *Scand J Clin Lab Invest* 19(suppl 99):160, 1967.

30. Dai WS, Gutai JP, Kuller LH, et al: Cigarette smoking and serum sex hormones in men, *Am J Epidemiol* 128:796, 1988.

31. Davidson JK, Alogna M, Goldsmith M, et al: Assessment of program effectiveness at Grady Memorial Hospital–Atlanta, in Steiner G, Lawrence PA, editors, *Educating diabetic patients*, New York, 1981, Springer-Verlag New York.

32. DeLaurentis DA: Do you know the treatment of choice in peripheral arterial occlusive disease? *Geriatrics* 34(10):33, 1979.

33. Delbridge L, Appleburg M, Reeve TS: Factors associated with the development of foot lesions in the diabetic, *Surgery* 93:78, 1983.

34. Dickhaut SC, Delee JC, Page CP: Nutritional status: importance in predicting wound-healing after amputation, *J Bone Joint Surg* 66:71, 1984.

35. Douglas PS: Gender and heart disease, *Hosp Pract* 25:8, 1990.

36. Drury TF, Danchik KM, Harris MI: Sociodemographic characteristics of adult diabetes, in Harris MI, Hammer RF, editors: *Diabetes in America*, Bethesda, 1985, NIH Pub no. 85-1468.

37. Dullaart RPF, Groener JEM, Dikkeschei BD, et al: Elevated cholesteryl ester transfer protein activity in IDDM men who smoke: possible factor for unfavorable lipoprotein profile, *Diabetes Care* 14:338, 1991.

38. Duncan HJ, Faris IB: Skin vascular resistance and skin perfusion pressure as predictors of healing of ischemic lesion of the lower limb: influences of diabetes mellitus, hypertension, and age, *Surgery* 99:432, 1986.

39. Ecker LM, Jacobs BS: Lower extremity amputation in diabetic patients, *Diabetes* 19189, 1970.

40. Edelman SV, Kosofsky EM, Paul RA, et al: Neuro-osteoarthropathy (Charcot's joint) in diabetes mellitus following revascularization surgery: three case reports and a review of the literature, *Arch Intern Med* 147:1504, 1987.

41. Edmonds ME, Blundell MP, Morris ME, et al: Improved survival of the diabetic foot: The role of a specialized foot clinic, *Q J Med* 60:763, 1986.

42. Evans DJ, Barth JH, Burke CW: Body fat topography in women with androgen excess, *Int J Obes* 12:157, 1988.

43. Fearon J, Campbell DR, Hoar CS Jr, et al: Improved results with diabetic below-knee amputations, *Arch Surg* 120:777, 1985.

44. Fisher DF Jr, Clagett GP, Brigham RA, et al: Dilemmas in dealing with the blue toe syndrome: aortic versus peripheral source, *Am J Surg* 148:836, 1984.

45. Ford Es, Newman J: Smoking and diabetes mellitus: findings from 1988 behavioral risk factor surveillance system, *Diabetes Care* 14:871, 1991.

46. Friedman AJ, Ravnikar VA, Barbieri RL: Serum steroid hormone profiles in postmenopausal smokers and non-smokers, *Fertil Steril* 47:398, 1987.

47. Gaskell P, Becker WJ: The erect posture as an aid to circulation in the feet in the presence of arterial obstruction, *Can Med Assoc J* 105:930, 1971.

48. Geiger M, Binder BR: Plasminogen activation in diabetes mellitus, *J Biol Chem* 259:2976, 1984.

49. Golbranson FL, Lurie L, Vance RM, et al: Multiple extremity amputations in hypotensive patients treated with dopamine, *JAMA* 243:1145, 1980.

50. Greene DA, Lattimer SA, Sima AAF: Sorbitol, phosphoinositides, and sodium-potassium-ATPase in the pathogenesis of diabetic complications, *N Engl J Med* 316:599, 1987.

51. Guy RJC, Clark CA, Malcolm PN, et al: Evaluation of thermal and vibration sensation in diabetic neuropathy, *Diabetologia* 28:131, 1985.

52. Haffner SM, Fong D, Hazuda HP, et al: Hyperinsulinemia, upper body adiposity and cardiovascular risk factors in non-diabetics, *Metabolism* 37:333, 1988.

53. Harati Y: Diabetic peripheral neuropathies, *Ann Intern Med* 107:546, 1987.

54. Janka HU, Standl E, Mehnert H: Peripheral vascular disease in diabetes mellitus and its relation to cardiovascular risk factors: screening with Doppler ultrasonic technique, *Diabetes Care* 3:207, 1980.

55. Jenkins AJ, Steele JS, Janus ED, et al: Increased plasma apollproprotein (a) levels in IDDM patients with microalbuminuria, *Diabetes* 40:787, 1991.

56. Jonason T, et al: Effect of physical training on different categories of patients with intermittent claudication, *Acta Med Scand* 206:253, 1979.

57. Kannel WB: Cigarette smoking and peripheral arterial disease, *Prim Cardiovasc* 12:(3):13, 1986.

58. Kaplan NM: The deadly quartet: upper body obesity, glucose intolerance, hypertriglyceridemia and hypertension, *Arch Intern Med* 149:1514, 1989.

59. Kaufman DW, Helmrich SP, Rosenberg L, et al: Nicotine and carbon monoxide content of cigarette smoke and the risk of myocardial infarction in young men, *N Engl J Med* 308:409, 1983.

60. Khaw KT, Tazuke S, Barrett-Conner E: Cigarette smoking and level of adrenal adrogens in postmenopausal women, *N Engl J Med* 318:1705, 1988.

61. Klamer TW, Towne JB, Bandyk DF, et al: The influence of sepsis and ischemia on the natural history of the diabetic foot, *Am Surg* 53:490, 1987.

62. Knighton DR, Ciresi K, Fiegel VD, et al: Stimulation of repair in chronic, nonhealing, cutaneous ulcers using platelet-derived wound healing formula, *Surg Gynecol Obstet* 170:56, 1990.

63. Kreines K, Johnson E, Albrink M, et al: The course of peripheral vascular disease in non-insulin dependent diabetes, *Diabetes Care* 8:235, 1985.

64. Laakso M, Pyorala K: Lipid and lipoprotein abnormalities in diabetic patients with peripheral vascular disease, *Atherosclerosis* 74:55, 1988.

65. Lapidus L, Bengtsson C, Larsson B, et al: Distribution of adipose tissue and risk of cardiovascular disease and death: a 12 year followup of participants in the population study of women in Gothenburg, Sweden, *Br Med J (Clin Res)* 289:1257, 1984.

66. Larson DM, Haudenschild CC: Activation of smooth muscle cell outgrowth from BB/Wor rat aortas, *Diabetes* 37:1380, 1988.

67. Leslie CA, Sapico FL, Ginunas VJ, et al: Randomized controlled trial of topical hyperbaric oxygen for treatment of diabetic foot ulcers, *Diabetes Care* 11:115, 1988.

68. Levin CM, Dealy FN: The surgical diabetic, a five year survey, *Ann Surg* 102:1029, 1935.

69. Levin ME, Sicard GA: Evaluating and treating diabetic peripheral vascular disease: part I, *Clin Diabetes* 5:62, 1987.

70. Levin ME, Spratt IL: To soak or not to soak, *Clin Diabetes* 4:44, 1986.

71. Levine PH: An acute effect of cigarette smoking on platelet function: a possible link between smoking and arterial thrombosis, *Circulation* 48:619, 1973.

72. Lineaweaver W, Howard R, Soucy D, et al: Topical antimicrobial toxicity, *Arch Surg* 120:267, 1985.

73. Lippmann HI: Must loss of limb be a consequence of diabetes mellitus? *Diabetes Care* 2:432, 1979.

74. Lipsky BA, Pecoraro RE, Larson SA, et al: Outpatient management of uncomplicated lower-extremity infections in diabetic patients, *Arch Intern Med* 150:790, 1990.

75. LoGerfo FW, Coffman JD: Vascular and microvascular disease of the foot in diabetes, *N Engl J Med* 311:1615, 1984.

76. Lower extremity amputations, in *Diabetes surveillance, 1980–1987*, Policy Program Research, Centers for Disease Control, US Department of Health and Human Services, Division of Diabetes Translation, 1990, Atlanta.

77. Malone JM, Snyder M, Anderson G, et al: Prevention of amputation by diabetic education, *Am J Surg* 158:520, 1989.

78. Mandelberg A, Sheinfeld W: Diabetic amputations: amputation of lower extremity in diabetes; analysis of one hundred twenty-eight cases, *Am J Surg* 71:70, 1944.

79. Mann SJ, James GD, Wang RS, et al: Elevation of ambulatory systolic blood pressure in hypertensive smokers: a case control study, *JAMA* 265:2226, 1991.

80. Marchel de Calvi CJ: Recherches sur les accidents diabetiques, Paris, 1864, Asselin.

81. Marigliano A, Tedde R, Sechi LA, et al: Insulinemia and blood pressure: relationships in patients with primary and secondary hypertension, and with or without glucose metabolism impairment, *Am J Hypertension* 3:521, 1990.

82. McDermott W, Rogers DE: Social ramifications of control of microbial disease, *Johns Hopkins Med J* 151:302, 1982.

83. McMillan DE: The role of blood flow in diabetic vascular disease, in Rifkin H, Porte Jr D, editors: *Ellenberg and Rifkin's diabetes mellitus: theory and practice*, ed 4, New York, 1990, Elsevier.

84. Mehigan JT, Stoney RJ: Lower extremity atheromatous embolization, *Am J Surg* 132:163, 1976.

85. Melton III LJ, Macken KM, Palumbo PJ, et al: Incidence and prevalence of clinical peripheral vascular disease in a population-based cohort of diabetic patients, *Diabetes Care* 3:650, 1980.

86. Miller LV: *Evaluation of patient education: Los Angeles County Hospital experience*, report of National Commission on Diabetes to the Congress of the United States, Washington, DC, 1975, US Department of Health, Education, and Welfare, DHEW Publ no (NIH) 76-1021, vol 3, part V.

87. Mitchell BD, Hawthorne VM, Vinik AI: Cigarette smoking and neuropathy in diabetic patients, *Diabetes Care* 13:434, 1990.

88. Modan M, Halkin H: Hyperinsulinemia or increased sympathetic drive as links for obesity and hypertension, *Diabetes Care* 14:470, 1991.

89. Moldveen-Geromimus M, Merriam JC Jr: Cholesterol embolization, from pathologic curiosity to clinical entity, *Circulation* 35:946, 1967.

90. Mulhauser I, Sawicki P, Berger M: Cigarette-smoking as a risk factor for macroproteinuria and proliferative retinopathy in type I (insulin-dependent) diabetes, *Diabetologia* 29:500, 1986.

91. Nadler JL, Velasco JS, Horton R: Cigarette smoking inhibits prostacyclin formation, *Lancet* 1:1248, 1983.

92. Nelson RC, Gohdes DM, Everhart JE, et al: Lower-extremity amputation in NIDDM: 12 year follow-up study in Pima Indians, *Diabetes Care* 11:8, 1988.

93. Oberg MS, Lindsey D: Do not put hydrogen peroxide or povidone iodine into wounds! [editorial], *Am J Dis Child* 141:27, 1987.

94. O'Brien IAD, Corrall RJM: Epidemiology of diabetes and its complications, *N Engl J Med* 318:1619, 1988.

95. Palmer JR, Rosenberg L, Shapiro MB: "Low yield" cigarettes and the risk of nonfatal myocardial infarction in women, *N Engl J Med* 320:1569, 1989.

96. Palumbo PJ, Melton LJ III: Peripheral vascular disease and diabetes, In *Diabetes in America*, Diabetes data compiled in 1984, NIH Publ no 85-1468, Washington, DC, 1985, US Government Printing Office.

97. Parkhouse N, LeQuesne PM: Impaired neurogenic vascular response in patients with diabetes and neurogenic foot lesions, *N Engl J Med* 318:1306, 1988.

98. Pecoraro RE, Ahroni JH, Boyko EJ, et al: Chronology and determinants of tissue repair in diabetic lower-extremity ulcers, *Diabetes* 40:1305, 1991.

99. Pecoraro RE, Reiber GE, Burgess EM: Pathways to diabetic limb amputation: basis for prevention, *Diabetes Care* 13:513, 1990.

100. Peiris AN, Sothmann MS, Hoffman RG, et al: Adiposity, fat distribution, and cardiovascular risk, *Ann Intern Med* 110:867, 1989.

101. Peterson GE: Exercise therapy "rediscovered" for diabetes, but what does it do? *JAMA* 242:1591, 1979.

102. Pirart J: Diabetes mellitus and its degenerative complications: a prospective study of 4,400 patients observed between 1947 and 1973: part II, *Diabetes Care* 1:252, 1978.

103. Pollin W: The role of the addictive process as a key step in causation of all tobacco-related diseases, *JAMA* 252:2874, 1984.

104. Poucher RL, Leahy JD, Howells G: Active healing of diabetic wounds utilizing growth factor therapy, *Wounds Compend Clin Res Pract* 3:65, 1991.

105. Prentice CRM, Lowe GDO: Blood viscosity and the complications of diabetes, *Adv Exp Med Biol* 164:99, 1984.

106. Rayman G, Hassan A, Tooke JE: Blood flow in the skin of the foot related to posture in diabetes mellitus, *Br Med J* 292:87, 1986.

107. Reaven GM: Banting lecture 1988: role of insulin resistance in human disease, *Diabetes* 37:1595, 1988.

108. Relationship of atherosclerosis in young men to serum lipoprotein cholesterol concentrations and smoking: a preliminary report from the pathobiological determinants of atherosclerosis in youth (PDAY) research group, *JAMA* 264:3018, 1990.

109. Rendell M, Bergman T, O'Donnell G, et al: Microvascular blood flow, volume, and velocity measured by laser Doppler techniques in IDDM, *Diabetes* 38:819, 1989.

110. Robillard R, Gagnon P, Alaries R: Diabetic neuroarthropathy: a report of four cases, *Can Med Assoc J* 91:895, 1964.

111. Rosenberg CS: Wound healing in the patient with diabetes mellitus, *Nurs Clin North Am* 25:247, 1990.

112. Sage R, Doyle D: Surgical treatment of diabetic foot ulcers: a review of forty-eight cases, *J Foot Surg* 23:102, 1984.

113. Sato Y, Shiraishi S, Oshida Y, et al: Experimental atherosclerosis-like lesions induced by hyperinsulinism in Wistar rats, *Diabetes* 38:91, 1989.

114. Shimokata H, Muller DC, Andres R: Studies in the distribution of body fat: III, effects of cigarette smoking, *JAMA* 261:1169, 1989.

115. Silbert S: Amputation of the lower extremity in diabetes mellitus: a follow-up study of 294 cases, *Diabetes* 1:297, 1952.

116. Soulier SM: The use of running shoes in the prevention of plantar diabetic ulcers, *J Am Podiatr Med Assoc* 76:395, 1986.

117. Taylor LM Jr, Porter JM: Drug treatment of claudication: vasodilators, hemorrheologic agents, and antiserotonin drugs, *J Vasc Surg* 3:374, 1986.

118. Taylor LM Jr, Porter JM: The clinical course of diabetics who require emergent foot surgery because of infection or ischemia, *J Vasc Surg* 6:454, 1987.

119. Tunick PA, Perez JL, Kronzon I: Protruding atheromas in the thoracic aorta and systemic embolization, *Ann Intern Med* 115:423, 1991.

120. Vaccaro O, Pauciullo P, Rubba P, et al: Peripheral arterial circulation in individuals with impaired glucose tolerance, *Diabetes Care* 8:594, 1985.

121. Vannini P, Ciavarella A, Mustacchio A, et al: Intra-arterial urokinase infusion in diabetic patients with rapidly progressive ischemic foot lesions, *Diabetes Care* 14:925, 1991.

122. Veves A, Masson EA, Fernando DJS, et al: Studies of experimental hosiery in diabetic neuropathic patients with high foot pressures, *Diabetes Med* 7:324, 1990.

123. Wald N, Howard S, Smith PG, et al: Association between atherosclerotic disease and carboxyhemoglobin levels in tobacco smokers, *Br Med J* I:761, 1973.

124. Walmsley D, Wales JK, Wiles PG: Reduced hyperaemia following skin trauma: evidence for an impaired microvascular response to injury in the diabetic foot, *Diabetologia* 32:736, 1989.

125. Warram JH, Laffel LMB, Valsania P, et al: Excess mortality associated with diuretic therapy in diabetes mellitus, *Arch Intern Med* 151:1350, 1991.

126. Weidmann P, Ferrari P: Central role of sodium in hypertension in diabetic subjects, *Diabetes Care* 14:220, 1991.

127. Weismann RE: Plaques and platelets: the vascular surgeon's challenge and dilemma, *Arch Surg* 118:1019, 1983.

128. Wheat LJ: Commentary on Lipsky, et al: outpatient management of uncomplicated lower-extremity infections in diabetic patients, *Diabetes Spect* 4(no 2):78. 1991.

129. Working group on hypertension in diabetes: statement on hypertension in diabetes mellitus, final report, *Arch Intern Med* 147:830, 1987.

130. Younger D: Infection in diabetes, *Med Clin North Am* 49:1005, 1965.

131. Zacharias FJ, Cowen KJ, Prestt J, et al: Propranolol in hypertension: a study of long-term therapy, 1964–1970, *Am Heart J* 83:755, 1972.

132. Zavaroni I, Bonora E, Pagliara M, et al: Risk factors for coronary artery disease in healthy persons with hyperinsulinemia and normal glucose tolerance, *N Engl J Med* 320:702, 1989.

# CHAPTER 3

# Dermatology

**J. E. Jelinek, M.D.**

Diabetes mellitus affects every organ system of the body. Thus it is not surprising that the skin, the largest organ, participates with numerous manifestations related to this disease.

Although there is uncertainty about the pathogenesis of many of the skin conditions affecting diabetic patients, in no small part because of our imperfect understanding of the metabolic abnormalities of diabetes itself, many cutaneous signs are easily recognizable so as to make them diabetic markers and a few (diabetic bullae, limited joint mobility and waxy skin, and diabetes dermopathy), when strict clinical criteria are observed, are virtually diagnostic of diabetes.

Some cutaneous conditions appear to be caused by the primary abnormalities of diabetes or by its major complications, vasculopathy and neuropathy. Others are linked to altered immunologic causes and to changes in collagen, and some are a consequence of treatment. Several dermatoses, not generally thought to be linked to abnormal glucose metabolism, appear with greater than expected frequency in diabetics. The numerous skin problems of the diabetic have recently been addressed in a text specifically devoted to that subject.[62]

Dermatologic disorders generally appear after diabetes has developed, but they may signal or appear coincidentally with its onset or even precede the disease by many years. Interestingly, many cutaneous signs and complications often occur on the lower parts of the legs and on the feet. It is the purpose of this chapter to review the major dermatologic manifestations of diabetes with particular emphasis to that region of the body.

## CUTANEOUS SIGNS ASSOCIATED WITH VASCULAR CHANGES IN DIABETES

### Atherosclerosis

Atherosclerosis occurs both frequently and earlier in diabetics. On the skin of the legs the condition is associated with atrophy, coldness of the toes, loss of hair, and dystrophy of the nails.[57] A waxy pallor of the feet when the legs are raised, with a delayed return of color and in the filling of the superficial veins, is a reliable sign of occlusive arterial disease.

### Periungual Telangiectasia

Periungual telangiectasia, seen often in connective tissue diseases, has been found more frequently in diabetics.[69] Although more apparent at the proximal nail folds of fingernails, they may be found affecting the toes as well. Detection of early morphologic changes in nail fold capillaries has also been reported in diabetic children.[128] The vascular dilatations appear to be not only a diabetic marker but also an indicator of functional microangiopathy and a measure of long-term control of glucose metabolism.[54]

One study claims that morphologic differences differentiate the dilated vessels in these areas caused by diabetes from those caused by connective tissue diseases.[40]

The value of this sign is challenged by Trapp et al.,[126] who found no statistical difference in capillaries of the nail folds of insulin-dependent diabetics and limited joint mobility, and by Trevisan et al.,[127] who found no connection between single modification of capillary loops and the levels of glucose in sera and urine in diabetic children or complex changes in nail fold capillaries in well-controlled patients.

### Erythema of the Feet

Lithner and Hietala[78] describe a cutaneous sign of vascular insufficiency in diabetics. This erythema without necrosis appears to be a sign of incipient gangrene in the diabetic foot. The well-demarcated redness correlates with underlying bone destruction, which can be confirmed by x-ray film. The erythema can involve the lower leg, as well as the foot. It is differentiated from erysipelas by the normal temperature of the patient and by the absence of a polymorphonuclear leucocytosis. Small vessel involvement appears to be important, although cardiac decompensation is the most common precipitating factor. The same author[77] noted the frequent nonpalpable purpura evident in both erythematous and nonerythematous areas on the legs of elderly diabetics.

## DIABETIC MARKERS IN SKIN

### Necrobiosis Lipoidica Diabeticorum

Necrobiosis lipoidica diabeticorum was first described in 1929 by Oppenheim[93] and received its current name from Urbach[129] 3 years later. The disease, which is quite distinct clinically and unusual but diagnostic histologically, has, however, no clearly explainable pathogenesis, and its very name poses difficulties. The word "necrobiosis" literally means a state of life and death, better discussed in a religious or philosophic treatise than a medical textbook. "Lipoidica" refers to deposits of extracellular fat that is neither a primary histologic event nor even a constant finding. Finally, "diabeticorum" could strictly be left out of the title

in as many as one third of newly diagnosed cases.

The name, nevertheless, is here to stay, and NLD remains the best-known cutaneous marker of diabetes. This is despite its relative rarity, even in diabetics, where it is reported to occur in between 0.3% and 1.2%.[88, 116] It is much less common in nondiabetics. At the time of diagnosis, two thirds of patients will have overt diabetes. Of the rest, all but 10% will either develop diabetes within 5 years, have abnormal glucose tolerance (some shown by cortisone challenge), or a history of the disease in at least one parent.[88] Although diabetes is usually the first of the two to be diagnosed, in as many as one third, necrobiosis lipoidica diabeticorum precedes diabetes, sometimes by several years.[2] Where the two conditions coexist, the diabetes is often more severe. There is a mean delay of 10 years of necrobiosis lipoidica diabeticorum developing in those having diabetes first.[116]

Necrobiosis lipoidica diabeticorum is four times more common in women; the sexual preferment is even more obvious in patients who are nondiabetic.[47] The condition may

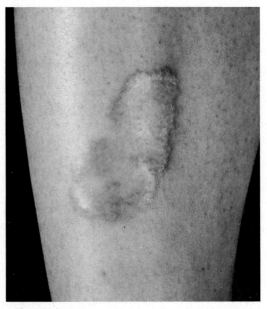

**FIG 3–1.**
Necrobiosis lipoidica diabeticorum. Plaque with an atrophic center and an active and geographic border. *(From Jelinek JE, editor: The skin in diabetes, Philadelphia, 1986, Lea & Febiger. Used by permission.)*

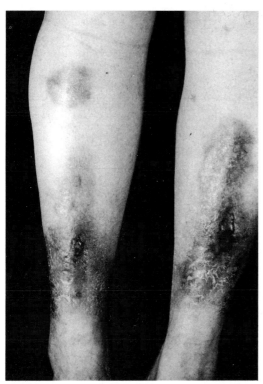

**FIG 3-2.**
Necrobiosis lipoidica diabeticorum. Multiple bilateral plaques on the pretibial region. *(From Jelinek JE, editor: The skin in diabetes, Philadelphia, 1986, Lea & Febiger. Used by permission.)*

appear at any age from infancy to septuagenarians but generally favors young adults. It is curiously selective of whites, although a few cases have been mentioned in the Japanese literature.[114]

The characteristic lesion of necrobiosis lipoidica diabeticorum is a slowly enlarging, irregularly contoured plaque. The border is often slightly elevated and has a reddish blue periphery. The central portion, at first erythematous, becomes yellow or sclerotic and resembles glazed porcelain (Fig 3-1). The plaque often atrophies further and may soften and become entirely brown. In the later stages of development, visible telangiectasias on the surface are common (Plate 4). Lesions vary in size from a few millimeters to several centimeters. Although initially single lesions herald the condition, most patients develop multiple plaques, usually more than four.[88] Eighty-five percent are in pretibial and medial malleolar loca-

tions (Fig 3-2), generally bilateral but not in perfect symmetry. Lesions of necrobiosis lipoidica may, however, appear elsewhere on the body, including the thighs, feet, arms, face and scalp, and even the penis, but in diabetics they almost always involve the classic area of the lower legs in addition to those less usual areas. Lesions may have decreased or absent sensation to pinprick and fine touch.[83] One third of lesions ulcerate sometimes spontaneously, sometimes as a result of trauma (Fig 3-3).[72] This may be because of local destruction of cutaneous nerves by inflammation.[10] Other findings are partial alopecia and significant hypohidrosis, within the lesions, a finding that may serve as a differential point of diagnosis in cases of granuloma annulare.[46] The sensory and sweating deficits may well be secondary to destruction of the nerves and sweat glands by the disease rather than pathogenic.

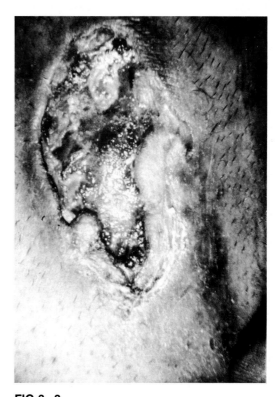

**FIG 3-3.**
Necrobiosis lipoidica diabeticorum. Ulceration, which indicates need for active treatment. *(From Jelinek JE, editor: The skin in diabetes, Philadelphia, 1986, Lea & Febiger. Used by permission.)*

Even though ulceration is fairly common and often long standing, squamous cell carcinoma as a complication is, happily, very rare. Only six such cases have been reported up to 1991, one half of these in diabetics.[99]

Among proposed causative factors are microangiopathy,[67] obliterative endarteritis,[48] immune-mediated vasculitis,[100] other immune factors,[16] delayed hypersensitivity,[118] nonenzymatic glycosylation and other defects in collagen,[10] trauma,[72] platelet aggregation,[124] defective mobility of neutrophils,[35] and vascular insufficiency.[12] It is uncertain whether any of these are primary or secondary, what relationship they bear to one another, and whether any are central, significant, or even relevant to the etiologic explanation of the disease.[60]

Necrobiosis lipoidica diabeticorum can usually be diagnosed by a dermatologist on clinical appearance alone. If the diagnosis is not certain, a biopsy should reveal characteristic changes. These are degeneration of collagen throughout the dermis, particularly in the lower two thirds, histocytes in a palisaded arrangement around the degenerated collagen, and obliterative granulomatous vasculitis. It should be stressed, however, that it is preferable to avoid, whenever possible, surgical procedures on the lower legs of these patients, particularly those who are diabetic.

The variety of suggested treatment for necrobiosis lipoidica diabeticorum betrays the efficacy of a single one. Where there is no ulceration and, as is most common, little in the way of subjective symptoms, the approach should be conservative. Protection from injury is important and patients should avoid crowds, wear shin pads if likely to be traumatized, and, if getting out of bed at night, put on the light to avoid collision with furniture. Topical corticosteroids, sometimes under occlusive dressings, may be helpful. Intralesional triamcinolone acetonide for both ulcerated and nonulcerated lesions has its advocates,[119] but this treatment is best reserved for the borders or just beyond the borders of either ulcerated, or symptomatic, or advancing lesions. The demonstration of inflammation extending beyond the clinical borders would suggest this therapy may be useful in these areas in these circumstances.[10]

Aspirin and dipyridamole modify aggregation of platelets and have been used, either alone or in combination, with reported success,[23, 49, 101] but others have found this treatment disappointing.[5] The efficacy of this treatment in preventing new lesions or stemming progression of old ones is still unproved. Pentoxitylline, which decreases the viscosity of blood by increasing fibrinolysis, in addition to inhibiting aggregation of platelets, has been reported as useful in the healing of ulcers.[79]

Other reported therapy, usually used in single or very few patients, includes nicotinamide[43] and seaweed-based (alginate) dressings.[113]

Active treatment is always called for when ulceration occurs. In addition to the previously mentioned approaches, attention should be given to the prevention and treatment of secondary infection by compresses and local and systemic antibiotics.[58] Topical administration of benzoyl peroxide has been found useful.[44] The new hydrocolloid occlusive dressings may prove helpful in treating noninfected ulcers. When conservative treatment fails, radical excision of the muscularis fascia, ligation of perforating vessels, and split-thickness grafting is a therapeutic option.[31]

## Granuloma Annulare

Granuloma annulare has several forms that are identical on histology. The classic and commonest type manifests as one or more localized annular or arciform lesions with flesh-colored papular borders and flat centers. These are seen most often on the dorsal and lateral aspects of the hands and feet of children and young adults (Fig 3–4). Granuloma annulare is a benign, usually asymptomatic, and generally self-limiting dermatosis.

Less common varieties include generalized, multiple, perforating, and subcutaneous forms. The generalized form may consist of multiple classic lesions or a type in which numerous, disseminated, flesh-colored papules are symmetrically distributed on the arms, neck, and upper half of the trunk and

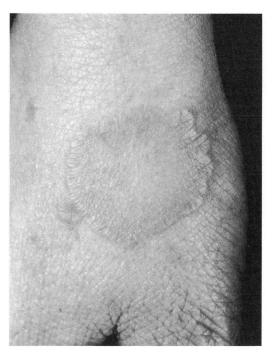

**FIG 3–4.**
Granuloma annulare. Flesh-colored plaque with papular border. *(From Jelinek JE, editor:* The skin in diabetes, *Philadelphia, 1986, Lea & Febiger. Used by permission.)*

less often on the legs (Plate 5). The cause of granuloma annulare is not known. Treatment is similar to the nonulcerated forms of necrobiosis lipoidica diabeticorum and meets with about equal success.

All forms of granuloma annulare share common histologic features, namely, focal degeneration of collagen in the upper and middermis, with histiocytic palisaded arrangement around collagen bundles, and abundant mucin.[73] These features, although distinguishable from necrobiosis lipoidica diabeticorum, bear enough resemblance to that disease to invite the question of the relationship of granuloma annulare to diabetes mellitus. (Rheumatoid nodules and necrobiosis lipoidica diabeticorum also show histologic similarities, yet no association of diabetes and rheumatoid arthritis exists.) Although there is considerable similarity under the microscope, the two conditions of granuloma annulare and necrobiosis lipoidica diabeticorum have only been reported to occur together in the same patient seven times.[1, 22]

Approximately 120 patients have indeed been reported to have coexistent diabetes and granuloma annulare in reported series of some 1,100 patients.[60, 87, 117] In most of these, no distinction was made as to the type of diabetes. Despite a natural bias in such reports and the usually transient course of granuloma annulare, there appears to be a greater than expected incidence of abnormal carbohydrate metabolism in these patients, particularly in the generalized disseminated and perforating forms.[28, 51, 56] Evidence for a link of diabetes and granuloma annulare in the localized form is much less firm, but it is appropriate to obtain glucose measurements on all patients with the dermatosis and to be particularly watchful for diabetes in adults with disseminated or generalized forms of the condition.

## DIABETIC DERMOPATHY

In 1964 Melin[84] noted that his chief, Nils Tornblom, pointed out characteristic, atrophic, circumscribed brown patches on the front and sides of the lower portions of the legs in diabetic subjects. It is probable that Kramer[68] described the same condition 30 years earlier. Binkley[9] coined the name "diabetic dermopathy" for the condition, and it is this term that is now generally used.[9] Others have written of this condition as "the spotted leg syndrome,"[89] shin spots,[24] and pigmented pretibial patches.[4] Despite the name "dermopathy," there is little evidence of angiopathy or a kinship to other diabetic angiopathies. It appears that microangiopathy, when present, reflects the underlying diabetes rather than the cutaneous problem itself.

The lesions are at first small, dull red, scaly papules and small plaques. They eventuate to the characteristic, multiple, bilateral, circumscribed, round of oval, shallow pigmented scars on the pretibial areas (Plate 6). Diabetic dermopathy is the commonest cutaneous sign of diabetes. Its relatively late recognition is explained by the absence of symptoms. The condition has been seen in nondiabetics,[24] but the majority of patients are adult diabetics. The incidence correlates reasonably with the severity of diabetes and its complications,[84] although it may precede that condition.[3] A recent report indicates that most patients with diabetic dermopathy have an increase in glycosylated hemoglobin levels and a long history of diabetes.[122] It is twice as common in men.

The predilection for the pretibial area invites speculation on the relationship of diabetic dermopathy to necrobiosis lipoidica diabeticorum; the matter is easily settled under the microscope. Necrobiosis lipoidica diabeticorum has diagnostic histologic features, whereas diabetic dermopathy is nonspecific. The second question, the role of trauma, is less easily answered. Although the history of repeated physical insults is usually not forthcoming, and attempts to produce the lesions by repeatedly striking the areas of the leg with a rubber hammer failed,[84] experimental thermal injuries[76] and reports linking the dermatosis to peripheral neuropathy[89] suggest that trauma may be a modifying factor.

Other pigmented lesions of the legs are differentiated from diabetic dermopathy by their localization, associated peripheral vascular disease, and the presence of purpura. Diabetic dermopathy, being asymptomatic, requires no treatment except for protection from trauma.

## DIABETIC BULLAE

Although not common, the sudden appearance of one or more tense blisters, generally on the acral portions of the body, is a clinically distinct diabetic marker. Referred to in 1930 by Kramer,[68] the recognition of it as a separate entity was made by Rocca and Pereyra in 1963.[103] The name "bullosis diabeticorum" was coined in 1967.[15] Fewer than 100 cases have been reported up to 1991.[94]

The characteristic history is spontaneous blisters appearing suddenly, most commonly on the dorsa or sides of the hands and feet (Fig 3–5), forearms, and lower legs. The bullae range from 0.5 to several cm, are often bilateral, and contain generally clear fluid, which is invariably sterile. There is no

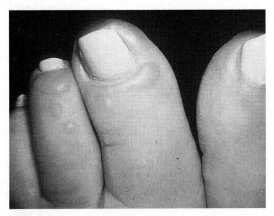

**FIG 3–5.**
Diabetic bullae. Spontaneous lesions appeared on the hands as well as the feet. *(From Jelinek JE, editor: The skin in diabetes, Philadelphia, 1986, Lea & Febiger. Used by permission.)*

surrounding erythema. The lesions are usually asymptomatic and heal by themselves in a few weeks, usually without scarring. They may recur.

The patients are always adults, more often men, and their diabetes is often, though not invariably, severe and long standing. The abnormalities of carbohydrate metabolism are not proportionate to the clinical manifestation. Outside of preventing secondary infection, no treatment is necessary.

Diabetic bullae are usually intraepidermal (explaining the lack of scarring), though a subepidermal location has also been reported. Heterogeneity of histologic appearance may be explained by different pathogenesis or by obtaining biopsy specimens at different stages of development. Although insulin-dependent diabetics appear to have a reduced threshold to blister formation,[8] the appearance at the same time of the bullae at widely separated sites argues against trauma as a pathogenic factor.

Diabetic bullae resemble those seen in patients in coma from overdosing on barbiturates or from poisoning with carbon monoxide, but the clinical picture is easily differentiated.

### Limited Joint Mobility and Waxy Skin Syndrome

A new clinical syndrome, originally described in insulin-dependent adolescent diabetics in 1974 by Rosenbloom and Frias,[108] consists of two major components: limitation of mobility, primarily of the small joints of the hands, and thickening and stiffness of the skin, most marked on the dorsa of the fingers. Apart from functional limitations of mobility, the condition is asymptomatic, and the lack of pain probably explains why it has only recently been delineated in spite of being evidently common. It appears to be the earliest clinically detectable complication of childhood and adolescent diabetics.[107]

The stiffness usually begins in the metacarpophalangeal and proximal interphalangeal joints, generally of the fifth digit, and then progressing to involve one or more other adjoining fingers.[105] It is bilateral, symmetric, and painless. The limitations of movement initially in active, and later even in passive, extension may less frequently involve larger joints of the wrist, elbow, and even the spine.[41] Flexion limitation occurs much later, if at all.

Recently the syndrome of limited joint mobility has become recognized as an important contributor to abnormal mechanics in the diabetic foot. Campbell et al.[13] first mentioned limitation of motion of the ankle, and subsequently Deldridge et al.[26] confirmed the presence of the entity in diabetics and commented on its relation to neuropathic ulceration. Similar findings were reported by Mueller et al.[86] Fernando et al.[32] pointed out the relationship of limitation of joint mobility to abnormal pressures in the feet in patients with diabetic neuropathy. In their group two thirds of the patients developed foot ulcers. Patients who had limited joint mobility without neuropathy also had abnormal foot pressures but did not develop ulcers.

Limited joint mobility of the hand can be demonstrated by the inability to flatten the affected hand on a table top (Fig 3–6) and by failure to approximate the two palms with the fingers fanned and the wrists maximally flexed (the prayer sign). The most accurate sign, however, is limitation of extension with the examiner passively testing the interphalangeal and metacarpophalangeal joints (Fig 3–7).[107] Skin thickening is assessed by palpation and can also be demonstrated by ultrasound-A scanning.[20]

Although in early reports the condition appeared to be found only in juvenile insulin-dependent diabetics, it is now apparent that it can also affect adult non-insulin-dependent diabetic patients.[33, 70, 111] Although clearly related to and much commoner in diabetics, both components of the syndrome have been described in nondiabetic controls.[70, 95] More than 4,500 diabetic patients have been assessed for this condition from 1974 to 1985. The incidence of the syndrome has ranged from 8% to 50%, with variation probably explainable by the age of the population studied, duration of diabetes, and different examination techniques.[107]

Although contractures of the joints seem related to duration of hyperglycemia, partic-

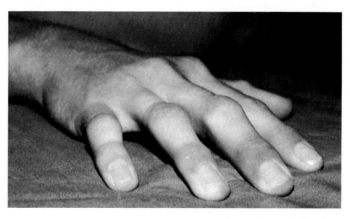

**FIG 3–6.**
Limited joint mobility. The patient could not flatten the hand on a table top. *(From Hempstead RW: J Assoc Milit Dermatol 9[2]:30, 1983. Used by permission.)*

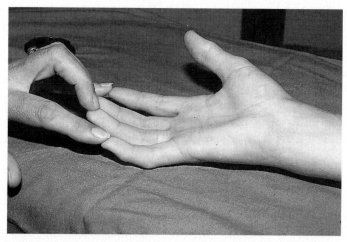

**FIG 3–7.**
Limited joint mobility. Resistance to passive extension. *(From Hempstead RW: J Assoc Milit Dermatol 9[2]:30, 1983. Used by permission.)*

ularly in those with insulin dependence,[121] it is probable that if a patient will develop this complication he or she will do so by the end of the first decade of disease.[17] There is less agreement as to the relationship of the syndrome to diabetic control. No such association was found in several studies,[110, 120] but a strong inverse correlation was reported in another.[14] The importance of strict control is certainly implied in a report of diminished thickness of the skin following careful control of levels of glucose by using an insulin infusion pump.[74] Recently Lyons et al.[82] also showed decrease in skin collagen glycation with improved glycemic control in insulin-dependent diabetes. Maintaining this control could potentially, therefore, limit subsequent long-term damage.

The abnormal waxiness and thickening of the skin appears in about one third of patients with limited joint mobility, more predictably in the more severe cases,[109] although at times evident without joint involvement.[115] Clinically the taut, shiny skin bears similarity to scleroderma, but that condition is excluded by the absence of Raynaud's phenomenon, ulceration, tapering and calcinosis of the fingers, and the lack of visceral involvement. Histologic appearance of waxy skin is marked by thickening of the dermal collagen and especially by a paucity of elastic fibers.[30]

The pathogenesis of the thickened skin and limitation of mobility of the joints seem interrelated. Despite the name, the joints themselves are not directly involved. The fault apparently is in the collagen of the periarticular tissues. The abnormal collagen of both components may be a reflection of nonenzymatic glycosylation of protein, an accompaniment of persistent hyperglycemia, although tissue glycosylation is not greater in diabetics with the syndrome than in those without it.[81] Because the condition occurs primarily in young patients, it appears not to be vascular in origin.[106]

The suggestion has been made that the syndrome is a harbinger of retinopathy with a threefold to fourfold increased chance of developing this complication in later years,[13, 65, 109, 121] especially in poorly controlled and younger patients.

In older patients, especially those with non-insulin-dependent diabetes, the association of limited joint mobility and microvascular disease is less marked.[70] Others, however, have questioned the syndrome as an indicator of future problems in all patients.[131]

## Scleredema Diabeticorum

Scleredema is a rare disorder of diffuse, symmetric induration, and thickening of the skin favoring the posterior side of the neck and upper half of the back. It has two forms. The classic type is known as "scleredema adultorum of Buschke," which, despite its name, more commonly affects children, is usually heralded by an acute infection (frequently streptococcal), followed a few weeks later by a progressive induration of the posterolateral portion of the neck, upper half of the back, and shoulders. The diagnosis is clinically evident by palpation, which demonstrates a hardened, nonpitted skin, often shiny, and with absent superficial markings, that can be neither wrinkled nor pressed together into folds. On rare occasions, the cutaneous involvement is much more widespread, and internal organs may be affected. The condition is painless, and symptoms, if any, are caused by limitation of movement. This type generally resolves spontaneously in about 18 months.

Histologically, the collagen bundles are separated by an accumulation of hyaluronic acid and glycosaminoglycans.[112]

Scleredema is also seen in diabetics and, although sharing certain characteristics with the "adultorum" type, has distinct differences. Like the classic type, the disease initially affects the upper half of the back and the neck but subsequently tends to involve a much greater part of the body, especially the trunk and sometimes the arms and legs.[104]

Demarcation from the normal skin may be obvious or imperceptible. Not infrequently there is diminished response to pain and light touch in affected areas.[19] There usually is no prodromal infection.

Some 140 patients with scleredema diabeticorum have now been described in the world's literature,[59, 125] about one half as many as of the classic type. The diabetic patients are normally middle-aged men, almost invariably obese, and although their diabetic state varies from mild to severe, most are in need of insulin and many have associated microvascular complications.[19] The cutaneous problem is not only generally more widespread than in the classic type but also has little tendency to resolution. The histology is identical in both types, and both also share a lack of effective treatment.

Although regarded as a rare disease, in a prospective study of 484 diabetics, scleredema had a incidence of 2.5%.[19] Collier et al.[21] found that patients who had diabetes for more than 10 years had thicker skin on their arms than either patients with a shorter duration of diabetes or nondiabetic controls. This thickening was found in another recent study and differentiated by both conventional and electron microscopic appearance from scleroderma.[45] Huntley and Walter[55] have shown thickness of the skin in diabetics not only of the hands but also of the feet. They considered this thickness independent of the syndromes of limited joint mobility and scleredema and found no correlation with retinopathy. The thickening that diabetics have on their extremities may be unapparent clinically but is measurable. In this study it was demonstrated with ultrasonography.[55]

## DERMATOSES REPORTED TO BE MORE FREQUENT IN DIABETICS

### Perforating Dermatoses

There are several acquired cutaneous disorders having as a common histologic denominator the transepidermal elimination of degenerative material, chiefly collagen and elastic fibers. Although these dermatoses have been reported independently of associated internal problems, many are in patients with chronic renal failure, particularly those on dialysis; approximately two thirds of these have been diabetic.[36]

Attempts to separate the perforating dermatoses, chief of which are Kyrle's disease, perforating folliculitis, and reactive perforating collagenosis, have been made on both clinical and histologic grounds. Their similarities, however, outweigh their differences, and the term "acquired perforating dermatoses" seems appropriate.[102]

Clinically, patients have multiple umbilicated keratotic papules, sometimes with a tendency to linear formation (Fig 3–8). They favor the extensor surface of the trunk and extremities. They are often very itchy, with little tendency to spontaneous resolution. Most patients are middle aged, and often black. Slightly more males than females are affected.

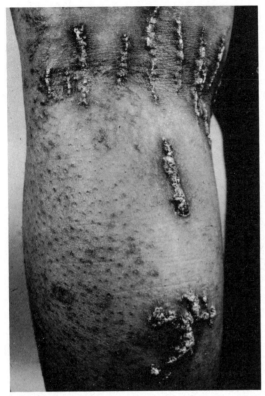

**FIG 3–8.**
Perforating disease, Kyrle's disease. Keratotic lesions showing the isomorphic (Koebner's) phenomenon. *(From Jelinek JE, editor: The skin in diabetes, Philadelphia, 1986, Lea & Febiger. Used by permission.)*

Improvement has been achieved with topical retinoic acid[7] and with protection from scratching, combined with diabetic control,[18] and ultraviolet therapy.[130]

Often, unfortunately, treatment is not too effective. The phenomenon of transepidermal elimination is probably multifactorial. Changes in epidermal keratinization, immunologic and inflammatory factors, alteration of the underlying glycosylation, and contributions from lysosomal enzymes released from leucocytes all have been suggested as being responsible.[27, 97, 133]

## Vitiligo

Vitiligo is a disease in which diminished or absent function of melanocytes results in macular depigmentation, most often seen periorificially and on the extensor aspects of the extremities (Plate 7). It is asymptomatic but emotionally stressful, particularly in people with darker skin. It is regarded as an autoimmune disorder. The higher than expected incidence of vitiligo in diabetics seems further evidence for an immunologic basis. Vitiligo, however, has been reported in maturity-onset diabetics,[25] as well as in insulin-dependent ones,[39] making it more difficult to advance autoimmune and genetic factors as the only explanation for their coexistence. The frequency of diabetes in patients with vitiligo, however, seems no higher than would be expected.[61]

A recent report from Japan[66] claims that vitiligo can be divided into types that are confined to a dermatome and others that are generalized and usually progressive. The latter form seems to be associated with conditions that have an allergic or immune basis.

## Lichen Planus

Lichen planus, a disease of unknown cause, has a distinctive morphologic and histologic appearance. Clinically it is characterized by itchy, flat-topped, violaceous papules, most often on the flexor aspects of the forearms and wrists, lower portions of the legs, and the lower back. Mucous membranes, including the mouth and genitalia, are involved in two thirds of cases. In the buccal mucosa, lichen planus forms a white lacework pattern that can become erosive.

An increased incidence of diabetes and abnormalities of insulin response to glucose challenge have been claimed in patients with lichen planus.[91] This is particularly true of adults and more so in those with the erosive oral form.[80]

Whether there is a relationship of diabetes to lichen planus, a usually transient condition, remains speculative. In one report, an increase of A28-HLA antigen among nondiabetic patients with lichen planus but not those with diabetes suggests that there may be two forms of this disease.[42] This concept of two types of lichen planus, one of an immunologic, the other of a metabolic defect linked to diabetes, is supported by the studies of Lisi and Giommoni.[75]

## Carotenoderma, Yellow Skin, and Yellow Nails

Carotenes are lipid-soluble pigments. All green vegetables, some fruits, and dairy products contain carotene, but the red and yellow vegetables have the richest content. Carotene contributes a yellow component to normal skin, and in excessive amounts imparts a deep yellow-orange tint, especially on the palms, soles, and the nasolabial folds, where there is either thicker keratin or an abundance of sebaceous or sweat glands. Carotenemia does not alter the color of the sclerae or that of urine. The normal value of carotene is 1 mg/mL in the serum, and levels have to be about 25 times that amount to give clinical evidence of carotenoderma.[71] Carotenoderma, which is asymptomatic, may appear in response to a variety of mechanisms, including excessive intake of foods rich in carotenes, defective conversion of carotene to vitamin A, and in hyperlipidemic conditions.[85] The most common cause is dietary. In preinsulin days, this probably accounted for the reported high incidence of this phenomenon in diabetics. Although diabetics frequently have a yellowish color,[53] there appears in most cases to be no correlation to elevations of carotene levels in the serum.[50] A possible explanation of the yellow color may lie in the consequences of nonenzymatic glycosylation and storage temperatures of the stratum corneum.[123] One of the advanced glycosylatious products that has been identified, 2-(2-furoyl)-4(5)-(2-furanyl)-1$H$-imadozole, has a distinctly yellow hue.[98]

As many as 50% of diabetics have been reported to have yellow nails, best seen on the distal hallux (Plate 8). One study of fingernails showed diabetics have high levels of fructose-lysine, another marker of nonenzymatic glycosylation.[92] Yellow nails are seen in association with onychomycosis and psoriasis and in the elderly but seem to be a common diabetic marker unassociated with these causes. The early sign is a yellow or brown color of the distal part of the hallux nail plate. Later a canary yellow color can affect nails on both toe and fingernails.

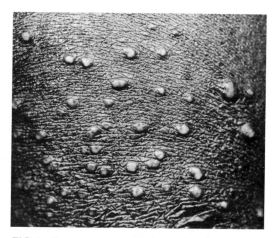

**FIG 3–9.**
Eruptive xanthoma. The condition resolves when metabolic control is established. *(From Jelinek JE, editor: The skin in diabetes, Philadelphia, 1986, Lea & Febiger. Used by permission.)*

## Eruptive Xanthomas

Eruptive xanthomas may appear when serum triglycerides rise to high levels. The majority of patients with this condition are diabetics in poor control. The eruption is of multiple, firm pink-yellow papules and nodules appearing in crops (Fig 3–9). There is often an erythematous halo surrounding individual papules. The favored sites are the extensor aspects of the extremities and trunk. The oral mucosa may be involved on occasion. The condition is pruritic. With the correction of the hyperlipidemia and control of diabetes, the lesions involute.

The mechanism of the formation of xanthomas is not known. There is some evidence that eruptive xanthomas in diabetes result from macrophages incorporating circulating plasma lipoproteins, forming foamy or xanthoma cells.[96]

## Kaposi's Sarcoma

Multiple idiopathic hemorrhagic sarcoma, first described by Kaposi in 1872,[64] is a neoplasm that usually begins on the lower parts of the legs, most often in elderly Jewish and Italian men. The lesions, usually multiple, are purple macules, nodules, or plaques. Later, other areas of the skin, mucous membranes, and internal organs may be involved. Edema of the legs is frequent and may even be a prodrome. The classic form of the disease is uncommon, generally indolent, and usually not aggressive. Histologic examination shows an accumulation of spindle cells forming vascular slits containing erythrocytes.

Diabetes mellitus has been reported with greater than expected frequency in Kaposi's sarcoma,[29, 34] but confirmation is still needed because others have not found a statistically significant association.[11] In a recent study from Sweden that found a 27% incidence of diabetes in 63 patients with Kaposi's sarcoma, the authors[6] related the pathogenesis to cardiac failure with edema in the elderly as the more important factor.

## Glucagonoma

Tumors of the α-cell, glucagon-secreting portion of the pancreas have a cutaneous component that may precede other evidence of its existence, sometimes by several years. The distinct skin eruption is necrolytic migratory erythema and is characterized by eczematous patches in annular and gyrate forms that eventuate in plaques, erosions, and crusts. Although preferring the lower abdomen, buttocks, and periorificial areas, the dermatosis may be found not infrequently on the lower portions of the legs (Fig 3–10). The condition fluctuates but is chronic and persistent. The histology resembles that found in pustular psoriasis with features of intracellular edema in the upper epidermis, acanthosis, subcorneal pustules, and dyskeratosis.[52]

Systemic accompaniments include weight loss, weakness, diarrhea, and, frequently, diabetes. Glossitis and paronychial candidiasis are frequent.

Diagnosis is confirmed by elevated plasma glucagon levels. Hypoaminoacidemia is often an associated finding. Several medications have been reported to ameliorate the cutaneous part of the syndrome, but in the majority of patients the cause is a pancreatic neoplasm, and its surgical removal is the definitive treatment.

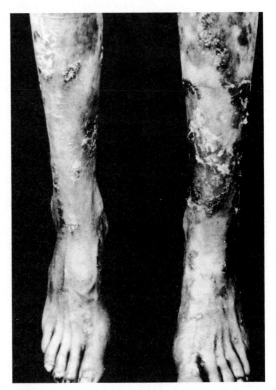

**FIG 3–10.**
Glucagonoma. Necrolytic migratory erythema. Serpigenous erosions with crusts, vesicles, and pustules at the periphery. *(From Shupack JL, Berczeller PH, Stevens DM: J Dermatol Surg Oncol 4:242–247, 1978. Used by permission.)*

## Werner's Syndrome

Werner's syndrome is a rare autosomal recessive disease remarkable for premature and accelerated aging. Approximately half of the patients have nonketotic, relatively insulin-resistant, mild diabetes. The skin becomes taut and thin, with loss of subcutaneous tissue and diminished sweat glands. This is most evident on the lower parts of the legs, where ulcers often supervene, and on the face, resulting in a birdlike appearance. Poikiloderma marked by both hypopigmentation and hyperpigmentation and telangiectasia, alopecia, hyperkeratoses, and skin cancers are common.[38, 132]

Patients with Werner's syndrome showed a reduction in the growth of skin fibroblasts when compared with subjects with diabetes and those with normal aging, and even more so in normal controls.[37]

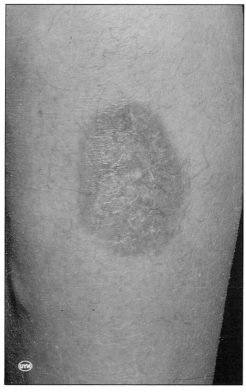

**PLATE 4.**
Necrobiosis lipoidica diabeticorum. Plaque on leg, with a yellow, atrophic, and telangiectatic center and an elevated red border. (From Jelinek JE, editor: *The skin in diabetes, Philadelphia, 1986, Lea & Febiger. Used by permission.)*

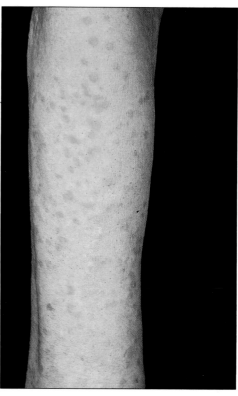

**PLATE 5.**
Granuloma annulare. Multiple papules of the disseminated form. (From Jelinek JE, editor: *The skin in diabetes, Philadelphia, 1986, Lea & Febiger. Used by permission.)*

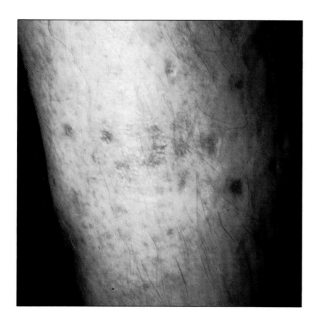

**PLATE 6.**
Diabetic dermopathy. Multiple brown, atrophic lesions on the anterior and lower portions of the legs. (From Jelinek JE, editor: *The skin in diabetes, Philadelphia, 1986, Lea & Febiger. Used by permission.)*

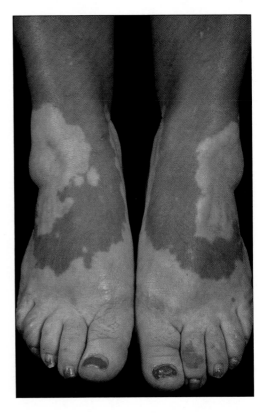

**PLATE 7.**
Vitiligo. Loss of pigment on the lower legs and feet. (From Jelinck JE, editor: *The skin in diabetes,* Philadelphia, 1986, Lea & Febiger. Used by permission.)

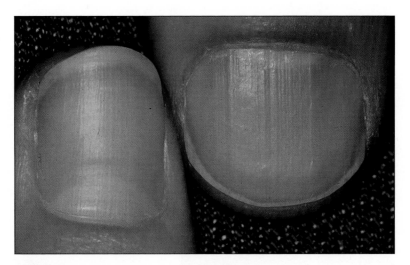

**PLATE 8.**
Yellow nail. Discoloration of the nails often is independent of dermatophytosis or vascular disease. *(Courtesy of Arthur C. Huntley, M.D.)*

## Pruritus

It is a commonly held belief that generalized itching is a symptom of diabetes mellitus. This relationship is highly questionable. In recent studies[63, 90] there was no statistical basis for this belief. Localized anogenital pruritus (particularly pruritus vulva associated with moniliasis) is, however, more common in diabetics.[90]

Itching on the legs in elderly diabetics is not a feature of hyperglycemia but a manifestation of xerosis. Simple lubricants or low-potency corticosteroid creams usually suffice to control this symptom.

## REFERENCES

1. Abraham Z, et al: Psoriasis, necrobiosis lipoidica, granuloma annulare, vitiligo and skin infection in the same diabetic patient, *J Dermatol* 17:440–447, 1990.

2. Abramova EA, Polyanskaya NP: Relationship between lipoid necrobiosis and diabetes mellitus, *Vestn Dermatol Venerol* (2):36–38, 1985.

3. Bauer M, Levan NE: Diabetic dermangiopathy: a spectrum including pretibial patches and necrobiosis lipoidica diabeticorum, *Br J Dermatol* 83:528–535, 1970.

4. Bauer MF et al: Pigmented pretibial patches: a cutaneous manifestation of diabetes mellitus, *Arch Dermatol* 93:282–286, 1966.

5. Beck HI, Bjerring P: Skin blood flow in necrobiosis lipoidica during treatment with low-dose acetylsalicylic acid, *Acta Derm Venereol (Stockh)* 68:364–365, 1988.

6. Bendsoe N, et al: Increased incidence of Kaposi sarcoma in Sweden before the AIDS epidemic, *Eur J Cancer* 26:699–702, 1990.

7. Berger RS: Reactive perforating collagenosis of renal failure—diabetes responsive to topical retinoic acid, *Cutis* 43:540–542, 1989.

8. Bernstein JE, et al: Reduced threshold to suction-induced blister formation in insulin-dependent diabetics, *J Am Acad Dermatol* 8:790–791, 1983.

9. Binkley, GW: Dermopathy in the diabetic syndrome, *Am Dermatol* 92:625–634, 1965.

10. Boulton AJM, et al: Necrobiosis lipoidica diabeticorum: a clinicopathologic study, *J Am Acad Dermatol* 18:530–537, 1988.

11. Brambilla L, et al: Sarcoma di Kaposi mediterraneo patologie associate in una casistica di 100 pazienti, *G Ital Dermatol Venereol* 123:477–480, 1988.

12. Brungger A: Transkutane Sauerstoff—und Kohlendioxiddruck-messung bei Necrobiosis Lipoidica, *Hautarzt* 40:231–232, 1989.

13. Campbell RR, et al: Limited joint mobility in diabetes mellitus, *Ann Rheumatol Dis* 44:93–97, 1985.

14. Canfield WK, Chase HP, Hambidge KM: Limited joint mobility (LJM) in insulin dependent diabetes mellitus (IDDM): relationship to glucose control and zinc nutriture, *Pediatr Res* 16(suppl):135A, 1982.

15. Cantwell AR, Martz W: Idiopathic bullae in diabetics: bullosis diabeticorum, *Arch Dermatol* 96:42–44, 1967.

16. Chambers B, Milligan A, Fletcher A: Epidermal dentric S100 positive cells in necrobiosis lipoidica and granuloma annulare, *Br J Dermatol* 123:765–768, 1990.

17. Chapple M, et al: Joint contracture and diabetic retinopathy, *Postgrad Med J* 59:291–294, 1983.

18. Cohen RW, Auerbach R: Acquired reactive perforating collagenosis, *J Am Acad Dermatol* 20:287–289, 1989.

19. Cole GW, Headley J, Skowsky R: Scleredema diabeticorum: a common and distinct cutaneous manifestation of diabetes mellitus, *Diabetes Care* 6:189–192, 1983.

20. Collier A, et al: Change in skin thickness associated with cheiroarthropathy in insulin dependent diabetes mellitus, *Br Med J* 292:936, 1986.

21. Collier A, et al: Relationship of skin thickness to duration of diabetes, glycemic control, and diabetic complications in male IDDM patients, *Diabetes Care* 12:309–312, 1989.

22. Crosby DL, Woodley DT, Leonard DP: Concomitant granuloma annulare and necrobiosis lipoidica: report of a case and review of the literature, *Dermatologica* 183:225–229, 1991.

23. Csaszar A, et al: Necrobiosis lipoidica without diabetes mellitus (diagnostic and therapeutic possibilities), *Orv Hetil* 130:2141–2145, 1989.

24. Danowski TS, et al: Skin spots and diabetes mellitus, *Am J Med Sci* 251:570–575, 1966.

25. Dawber RPR: Vitiligo in mature onset diabetes mellitus, *Br J Dermatol* 80:275–278, 1968.

26. Deldridge L, et al: Limited joint mobility in the diabetic foot: relationship to neuropathic ulceration, *Diabetic Med* 5:333–337, 1988.

27. Detmar M, et al: Kyrle disease in juvenile diabetes and chronic renal failure, *Z Hautkr* 65:53–61, 1990.

28. Dicken CH, Carrington SG, Winkelmann RK: Generalized granuloma annulare, *Arch Dermatol* 99:556–563, 1969.

29. Digiovanna JJ, Safai B: Kaposi's sarcoma: retrospective study of 90 cases with particular emphasis on the familial occurrence, ethnic background

and prevalence of other diseases, *Am J Med* 71:779–783, 1981.

30. Dowd PM, et al: Diabetic sclerodactyly, *Br J Dermatol* 115:21, 1986.

31. Dubin BJ, Kaplan EN: The surgical treatment of necrobiosis lipoidica diabeticorum, *Plast Reconstr Surg* 60:421–427, 1977.

32. Fernando DJS, et al: Relationship of limited joint mobility to abnormal foot pressures and diabetic foot ulceration, *Diabetes Care* 14:8–11, 1991.

33. Fitzcharles MA, et al: Limitation of joint mobility (cheiroarthropathy) in adult non-insulin dependent diabetic patients, *Ann Rheum Dis* 43:251–257, 1984.

34. Friedman-Birnbaum R, Weltfriend S, Katz I: Kaposi's sarcoma: retrospective study of 67 cases with the classical form, *Dermatologica* 180:13–17, 1990.

35. Grange RW, Black MM, Carrington P: Defective neutrophil migration in granuloma annulare, necrobiosis lipoidica and sarcoidosis, *Arch Dermatol* 155:32–35, 1979.

36. Goette DK: Transepithelial elimination disorders, *J Assoc Miliary Dermatol* 11:28–46, 1985.

37. Goldstein S: Studies on age-related diseases in cultured skin fibroblasts, *J Invest Dermatol* 73:19–23, 1979.

38. Goto M, et al: Family analysis of Werner's syndrome: a survey of 42 Japanese families with a review of the literature, *Clin Genet* 19:8–15, 1981.

39. Gould IM, et al: Vitiligo in diabetes mellitus, *Br J Dermatol* 113:153–155, 1985.

40. Grassi W, Gasparini M, Cervini C: Nail fold computed videomicroscopy in morphofunctional assessment of diabetic microangiopathy, *Acta Diabetol Lat* 22:213–228, 1985.

41. Grgic A, et al: Joint contracture in childhood diabetes, *N Engl J Med* 292:372, 1975.

42. Halevy S, et al: HLA system in relation to carbohydrate metabolism in lichen planus, *Br J Dermatol* 100:683–686, 1979.

43. Handfield-Jones S, Jones S, Peachey R: High dose nicotinamide in the treatment of necrobiosis lipoidica, *Br J Dermatol* 118:693–696, 1988.

44. Hanke CW, Bergfeld WF: Treatment with benzoyl peroxide of ulcers on legs within lesions of necrobiosis lipoidica diabeticorum, *J Dermatol Surg Oncol* 4:701–704, 1978.

45. Hanna W, et al: Pathologic features of diabetic thick skin, *J Am Acad Dermatol* 16:546–553, 1987.

46. Hatzis J, et al: Sweat gland disturbances in granuloma annulare and necrobiosis lipoidica, *Br J Dermatol* 108:705–709, 1983.

47. Heite HJ, Scharwenka HX: Erythema elevatum diutinum Granuloma annulare, Nekrobiosis lipoidica und Granulomatosis disciformis Gottron-Miescher, *Arch Klin Exp Dermatol* 208:260–290, 1959.

48. Heng MCY, et al: Focal endothelial cell degeneration and proliferative endarteritis in trauma-induced early lesions of necrobiosis lipoidica diabeticorum, *Am J Dermatopathol* 13:108–114, 1991.

49. Heng MCY, Song MK, Heng MK: Healing of necrobiotic ulcers with antiplatelet therapy correlation with plasma thromboxane levels, *Int J Dermatol* 28:195–197, 1989.

50. Hoerer D, Dreyfuss F, Herzberg M: Carotenemia, skin colour and diabetes mellitus, *Acta Diabetol Lat* 12:202–207, 1975.

51. Horikawa S, Ono T: Generalized granuloma annulare, *Nishinihon J Dermatol* 42:587–591, 1980.

52. Hunt SJ, Narus VT, Abell E: Necrolytic migratory erythema: dyskeratotic dermatitis, a clue to early diagnosis, *J Am Acad Dermatol* 24:473–477, 1991.

53. Huntley AC: Diabetes mellitus and miscellaneous metabolic conditions affecting the skin, in Jelinek JE, editor: *The skin and diabetes*, Philadelphia, 1986, Lea & Febiger, pp 136–137.

54. Huntley AC: Cutaneous manifestations of diabetes mellitus, in Sammarco GJ, editor: *The foot in diabetes*, Philadelphia, 1991, Lea & Febiger, pp 124–125.

55. Huntley AC, Walter RM, Jr: Quantitative determination of skin thickness in diabetes mellitus: relationship to disease parameters, *J Med* 21:257–264, 1990.

56. Husz S, et al: Disseminated atypical granuloma annulare, *J Dermatol* 14:67–69, 1987.

57. Jelinek, JE: The skin in diabetes mellitus: cutaneous manifestations, complications and associations, in *Yearbook of Dermatology*, Chicago, 1970, Mosby-Year Book, pp 5–35.

58. Jelinek JE: Necrobiosis lipoidica diabeticorum, in Maddin S, editor: *Current dermatologic therapy*, Philadelphia, 1982, WB Saunders, p 325.

59. Jelinek JE: Collagen disorders in which diabetes and cutaneous features co-exist, in *The skin in diabetes*, Philadelphia, 1986, Lea & Febiger, pp 155–173.

60. Jelinek JE: Cutaneous markers of diabetes mellitus and the role of microangiopathy, in *The skin in diabetes*, Philadelphia, 1986, Lea & Febiger, pp 31–72.

61. Jelinek JE: Dermatoses reported to be more frequent in diabetes, *The skin in diabetes*, Philadelphia, 1986, Lea & Febiger, pp 175–202.

62. Jelinek JE: *The skin in diabetes*, Philadelphia, 1986, Lea & Febiger.

63. Kantor GA, Lookingbill DP: Generalized pruritus

and systemic disease, *J Am Acad Dermatol* 9:375–382, 1983.

64. Kaposi M: Idiopathisches multiples Pigmentsarkom der Haut, *Arch Dermatol Syphilol* 4:265–273, 1872.

65. Kennedy L, et al: Limited joint mobility in type I diabetes mellitus, *Postgrad Med J* 58:481–484, 1982.

66. Koga M, Tango T: Clinical features and course of type A and type B vitiligo, *Br J Dermatol* 118:223–228, 1988.

67. Koh MS, et al: Increased plasma fibronectin in diabetes mellitus, necrobiosis lipoidica and widespread granuloma annulare, *Clin Exp Dermatol* 9:293–297, 1984.

68. Kramer DW: Early or warning signs of impending gangrene in diabetes, *Med J Rec* 132:338–342, 1930.

69. Landau J, Davis E: The small blood vessels of the conjunctiva and nail bed in diabetes mellitus, *Lancet* 2:731–734, 1960.

70. Larkin JG, Frier BM: Limited joint mobility and Dupuytren's contracture in diabetic hypertensive and normal populations, *Br Med J* 292:1494, 1986.

71. Lascari AD: Carotenemia: a review, *Clin Pediatr* 20:25–29, 1981.

72. Laukkanen A, et al: Necrobiosis lipoidica: clinical and immunofluorescent study, *Dermatologica* 172:89–92, 1986.

73. Lever WF, Schaumberg-Lever G: *Histopathology of the skin*, ed 6, Philadelphia, 1983, JB Lippincott, pp 234–236.

74. Lieberman LS, et al: Reduced skin thickness with pump administration of insulin, *N Engl J Med* 303:940–941, 1980.

75. Lisi P, Giommoni V: A study on the carbohydrate metabolism in lichen planus patients in time, *Ann Ital Dermatol Clin Sper* 37:29–33, 1983.

76. Lithner F: Cutaneous reactions of the extremities of diabetics to local thermal trauma, *Acta Med Scand* 198:319–325, 1975.

77. Lithner F, Hallmans G, Hietala S-O: Cutaneous hemorrhages and gangrenes localized to the lower limbs in patients with collagen diseases and in diabetes, *Upsala J Med Sci* 83:141–151, 1978.

78. Lithner F, Hietala S-O: Skeletal lesions of the feet in diabetes and their relationship to cutaneous erythema with or without necrosis of the feet, *Acta Med Scand* 200:155–161, 1976.

79. Littler CM, Tschen EH: Pentoxifylline for necrobiosis lipoidica diabeticorum, *J Am Acad Dermatol* 17:314–315, 1987.

80. Lundström IM: Incidence of diabetes mellitus in patients with oral lichen planus, *Int J Oral Surg* 12:147–152, 1983.

81. Lyons TJ, Kennedy L: Non-enzymatic glycosylation of skin collagen in patients with type 1 (insulin-dependent) diabetes mellitus and limited joint mobility, *Diabetologia* 28:2–5, 1985.

82. Lyons TJ, et al: Decrease in skin collagen glycation with improved glycemic control in patients with insulin-dependent diabetes mellitus, *J Clin Invest* 87:1910–1915, 1991.

83. Mann RJ, Harman RRM: Cutaneous anaesthesia in necrobiosis lipoidica, *Br J Dermatol* 110:323–325, 1984.

84. Melin H: An atrophic circumscribed skin lesion in the lower extremities of diabetics, *Acta Med Scand* 176(suppl 423):9–75, 1964.

85. Monk B: Carotenemia, *Int J Dermatol* 22:376–377, 1983.

86. Mueller MJ, et al: Insensitivity, limited joint mobility and plantar ulcers in patients with diabetes mellitus, *Phys Ther* 69:453–462, 1989.

87. Muhlemann MF, Williams DRR: Localized granuloma annulare is associated with insulin-dependent diabetes mellitus, *Br J Dermatol* 111:325–329, 1984.

88. Muller SA, Winkelmann RK: Necrobiosis lipoidica diabeticorum, a clinical and pathological investigation of 171 cases, *Arch Dermatol* 93:272–281, 1966.

89. Murphy R: Skin lesions in diabetic patients: the "spotted leg" syndrome, *Lahey Clinic Found Bull* 14:10–14, 1965.

90. Neilly JB, et al: Pruritus in diabetes mellitus: investigation of prevalence and correlation with diabetes control, *Diabetes Care* 9:273–275, 1986.

91. Nigam PK, Singh G, Agrawal JK: Plasma insulin response to oral glycemic stimulus in lichen planus, *Br J Dermatol* 19:128–129, 1988.

92. Oimomi M, et al: Glycosylation levels of nail proteins in diabetic patients with retinopathy and neuropathy, *Kobe J Med Sci* 31:183–188, 1985.

93. Oppenheim M: Eigentümliche disseminerte Degeneration des Bindegewebes der Haut bei einem Diabetiker, *Zentralbl Haut Geschlechtskr* 32:179, 1930.

94. Oursler JR, Goldblum OM: Blistering eruption in a diabetic, *Arch Dermatol* 127:247, 1991.

95. Pal B, et al: Limitation of joint mobility and shoulder capsulitis in insulin and ono-insulin dependent diabetes mellitus, *Br J Rheumatol* 25:147–151, 1986.

96. Parker F, et al: Evidence for the chylomicron origin of lipids accumulating in diabetic eruptive xanthomas: a correlative lipid biochemical, histochemical and electron microscope study, *J Clin Invest* 49:2172–2187, 1970.

97. Patterson JW: The perforating disorders, *J Am Acad Dermatol* 10:561–581, 1984.

98. Pongor S, et al: Aging of proteins and identifica-

tion of a fluorescent chromophore from the reactions of polypeptides with glucose, *Proc Natl Acad Sci USA* 81:2684–2688, 1984.

99. Porneuf M, et al: Carcinoma cuniculatum arising in necrobiosis lipoidica, *Ann Dermatol Venereol* 118:461–464, 1991.

100. Quimby SR, Muller SA, Schroeter AL: The cutaneous immunopathology of necrobiosis lipoidica diabeticorum, *Arch Dermatol* 124:1364–1371, 1988.

101. Quimby SR, et al: Necrobiosis lipoidica diabeticorum: platelet survival and response to platelet inhibitors, *Cutis* 43:213–216, 1989.

102. Rapini RP, Hebert AA, Drucker CR: Acquired perforating dermatosis, *Arch Dermatol* 125:1074–1078, 1989.

103. Rocca FF, Pereyra E: Phlyctenar lesions in the feet of diabetic patients, *Diabetes* 12:220–223, 1963.

104. Roenigk HH Jr, Taylor JS, Binkley GW: Scleredema adultorum of Buschke (case in society transactions), *Arch Dermatol* 99:124–125, 1969.

105. Rosenbloom AL: Skeletal and joint manifestations of childhood diabetes, *Pediatr Clin North Am* 31:569–589, 1984.

106. Rosenbloom AL: Diabetic thick skin and stiff joints [letter], *Diabetologia* 32:74–75, 1989.

107. Rosenbloom AL: Limited joint mobility in insulin dependent childhood diabetes, *Eur J Pediatr* 149:380–388, 1990.

108. Rosenbloom AL, Frias JL: Diabetes, short stature and joint stiffness—a new syndrome, *Clin Res* 22:92A, 1974.

109. Rosenbloom AL, et al: Limited joint mobility in childhood diabetic mellitus indicated increased risk for microvascular disease, *N Engl J Med* 305:191–194, 1981.

110. Rosenbloom AL, et al: Limited joint mobility in diabetes mellitus of childhood: natural history and relationship to growth impairment, *J Pediatr* 101:874–878, 1982.

111. Rosenbloom AL, et al: Limited joint mobility in childhood diabetes: family studies, *Diabetes Care* 6:370–373, 1983.

112. Roupe G, et al: Biochemical characterization and tissue distribution of the scleredema in a case of Buschke's disease, *Acta Derm Venereol (Stockh)* 67:193–198, 1987.

113. Rowe BR, et al: Wound healing of ulcerated necrobiosis lipoidica with optimum glycaemic control and seaweed-based dressings [letter], *Br J Dermatol* 125:603, 1991.

114. Sawada Y: Successful treatment of ulcerated necrobiosis lipoidica diabeticorum with prostaglandin E and skin flap transfer: a case report, *J Dermatol* 12:449–454, 1985.

115. Seibold J: Digital sclerosis in children with insulin dependent diabetes mellitus, *Arthritis Rheum* 25:1357–1361, 1982.

116. Shall L, et al: Necrobiosis lipoidica: "The footprint not the footstep," *Br J Dermatol* 123(suppl 37):47, 1990.

117. Shimizu H, et al: Perforating granuloma annulare, *Int J Dermatol* 24:581–583, 1985.

118. Smolle, J: T-zone histiocytes in granulomatous skin disorders, *Dermatologica* 171:316–320, 1985.

119. Sparrow G, Abell E: Granuloma annulare and necrobiosis lipoidica treated by jet injector, *Br J Dermatol* 93:85–89, 1975.

120. Starkman H, Brink S: Limited joint mobility of the hands in type I diabetes mellitus, *Diabetes Care* 5:534–536, 1982.

121. Starkman HS, et al: Limited joint mobility (LJM) of the hand in patients with diabetes mellitus: relation to chronic complications, *Ann Rheum Dis* 45:130–135, 1986.

122. Sueki H, Fujisawa R: Pigmented pretibial patches with special references to the clinical classification and the correlation to HbA1 which serves as an index of diabetic control, *Jpn J Dermatol* 96:157–163, 1986.

123. Sueki H, et al: Effects of non-enzymatic glycosylation and heating on browning of human stratum corneum and nail, *Dermatologica* 183:197–202, 1991.

124. Tkach JR: Platelet-inhibition therapy of ulcerated necrobiosis lipoidica diabeticorum, *Dermatol Allergy* 5:9–12, 1982.

125. Toyota T, et al: Diabetic scleredema, *Tohoku J Exp Med* 141:457–461, 1983.

126. Trapp RG, Soler NG, Spencer-Green G: Nail fold capillaroscopy in type I diabetics with vasculopathy and limited joint mobility, *J Rheumatol* 13:917–920, 1986.

127. Trevisan G, Rizzi MG, Tonini G: Capillaroscopia del vallo ungueale e diabete insulino-dipendente osservazioni in ambiente pediatrico, *Giornale Ital Dermatol Venereol* 122:621–624, 1987.

128. Tubiana-Rufi N, et al: Detection by nail fold capillary microscopy of early morphologic capillary changes in children with insulin dependent diabetes mellitus, *Diabete Metab* 15:118–122, 1989.

129. Urbach E: Beitrage zu einer physiologischen und pathologischen Chemie der Haut. Eine neue diabetische Stoff wechseldermatose: Nekrobiosis lipoidica diabeticorum, *Arch Derm Syph* 166:273–285, 1932.

130. Vion B, Frenk E: Erworbene reaktive kollagenose des Erwachsenen: erfolgreiche behandlung durch UV-B Licht, *Hautarzt* 40:448–450, 1989.

131. Weber B: Pathophysiology of diabetes mellitus, in Brook CGD, editor: *Clinical paediatric endocrinology*, Cambridge, Mass, Blackwell Scientific Publications, 1989, pp 579–581.

132. Zalla JA: Werner's syndrome, *Cutis* 25:275–278, 1980.

133. Zelger B, et al: Acquired perforating dermatosis: transepidermal elimination of DNA material and possible role of leukocytes in pathogenesis, *Arch Dermatol* 127:695–700, 1991.

# CHAPTER 4

# New Concepts About the Pathogenesis of Atherosclerosis and Thrombosis in Diabetes Mellitus

**John A. Colwell, M.D., Ph.D.**

**Timothy J. Lyons, M.D.**

**Richard L. Klein, M.D.**

**Maria F. Lopes-Virella, M.D.**

The development of atherosclerosis is accelerated in diabetes mellitus, leading to increased morbidity and mortality and excessive health care costs. Virtually all of the large vessels are involved in this process, and clinical manifestations are apparent as a result of atherosclerotic narrowing and thrombosis of coronary, cerebral, and leg vessels.

These factors have led to a renewed interest in factors present in the diabetic state that may help to explain the acceleration of this process. Work in diabetes has been facilitated by new concepts about the pathophysiology of the process of atherosclerosis in the nondiabetic state.

Review articles, and our previous chapter in this text,[60] have considered atherosclerosis in depth and should be consulted for older references.[56, 59, 60] This chapter provides updated information about the factors associated with the diabetic state that may underlie accelerated atherosclerosis and thrombosis and suggests a pathogenetic scheme that builds on knowledge of these processes in the nondiabetic state. The emphasis is on changes in the endothelium, on qualitative and quantitative changes in lipids and lipoproteins, on glycation and glycooxidation, and on altered coagulation in diabetes mellitus.

## HISTORICAL PERSPECTIVE

Clinicians have long recognized that peripheral vascular disease is an extremely serious medical complication. Advanced calcification of the aorta was found in a mummy from ancient Egyptian times (approximately 2500 B.C.), and calcific atherosclerosis was found in the vessels of the lower extremities in the mummy of Ramses II (approximately 1290–1223 B.C.[156]). It is reported that Hippocrates, in 400 B.C., "cut away the mortified parts," presumably in patients with gangrene after trauma or vascular occlusion. The first evidence of an amputation was a picture in the *Field Book of Wound Surgery* in 1517, showing the technique of Hans von Gersdorff. It was clear by the 17th century that amputations were indicated not only after traumatic injury but also for foot ulcers and abscesses. In the mid-1800s, Syme performed his celebrated amputation at the ankle joint, ether anesthesia was introduced, and an association of diabetes with gangrene was described by Marchal. By 1891, Heidenhain had published a thorough review of diabetes and arteriosclerosis of the legs and had recommended levels for amputation if gangrene was found.[68, 154]

Autopsy studies prior to 1930 in diabetic patients showed that 29% of them had gangrene at the time of death, and data from the Joslin Clinic between 1923 and 1969 indicated that amputations accounted for 22% to 40% of major surgical operations in their diabetic patients.[296] In Bell's classic autopsy study of 2,130 diabetic persons who had died from 1911 through 1955, gangrene was found in 21% and was 53 to 71 times more common than in nondiabetic individuals.[22]

As time has progressed, diagnostic techniques have improved. Cross-sectional (prevalence) studies have indicated that about 15% to 30% of a heterogenous group of noninsulin-dependent diabetes mellitus (NIDDM) patients may have evidence of peripheral vascular disease when studied by noninvasive techniques.[21, 56, 83, 127, 185] The disease appears to progress as a function of age, duration of diabetes, or both when extrapolation from cross-sectional data is done. Longitudinal data are limited but suggest that the rate of progression may be about 2.5% per year in newly diagnosed white NIDDM subjects in the United States, whereas it may reach 5% to 7% per year in such NIDDM populations who are followed up after the disease is present.[205] In any case, longitudinal studies agree that macrovascular complications involving both the leg and coronary vessels progress with increasing duration of diabetes. Whether this is related to hyperglycemia or other factors is not clear.

## RISK FACTORS FOR PERIPHERAL VASCULAR DISEASE IN DIABETES

Studies of risk factors provide insight into the pathogenesis of peripheral vascular atherosclerosis in diabetes and have been reviewed elsewhere in this edition (see Chapter 2). In addition to the influences of age and duration of diabetes, several studies have indicated that hypertension and cigarette smoking, two classical risk factors for coronary artery disease, are also operative for peripheral vascular disease.[56] These correlations have been seen in populations as geographically diverse as Rochester, Minnesota,[213] Seattle, Washington,[21] Munich, Germany,[127] Kuopio, Finland,[276] and Framingham, Massachusetts.[96] It is not clear whether hyperglycemia is an independent risk factor for peripheral vascular disease. Indeed, in some populations, such as Japan, peripheral vascular disease is rarely seen in NIDDM, despite long-standing hyperglycemia.[56] Studies in the United States and Germany have not established that either fasting glucose or hemoglobin $A_{1c}$ values are good predictors of progression of peripheral vascular disease in NIDDM.[21, 127]

Altered lipid and lipoprotein profiles are frequently seen in NIDDM subjects, with or without peripheral vascular disease. Several large-scale studies indicate that certain lipid-lipoprotein changes may be important risk factors for peripheral vascular disease in diabetes mellitus. In a cross-sectional study of 252 individuals with NIDDM, elevated plasma triglyceride levels and decreased high density lipoprotein (HDL) cholesterol levels emerged as possible risk factors for peripheral vascular disease.[21] In a 5-year prospective study in Finland, claudication was associated with increased plasma cholesterol, very low density lipoprotein (VLDL) cholesterol, decreased HDL cholesterol, and increased VLDL triglyceride and LDL triglyceride levels.[276] Multivariate analysis revealed that high LDL triglyceride and VLDL cholesterol levels had independent associations with claudication. On the other hand, negative correlations with lipids and either prevalence or incidence of peripheral vascular disease has been reported in some studies.[213]

Hyperinsulinemia has emerged as an independent vascular risk factor in many epidemiologic studies.[76, 87, 221, 294] Generally, prospective studies have used ischemic heart disease and vascular deaths as the vascular endpoints of interest rather than peripheral vascular disease. In one large cross-sectional study, the greatest risk for coronary heart disease and peripheral vascular disease was seen in diabetic and nondiabetic subjects with the highest plasma c-peptide levels.[256] Thus, although data in diabetic subjects with peripheral vascular disease are limited, it is possible that endogenous hyperinsulinemia may interact with other risk factors to accelerate macrovascular disease. There are many reviews of this issue, which should be consulted for details.[58, 261, 262]

Thus there are mixed messages from epidemiologic studies of peripheral vascular disease in diabetes. It is likely that this state of affairs is caused by confounding factors, including: (1) insensitive endpoints such as claudication and amputation; (2) the likelihood that pathogenesis may differ in IDDM and in the many stages of impaired glucose tolerance (IGT) and NIDDM; (3) the probability that multiple risk factors such as hyperglycemia, lipid disturbances, hypertension, and cigarette smoking interact; and (4) the frequent association of diabetic neuropathy with vascular insufficiency in many patients with diabetes. Nevertheless, epidemiologic data suggest that an atherogenic mix of lipids and lipoproteins may, in particular, contribute to peripheral vascular disease and that hypertension, smoking, and perhaps hyperglycemia may interact in many subjects to accelerate the process. Such leads from epidemiologic studies have stimulated research on precise mechanisms that may be involved in the pathogenesis of atherosclerosis in diabetes mellitus.

## PATHOGENESIS OF ATHEROSCLEROSIS

One of the accepted theories to explain the development of arteriosclerosis is the response to injury hypothesis, which was formulated by Ross and Glomset[233] in 1976. The hypothesis in its initial formulation postulated that injury to the endothelium could occur by mechanical, chemical, toxic, viral, or immunologic mechanisms that promoted endothelial denudation, followed by platelet adhesion, aggregation, and release of platelet-derived growth factor (PDGF), which, in

turn, would stimulate the migration and proliferation of smooth muscle cells within the intima. This process and how it is modified in the diabetic state were illustrated in our previous chapter in this text.[60]

In recent years this hypothesis has undergone several modifications. The most important is the focus on the endothelium. The endothelium can respond to a variety of stimuli and suffer subtle alterations in its functional capacity and integrity, which, in turn, induce a series of cellular responses. These cellular responses include interactions among the cells involved in the arteriosclerotic process and the release by these cells of growth factors, cytokines, and in certain cases toxic substances. Such interactions may play a crucial role in determining the fate of the early lesions of arteriosclerosis and whether or not they will progress to advanced lesions.

How injury to the endothelium may occur in patients with hyperlipidemia, hypertension, diabetes, or a history of cigarette smoking is in the process of being defined. This has been one of the most exciting areas of research in the past decade. Although a considerable amount of knowledge has been accumulating, our understanding of the pathways that may induce endothelial cell injury is far from complete. Injury to the endothelium may result in very subtle changes in the endothelial cell. Examples of a mild injury would include minor changes in the lipid composition of the endothelial cell membrane that may lead to an increased rigidity of the membrane or to alterations in its permeability, thus altering its functional behavior. More profound changes include alterations in the cell surface glycoproteins or the expression of adhesion molecules, which would determine adherence of circulating cells to the endothelium. Clear damage to the endothelium may be induced by modified lipoproteins and/or activation of phagocytic cells, with release of such cytokines as tumor necrosis factor alpha and interleukin-1.

A group of substances that may induce functional changes of the endothelium are minimally modified lipoproteins. These lipoproteins have been shown to stimulate the adherence of monocytes to endothelial cells,[24] to induce the expression of monocyte chemotactic protein 1 in human endothelial and smooth muscle cells,[66] to promote the expression of adhesion molecules, specifically vascular cell adherence molecules (VCAMs) and endothelial-leukocyte adherence molecules (ELAMs) in endothelial cells, and to induce tissue factor expression in cultured human endothelial cells.[75] Limited information is yet available concerning the role of glycated or "glycoxidized" LDL in inducing the expression of adhesion molecules. These studies are of great theoretical importance in diabetes mellitus. In the group of substances that are toxic to the endothelial cells, oxidized LDL plays an important role. It has been shown that oxidized LDL is cytotoxic to the endothelial cell[192] and can also act as a chemotactic factor for peripheral blood monocytes.[222] Furthermore, both oxidized and glycated LDL have been shown to be immunogenic and promote the formation of autoantibodies. Thus, in addition to the direct effects of oxidized LDL on the endothelium, it could be argued that immune complexes formed as a consequence of the autoimmune response to oxidized or glycated (or both) LDL could also have a direct pathogenic effect on endothelial cells. The interaction between LDL–immune complexes (LDL-IC) and endothelial cells would be likely if these cells expressed Fcγ receptors (receptors that recognize the Fc fragment of immunoglobulin G), but this is a point that has been the object of controversy. Some authors claim that Fcγ receptors are expressed only by previously damaged endothelial cells or by endothelial cells infected by latent viruses[54] or bacteria.[23] Thus it is not clear whether immune complexes can play an initial role in damaging endothelial cells or whether they are involved solely in the evolution of a lesion initiated by some other insult. It is interesting to note that the role of infectious agents in the onset of atherosclerosis has been postulated and has received some attention.[184] In either case, the binding of immune complexes to endothelial cells can have deleterious consequences by promoting endothelial binding and activation of phagocytic cells.

Furthermore, if the endothelial cell–bound immune complexes are able to activate complement and release C5a, this complement fragment can attract and activate neutrophils, further contributing to the recruitment of cells potentially able to damage the endothelium.[28, 272] This mechanism may be particularly relevant to diabetes, because it is well known that immune complexes are present in diabetes in increased levels, and it has been proposed that in diabetes the immune system is in a state of polyclonal activation, underlying the production of autoantibodies and the subsequent formation of immune complexes.

Injury to the endothelium may also occur indirectly through activation of phagocytic cells. Macrophages, when activated, secrete a number of enzymes and factors known to possess chemoactractant activity for leukocytes, including complement C5a, leukotriene $B_4$, 12-hydroxy-eicosatetraenoic acid (12-HETE), interleukin 1 (IL-1), tumor necrosis factor α (TNF-α) and PDGF. Data generated in our laboratory also demonstrated (unpublished observations) that the uptake of the LDL-immune complexes by macrophages leads to their activation and to the release of TNF-α and IL-1. Actually, LDL-IC appear to be more potent activators of TNF-α than endotoxin (lipopolysaccharide [LPS]) or any other type of immune complex. This could reflect the fact that LDL-IC have the potential to interact simultaneously with two different macrophage receptors (Fcγ receptor and LDL receptor), a situation that appears to fulfill the conditions required for maximal macrophage activation.[175] Both TNF-α and IL-1 can enhance the expression of vascular cell adherence molecules (VCAMs) on endothelial cells.[166] Interleukin 1 and TNF-α-activated endothelial cells, on the other hand, release factor or factors that enhance the expression of leukocyte function–associated antigen 1 (LFA-1) molecules on neutrophils,[219] one of the molecules of the integrin family that promotes leukocyte–endothelial cell interaction. Regardless of the molecules and receptors involved, the adherence of activated leukocytes to the endothelium is usually followed by endothelial cell damage[219] probably caused by the release of superoxide radicals, which among other effects can cause increased peroxidation of cell membrane lipids.[193]

Once monocytes have come into contact with and adhered to the endothelium, they may be chemotactically induced to migrate between endothelial cells and become localized subendothelially, where they become active and undergo conversion to macrophages. Activation of macrophages leads to the release of the mediators mentioned previously, which may contribute to further damage the endothelium and as chemotactic stimuli. Thus, it has been postulated that in certain conditions (e.g., hypercholesterolemia) macrophages once present in the vessel wall can initiate an amplification loop by further directing monocyte migration into the vessel wall and thus sustaining local accumulation of macrophages. These cells will eventually be transformed into foam cells by ingestion of modified lipoproteins, and fatty streaks form and expand with the continued accumulation of these cells.

It is believed that foam cell formation is a key event in atherosclerosis, and there has been considerable interest in defining mechanisms responsible for the accumulation of cholesteryl esters (CEs) in macrophages, which eventually leads to the formation of foam cells. Modified lipoproteins, including glycated and oxidized LDL, have been shown to induce foam cell formation. Oxidized LDL promotes the transformation of macrophages into foam cells by well-known mechanisms involving its uptake by these cells via the scavenger receptor.[222] We have shown that there is increased accumulation of CE in macrophages exposed to lipoproteins isolated from diabetic patients[146, 172] or to in vitro glycated LDL even when the degree of glycation is minimal.[146] We have also shown that the degree of CE synthesis in macrophages exposed to glycated LDL is directly proportional to the degree of LDL glycation.[146] Thus, diabetic patients with poor glycemic regulation are likely to accumulate CEs in macrophages to a greater extent than well-controlled diabetic or nondiabetic subjects. This accumulation of CE may contribute to foam cell formation. It is important to

point out, however, that if foam cell formation occurs secondarily to the uptake of glycated LDL, the mechanism is different from that described for other modified lipoproteins because it is not mediated by the scavenger receptor.[164] Our work actually suggests that glycated LDL is taken up by the macrophages through a separate receptor of lower affinity and higher capacity.[164]

Both glycated and oxidized LDL can induce transformation of macrophages into foam cells by mechanisms other than by their uptake by the receptors mentioned earlier. As stated previously, glycation and oxidation render LDL immunogenic and may trigger antibody and IC formation. Low density lipoprotein IC have been shown by us[103, 109] and others [147] to induce foam cell formation, particularly when presented to the monocytes as either large-sized (insoluble) aggregates or as erythrocyte-adsorbed LDL-IC. Both types of IC induce profound alterations in cholesterol metabolism of normal monocyte-derived macrophages, leading to marked intracellular accumulation of CE and foam cell formation.[103, 109, 147] In general, immune complexes are taken up by macrophages predominantly via Fc receptors and also through nonspecific endocytosis as a result of conformational changes of the protein's surface.[103, 109, 147] Macrophages exposed to LDL-IC also take up increased amounts of LDL because of an increased expression of LDL receptors, apparently reflecting a profound imbalance of cholesterol metabolism, which leads to a depletion of the intracellular free cholesterol regulatory pool while the cell is accumulating large amounts of CEs.[103b] The precise mechanism responsible for this deregulation has not yet been fully elucidated. It should be stressed that these effects are specific for LDL-IC and cannot be duplicated with any other immune complexes, suggesting that the alteration of cholesterol metabolism is caused by the delivery of LDL to the cell through an abnormal pathway rather than by nonspecific stimulation of macrophages as a consequence of the occupancy of Fc receptors with immune complexes. Thus strong evidence suggests that both glycated and oxidized LDL, by becoming immunogenic and triggering an autoimmune response, could subsequently be involved in immune complex formation and induce macrophage activation and foam cell formation.

Subsequent to intimal macrophage accumulation, smooth muscle cells appear to be attracted from the media into the intima, and many of these cells multiply, leading to the formation of a fibrofatty lesion. With continuing smooth muscle cell migration and proliferation in the intima, connective tissue is formed by the smooth muscle cells, and fibrous plaque formation occurs. The components responsible for the migration and proliferation of smooth muscle cells into the intima are cytokines and growth factors such as IL-1, TNF-α, and PDGF, which are released by activated macrophages, activated endothelium, the smooth muscle cells, and perhaps platelets.

Interleukin 1 and TNF-α are known to affect both endothelial cells and smooth muscle cells. Interleukin 1 has been shown to induce synthesis and cell surface expression of procoagulant activity in endothelial cells,[25] to increase vascular permeability,[177] to induce IL-1 release from ECs by a positive feedback mechanism,[291] and to stimulate the release of platelet-aggregating factor (PAF) by endothelial cells. Platelet-aggregating factor, in turn, activates platelets and neutrophils, stimulating platelet aggregation, and enhancing the adhesiveness of neutrophils.[34] Also, IL-1 can be indirectly responsible for fibroblast and neutrophils[34] and can be indirectly responsible for fibroblast and smooth muscle cell proliferation by inducing the production of PDGF-AA by these cells, activating what appears to be an autocrine growth-regulating mechanism.[224] However because IL-1 induces secretion of prostanoids by smooth muscle cells,[158] and prostanoids are known to have growth-inhibiting properties, the in vivo effect of IL-1 release in the arterial wall is unclear. Tumor necrosis factor α, which can be produced not only by macrophages but also by smooth muscle cells, shares with IL-1 the ability to stimulate IL-1 secretion, as well as cell surface expression of procoagulant activity.[25, 195] Another potentially important role of TNF-α is the ability to suppress lipoprotein lipase (LPL) activity.[45] It has been shown that LPL is secreted by macrophages in culture,[52] and it has been proposed that macrophages induce lipolysis in the arteriosclerotic plaque by secreting LPL. However recent studies by Jonasson et al.[129] were not able to detect immunoreactive LPL in the macrophages of arteriosclerotic lesions, and this may reflect local TNF-α-induced inhibition of LPL production.

Platelet-derived growth factor will derive from at least four sources in the intimal lesion: platelets, macrophages, endothelial cells and smooth muscle cells. It is known to induce both smooth muscle cell and fibroblast proliferation. The susceptibility of a given cell to respond to PDGF depends on the type of PDGF receptor subunits present in the cell. For instance, it is well known that fibroblasts respond poorly to PDGF-AA, but they respond well to PDGF-BB.[237] In contrast, smooth muscle cells respond equally well to both PDGF-AA and PDGF-BB. Macrophages and endothelial cells can make both.

In addition to IL-1, TNF, and PDGF, transforming growth factor β (TGF-β), which is usually formed by macrophages but can also be formed by smooth muscle cells, is also responsible for new connective tissue matrix formation.[232] Furthermore, it seems to be also markedly chemotactic for monocytes and smooth muscle cells. However, TGF-β may also play a role in lesion regression, because it can inhibit cell proliferation. Interferon γ, which is released by T cells, is also known to inhibit proliferation and thus to contribute to lesion regression.[232] Thus, the balance between growth factors and growth inhibitors may be crucial to the development of the atheromatous lesions.

Platelets are also a source for growth factors. Platelets release numerous growth factors (PDGF, epidermal growth factor [EGF]/TGF-α, TGF-β and possibly others) when aggregation and the release reaction occur. Platelet-mediated smooth muscle cell proliferation appears to occur frequently in humans in two particular circumstances: after coronary bypass and after percutaneous transluminal coronary angioplasty. It is also

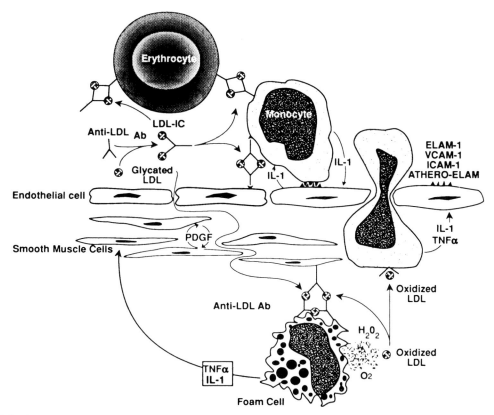

**FIG 4–1.**
New concepts about the pathogenesis of atherosclerosis, with emphasis on the roles of monocyte-derived macrophages, cytokines, immune complexes, glycation and oxidation of LDL, and endothelial adhesion proteins.

likely that platelets may interact with the vessel wall at particular anatomic sites where exposure of macrophages and connective tissue may occur as a result of gross endothelial damage. When this occurs, platelet adhesion and aggregation may aggravate the response and further enhance the development of the atheromatous lesion.

Figure 4–1 illustrates some of these newer concepts of the pathogenesis of atherosclerosis. Alterations that may be important in the diabetic state are discussed in the sections that follow.

Whatever the precise pathologic sequence of events, it is clear that advanced atherosclerotic lesions may result from altered function of endothelium, monocytes and macrophages, platelets, smooth muscle cells, lipids, and lipoproteins. Thrombosis may be the final event that leads to vascular occlusion and ischemic injury. This chapter reviews recent ideas about the effect of the diabetic state of these variables. It updates and extends observations made in the previous edition of this text. Hopefully insights into the mechanisms by which diabetes may alter the function of the vascular wall, its various components, as well as the hemorheologic factors involved in vascular thrombosis, will emerge. An understanding of these events should lead to improved preventive and therapeutic measures for individuals with diabetes.

## ENDOTHELIUM

Vascular endothelial cells participate in a number of important homeostatic and cellular functions such as the coagulation of blood, the activity of leucocytes, the reactivity of platelets, capillary permeability, and regulation of vascular smooth muscle tone. The tonic regulation of vascular smooth muscle cells may be influenced by the endothelium through the release of potent vasorelaxing agents, such as endothelium-derived relaxing factor (EDRF) and prostacyclin (PGI$_2$), and vasoconstrictors, including thromboxane and endothelin.

## Endothelium-Derived Relaxing Factor

The potent vasorelaxation action of EDRF was first demonstrated by Furchgott and Zawadzki.[92] The active constituent of EDRF recently has been identified to be the free radical species nitric oxide.[122, 212] Endothelial cells in culture synthesize nitric oxide from the terminal guanidino nitrogen or atoms of the amino acid L-arginine.[187, 211]

The demonstration that nitric oxide is the mediator of EDRF has stimulated new investigations into abnormal vascular physiology. Defective endothelium-dependent relaxation characterizes many pathophysiologic states, including atherosclerosis. Several studies have demonstrated depressed release or diminished activity of EDRF from atherosclerotic arteries[32, 250] and in patients with heart failure.[150] Dietary-induced hypercholesterolemia[203, 204, 281] and LDL, but not HDL,[7, 264] inhibit endothelium-dependent relaxation in rabbit and porcine[271] arteries. Arteries and arterioles from humans with atherosclerosis or hypercholesterolemia[32, 63] are also relatively unresponsive to endothelium-dependent vasodilators.

Defective endothelium-dependent relaxation is also a feature of both experimental and human diabetes.[1, 74, 186, 208] The factor or factors responsible for the diabetes-induced alterations in endothelium-dependent relaxation are not presently known. However, recent evidence suggests that lipoproteins, especially LDL, may play an important role. As discussed elsewhere in this chapter, diabetes may modify LDL by oxidation or by glycation. Oxidized LDL markedly inhibits the endothelium-dependent relaxation of rabbit aorta[152] and pig coronary artery[251, 268] and may potentiate agonist-induced vasoconstriction by a direct effect on vascular smooth muscle.[94] Recent studies suggest that oxidized LDL may decrease endothelium-dependent relaxation by inactivation of EDRF after its release from ECs.[53, 95, 239] This appears to be caused mainly by the lipid component, especially lysophosphatidylcholine,[53, 152] of the oxidized LDL. Additional studies have also shown that advanced glycosylation products quench nitric oxide and mediate the defective endothelium-dependent vasodilation in experimental diabetes.[42] A role of lipoprotein oxidation and glycation in the alteration of endothelium-derived vascular relaxation in atherogenesis in diabetes mellitus may therefore be postulated but remains to be investigated in more detail.

Several recent studies have attempted to ameliorate the inhibitory effects of the several factors on endothelium-derived relaxation. Administration of L-arginine, a precursor for EDRF, returns endothelial function to normal in hypercholesterolemic rabbits.[61, 234] There are no comparable studies in hypercholesterolemic or diabetic individuals, and the levels of EDRF in plasma obtained from diabetic patients have not been investigated.

## Prostacyclin

The release from endothelial cells of EDRF and PGI$_2$, another potent vasorelaxant, are coupled.[73, 121] Previous studies, extensively reviewed in our previous chapter of this text,[60] have concluded that the synthesis of PGI$_2$ by the vasculature of diabetic patients is reduced.[60] Thus, one might anticipate that the release of EDRF by the vasculature of diabetic patients would also be reduced. Both PGI$_2$ and EDRF act synergistically and influence many functions that control intravascular homeostasis. Nitric oxide and PGI$_2$ inhibit platelet aggregation[174, 223, 253]; thus, the combined decrease in the release of both products in diabetic patients may contribute to a thrombogenic endothelial surface in these patients. Monocyte adhesion to the endothelial cell surface is one of the earliest events in atherogenesis. Nitric oxide inhibits monocyte adhesion to endothelial cell monolayers, whereas PGI$_2$ has no effect[17]; thus, decreased EDRF levels in diabetic patients could contribute to monocyte adhesion to the endothelium and, thus, to atherogenesis in diabetes mellitus.

The decrease in $PGI_2$ concentrations in plasma from diabetic patients may result from a factor described in plasma obtained from type II diabetic patients and streptozotocin-induced diabetic rats.[123, 273] Rat and human plasma–derived serum contained significantly less of a factor that stimulates $PGI_2$ production by the vascular wall. In addition, plasma-derived serum showed less of the $PGI_2$ stimulatory activity in samples obtained from diabetic patients before the clinical onset of vascular complications such as retinopathy and proteinuria. Analysis of the plasma-derived serum indicated that the factor was heat stable, nondialysable, not extractable with lipid solvents, and precipitable with trichloroacetic acid. The reduction in the $PGI_2$ stimulatory activity in plasma from diabetic patients may cause a reduction of $PGI_2$ production by the vascular wall and thus contribute to the development of diabetic vascular complications.

## Thromboxane $A_2$

The endothelium also contributes to the local regulation of vascular smooth muscle function by releasing endothelium-derived contracting factors. Recent studies indicate that the aorta from alloxan-induced diabetic rabbits releases a major vasoconstrictor cyclo-oxygenase product that either directly counteracts the relaxation caused by or selectively interferes with the release of endothelium-derived relaxing factors.[269] The vasoconstrictor is most likely thromboxane $A_2$ or possibly its precursor, prostaglandin $H_2$ ($PGH_2$). Additional studies demonstrated that elevated glucose levels per se, not the hyperlipidemia associated with the experimental diabetic model, promoted the generation of the endothelium-derived vasoconstrictor prostanoids.[270] Thus, hyperglycemia per se may contribute to the endothelial dysfunction in diabetes mellitus. The diabetic state was also shown to enhance the contractile response of rat mesenteric veins induced by the prostanoids $PGE_2$ and $PGF_{2\alpha}$ and the prostacyclin derivatives $PGI_2$-Na and TRK-100.[142] The diabetic state also significantly decreased the vasorelaxation response of cerebral arteries exposed to the platelet vaso-

active compound adenosine diphosphate (ADP) and significantly increased vasoconstriction in arteries exposed to serotonin and the thromboxane analogue U-46619.[178]

## Endothelin

Endothelin is a 21-amino acid polypeptide, which is the most potent natural vasoconstrictor substance yet discovered. The immunoreactive-endothelin concentrations in plasma were found to be significantly increased in patients with diabetes mellitus compared with healthy subjects.[263] Endothelin levels did not correlate with the presence of diabetic retinopathy, duration of diabetes, fasting blood glucose levels, or fructosamine concentrations. To further investigate these findings, Takahashi et al.[265] determined immunoreactive-endothelin levels in rat models with diabetes mellitus. Short-term dexamethasone treatment increased plasma levels of endothelin, whereas streptozotocin treatment decreased the levels. In contrast, an additional study concluded that plasma levels and the rate of release of endothelin from mesenteric arteries are significantly increased in streptozotocin-induced diabetic rats.[266] Diabetes may also influence the action of endothelin on vascular tissue because the effect of endothelin-1 on regional hemodynamics differed in streptozotocin-induced and control rats.[140] These studies suggest that multiple factors may influence endothelin plasma concentrations and actions in diabetes.

## Adhesion Proteins

Studies of adhesion proteins are limited in diabetes mellitus. Nevertheless, it is likely that future work will show alterations in the diabetic state. Therefore, a brief review of this rapidly changing area is indicated. As previously noted, monocyte adhesion to the endothelium is thought to be the first event in the development of fatty streaks during atherogenesis. After adhesion, the monocytes may migrate into the subendothelium, differentiate into macrophages, take up lipids, and become foam cells. Granule membrane protein-140 (GMP-140) is a membrane-associated glycoprotein that can be translocated from its intracellular storage pool to the surface of endothelial cells, where it acts as a ligand for leukocyte adhesion.[100] Another protein with similar properties, termed "platelet activation–dependent granule to external membrane" (PADGEM), was eventually determined to be identical to GMP-140.[180] GMP-140 is located in membranes of Weibel-Palade bodies of endothelial cells.[44, 179] After stimulation of the endothelial cell, GMP-140 is rapidly but transiently redistributed to the cell surface.[115] Experimentally, activators of GMP-140 secretion from endothelial cells include thrombin, histamine, and aqueous or lipid-soluble oxidants.[217] The mechanism by which oxidants induced the translocation of GMP-140 to the endothelial cell surface is not known; however, free radicals were essential components. The ability of LDL modified by glycation, oxidation, or glycoxidation to stimulate GMP-140 translocation is unknown but presents an intriguing scenario for study in diabetes. In vivo, the continual stimulated expression of GMP-140 could result in monocyte recruitment, the additional production of oxygen radicals by the recruited monocytes adhering to the endothelium and eventual endothelial damage. Support for this hypothesis comes from the observation that LDL, minimally modified by prolonged storage or by mild iron oxidation, stimulates the production of an endothelial cell chemotactic factor for monocytes and increased monocyte binding.[24] The minimally modified LDL has been shown to stimulate the expression of MCP-1, a monocyte chemotactic factor.[66] It is not known if the minimally modified LDL can stimulate GMP-140 translocation or if LDL modified by the diabetic milieu can exert effects on endothelial cells similar to those of modified LDL.

Recent studies have identified an inducible endothelial cell adhesion molecule that is selective for mononuclear leukocytes.[67] The adhesion protein is expressed on the surface of activated cultured endothelial cells and also in hypercholesterolemic and Watanabe heritable hyperlipidemic rabbits

in a localized fashion on the aortic endothelium that overlies early foam cell lesions. Thus, this adhesion molecule may be a molecular marker for early atherogenic changes in endothelial cells. In studies conducted in humans, monocytes obtained from patients with combined hypercholesterolemia-hypertriglyceridemia exhibited increased adhesion to ECs compared with monocytes isolated from heterozygotic familial hypercholesterolemic patients or healthy subjects.[72] This study also suggested that an increased level of plasma TGs was the major determinant of the increased monocyte adhesion to endothelial cells because hypercholesterolemia alone did not induce adhesion. Thus, factors involved during the early stages of atherogenesis may modify not only endothelial cells but also monocytes and result in increased endothelial cell–monocyte interactions that potentially may further escalate the atherogenic process. The usual alterations in lipid and lipoprotein levels accompanying poor glycemic control in diabetic patients may put these individuals at greater risk and contribute to the increased prevalence of atherosclerosis in diabetic patients.

## von Willebrand Factor

von Willebrand factor (vWF) is a complex glycoprotein synthesized by vascular endothelium and megakaryocytes. It is one of the most important adhesion molecules mediating hemostatic interactions between blood and the vessel wall. Increased plasma concentrations of vWF have been observed in most studies in both IDDM and NIDDM patients and are completely reviewed in our previous chapter in the fourth edition of this text.[60] vWF is a cofactor of platelet function and its increased levels may be involved in the increased platelet adhesiveness observed in diabetic patients. vWF deposited by endothelial cells in the extracellular matrix may be the most active form in platelet adhesion, whereas plasmatic vWF may play only a secondary role.[15] It is a possible marker of endothelial cell damage in diabetes, and its plasma levels are increased in patients with diabetic microangiopathy.[60, 220] The basic subunit of vWF is made up of 2,050 amino acid residues and has a molecular weight of 260,000 daltons. Circulating vWF is composed of multimers forms of the subunit, with the highest molecular weight multimers the most active biologically. A recent study of 22 type I and type II diabetic patients demonstrated that 14 of the subjects showed abnormal patterns of vWF multimer structure when plasma was analyzed by crossed immunoelectrophoresis, suggesting that the proportion of the different molecular forms of vWF were altered.[216] The vWF antigen abnormalities disappeared in six of seven patients studied after a 3-month period of improved glycemic control. In addition, some of the structural abnormalities in vWF antigen were accompanied by loss of vWF functional activity. Changes in plasma vWF levels after short-term insulin administration have been previously reported.[60]

As discussed elsewhere in this chapter, immunologic factors may play an important role in atherogenesis. Evidence regarding the effect of cytokines on vWF release from endothelial cells is conflicting. De Groot et al.[71] reported that pretreatment of endothelial cells with recombinant human or murine IL-1 decreased both constitutive and stimulated release of vWF with a concomitant reduction in the amount of vWF stored in Weibel-Palade organelles. Zavoico et al[305] failed to observe any effect of IL-1 treatment on either basal or agonist-induced secretion of vWF. In contrast, Giddings et al.[102] reported that IL-1 significantly increased the release of vWF from endothelial cells.[102] The effect of cytokines on vWF release may be even more complex, however, because even though IL-1 and TNF may have little or no direct effect on vWF release from endothelial cells, these cytokines can modulate the acute release of vWF in response to other stimuli.[209] The results on the stimulation of vWF secretion by TNF are also controversial, however.[267] Clearly more research is needed to resolve the question of the effect of inflammatory cytokines on endothelial cell vWF release and possible effects on atherogenesis.

It is therefore evident that altered endothelial function occurs in the diabetic state (Table 4-1). In view of the apparent relationship of these findings to accelerated atherosclerosis in diabetes mellitus, it is clear that this is a fertile area for continued research. Such research could theoretically lead to the development of pharmacologic or physiologic approaches that would prevent or retard the earliest lesions of atherosclerosis.

**TABLE 4-1.**

Altered Endothelial Function in Diabetes

| |
|---|
| ↓ Endothelium-dependent relaxation |
| ↓ Prostacyclin release |
| ↑ Thromboxane release |
| ↑ Plasma endothelin levels |
| ↑ Plasma von Willebrand's factor levels |
| ↑ Adhesion proteins (?) |

## LIPIDS AND LIPOPROTEINS

### Plasma Levels of Lipoproteins in Diabetes

In poorly controlled diabetic patients, plasma LDL, intermediate-density lipoproteins (IDLs) and VLDL levels are elevated.[134, 153, 160, 161, 163, 229, 254] The increase in VLDL levels has been attributed to increased hepatic production or decreased clearance of VLDL[225] and may be more significant in women.[276] High-density lipoprotein levels in diabetes vary with the type of diabetes and, in some groups, with glycemic control. In type II diabetic patients, HDL levels are usually low and do not necessarily increase with improved metabolic control.[134, 160, 197] The low HDL levels are thought to be caused by an increased rate of clearance by hepatic triglyceride lipase[138] and may be more significant in men.[275] In type I diabetic patients HDL cholesterol levels are low during poor glycemic control and increase to normal or even above normal concentration when adequate control is achieved.[134, 161, 163, 248] Changes in HDL cholesterol levels with improved glycemic control are less marked in women than in men,[161, 163] and in black women with type 1 diabetes, there seems to be little association between any plasma lipid levels and glycemic control.[248]

## Qualitative Lipid Abnormalities

Regardless of the association between lipid levels and atherosclerosis, it is well known that even when lipid levels are similar, the mortality and morbidity from atherosclerotic disease in diabetic patients is higher than in nondiabetic individuals. It is also well known that even normolipemic diabetic subjects are more prone to develop atherosclerosis than nondiabetic individuals. In fact, only a small portion of the increased risk for atherosclerotic disease in diabetes can be explained by consideration of the quantitative abnormalities of plasma lipids.[229] To explain the increased prevalence of atherosclerosis in diabetes, several postulates have been advanced. One of them considers the formation of atherogenic, qualitatively abnormal lipoprotein particles in the diabetic state. Qualitative abnormalities resulting from abnormal lipoprotein glycation, oxidation and immune-complex formation are considered. Other qualititative abnormalities involve compositional alterations in the particles.

## Very Low-Density Lipoprotein

Hypertriglyceridemia is a common lipid abnormality in diabetic patients because of both an increase in VLDL synthesis and an impaired catabolism of triglyceride-rich lipoproteins. Impaired VLDL catabolism, which results from decreased peripheral lipoprotein lipase activity, leads to accumulation of remnant particles and may respond to improved glycemic control.[293] The possible roles of glycation and oxidation in altering VLDL metabolism are considered later on. Compositional abnormalities may also be important. In poorly controlled diabetes, the VLDL remnants are enriched with both free and esterified cholesterol and with apolipoprotein B.[293] The relative proportions of other apoprotein components of triglyceride-rich lipoproteins may also be abnormal. It is known that apolipoprotein E facilitates the

uptake of triglyceride-rich lipoprotein remnants by the liver, whereas apolipoprotein CIII inhibits this process.[116, 298] It is also established that apolipoprotein E plays a role in the recognition of VLDL by human macrophages.[290] As discussed later on, we found at least some groups of diabetic patients that the ratio of apoC/apoE was decreased.[145, 146] This might be expected to enhance hepatic clearance, but any such effect may be overwhelmed by impaired peripheral clearance or unknown effects because of apoprotein glycation or oxidation. Although quantitative abnormalities of VLDL improve with improved glycemic control, at least some of the qualitative abnormalities in this and other lipoproteins persist. In the case of VLDL, these include altered surface rigidity, mediated by an abnormal sphingomyelin/lecithin ratio.[13]

The possibility that abnormal VLDL may contribute to the acceleration of atherosclerosis in diabetes has stimulated a number of studies investigating the metabolism, by cultured cells, of TG-rich lipoproteins isolated from diabetic patients. In the presence of hypertriglyceridemia and diabetes, VLDL and remnant particles are preferentially taken up by murine macrophages, leading to intracellular accumulation of CE or triglycerides.[101, 149] We studied the interaction of VLDL isolated from a group of very well-controlled type II diabetic patients with human monocyte-macrophages (the precursors of foam cells).[145] No increase in CE synthesis by the cells was observed, though with VLDL from a subset of less well-controlled patients, there was a tendency towards increased CE synthesis. VLDL from these type II diabetic patients differed from that from controls in having a decreased apoC/apoE ratio, with a tendency toward higher apoE and apoCI levels, and lower apoCIII levels. In contrast, VLDL from a group of type I diabetic patients, who were not so well-controlled as the type II patients just discussed, did stimulate enhanced CE synthesis in the human macrophages.[146] In this study, VLDL from the diabetic patients was significantly enriched in free cholesterol but otherwise did not differ significantly in composition from that obtained from control patients. Whether the altered VLDL metabolism was the result of altered lipoprotein composition, glycation, or some other undetected alteration (e.g., oxidation) is unknown.

## Low-Density Lipoprotein

Qualitative abnormalities of LDL isolated from diabetic patients may alter their cellular recognition. We demonstrated that LDL isolated from IDDM patients in poor metabolic control was taken up and degraded less efficiently by human fibroblasts than normal LDL or LDL isolated from the same patients after metabolic control was attained.[162] In these studies, in addition to its presumed increased glycation, the LDL isolated from the diabetic patients was triglyceride enriched. Hiramatsu et al.[119] confirmed our studies and demonstrated that triglyceride-enriched LDL isolated from both diabetic and nondiabetic subjects with hypertriglyceridemia was poorly recognized by fibroblasts. Triglyceride enrichment of LDL may therefore, in addition to increased glycation, lead to poor recognition of LDL by the classical LDL receptor in diabetes. Lipoprotein surface lipid composition may also be abnormal even in "normolipemic" type I diabetic patients. Bagdade et al.[11] demonstrated altered free cholesterol/lecithin ratios in the combined LDL and VLDL fractions, and these may result in altered lipoprotein metabolism. Similar observations were made in type II diabetic patients, and the abnormalities did not respond to improved glycemic control.[13] Recently, the presence of "polydisperse" LDL, that is, LDL particles that are abnormally large and abnormally small, has been described in diabetes.[126] Large quantities of small, dense LDL may enhance the atherogenicity of diabetic plasma and may also imply higher than expected apolipoprotein B levels for a given LDL cholesterol level.

## High-Density Lipoprotein

High density lipoprotein, because of its role in reverse cholesterol transport, plays an important role in controlling intracellular lipid accumulation.[16, 258] HDL seems to prevent lipid accumulation in macrophages exposed to modified lipoproteins, though the mechanisms for this action are unknown. Recently the existence of an HDL receptor on human fibroblasts, smooth muscle cells, and aortic endothelial cells has been described; it has been postulated that this receptor may be important in promoting cholesterol efflux.[35, 36] Although cellular binding of HDL does not seem to be essential for the transport of cholesterol from the cells to HDL, it does appear to facilitate the removal of cholesterol from cells that are overloaded.[35] Whether an identical receptor is present in human macrophages is not known. Foam cells in arterial walls seem, however, to retain large quantities of cholesterol ester even in the presence of a medium containing HDL.[218] The loss of the ability to release accumulated cholesterol ester could be an important difference between foam cells derived from atherosclerotic lesions and those induced in vitro by incubation of abnormal lipoproteins with macrophages.

HDL composition can also be markedly affected by diabetes, and this may impair reverse cholesterol transport. Fielding et al.[84, 85] observed that cholesterol efflux from normal fibroblasts was inhibited when the cells were incubated with plasma from poorly controlled type II diabetic patients compared with normal plasma. The defect in cholesterol transport was caused by a spontaneous transfer of free cholesterol from VLDL and LDL to HDL, induced by free cholesterol (and phospholipid) enrichment of both VLDL and LDL present in diabetic plasma. An increase in the triglyceride content of HDL has also been noted in type II diabetic patients with hypertriglyceridemia and low levels of HDL cholesterol[13, 26, 27, 275] and cannot be fully corrected by improved glycemic control.[13] The ability of such triglyceride-enriched HDL to remove cholesterol from tissues is not known. Although HDL levels may be normal or increased in type I diabetes, the proportion of the less favorable fraction, $HDL_3$, tends to be increased at the expense of the antiatherogenic $HDL_2$ fraction.[11] As with VLDL and LDL, the composition of surface lipids in HDL is abnormal in diabetes and, at least in $HDL_3$, remains so despite improvements in glycemic control.[13]

Alterations in the apoprotein content of HDL in diabetes have been described. Plasma apoprotein AI levels are increased in diabetic patients,[134] and consequently the HDL cholesterol/apo A-I ratio is reduced,[229] diminishing the particle's antiatherogenic potential. Only some of the abnormalities in apo A-I, apo A-II, and apo E in $HDL_2$ and $HDL_3$ could be corrected by improved glycemic control in type II diabetes.[13]

### Other Factors in Diabetic Plasma That May Alter Lipoprotein Metabolism

Factors other than those inducing alterations of lipoprotein particles may induce a metabolic alteration in cells involved in the arteriosclerotic process. A marked decrease in uptake and intracellular degradation by fibroblasts of LDL isolated from normal and diabetic subjects was observed when the cells were exposed to lipoprotein-deficient serum (LPDS) isolated from poorly controlled diabetic patients.[162] Comparative studies of the composition of LPDS obtained from normal donors and poorly controlled diabetic patients showed an increase in saturated and total unesterified fatty acids, lecithin, apo A-I, and immunoreactive insulin in the LPDS from diabetic patients. Addition of palmitic acid, oleic acid, and lecithin to a pooled LPDS to obtain concentrations similar to those found in the diabetic LPDS led to a decrease in LDL degradation. It is possible that exposure of cells to LPDS obtained from poorly controlled diabetic patients may induce changes in the composition of the fibroblast membrane and alter its fluidity, leading to a decrease in the uptake and degradation of LDL. When diabetic patients are in poor metabolic control, cell membrane changes and modification of LDL composition are likely to act either additively or synergistically to induce an abnormal LDL-cell interaction.

It is therefore apparent that alterations of lipids and lipoproteins are frequently present in diabetes and that insights into mechanisms by which they may accelerate atherosclerosis are emerging. In addition to these critical observations, evidence is accumulating that glycation and glycoxidation of lipoproteins and of other proteins may influence accelerated atherosclerosis in diabetes.

## GLYCATION AND GLYCOXIDATION

In diabetes, increased glycation (nonenzymatic glycosylation) affects any protein exposed to elevated glucose concentrations. Glucose is covalently bound, principally to lysine residues in protein molecules, forming fructose-lysine (FL). The name of the sugar residue changes because of rearrangement of its double bond in the course of the reaction. Subsequently, especially in long-lived proteins, further (Maillard) reactions occur, leading to the development of unreactive end products, many of which are cross-linked, brown, or fluorescent.[155] These end products have been variously termed "browning products," "Maillard reaction products," or "advanced glycation end products" (AGE). Although many of these end products exist, the structures of only two, carboxymethyl-lysine (CML)[3] and pentosidine,[246] have been established (Fig 4–2). Recently it has been demonstrated that the formation of these end products, and indeed all manifestations of the Maillard reaction, including increased protein fluorescence, are mediated by free radical oxidation reactions.[90] Thus, the process involves sequential glycation and oxidation reactions, and accordingly the products have been termed "glycoxidation products."[18]

In diabetic patients, elevated levels of FL (the initial product of glycation) in long-lived proteins such as collagen can be decreased with improved glycemic control, but those of the glycoxidation products (CML and pentosidine) and total protein fluorescence cannot be reduced.[173] Free radical–mediated oxidation may therefore be regarded as a "fixative" for "glycative" damage: like rust on a car, the oxidative damage cannot be reversed once it has occurred. Theoretically at least, oxidative damage may be enhanced by the process of glycation itself, because glycation may generate free radicals.[302]

The hypothesis that enhanced glycation

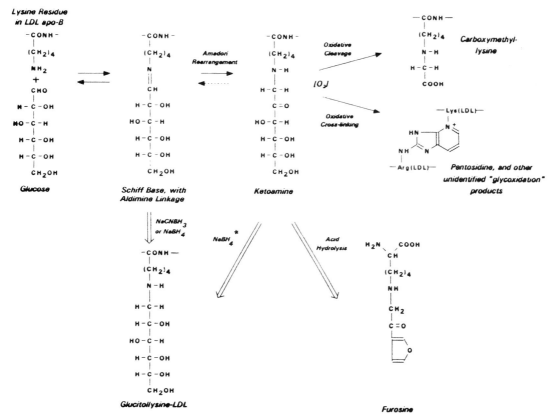

**FIG 4–2.**
Biochemistry of protein glycation and glycoxidation. *(From Lyons TJ:* Diabetes 41(suppl 2), 1992. Used by permission.)

and glycoxidation may underlie the development of diabetic complications is attractive. If the accumulation of glycoxidation products is the crucial issue, the hypothesis provides an explanation for the common observation that there is no simple relationship between glycemic control and the risk of complications. Individual variations in antioxidant defenses, which may or may not be affected by the presence of diabetes, may modulate the effects of hyperglycemia, explaining, at least in part, the differing propensities of individuals to develop complications in the face of similar long-term glycemic control. Initial investigations seeking a role for glycation in the development of complications centered around the early stage of the glycation reaction, namely, FL formation.[139] More recently, the role of browning (glycoxidation) has been investigated.[176, 190] Evidence is presented that both glycation (particularly in short-lived plasma proteins) and glycoxidation (particularly in long-lived vascular structural proteins) may be relevant to the accelerated development of atherosclerosis in diabetic patients.

## Low-Density Lipoprotein Glycation

### Effect on Lipoprotein Metabolism

It is now established that increased glycation of plasma apolipoproteins occurs from the time of onset of diabetes mellitus,[238] that it correlates with other indices of recent glycemic control,[171] and that for a number of reasons, it may contribute to the acceleration of atherosclerosis. Recognition of glycated LDL by the classic LDL receptor is impaired (whether glycated in vitro[104, 236, 301] or in vivo[162]). This may contribute to hyperlipidemia in poorly controlled diabetes. In contrast, uptake of glycated LDL by human monocyte-macrophages is enhanced, and this may accelerate foam cell formation, which is characteristic of the early atherosclerotic plaque.[164, 172]

Recent studies in our laboratory further support the enhanced atherogenicity of glycated LDL in diabetes. We isolated two fractions of *intact* LDL using boronate affinity chromatography[125] to separate "bound" and "nonbound" (i.e., more and less glycated) LDL. We isolated these LDL fractions from type I diabetic patients and nondiabetic control subjects. Glycation of the bound fractions was increased twofold in control and threefold in diabetic patients, suggesting that in diabetes, glycation per particle in this fraction is increased. We studied the metabolic behavior of the fractions using human fibroblasts and human monocyte-derived macrophages. Recognition of the bound (heavily glycated) LDL by fibroblasts was impaired, again regardless of the source of the particles, confirming the results of previous studies.[104, 162, 236, 299]

In macrophages, LDL receptor–mediated degradation of bound LDL isolated from diabetic patients was mildly impaired, while non-LDL receptor–mediated degradation was significantly increased. Thus, the higher levels of glycation of LDL from diabetic patients impairs its recognition by the macrophage LDL receptor but stimulates its recognition by non-LDL receptor–mediated mechanisms. These data confirm that in humans, although glycated LDL is poorly recognized by the classical LDL receptor on fibroblasts, it is recognized by another high-capacity, low-affinity pathway on monocyte-macrophages, enhancing uptake by these cells and thereby enhancing foam cell formation.

### Effect on Platelet Function

Watanabe et al.[292] isolated LDL from young type I diabetic patients, and from matched nondiabetic controls. Glycation of LDL from the diabetic patients was increased, whereas LDL composition was similar in the two groups. LDL from diabetic patients and also in vitro–glycated LDL were more potent stimulators of thromboxane $B_2$ release and thrombin-induced platelet aggregation. It appeared, however, that this effect was not linearly related to the extent of LDL glycation. We proposed that subtle alterations in the composition of platelet membranes, induced by interaction with glycated LDL, may underlie the effects on platelet behavior. Finally, when LDL from type I diabetic patients was subfractionated by affinity chromatography into bound and nonbound fractions, using the method described earlier, platelet aggregation was enhanced to a significantly greater extent by the bound (highly glycated) fraction.[144]

### Glycation of Very Low-Density Lipoprotein and High-Density Lipoprotein

Increased glycation affects other apolipoproteins apart from apo B100 in LDL. Elevated levels in VLDL and HDL apoproteins have been demonstrated by Curtiss and Witztum[65] and may affect their cellular interactions, function, and metabolism. Recently, VLDL isolated from normolipemic patients with both type I and II diabetes was found to interact abnormally with cultured human monocyte-macrophages,[145, 146] stimulating increased CE synthesis and accumulation. However, the effect was not as marked as with LDL. Also, subtle alterations in lipid and apoprotein composition were observed and may account for some of the findings. Nevertheless, increased glycation of the apoproteins of VLDL may be important. Investigations are hampered by the difficulty of measuring the extent of glycation of the individual apoproteins of VLDL.

Glycation of HDL in vitro was found to accelerate its clearance from the circulation of guinea pigs[298] (in contrast to LDL, whose catabolic rate was reduced). The effect was seen even with mild degrees of glycation and may lower plasma HDL levels in diabetic patients and hence to increased cardiovascular risk. Increased glycation of apo AI has been shown to facilitate its dissociation from HDL, thus compromising the structural cohesion of the particle.[43] Recently, Duell et al.[77] have shown that high-affinity binding of glycated HDL to fibroblasts is impaired and that this reduces its capacity to remove cholesterol from peripheral cells.

## Lipoprotein Glycation and the Immune System

Modification of proteins, such as glycation and glycoxidation, may alter their structure sufficiently to render them immunogenic. Curtiss and Witztum[64] found that LDL glycated to the extent that occurs in vivo is a relatively weak antigen and that antibodies against it had no effect on its rate of clearance. However, the existence of even low levels of antibodies against glycated LDL may have pathophysiologic relevance because it may imply the presence of circulating antigen-antibody complexes, which are known to be potentially atherogenic. In addition, the more severely modified ("glycoxidized") lipoproteins that may be present in vessel walls may behave as more potent antigens stimulating the in situ formation of immune complexes.[38]

## Lipoprotein Glycation and Oxidation

Lipoproteins, containing unsaturated fatty acids in their cores, are particularly vulnerable to oxidative damage, and the role of oxidized lipoproteins in the pathogenesis of atherosclerosis in diabetes has been reviewed recently.[168] Oxidized LDL is a potent stimulator of foam cell formation, and theoretically at least, glycation may enhance oxidative damage.[193, 302] Despite this, there is little evidence that oxidation of plasma lipoproteins is increased in uncomplicated diabetes, whereas glycation clearly is. Also no studies have shown a correlation between lipoprotein oxidation and glycemic control in diabetic patients, and there is some evidence that lipid peroxidation, at least in some tissues, is actually reduced in diabetes.[214] However, in the vessel wall, glycation enhances covalent binding of lipoproteins to structural proteins, increasing half-life and the likelihood of oxidative damage. Here the processes of glycation, oxidation, and browning may be closely interwoven, causing vicious cycles of vascular injury.

## Browning of Vascular Structural Proteins

Glycation and browning, or glycoxidation, of vascular wall structural proteins may also be important in atherogenesis, and these processes may not only alter the characteristics of the vessel wall itself, but also influence its interaction with circulating plasma constituents. With advancing age, collagen becomes increasingly insoluble, thermally stable and resistant to enzymatic attack.[110] Evidence is accumulating that these changes result from glucose-derived cross-links, formed via the browning or glycoxidation process. As mentioned already, these changes are irreversible once they have occurred.[173] This is consistent with the exaggeration of aging changes in collagen in the presence of diabetes. Glycoxidation of vascular connective tissues may contribute to accelerated atherosclerosis in various ways.

### Abnormal Vascular Rigidity and Tone

Monnier et al.[190] showed that increased collagen fluorescence is associated with increased arterial stiffness (assessed in vivo) and with elevated systolic and diastolic blood pressures. Increased aortic stiffness in autopsy studies of patients with type I diabetes was confirmed by Oxlund et al.,[207] but the level of glycoxidation products was not determined. Loss of the normal elasticity and compliance of arteries and arterioles in diabetes may be at least partially caused by increased glucose-mediated cross-linking. This may contribute directly to the development of hypertension, whereas arterial stiffness and hypertension together may result in abnormal shear stresses on the endothelium, predisposing it to injury and the development of atherosclerosis. Also, recent evidence suggests that collagen glycoxidation products quench the activity of nitric oxide (EDRF) both in vitro and in vivo.[42] This leads to an impairment of endothelium-mediated vasodilation and therefore may cause abnormalities in vascular tone. It is possible that local abnormalities of flow, perfusion, and blood pressure may result, which may be injurious to arteries and arterioles.

### Covalent Binding of Plasma Constituents

Endothelial injury allows increased permeation of plasma constituents into the vessel wall, where they come into contact with elevated levels of connective tissue glycoxidation products. Brownlee et al.[40] demonstrated there is increased LDL-collagen cross-linking when the lipoprotein was exposed to modified collagen (containing browning products) compared with control collagen. In diabetic compared with nondiabetic animals, cross-linking of LDL to aortic collagen was increased 2.5-fold. Trapped in a high-glucose environment in the vessel wall, the LDL particles may undergo extensive glycative and oxidative modification, with further increases in particle atherogenicity. Free radical chain reactions in the trapped LDL may damage not only the lipids within the particle but also neighboring structural proteins and cells. It has been shown, for instance, that products of lipid peroxidation stimulate cross-linking of collagen.[118] In diabetes, these interrelated mechanisms are likely to result in various vicious cycles, leading to damage of the arterial wall and in situ formation of lipoprotein-immune complexes,[38] further accelerating foam cell formation.

### Macrophage AGE Receptor

Monocyte-macrophages possess a specific receptor that recognizes glycoxidation products; this has been termed the AGE receptor and has been shown to be distinct from other scavenger receptors.[284] Macrophages expressing this receptor are capable of engulfing not just protein molecules but even entire cells that have glycoxidation products on their surface.[285] Glycoxidation (or AGE) products in vessel walls are chemotactic to circulating monocyte-macrophages, inducing them to migrate through the vascular endothelium.[143] Also, the interaction of AGE proteins with the AGE receptor has been shown to be accompanied by release of TNF and IL-1.[286] These are known to mediate growth and remodeling processes, which, as previously discussed, may accelerate the atherosclerotic process.

### Renal Impairment

Increased collagen fluorescence and pentosidine content is associated with renal im-

pairment in diabetes.[176, 190] Recently we have found a correlation between glycoxidation products in skin collagen and microalbuminuria, the earliest manifestation of renal disease (unpublished observations, 1992). This suggests that a generalized collagen abnormality may underlie the development of microalbuminuria, and this may partly explain the association of microalbuminuria with the subsequent development of macrovascular disease, glycoxidation being the underlying common denominator.

Table 4–2 lists the findings of glycation and glycoxidation in diabetes and how these may affect processes of atherosclerosis and thrombosis.

If the gradual (and irreversible) accumulation of glycoxidation products in vascular structural proteins is indeed harmful, it would clearly be desirable to inhibit the process, particularly in diabetic patients. Ways to inhibit the "glycosylative" and "oxidative" arms of the process may be considered separately.

**TABLE 4–2.**

Glycation and Glycoxidation in Diabetes: Atherosclerosis

| |
|---|
| Skin collagen |
| ↑ Fructose-lysine |
| ↑ Carboxymethyllysine |
| ↑ Pentosidine |
| Plasma proteins |
| ↑ Glycated LDL |
| ↓ Uptake by classical receptors |
| ↑ Uptake by macrophages |
| ↑ Platelet aggregation and release |
| ↑ Glycated VLDL |
| ↑ Cholesterol ester synthesis by macrophages |
| ↑ Glycated HDL |
| ↑ Clearance from circulation |
| ↓ Binding to fibroblasts |
| ↓ Cholesterol ester transport |
| Vascular wall proteins |
| ↑ Arterial stiffness |
| ↓ EDRF activity |
| ↑ LDL-collagen binding |
| ↑ Binding plus interactions with macrophages |
| Correlation with renal impairment in diabetes |
| Other findings |
| ↑ LDL immune complexes |
| ↑ Thrombogenesis |

*LDL = low-density lipoprotein; VLDL = very low-density lipoprotein; HDL = high-density lipoprotein; EDRF = endothelium-derived relaxing factor.*

**Reducing Glycosylative Stress.**—The most obvious measure is to optimize glycemic control to minimize FL formation. Also, the existing levels of FL may be reduced; even a short-term improvement in glycemic control can reduce the FL content of insoluble skin collagen[173] and presumably that of arterial collagens as well. This should decrease the subsequent formation of glycoxidation products. In the future, pharmacologic intervention may be possible. Aminoguanidine, a hydrazine that binds to reactive carbonyl groups, has been the subject of intensive study by Brownlee et al.[41] It is thought to act by blocking the open-chain form of glucose or reactive dicarbonyl browning intermediates derived from the dissociation of FL (or both).[227] Aminoguanidine has been successful in preventing the browning process both in vitro and in vivo.[41] However, there are no studies in humans with diabetes.

**Reducing Oxidative Stress.**—Currently there is little evidence concerning the efficacy of any treatment aimed to reduce oxidative damage to proteins in diabetes. Probucol may be effective in reducing lipid peroxidation[215] and may therefore have a protective effect in the vessel wall. Another approach involves the supplementation of free radical scavengers. Of these, ascorbate is believed to be the most important[89] and plasma levels of this and platelet levels of vitamin E, another free radical scavenger, tend to be abnormally low in diabetic patients.[128, 137] However, no studies exist to demonstrate that supplementation of these vitamins will affect the progress of atherosclerosis in diabetic patients.

## Discussion

It is apparent that quantitative and qualitative alterations of lipoproteins frequently occur in diabetes mellitus and presumably are major contributors to accelerated atherosclerosis. In the fourth edition of this text, we[60] showed a simplified scheme that illustrated some of these effects of altered lipoproteins on the process of atherosclerosis in diabetes. Knowledge has increased to the point where it is not possible to show all potential influences of the diabetes state on the process of atherosclerosis in one simple figure. Some of the newer concepts, with an emphasis on possible immune mechanisms, adhesion proteins, local mediators, and monocyte-macrophage metabolism are shown in Figure 4–1. Figure 4–3 summarizes the major points of the sections on lipoproteins and glycoxidation and illustrates how these changes could accelerate the atherosclerotic process in diabetes.

## THROMBUS FORMATION

### Mechanisms

Thrombi may form in atherosclerotic vessels, leading to tissue ischemia, death, or both. Platelets may adhere at areas of endothelial damage or destruction, leading to a local accumulation of platelets at sites of vascular injury. Platelet aggregation occurs, with release of intraplatelet materials, and a platelet mass may form that can impede flow and lead to platelet microemboli. This process may be reversible, and its activity and extent depends on the type, size, and configuration of the involved vessels, as well as the local blood flow.

Platelet-fibrin masses are then formed at the next step. It is likely that local fibrinolytic activity is a major determinant of whether the platelet-fibrin masses will break up or will organize further. As thrombi grow, conditions favorable for intravascular coagulation may proceed. Platelets may degenerate, leading to fibrinous transformation. The organizing thrombus may be infiltrated by leucocytes, macrophages, and smooth muscle cells, and thrombin may be incorporated into the vascular wall, contributing to intimal plaque formation.[33]

Recognition of this process has stimulated research into platelet function, the coagulation system, and fibrinolysis in individuals with diabetes mellitus, where thrombosis in large and small vessels often accompanies accelerated atherosclerosis. Atherosclerosis and thrombus formation is a dynamic process that can be reversible and may occur at multiple sites, and it has been difficult to describe the exact sequence of events that may

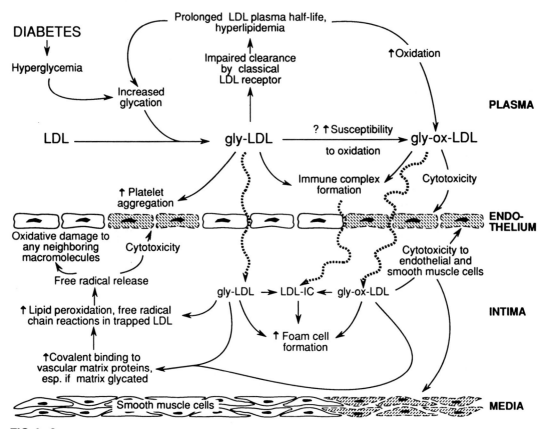

**FIG 4–3.**
A postulated scheme for the mechanism of atherosclerosis in diabetes. *(From Lyons TJ: Diabetes 41(suppl 2), 1992. Used by permission.)*

occur in diabetes. Nevertheless, there is evidence that various aspects of platelet function, coagulation, and fibrinolysis are affected by diabetes and that such alterations may help explain thrombotic events in some individuals with diabetes. Further, there is evidence that certain aspects of this process are under metabolic control and that insulin may play a key role in that regulation. For these reasons, a review of platelet function, coagulation, and fibrinolytic activity in diabetes is provided.

## Platelets

Many alterations in platelet function are seen in diabetes mellitus. Some of these are summarized in Table 4–3. There have been numerous publications on this subject, and altered platelet function has been the source of many reviews in previous volumes of this text and in the scientific literature.[57, 59, 60, 206] These reviews should be consulted for complete references. Studies have shown that platelets from diabetic subjects are more sensitive in vitro to platelet-aggregating agents and that the synthesis of thromboxane is increased. These findings have been reported in IDDM individuals shortly after the onset of the disease, as well as in diabetic animals, suggesting that altered platelet function may be the consequences of metabolic changes in the diabetic state rather than resulting from the presence of vascular disease. Insulin therapy will decrease platelet thromboxane release in IDDM, supporting this concept. On the other hand, there is ample evidence that platelets may be hypersensitive to aggregating agents and may release increased amounts of thromboxane in nondiabetic and diabetic individuals with vascular disease. These observations suggest that platelet damage may occur as a result of diabetic vascular disease, as well possibly contributing to the development of that process.

**TABLE 4–3.**

Alterations of Platelet Function in Diabetes

| In Vitro | In Vivo |
|---|---|
| ↑ Adhesiveness (vWF?) | ↑ Turnover |
| ↑ Aggregability | ↓ Survival |
| ↑ Thromboxane release | ↑ β-Thromboglobulin |
| Platelet-plasma interactions | ↑ Plasma factor 4 |
| vWF | ↑ Platelet-derived growth factor |
| Fibrinogen | |
| Immune complexes | ↑ Circulating platelet aggregates |
| Glycosylated LDL | ↑ Platelet-derived urinary $TxB_2$ |
| ↑ LDL oxidation | Vessel wall interaction |
| ↓ Phosphoinositide turnover | |
| ↓ Membrane fluidity | |

*vWF = von Willebrand's factor; LDL = low-density lipoprotein; $TxB_2$ = thromboxane $B_2$.*

## Coagulation

During the process of platelet adhesion and aggregation, the clotting mechanism is activated and thrombin is generated. This leads to further platelet aggregation and the polymerization of thrombin, which maintains the stability of the thrombus. This activation of the intrinsic coagulation system may occur by platelet stimulation of coagulation factors. In addition, through the extrinsic coagulation pathway, tissue thromboplastin generation from the injured vessel wall may also promote coagulation.

A simplified scheme of the intrinsic and extrinsic coagulation systems is shown in Figure 4–4. Various aspects of the coagulation processes have been studied in diabetic individuals. In older studies, elevated levels of factors IX and XII were reported,[82] and more recently, elevated levels of factor VII have been reported in diabetes.[91] Evidence is accumulating that the plasma levels of certain coagulation factors may be under acute control by plasma glucose levels, insulin levels, or both. Thus, Ceriello et al.[49] have demonstrated that factor VII levels are elevated in patients with IDDM and that these are directly related to plasma glucose levels in normal and diabetic individuals. Further, plasma levels of factor VII rise during a glucose infusion, fall when the infusion is stopped in nondiabetic subjects, and fall toward normal with an insulin infusion in IDDM individuals.[49] In NIDDM individuals, glycemic regulation with diet is associated with a fall in factor VII levels.

Activated protein C is a vitamin K–dependent plasma protein that is a potent anticoagulant. It acts at the levels of factor V and VIII in the intrinsic coagulation scheme (see Fig 4–4). Several investigators have reported decreased protein C antigen and activity levels in IDDM,[51, 288] and such changes could theoretically promote co-

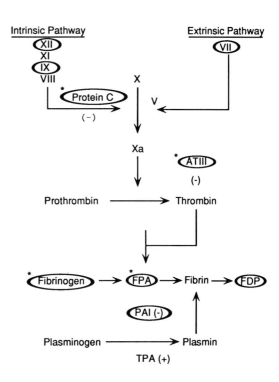

**FIG 4–4.**

Pathways of blood coagulation, with emphases on alterations that may occur in the diabetic state.

agulation. Glucose-induced hyperglycemia will lead to a fall in protein C levels and activity in normal and diabetic individuals. Depressed plasma levels and activity of protein C will rise with insulin-induced normoglycemia in IDDM.[51]

### Fibrinogen

Attention has been directed at fibrinogen levels and dynamics in diabetes for a variety of reasons. It is now clear that the plasma level of fibrinogen is an independent risk factor for thrombotic events in population-based studies.[136, 182, 297] There have been many studies of fibrinogen levels and dynamics in diabetes mellitus. Generally plasma fibrinogen levels are found to be elevated in diabetic individuals, particularly in those with previous hyperglycemia.[88, 91, 130, 132, 206] Insulin deficiency results in an increase in fibrinogen synthesis in IDDM, and an insulin infusion will decrease fibrinogen synthetic rate.[69] Fibrinogen survival has been reported to be decreased in diabetes, and this abnormality is quickly reversed when euglycemia is achieved with insulin.[130, 132] Decreased fibrinogen survival in diabetes is also reversed by heparin, suggesting that intravascular fibrin formation may be taking place.[130] Fibrinogen is glycated in diabetic subjects, and cross-linking of the α-chains of fibrinogen is impaired.[167] Exercise conditioning will lower plasma fibrinogen levels in NIDDM individuals.[120]

These findings suggest that there may be increased fibrin formation in vivo in individuals with diabetes. Because fibrinogen to fibrin formation may be catalyzed by thrombin, investigations have centered on the regulation of thrombin activity in diabetes and on an in vivo index of thrombin activity, fibrinopeptide A.[131]

### Fibrinopeptide A

As indicated in Figure 4–1, a product of thrombin activity is fibrinopeptide A (FPA). Fibrinopeptide A is cleaved from the α-chain of fibrinogen by the action of thrombin. This forms the first step in the conversion of fibrinogen to fibrin. Studies of plasma FPA levels in diabetes have yielded conflicting results. Although elevated levels may be found in some patients, in others the mean FPA levels in plasma in diabetes have been found to be normal.[131] Fibrinopeptide A is rapidly cleared from the circulation and excreted in the urine, and in the presence of normal renal function, urinary levels give an estimate of FPA turnover in vivo. Increased urinary FPA levels have been reported in diabetes mellitus.[88] A relation between plasma and urinary FPA with hyperglycemia in diabetes has been reported.[131] Further, recent studies have indicated that elevated FPA levels may be seen in diabetic individuals before vascular complications are present, suggesting that increased thrombin activity and fibrinogen degradation may contribute to, rather than be the result of, vascular complications.[88]

These studies suggest that there may be increased thrombin activity in diabetes. Such observations are supported by studies of inhibitors of thrombin activity such as antithrombin III (AT III).

### Antithrombin III

This is a physiologically important inhibitor of thrombin. Elevated plasma levels of this inhibitor are correlated with diminished thrombin activity, whereas depressed levels indicate increased thrombin activity. Studies of plasma AT III concentrations in children with IDDM showed elevated levels, perhaps reflecting counterregulation in response to activation of the coagulation system. More recent studies have indicated that AT III activity, as distinct from AT III concentration, is depressed in adults with IDDM.[47, 48]

Functional depression of AT III activity in diabetes may be caused by nonenzymatic glycation of the AT III molecule. In vitro glycation of AT III results in activity that is three times weaker than normal AT III, as an in vitro inhibitor of thrombin.[39, 282] If comparable findings were to exist in vivo, accumulation of fibrin could result because of defective inhibition of the coagulation cascade.

Studies suggest that this system is under physiologic control in vivo by glucose and insulin. Hyperglycemia will cause a decrease in AT III activity (but not AT III concentration) in nondiabetic subjects, and activity returns to normal after a glucose infusion is stopped.[48] Depressed levels of AT III activity are found in adult IDDM subjects, and infusion of insulin to produce normoglycemia will return AT III activity to normal.[50] There is an inverse correlation between AT III levels and plasma glucose, as well as the labile component of hemoglobin $A_1$ in adults with IDDM.[47]

Thus, one can make a case that depressed AT III activity may result in increased thrombin activity in diabetes and that this may contribute to the tendency to vascular thrombosis seen in diabetes mellitus.

### Fibrinolytic System

The fibrinolytic system consists of a group of activators and inhibitors that convert plasminogen to plasmin (see Fig 4–1). Because plasmin production leads to the lysis of fibrin, this is a critical system for maintenance of vascular patency. Theoretically, disturbances of plasminogen, tissue-type plasminogen activator (t-PA), or either of the physiologic inhibitors of the system, plasminogen activator inhibitor-1 (PAI-1) or PAI-2, could occur in diabetes and could compromise clot lysis.

Plasminogen activation may be impaired in diabetes. In vitro glycation of plasminogen impairs activation by t-PA, and glycation of t-PA can affect its action on plasminogen.[98, 99] Further, when plasminogen and t-PA are harvested from diabetic patients, plasminogen activation is impaired when either is used in in vitro systems.[98, 99]

Lipoprotein(a) (Lp[a]) may have an important role in the fibrinolytic system.[165, 237] Further, there is evidence that Lp(a) may be a risk factor for atherosclerosis and that plasma levels may be lowered by insulin therapy in IDDM subjects. Lp(a) is an LDL-like particle with a unique apoprotein, apo(a), which is remarkably similar to plasminogen in its structure, and may compete with plasminogen in the fibrinolytic system. In vitro, Lp(a) will inhibit plasminogen activation, perhaps by competing with t-PA in converting plasminogen to plasmin or by competing with plasminogen for high-affinity binding sites.[165, 237] Additional studies of Lp(a) in individuals with diabetes are clearly indicated.

Estimates of the activity of the fibrinolytic system in diabetes have yielded conflicting results. In the previous edition of this text, we[60] reviewed 23 separate studies of fibrinolytic activity in diabetes, as assessed by a variety of in vitro techniques. Depending on the populations studied and the methods used, activity has been found to be low, normal, or elevated in individuals with diabetes.

Recent studies have shed insight into some reasons for these discrepancies. Many of the older studies used the euglobulin lysis time as a global estimate of fibrinolytic activity. This test appears to estimate the balance between t-PA and PAI-1 in the specimen assayed. More recently, investigators have separately measured t-PA and PAI-1 in individuals with diabetes mellitus. Generally subjects with IDDM are found to have elevated t-PA levels, and levels of PAI-1 are generally normal to slightly elevated.[106, 289] Presumably this leads to normal or high fibrinolytic activity in most individuals with uncomplicated IDDM. However, activity may be depressed by neuropathy, cigarette smoking, and extensive microvascular disease. Thus, a family of responses may be seen, depending on methods used or clinical state of patients studied.

Consensus is emerging that increased PAI-1 activity often occurs in NIDDM[106, 289] and that this may be responsible for the many reports of diminished fibrinolytic activity in that disease.[60, 206] There appears to be hormonal regulation of PAI-1 gene expression and protein synthesis. Insulin has been shown to induce PAI-1 mRNA expression in hepatocytes, leading to an increased release of this protein by liver cells.[5, 108] Some evidence for this effect of insulin has been shown in in vivo studies[135] but not in others.[278] There is a correlation between PAI-1 and plasma insulin levels in obese individuals.[279, 280] Studies have shown a correlation between PAI-1 and plasma triglyceride levels.[31, 183] Longitudinal studies are needed on the relationships of obesity, plasma glucose, insulin, triglycerides, and PAI-1 in the syndrome of centripetal obesity and insulin resistance.

In vitro studies with cultured endothelial cells have provided some insights into regulation of t-PA and PAI-1 release by lipoproteins. Very low density lipoproteins harvested from normal individuals will cause release of t-PA and PAI-1 from cultured endothelial cells, whereas VLDLs from hypertriglyceridemic individuals will not.[31] Similar studies showed that endothelial production of PAI-1 is increased by incubation in vitro with VLDL obtained from hyperglycemic patients.[260] Stimulation of endothelial release of t-PA and PAI-1 with desmopressin acetate in NIDDM subjects with hypertriglyceridemia causes a decreased plasma t-PA activity and an elevated PAI-1 response when compared with normal controls.[37] These studies provide some in vivo evidence to support the in vitro reports of increased PAI-1 activity in NIDDM.

The source of physiologically active PAI-1 in plasma is probably the endothelium. Elevated levels may reflect endothelial damage. On the other hand, liver cells synthesize and release PAI-1,[5, 108] and studies of PAI-1 in plasma, serum, and platelets have shown that the concentration of PAI-1 antigen in platelets is very high and that platelets account for 93% of PAI-1 antigen in whole blood.[30] Platelet PAI-1 exists primarily in an inactive form.

## DISCUSSION

What does all of this mean? Is diabetes characterized by a hypercoagulable state? If so, could this underlie the predisposition toward thrombosis often seen in diabetes? What is the effect of therapy? Can we prevent macrovascular thrombosis?

Clearly the final answers to all of these questions are not apparent. There is still a lot of work to do. Generalization is dangerous for a number of reasons. First, in clinical studies it is important to differentiate data obtained from IDDM and NIDDM subjects in view of the major differences in pathophysiology between these two syndromes. Second, there is great heterogeneity within IDDM populations. In some cases, studies are done in prepubertal children; in others, adults of short duration; in others, IDDM individuals with nephropathy, retin-

opathy, neuropathy, or macrovascular disease. Third, there is even greater heterogeneity within NIDDM populations. Thus, individuals may be obese or nonobese, have low, normal, or elevated plasma insulin or lipid levels, be free from microvascular or macrovascular disease, be treated with diet, oral agents, or insulin, or have clinically apparent or in apparent microvascular or macrovascular disease. Further, the majority of studies are cross-sectional in nature, and this may give misleading data because of patient selection. Longitudinal data are limited and extremely difficult and costly to pursue.

Nevertheless, from the studies cited in this review and in other sources,[56–60, 206] some trends are apparent. First, even when an abnormal mean value for platelet function or index of coagulation is found and the subjects are well defined (e.g., IDDM free from clinical vascular disease), there are many patients with normal activity or levels no matter what parameter is measured. On the other hand, there is a certain consistency in reported results in uncomplicated IDDM subjects with hyperglycemia, and there is increasing evidence that in these individuals, insulin therapy may return altered values to or toward normal. The evidence to support this statement is given in Table 4–4. By probing results from a number of different studies in different IDDM populations, some interesting findings emerge. In all cases, when studied in vivo, insulin administration to hyperglycemic IDDM subjects has been found to produce changes in platelet function, the intrinsic coagulation system, and in fibrinogen dynamics that could reduce the tendency toward intravascular thrombosis. These findings provide a theoretical basis for intensive insulin therapy in IDDM subjects. On the other hand, studies in NIDDM are limited, and a role of hyperinsulinism in increasing PAI-1 activity may be postulated. It must be recognized that it will require properly designed, multicenter collaborative trials, such as the Diabetes Control and Complications Trial[70] and the VA Cooperative Study in NIDDM,[277] to definitely answer the question as to whether intensive insulin therapy will

**TABLE 4–4.**
Effect of Insulin Therapy on Platelet Function and Coagulation in IDDM
Subjects With Hyperglycemia

| Measurement | Finding: IDDM | Effect of Insulin | Theoretical Result |
|---|---|---|---|
| Platelet TxA$_2$ release | ↑ | ↓ | ↓ Platelet aggregation |
| VIII R: WF (or Ag) | ↑ | ↓ | ↓ Platelet adhesion |
| Factor VII | ↑ | ↓ | ↓ Coagulation |
| Protein C | ↓ | ↑ | Same |
| Plasma fibrinogen | ↑ | ↓ | ↓ Fibrin formation |
| Fibrinogen synthesis | ↑ | ↓ | Same |
| Fibrinogen survival | ↓ | ↑ | Same |
| Plasma and urine FPA | ↑ | ↓ | Same |
| AT III activity | ↓ | ↑ | ↓ Thrombin activity |

*IDDM = insulin-dependent diabetes mellitus; TxA$_2$ = thromboxane A$_2$; FPA = fibrinopeptide A; AT III = antithrombin III.*

alter thrombotic events in IDDM or NIDDM individuals.

In light of current knowledge, however, it is generally accepted that one reasonable approach to the prevention of thrombotic events is the use of agents such as aspirin, which irreversibly acetylates platelet cyclooxygenase and thereby inhibits platelet thromboxane production. Presently, there are more than 200 studies with antiplatelet agents in nondiabetic and in diabetic individuals, in which major vascular events such as strokes, myocardial infarctions, and vascular death have been monitored before and after antiplatelet therapy. Results have been compared with those obtained in individuals receiving placebo therapy. There is general agreement, as indicated by metanalyses of published data, that antiplatelet therapy is a safe and effective way to prevent future cardiovascular events in diabetic or nondiabetic individuals who have had one vascular event.[9] Thus, pooled data suggest that vascular morbidity can be lowered about 25%, nonfatal myocardial infarctions about 30%, and vascular mortality approximately 15% after antiplatelet therapy when it is used as a secondary prevention strategy.[9] Although there is an increased risk of gastrointestinal bleeding and hemorrhagic stroke in some studies, it is generally believed that the benefits of antiplatelet therapy outweigh the risks. There is no evidence that aspirin therapy will accentuate diabetic retinopathy or vitreous hemorrhage. Although use of aspirin as a primary prevention strategy is still controversial, some studies in nondiabetic individuals suggest that this may be effective in reducing myocardial infarction incidence.[257]

## SUMMARY

Is it presumptuous to attempt to define the pathogenesis of atherosclerosis in diabetes mellitus? One could adopt this view because the pathogenesis in nondiabetic individuals is a subject of active research and therefore is open to changing views. Extrapolation from these current postulates to a disease state as complicated and heterogeneous as diabetes mellitus could therefore be dangerous, inaccurate, and misleading. In addition, investigators are limited by a variety of factors in their search to delineate mechanisms involved in the atherosclerotic process in humans. Access to normal arterial tissue for in vitro studies has been limited, and noninvasive techniques for assessing the degree and extent of early lesions of atherosclerosis in vivo are limited. Longitudinal studies are compromised by these limitations in technique and by the slow progression of the process. These factors have led investigators to rely on correlative relationships and studies using cell systems that may not be directly transferable to the atherosclerotic process in humans. The issue is further complicated by the fact that animal models are limited; much of the work has been done in animal species in which atherosclerosis is a difficult lesion to produce. Clinical trials in diabetes that could provide useful indirect information have been sparse and usually have been secondary prevention trials in patients with very advanced vascular disease. Of course, primary prevention of atherosclerosis is of greatest importance.

Nevertheless, the situation is improving. Advances in surgical technique in humans, with close coordination of investigators from various disciplines, have led to the availability of fresh human tissue from coronary bypass patients and other individuals who undergo major surgery. Tissue culture techniques allow investigators to directly study the metabolism and function for critical components of the human arterial tree and to objectively manipulate variables involved in the atherosclerotic process. Noninvasive techniques for assessing the vascular system in humans are undergoing refinement and are becoming more available to clinical investigators. Techniques of molecular biology are opening up new approaches to the genetic influences on atherosclerosis. An explosion of biochemical and physiologic information about prostanoids and their derivatives and about lipids, lipoproteins, and apolipoproteins has occurred in recent years. Improved animal models of atherosclerosis and diabetes mellitus exist, and work using animals such as monkeys and pigs is beginning to appear. Clinical trials are moving in the direction of primary rather than secondary prevention trials and involve lipids, lipoproteins, platelets, and prostanoids, which are postulated to be operative in atherosclerosis associated with diabetes mellitus.

An explosion of information on endothelial function, immune complexes, cytokines, adhesion proteins, glycation, and glycoxidation has occurred and has led to newer concepts. Figures 4–1 and 4–3 give some of these new concepts of the pathogenesis of atherosclerosis in diabetes, and Figure 4–4 shows alterations in the coagulation and fibrinolytic systems that may predispose diabetic subjects to vascular thrombosis. As work in this very active area of research continues, it is likely that improved methods of preventing or forestalling the development of accelerated macrovascular disease in diabetes will emerge.

## Acknowledgments

Supported by the Research Service of the Department of Veterans Affairs. Dr. Lyons is a recipient of a Research Career Development Award for the American Diabetes Association.

We thank Mrs. Susan Morosko for excellent editorial assistance.

## REFERENCES

1. Abiru T, et al: Decrease in endothelium-dependent relaxation and levels of cyclic nucleotides in aorta from rabbits with alloxan-induced diabetes, *Res Commun Chem Pathol Pharmacol* 68:13, 1990.

2. Agardh CD, et al: Plasma lipids and plasma lipoproteins in diabetics with and without proliferative retinopathy, *Acta Med Scand* 223:165–169, 1988.

3. Ahmed MU, Thorpe SR, Baynes JW: Identification of carboxymethyllysine as a degradation product of fructose-lysine in glycosylated protein, *J Biol Chem* 261:4889–4994, 1986.

4. Ahmed MU, et al: Oxidative degradation of glucose adducts to protein. Formation of 3-(N epsilon-lysino)-lactic acid from model compounds and glycosylated proteins, *J Biol Chem* 263:8816–8821, 1988.

5. Alessi MC, et al: Insulin stimulates the synthesis of plasminogen activator 1 by hepatocellular cell line Hep G2, *Thromb Haemost* 60:491–494.

6. American Diabetes Association: Role of cardiovascular risk factors in prevention and treatment of macrovascular disease in diabetes, *Diabetes Care* 12:573–579, 1989.

7. Andrews HE, et al: Low-density lipoproteins inhibit endothelium-dependent relaxation in rabbit aorta, *Nature* 327:237, 1987.

8. Annuzzi G, et al: A controlled study on the effects of ω-3 fatty acids on lipid and glucose metabolism in non-insulin-dependent diabetic patients, *Atherosclerosis* 87:65–73, 1991.

9. Antiplatelet Trialists' Collaboration: Secondary prevention of vascular disease by prolonged antiplatelet treatment, *Br Med J* 296:320–331, 1988.

10. Bagdade JD, Porte D Jr, Bierman EL: Acute insulin withdrawal and the regulation of plasma triglyceride removal in diabetic subjects, *Diabetes* 17:127, 1968.

11. Bagdade JD, Subbaiah PV: Whole-plasma and high-density lipoprotein subfraction surface lipid composition in IDDM men, *Diabetes* 38:1226–1230, 1989.

12. Bagdade JD, et al: Effects of omega-3 fish oils on plasma lipids, lipoprotein composition, and post-

heparin lipoprotein lipase in women with IDDM, *Diabetes* 39:426–431, 1990.

13. Bagdade JD, et al: Persistent abnormalities in lipoprotein composition in noninsulin-dependent diabetes after intensive insulin therapy, *Arteriosclerosis* 10:232–239, 1990.

14. Bailey AJ, Kent MJC: Non-enzymatic glycosylation of fibrous and basement membrane collagens, in Baynes JW, Monnier VM, editors: *The Maillard reaction in aging, diabetes and nutrition*, New York, 1989, Alan R Liss, pp 109–122.

15. Baruch D, et al: Role of von Willebrand factor associated to extracellular matrices in platelet adhesion, *Blood* 77:519, 1991.

16. Bates SR, Rothblatt GH: Regulation of cellular sterol flux and synthesis by human serum lipoproteins, *Biochim Biophys Acta* 360:38, 1974.

17. Bath PMW, et al: Nitric oxide and prostacyclin: divergence of inhibitory effects on monocyte chemotaxis and adhesion to endothelium in vitro, *Arterioscler Thromb* 11:254, 1991.

18. Baynes JW: Role of oxidative stress in development of complications in diabetes, *Diabetes* 40:405–412, 1991.

19. Baynes JW, Monnier VM, editors:. *The Maillard reaction in aging, diabetes and nutrition*, New York, 1989, Alan R Liss.

20. Baynes JW, et al: Accumulation of Maillard reaction products in skin collagen in diabetes and aging, *Diabetologia* 34(suppl 2):A7, 1991.

21. Beach KW, et al: The correlation of arteriosclerosis obliterans with lipoproteins in insulin-dependent and noninsulin-dependent diabetes, *Diabetes* 28:836–840, 1979.

22. Bell ET: Incidence of gangrene of the extremities in non-diabetic and diabetic persons, *Arch Pathol Lab Med* 49:469–473, 1950.

23. Bengualid V, et al: *Staphylococcus aureus* infection of human endothelial cells potentiates Fc receptor expression, *J Immunol* 1990, 145:4279.

24. Berliner JA, et al: Minimally modified low density lipoprotein stimulates monocyte-endothelial interactions, *J Clin Invest* 85:1260, 1990.

25. Bevilacqua MP, et al: Interleukin-1 induces biosynthesis and cell surface expression of procoagulant activity in human vascular endothelial cells, *J Exp Med* 160:618–622, 1984.

26. Biesbroeck RC, et al: Abnormal composition of high-density lipoproteins in non-insulin-dependent diabetics, *Diabetes* 31:126, 1982.

27. Biesbroeck RC, et al: Specific high affinity binding of HDL to cultured human skin fibroblasts and arterial smooth muscle cells, *J Clin Invest* 71:525, 1983.

28. Boackle R: The complement system, in Virella G, Goust JM, Fudenberg HH, editors: *Introduction to medical immunology*, ed 2, New York, 1990, Marcel Dekker, pp 143–168.

29. Bonanome A, et al: Carbohydrate and lipid metabolism in patients with non-insulin-dependent diabetes mellitus: effects of a low-fat, high-carbohydrate diet vs. a diet high in monounsaturated fatty acids, *Am J Clin Nutr* 54:586–590, 1991.

30. Booth, NA, et al: Plasminogen activator inhibitor (PAI-1) in plasma and platelets, *Br J Haematol* 70:327–333, 1988.

31. Booyse FM, et al: Normal but not hypertriglyceridemic very low-density lipoprotein induces rapid release of tissue plasminogen activator from cultured human umbilical vein endothelial cells, *Semin Thromb Hemost* 14:175–179, 1988.

32. Bossaler C, et al: Impaired muscarinic endothelium-dependent relaxation and cyclic guanosine 5′-monophosphate formation in atherosclerotic human coronary artery and rabbit aorta, *J Clin Invest* 79:170, 1987.

33. Bowie EJ, Owen CA: The hemostatic mechanism, in Kwaan H, Bowie EJ, editors: *Thrombosis*, Philadelphia, 1982, WB Saunders, pp 7–22.

34. Breviario F, et al: IL-1 induced adhesion of polymorphonuclear leukocytes to cultured human endothelial cells: role of platelet-activating factor, *J Immunol* 141:3391–3397, 1988.

35. Brinton EA, et al: Binding of HDL to cultured fibroblasts after chemical alteration of apoprotein amino-acid residues, *Arteriosclerosis* 5:329, 1985.

36. Brinton EA, et al: Binding of HDL to cultured fibroblasts after chemical alteration of apoprotein amino-acid residues, *J Biol Chem* 261:495, 1986.

37. Brommer EJP, et al: Response of fibrinolytic activity and factor VIII-related antigen to stimulation with desmopressin in hyperlipoproteinemia, *J Lab Clin Med* 100:105–114, 1982.

38. Brownlee M, Pongor S, Cerami A: Covalent attachment of soluble proteins by non-enzymatically glycosylated collagen: role in the *in situ* formation of immune complexes, *J Exp Med* 158:1739–1744, 1983.

39. Brownlee M, Vlassara H, Cerami A: Inhibition of heparin-catalyzed human antithrombin III activity by nonenzymatic glycosylation, *Diabetes* 33:532–535, 1984.

40. Brownlee M, Vlassara H, Cerami A: Nonenzymatic glycosylation products on collagen covalently trap low-density lipoprotein, *Diabetes* 34:938–941, 1985.

41. Brownlee M, et al: Aminoguanidine prevents diabetes-induced arterial wall protein cross-linking, *Science* 232:1629–1632, 1986.

42. Bucala R, Tracey KJ, Cerami A: Advanced glycosylation products quench nitric oxide and mediate defective endothelium-dependent vasodilatation in experimental diabetes, *J Clin Invest* 87:432–438, 1991.

43. Calvo C, et al: Non enzymatic glycation of apolipoprotein A—I: effects on its self-association and

lipid binding properties, *Biochem Biophys Res Commun* 153:1060–1067, 1988.

44. Celi A, Furie B, Furie BC: PADGEM: an adhesion receptor for leukocytes on stimulated platelets and endothelial cells, *Proc Soc Exp Biol Med* 198:703, 1991.

45. Cerami A, Beutler B: The role of cachectin/TNF in endotoxic shock and cachexia, *Immunol Today* 9:28, 1988.

46. Cerami A, Vlassara H, Brownlee M: Glucose and aging, *Sci Am* 256:90–96, 1987.

47. Ceriello A, et al: Daily rapid blood glucose variations may condition antithrombin biological activity but not its plasma concentration in insulin dependent diabetes: a possible role for labile non-enzymatic glycation, *Diabetes Metab* 13:16–19, 1987.

48. Ceriello A, et al: Induced hyperglycemia alters antithrombin III activity but not its plasma concentration in healthy normal subjects, *Diabetes* 36:320–323, 1987.

49. Ceriello A, et al: Blood glucose may condition factor VII levels in diabetic and normal subjects, *Diabetologia* 31:889-891, 1988.

50. Ceriello, A, et al: Evidence for a hyperglycaemia-dependent decrease of antithrombin III-thrombin complex formation in humans, *Diabetologia* 33:163–167, 1990.

51. Ceriello A, et al: Protein C deficiency in insulin-dependent diabetes: a hyperglycemia-related phenomenon, *Thromb Haemost* 64:104–107, 1990.

52. Chait A, Iverius PH, Brunzell JD: Lipoprotein lipase secretion by human monocyte-derived macrophages, *J Clin Invest* 69:490, 1982.

53. Chin JH, Azhar S, Hoffman, BB: Inactivation of endothelial derived relaxing factor by oxidized lipoproteins, *J Clin Invest* 89:10, 1992.

54. Cines DB, Lyss AP, Bina M: Fc and C3 receptors induced by herpes simplex virus in cultured human endothelial cells, *J Clin Invest* 69:123, 1982.

55. Cohen MP, et al: Increased glycosylation of glomerular basement membrane collagen in diabetes, *Biochem Biophys Res Commun* 95:765–769, 1980.

56. Colwell JA: Peripheral vascular disease in diabetes mellitus, in Davidson J, editor: *Clinical diabetes mellitus*, New York, 1986, Thieme Medical Publishers, pp 357–375.

57. Colwell, JA, Halushka PV: Platelet function in diabetes mellitus, *Br J Haematol* 44:521–526, 1980.

58. Colwell JA, Lopes-Virella ML, Mayfield R, et al, editors: Workshop on insulin and atherogenesis, *Metabolism* 12(suppl 1):1–91, 1985.

59. Colwell JA, Winocour PD, Lopes-Virella MF: Platelet function and platelet interactions in atherosclerosis and diabetes mellitus, in Rifkin H,

Porte D, editors: *Diabetes mellitus: theory and practice*, New York, 1989, Elsevier, pp 249–256.

60. Colwell JA, et al: New concepts about the pathogenesis of atherosclerosis in diabetes mellitus, in Levin ME, O'Neal LW, editors: *The diabetic foot*, ed 4, St Louis, 1988, Mosby–Year Book, pp 51–70.

61. Cooke JP, et al: Arginine restores cholinergic relaxation of hypercholesterolemic rabbit thoracic aorta, *Circulation* 83:1057, 1991.

62. Cornacoff JB, et al: Primate erythrocyte-immune complex-clearing mechanism, *J Clin Invest* 71:236–247, 1983.

63. Creager MA, et al: Impaired vasodilation of forearm resistance vessels in hypercholesterolemic humans, *J Clin Invest* 86:228, 1990.

64. Curtiss LK, Witztum JL: A novel method of generating region-specific monoclonal antibodies to modified proteins: application to the identification of human glucosylated low density lipoproteins, *J Clin Invest* 72:1427–1438, 1983.

65. Curtiss LK, Witztum JL: Plasma apo-lipoproteins A-I, A-II, B, C-I and E are glucosylated in hyperglycemic diabetic subjects, *Diabetes* 34:452–461, 1985.

66. Cushing SD, et al: Minimally modified LDL induces monocyte chemotactic proteins I in human endothelial and smooth muscle cells, *Proc Natl Acad Sci USA* 87:5134, 1990.

67. Cybulsky MI, Gimbrone MA: Endothelial expression of a mononuclear leukocyte adhesion molecule during atherogenesis, *Science* 251:788, 1991.

68. Davis NS Jr: Diabetic gangrene, *JAMA* 31:103–105, 1898.

69. De Feo P, Gaisano MG, Haymond MW: Differential effects of insulin deficiency on albumin and fibrinogen synthesis in humans, *J Clin Invest* 88:833–840, 1991.

70. DCCT Research Group: Epidemiology of severe hypoglycemia in the Diabetes Control and Complications Trial (DCCT), *Am J Med* 90:450–459, 1991.

71. De Groot PG, et al: Interleukin 1 inhibits the synthesis of von Willebrand factor in endothelial cells which results in a decreased reactivity of their matrix towards platelets, *Atherosclerosis* 7:605, 1987.

72. de Gruijter M, et al: Patients with combined hypercholesterolemia-hypertriglyceridemia show an increased monocyte-endothelial cell adhesion in vitro: triglyceride level as a major determinant, *Metabolism* 40:1119, 1991.

73. de Nucci G, et al: Receptor-mediated release of endothelium-derived relaxing factor and prostacyclin from bovine aortic endothelial cells is coupled, *Proc Natl Acad Sci USA* 85:2334, 1988.

74. de Tejada IS, et al: Impaired neurogenic and

endothelium-mediated relaxation of penile smooth muscle in diabetic men with impotence, *N Engl J Med* 320:1025, 1989.

75. Drake TA, et al: Minimally oxidized LDL induces tissue factor expression in cultured human endothelial cells, *Am J Pathol* 138:601, 1991.

76. Ducimetier P, et al: Relationship of plasma insulin levels to the incidence of myocardial infarction and coronary heart disease mortality in a middle-aged population, *Diabetologia* 19:205–210, 1980.

77. Duell PB, Oram JF, Bierman EL: Nonenzymatic glycosylation of HDL and impaired HDL-receptor-mediated cholesterol efflux, *Diabetes* 40:377–384, 1991.

78. Dunn FL: Treatment of lipid disorders in diabetes mellitus, *Med Clin North Am* 72:1379–1398, 1988.

79. Dunn JA, et al: Reaction of ascorbate with lysine and protein under autoxidizing conditions: formation of $N^\epsilon$-(carboxymethyl)lysine by reaction between lysine and products of autoxidation of ascorbate, *Biochemistry* 29:10964–10970, 1990.

80. Dunn JA, et al: Age-dependent accumulation of $N^\epsilon$-(carboxymethyl)lysine and $N^\epsilon$-(carboxymethyl)hydroxylysine in human skin collagen, *Biochemistry* 30:1205–1210, 1991.

81. Dyer DG, et al: Formation of pentosidine during nonenzymatic browning of proteins by glucose: identification of glucose and other carbohydrates as possible precursors of pentosidine *in vivo*, *J Biol Chem* 266:11654–11660, 1991.

82. Egebert O: The blood coagulability in diabetic patients, *J Clin Lab Med* 15:833–838, 1963.

83. Epstein FH, et al: Epidemiological studies of cardiovascular diseases in a total community—Tecumseh, Michigan, *Ann Intern Med* 62:1170–1187, 1965.

84. Fielding DF, Reaven GM, Fielding PE: Human noninsulin-dependent diabetes: identification of a defect in plasma cholesterol transport normalized in vivo by insulin and in vitro by immunoadsorption of apolipoprotein E, *Proc Natl Acad Sci USA* 79:6365, 1982.

85. Fielding DF, et al: Increased free cholesterol in plasma low and very low density lipoproteins in noninsulin-dependent diabetes mellitus: its role in the inhibition of cholesteryl ester transfer, *Proc Natl Acad Sci USA* 81:2512, 1984.

86. Floren CH, Albers JJ, Bierman EL: Uptake of chylomicron remnants causes cholesterol accumulation in cultured human arterial smooth muscle cells, *Biochim Biophys Acta* 663:336, 1981.

87. Fontbonne AM, et al: Insulin and cardiovascular disease—Paris prospective study, *Diabetes Care* 6:461–469, 1991.

88. Ford I, et al: Activation of coagulation in diabetes mellitus in relation to the presence of vascular complications, *Diabetic Med* 8:322–329, 1990.

89. Frei B, England L, Ames BN: Ascorbate is an outstanding antioxidant in human plasma, *Proc Natl Acad Sci USA* 86:6377–6381, 1989.

90. Fu M-X, et al: Role of oxygen in the cross-linking and chemical modification of collagen by glucose: proceedings of IDF satellite symposium, *Diabetes* 40 (in press).

91. Fuller JH: Haemostatic variables associated with diabetes and its complications, *Br Med J* 2:964–966, 1979.

92. Furchgott RF, Zawadzki JV: The obligatory role of endothelial cells in the relaxation of arterial smooth muscle by acetylcholine, *Nature* 299:373, 1980.

93. Gabor J, Spain M, Kalant N: Composition of serum very low density lipoproteins in diabetes, *Clin Chem* 26:1261, 1980.

94. Galle J, Bassenge E, Busse R: Oxidized low density lipoproteins potentiate vasoconstrictions to various agonists by direct interaction with vascular smooth muscle, *Circ Res* 66:1287, 1990.

95. Galle J, et al: Effects of native and oxidized low density lipoproteins on formation and inactivation of endothelium-derived relaxing factor, *Arterioscler Thromb* 11:198, 1991.

96. Garcia ML, et al: Morbidity and mortality in diabetics in Framingham population: sixteen year follow-up study, *Diabetes* 23:105–111, 1974.

97. Garlick RL, Bunn HF, Spiro RG: Non-enzymatic glycosylation of basement membranes from human glomeruli and bovine sources, *Diabetes* 37:1144–1150, 1988.

98. Geiger M, Beckmann R, Binder BR, in Davidson JF, Bachmann F, Bouvier CA, et al, editors: *Progress in fibrinolysis*, New York, 1983, Churchill Livingstone, pp 286–291.

99. Geiger M, Binder BR: Plasminogen activation in diabetes mellitus, *J Biol Chem* 259:2976–2981, 1984.

100. Geng JG, et al: Rapid neutrophil adhesion to activated endothelium mediated by GMP-140, *Nature* 343:757, 1990.

101. Gianturco SH, et al: Hypertriglyceridemic very low density lipoproteins induce triglyceride synthesis and accumulation in mouse peritoneal macrophages, *J Clin Invest* 70:168, 1982.

102. Giddings JC, Shall L: Enhanced release of von Willebrand factor by human endothelial cells in culture in the presence of phorbol myristate acetate and IL-1, *Thromb Res* 47:259, 1987.

103a. Gisinger C, Virella GT, Lopes-Virella MF: Erythrocyte-bound low density lipoprotein (LDL) immune complexes lead to cholesteryl ester accumulation in human monocyte derived macrophages, *Clin Immunol Immunopathol* 59:37–52, 1991.

103b. Gisinger C, Lopes-Virella MF: Lipoprotein immune complexes and diabetic vascular complications. *Diabetes* 40 (in press).

104. Gonen B, et al: Non-enzymatic glycosylation of low-density lipoproteins *in vitro*, *Diabetes* 30:875–878, 1981.

105. Gordon T, et al: Diabetes, blood lipids and the role of obesity in coronary heart disease risk in women, *Ann Intern Med* 87:393, 1977.

106. Gough SCL, Grant PJ: The fibrinolytic system in diabetes mellitus, *Diabetic Med* 8:898–905, 1991.

107. Grandhee SK, Monnier VM: Mechanism of formation of the Maillard protein cross-link pentosidine: glucose, fructose and ascorbate as pentosidine precursors, *J Biol Chem* 266:11649–11653, 1991.

108. Grant PJ, Ruegg M, Medcalf RL: Basal expression and insulin-mediated induction of PAI-1 mRNA in Hep G2 cells, *Fibrinolysis* 5:81–86, 1991.

109. Griffith RL, et al: LDL metabolism by macrophages activated with LDL immune complexes: a possible mechanism of foam cell formation, *J Exp Med* 168:1041–1059, 1988.

110. Hamlin CR, Kohn RR: Evidence for progressive, age-related structural changes in post-mature human collagen, *Biochim Biophys Acta* 236:458–467, 1971.

111. Hamlin CR, Kohn RR: Determination of human chronological age by study of a collagen sample, *Exp Gerontol* 7:377–379, 1972.

112. Hamlin CR, Kohn RR, Luschin JH: Apparent accelerated aging of human collagen in diabetes mellitus, *Diabetes* 24:902–904, 1975.

113. Harman D: The aging process, *Proc Natl Acad Sci USA* 78:7124–7128, 1981.

114. Harris JE, Weeks KR: *X-raying the pharaohs*, New York, 1973, Charles Scribner & Sons.

115. Hattori R, et al: Stimulated secretion of endothelial von Willebrand factor is accompanied by rapid redistribution to the cell surface of the intracellular granule membrane protein GMP-140, *J Biol Chem* 264:7768, 1989.

116. Havel RJ, et al: Isoprotein specificity in the hepatic uptake of apolipoprotein E and the pathogenesis of familial dysbetalipoproteinemia, *Proc Natl Acad Sci USA* 77:4349, 1980.

117. Hendra TJ, et al: Effects of fish oil supplements in NIDDM subjects: controlled study, *Diabetes Care* 13:821–829, 1990.

118. Hicks M, et al: Increase in crosslinking of nonenzymatically glycosylated collagen induced by products of lipid peroxidation, *Arch Biochem Biophys* 268:249–254, 1989.

119. Hiramatsu K, Bierman EL, Chait A: Metabolism of LDL from patients with diabetic hypertriglyceridemia by cultured human skin fibroblasts, *Diabetes* 34:8, 1985.

120. Hornsby WG, Lyons, TJ, Boggess K, et al: The effect of an exercise program on risk factors for vascular disease in type II diabetes, *Diabetes Care* 13:87–92, 1990.

121. Hyslop S, de Nucci G: The mechanisms and significance of the coupled release of endothelium-derived relaxing factor (EDRF) and prostacyclin (PGI$_2$) from endothelial cells, *Wein Klin Wochenschr* 103:422, 1991.

122. Ignarro LJ, et al: Endothelium-derived relaxing factor produced and released from artery and vein is nitric oxide, *Proc Natl Acad Sci USA* 84:9265, 1987.

123. Inoguchi T, et al: Abnormality in prostacyclin-stimulatory activity in sera from diabetics, *Metabolism* 38:837, 1989.

124. Ishibashi S, et al: Composition of very-low-density lipoproteins in non-insulin-dependent diabetes mellitus, *Clin Chem* 35:808–812, 1989.

125. Jack CM, et al: Non-enzymatic glycosylation of low-density lipoprotein: results of an affinity chromatography method, *Diabetologia* 31:126–128, 1988.

126. James RW, Pometta D: The distribution profiles of very low density and low density lipoproteins in poorly-controlled male, type 2 (non-insulin-dependent) diabetic patients, *Diabetologia* 34:246–252, 1991.

127. Janka HU, Standl E, Mehnert H: Peripheral vascular disease in diabetes mellitus and its relation to cardiovascular risk factors: screening with the Doppler ultrasonic technique, *Diabetes Care* 3:207–213, 1980.

128. Jennings PE, et al: Vitamin C metabolites and microangiopathy in diabetes mellitus, *Diabetes Res* 6:151–154, 1987.

129. Jonasson L, Bondjers G, Hansson GK: Lipoprotein lipase in atherosclerosis: its presence in smooth muscle cells and absence from macrophages, *J Lipid Res* 28:437, 1987.

130. Jones RL, Peterson CM: Reduced fibrinogen survival in diabetes mellitus, *J Clin Invest* 63:485–493, 1979.

131. Jones RL: Fibrinopeptide-A in diabetes mellitus, *Diabetes* 34:836–843, 1985.

132. Jones RL, et al: Time course of reversibility of accelerated fibrinogen disappearance in diabetes mellitus: association with intravascular volume shifts, *Blood* 63:22–30, 1984.

133. Jones SL, et al: Plasma lipid and coagulation factor concentrations in insulin dependent diabetics with microalbuminuria, *Br Med J* 298:487–490, 1989.

134. Joven J, et al: Concentrations of lipids and apolipoproteins in patients with clinically well-controlled insulin-dependent and non-insulin-dependent diabetes, *Clin Chem* 35:813–816, 1989.

135. Juhan-Vague I, et al: Effect of 24 hours of nor-moglycaemia on tissue-type plasminogen activator plasma levels in insulin-dependent diabetes, *Thromb Haemost* 51:97–98, 1984.

136. Kannel, WB, et al: Fibrinogen and risk of cardiovascular disease: the Framingham study, *JAMA* 258:1183–1186, 1987.

137. Karpen CW, et al: Production of 12 HETE and vitamin E status in platelets from type 1 human diabetic subjects, *Diabetes* 34:526–531, 1985.

138. Kasim SE, et al: Significance of hepatic triglyceride lipase activity in the regulation of serum high density lipoproteins in type II diabetes mellitus, *J Clin Endocrinol Metab* 65:183–187, 1987.

139. Kennedy L, Baynes JW: Non-enzymatic glycosylation and the chronic complications of diabetes: an overview, *Diabetologia* 6:93–98, 1984.

140. Kiff RJ, et al: The effects of endothelin-1 and $N^G$-nitro-L-arginine methyl ester on regional haemodynamics in conscious rats with streptozotocin-induced diabetes mellitus, *Br J Pharmacol* 103:1321, 1991.

141. Kilpatrick JM, Hyman B, Virella G: Human endothelial cell damage induced by interactions between polymorphonuclear leukocytes and immune complex–coated erythrocytes, *Clin Immunol Immunopathol* 44:335–347, 1987.

142. Kimura I, et al: Diabetes-induced enhancement of prostanoid-stimulated contraction in mesenteric veins of mice, *Jpn J Pharmacol* 51:403, 1989.

143. Kirstein M, et al: Advanced protein glycosylation induces transendothelial human monocyte chemotaxis and secretion of platelet-derived growth factor: role in vascular disease of diabetes and aging, *Proc Natl Acad Sci USA* 87:9010–9014, 1990.

144. Klein RL, Lopes-Virella MF, Colwell JA: Enhancement of platelet aggregation by the glycosylated subfraction of low density lipoprotein (LDL) isolated from patients with insulin-dependent diabetes mellitus (IDDM), *Diabetes* 39(suppl 1):173a, 1990.

145. Klein RL, Lyons TJ, Lopes-Virella MF: Metabolism of very low- and low density lipoproteins isolated from normolipidaemic type 2 (non-insulin-dependent) diabetic patients by human monocyte-derived macrophages, *Diabetologia* 33:299–305, 1990.

146. Klein RL, et al: Interaction of VLDL isolated from type I diabetic subjects with human monocyte-derived macrophages, *Metabolism* 38:1108–1114, 1989.

147. Klimov AN, Denisenko AD, Popov AV, et al: Lipoprotein-antibody immune complexes: their catabolism and role in foam cell formation, *Atherosclerosis* 58:1–15, 1985.

148. Kobbah M, Vessby B, Tuvemo T: Serum lipids and apolipoproteins in children with type 1 (insulin-dependent) diabetes during the first two years of the disease, *Diabetologia* 31:195–200, 1988.

149. Kraemer FB, et al: Effects of noninsulin-dependent diabetes mellitus on the uptake of very low density lipoproteins by thioglycolate-elicited mouse peritoneal macrophages, *J Clin Endocrinol Metab* 61:335, 1985.

150. Kubo SH, et al: Endothelium-dependent vasodilation is attenuated in patients with heart failure, *Circulation* 84:1589, 1991.

151. Kuebler TW, et al: Diabetes mellitus and cerebrovascular disease: prevalence of carotid artery occlusive disease and associated risk factors in 482 adult diabetic patients, *Diabetes Care* 6:275, 1983.

152. Kugiyama K, et al: Impairment of endothelium-dependent arterial relaxation by lysolecithin in modified low-density lipoproteins, *Nature* 344:160, 1990.

153. Laakso M, Pyorala K: Lipid and lipoprotein abnormalities in diabetic patients with peripheral vascular disease, *Atherosclerosis* 74:55–63, 1988.

154. Lawson RA: Amputations through the ages, *Aust NZ J Med* 42:221–230, 1973.

155. Ledl F, Schleicher E: New aspects of the Maillard reaction in foods and in the human body, *Angew Chem Int Ed Engl* 29:565–594, 1990.

156. Levin ME, Powers MA: Hypertension and diabetes: then and now, *Diabetes Spectrum* 3:274, 1990.

157. Lewis B, et al: Plasmatriglyceride and fatty acid metabolism in diabetes mellitus, *Eur J Clin Invest* 2:445, 1972.

158. Libby P, Warner SJC, Friedman GB: Interleukin 1: a mitogen for human vascular smooth muscle cells that induces the release of growth inhibitory prostanoids, *J Clin Invest* 81:487–498, 1988.

159. Lisch HJ, Sailer S: Lipoprotein patterns in diet, sulphonylurea and insulin-treated diabetics, *Diabetologia* 20:118, 1981.

160. Lopes-Virella MF, Stone PG, Colwell JA: Serum high density lipoprotein in diabetes, *Diabetologia* 13:285, 1977.

161. Lopes-Virella MF, et al: Plasma lipids and lipoproteins in young insulin-dependent diabetic patients: relationship with control, *Diabetologia* 21:216, 1981.

162. Lopes-Virella MF, et al: Surface binding, internalization and degradation by cultured human fibroblasts of low density lipoproteins isolated from type I (insulin-dependent) diabetic patients: changes with metabolic control, *Diabetologia* 22:430–436, 1982.

163. Lopes-Virella MF, et al: Effect of metabolic control on lipid, lipoprotein and apolipoprotein levels in 55 insulin-dependent diabetic patients: a longitudinal study, *Diabetes* 32:20, 1983.

164. Lopes-Virella MF, et al: Glycosylation of LDL enhances CE synthesis in human monocyte-derived macrophages, *Diabetes* 37:550–557, 1988.

165. Loscalzo J: Lipoprotein(a): a unique risk factor for atherothrombotic disease, *Arteriosclerosis* 10:672–679, 1990.

166. Luscinskas FW, et al: Endothelial-leukocyte adhesion molecule-1-dependent and leukocyte (CD11/CD18)-dependent mechanisms contribute to polymorphonuclear leukocyte adhesion to cytokine-activated human vascular endothelium, *J Immunol* 142:2257–2263, 1989.

167. Lütjens A, et al: Polymerisation and crosslinking of fibrin monomers in diabetes mellitus, *Diabetologia* 31:825–830, 1988.

168. Lyons TJ: Oxidized low density lipoproteins—a role in the pathogenesis of atherosclerosis in diabetes? *Diabetic Med* 8:411–419, 1991.

169. Lyons TJ, Kennedy L: Effect of in vitro non-enzymatic glycosylation of human skin collagen on susceptibility to collagenase digestion, *Eur J Clin Invest* 15:128–131, 1985.

170. Lyons TJ, Kennedy L: Non-enzymatic glycosylation of skin collagen in patients with limited joint mobility, *Diabetologia* 28:2–5, 1985.

171. Lyons TJ, et al: Glycosylation of low density lipoprotein in patients with type 1 diabetes: correlations with other parameters of glycaemic control, *Diabetologia* 29:685–689, 1986.

172. Lyons TJ, et al: Stimulation of CE synthesis in human monocyte-derived macrophages by LDL from type I diabetic patients: the influence on non-enzymatic glycosylation of LDL, *Diabetologia* 30:916–923, 1987.

173. Lyons TJ, et al: Decrease in skin collagen glycosylation with improved glycemic control in patients with insulin-dependent diabetes mellitus, *J Clin Invest* 87:1910–1915, 1991.

174. Macdonald PS, Read MA, Dusting GJ: Synergistic inhibition of platelet aggregation by endothelium-derived relaxing factor and prostaglandin, *Thromb Res* 49:437, 1988.

175. MacIntyre, EA, et al: Activation of human monocytes occurs on cross-linking monocytic antigens to an Fc receptor, *J Immunol* 142:2377, 1989.

176. Makita Z, et al: Advanced glycosylation end products in patients with diabetic nephropathy, *N Engl J Med* 325:836–842, 1991.

177. Martin S, et al: IL-1 and INF-γ increase vascular permeability, *Immunology* 64:301–305, 1988.

178. Mayham, WG: Impairment of endothelium-dependent dilatation of cerebral arterioles during diabetes mellitus, *Am J Physiol* 256(3 part 2):H621, 1989.

179. McEver RP: GMP-140: a receptor for neutrophils and monocytes on activated platelets and endothelium, *J Cell Biochem* 45:156, 1991.

180. McEver RP, Martin MN: A monoclonal antibody to a membrane glycoprotein binds only to activated platelets, *J Biol Chem* 259:9799, 1984.

181. McVerry VA, et al: Non-enzymatic glycosylation of fibrinogen, *Haemostasis* 10:261–270, 1981.

182. Meade TW, et al: Hemostatic function and cardiovascular death: early results of a prospective study, *Lancet* 1:1050–1054, 1980.

183. Mehta J, et al: Plasma tissue plasminogen activator inhibitor levels in coronary artery disease; correlation with age and serum triglyceride levels, *J Am Coll Cardiol* 9:263–268, 1987.

184. Melnick JL, et al: Cytomegalovirus antigen within human arterial smooth muscle cells, *Lancet* 2:644, 1983.

185. Melton LJ, et al: Incidence and prevalence of clinical peripheral vascular disease in a population-based cohort of 56 diabetic patients, *Diabetes Care* 3:650–654, 1980.

186. Meraji S, et al: Endothelium-dependent relaxation in aorta of BB rat, *Diabetes* 36:978–981, 1987.

187. Moncada S, Palmer RMJ, Higgs EA: Biosynthesis of nitric oxide from L-arginine: a pathway for the regulation of cell function and communication, *Biochem Pharmacol* 38:1709, 1989.

188. Monnier VM: Toward a Maillard reaction theory of aging, *Prog Clin Biol Res* 304:1–22, 1989.

189. Monnier VM, Cerami A: Non-enzymatic browning *in vivo*: possible process for aging of long-lived proteins, *Science* 211:491–493, 1981.

190. Monnier VM, et al: Relations between complications to type I diabetes mellitus and collagen-linked fluorescence, *N Engl J Med* 314:403–408, 1986.

191. Monnier VM, et al: Collagen browning and cross-linking are increased in chronic experimental hyperglycemia: relevance to diabetes and aging, *Diabetes* 37:867–872, 1988.

192. Morel DW, et al: Endothelial and smooth muscle cells alter LDL in vitro by free radical oxidation, *Arteriosclerosis* 4:357–364, 1984.

193. Mullarkey CJ, et al: Free radical generation by early glycation products: a mechanism for accelerated atherogenesis in diabetes, *Biochem Biophys Res Commun* 173:932–939, 1990.

194. Mykkanen L, et al: Asymptomatic hyperglycemia and cardiovascular risk factors in the elderly, *Atherosclerosis* 88:153–161, 1991.

195. Nawroth PP, et al: Tumor necrosis factor/cachectin interacts with endothelial cell receptors to induce release of interleukin-1, *J Exp Med* 165:1363–1375, 1986.

196. Nievelstein PFEM, et al: Platelet adhesion and aggregate formation in type 1 diabetes under flow conditions, *Diabetes* 40:1410–1417, 1991.

197. Nikilla EA: High density lipoproteins in diabetes, *Diabetes* 30(suppl 2):82, 1981.

198. Nilsson TK, Johnson O: The extrinsic fibrinolytic system in survivors of myocardial infarction, *Thromb Res* 48:621–630, 1987.

199. Niskanen L, et al: Microalbuminuria predicts the development of serum lipoprotein abnormalities favouring atherogenesis in newly diagnosed type 2 (non-insulin-dependent) diabetic patients, *Diabetologia* 33:237–243, 1990.

200. Niskanen LK, et al: Aortic and lower limb artery calcification in type 2 (non-insulin-dependent) diabetic patients and non-diabetic control subjects: a five year follow-up study, *Atherosclerosis* 84:61–71, 1990.

201. Njoroge FG, Monnier VM: The chemistry of the Maillard reaction under physiological conditions: a review, *Prog Clin Biol Res* 304:85–107, 1989.

202. Ohta T, et al: Lipid and apolipoprotein compositions of two species of ApoA-I containing lipoproteins in young girls with insulin-dependent diabetes mellitus, *Pediatr Res* 28:42–45, 1990.

203. Osborne JA, et al: Cardiovascular effects of acute hypercholesterolemia in rabbits, *J Clin Invest* 83:465, 1989.

204. Osborne JA, et al: Lack of endothelium-dependent relaxation in coronary resistance arteries of cholesterol-fed rabbits, *Am J Physiol* 256(3 part 1):C591, 1989.

205. Osmundson PJ, et al: Course of peripheral occlusive arterial disease in diabetes, *Diabetes Care* 2:143–152, 1990.

206. Ostermann H, van de Loo J: Factors of the haemostatic system in diabetic patients: a survey of controlled studies, *Haemostasis* 16:386–416, 1986.

207. Oxlund H, et al: Increased aortic stiffness in patients with type 1 (insulin-dependent) diabetes mellitus, *Diabetologia* 32:748–752, 1989.

208. Oyama Y, et al: Attenuation of endothelium-dependent relaxation in aorta from diabetic rats, *Eur J Pharmacol* 131:75, 1986.

209. Paleolog EM, et al: Differential regulation by cytokines of constitutive and stimulated secretion of von Willebrand factor from endothelial cells, *Blood* 75:688, 1990.

210. Palinski W, et al: Low density lipoprotein undergoes oxidative modification *in vivo*, *Proc Natl Acad Sci USA* 86:1372–1376, 1989.

211. Palmer RMJ, Ashton DS, Moncada S: Vascular endothelial cells synthesize nitric oxide from L-arginine, *Nature* 333:664, 1988.

212. Palmer RMJ, Ferrige AF, Moncada S: Nitric oxide release accounts for the biological activity of endothelium-derived relaxing factor, *Nature* 327:524, 1987.

213. Palumbo PJ, et al: Progression of peripheral occlusive arterial disease in diabetes mellitus—what factors are predictive? *Arch Intern Med* 151:717–721, 1991.

214. Parinandi NL, Thompson EW, Schmid HH: Diabetic heart and kidney exhibit increased resistance to lipid peroxidation, *Biochim Biophys Acta* 1047:63–69, 1990.

215. Parthasarathy S, et al: Probucol inhibits oxidative modification of low density lipoprotein, *J Clin Invest* 77:641–644, 1986.

216. Pasi KJ, et al: Qualitative and quantitative abnormalities of von Willebrand antigen in patients with diabetes mellitus, *Thromb Res* 59:581, 1990.

217. Patel KD, et al: Oxygen radicals induce human endothelial cells to express GMP-140 and bind neutrophils, *J Cell Biol* 112:749, 1991.

218. Pitas RE, Innerarity TL, Mahley RW: Foam cells in explants of atherosclerotic rabbit aortas have receptors for β—very low density lipoproteins and modified low density lipoproteins, *Arteriosclerosis* 3:1, 1983.

219. Pohlman TH, et al: An endothelial cell surface factor(s) induced *in vitro* by lipopolysaccharide, interleukin-1 and tumor necrosis factor a increases neutrophil adherence by a CDw18-dependent mechanism, *J Immunol* 136:4548–4553, 1986.

220. Porta M, La Selva M, Molinatti PA: von Willebrand factor and endothelial abnormalities in diabetic microangiopathy, *Diabetes Care* 14(suppl 1):167, 1991.

221. Pyorala K: Relationship of glucose tolerance and plasma insulin to the incidence of coronary heart disease: results from two population studies in Finland, *Diabetes Care* 2:131–141, 1979.

222. Quinn MT, et al: Oxidatively modified low density lipoproteins: a potential role in recruitment and retention of monocyte/macrophages during atherogenesis, *Proc Natl Acad Sci USA* 84:2995, 1987.

223. Radomski MW, Palmer RMJ, Moncada S: Comparative pharmacology of endothelium-derived relaxing factor, nitric oxide and prostacyclin in platelets, *Br J Pharmacol* 92:181, 1987.

224. Raines EW, Dower SK, Ross R: Interleukin-1 mitogenic activity for fibroblasts and smooth muscle cells is due to PDGF-AA, *Science* 243:393–396, 1989.

225. Reaven GM, Javorski WC, Reaven EP: Diabetic hypertriglyceridemia, *Am J Med Sci* 269:382, 1975.

226. Reaven GM, et al: Effect of acarbose on carbohydrate and lipid metabolism in NIDDM patients poorly controlled by sulfonylureas, *Diabetes Care* 13(suppl 3):32–36, 1990.

227. Requena JR: The main mechanism of action of aminoguanidine, *Diabetologia* 34(suppl 2):A162, 1991.

228. Rillaerts EG, et al: Effect of omega-3 fatty acids in diet of type I diabetic subjects on lipid values and hemorheological parameters, *Diabetes* 38:1412–1416, 1989.

229. Ronnemaa T, et al: Serum lipids, lipoproteins, and apolipoproteins and the excessive occurrence of coronary heart disease in non-insulin-dependent diabetic patients, *Am J Epidemiol* 130:632–645, 1989.

230. Rosenberg H, et al: Glycosylated collagen, *Biochem Biophys Res Commun* 91:498–501, 1979.

231. Rosove MH, Frank HJL, Harwig SL, et al: Plasma b-thromboglobulin is correlated with platelet adhesiveness to bovine endothelium in patients with diabetes mellitus, *Thromb Res* 37:251–258, 1985.

232. Ross R: Mechanisms of atherosclerosis—a review, *Adv Nephrol* 19:79–86, 1990.

233. Ross RN, Glomset JA: The pathogenesis of atherosclerosis, *N Engl J Med* 295:369, 1976.

234. Rossitch E, et al: L-Arginine normalizes endothelial function in cerebral vessels from hypercholesterolemic rabbits, *J Clin Invest* 87:1295, 1991.

235. Santen RJ, Willis PW, Fajans SS: Atherosclerosis in diabetes mellitus, *Arch Intern Med* 130:833, 1972.

236. Sasaki J, Cottam GL: Glycosylation of LDL decreases its ability to interact with high-affinity receptors of human fibroblasts *in vitro* and decreases its clearance from rabbit plasma *in vivo*, *Biochem Biophys Acta* 713:199–207, 1982.

237. Scanu AM, Scandiani L, in Stollerman GH, editor: *Lipoprotein(a). Structure, biology and clinical relevance*, St Louis, 1991, Mosby–Year Book, pp 249–270.

238. Schleicher E, Deufel T, Wieland OH: Non-enzymatic glycosylation of human serum lipoproteins, *FEBS Lett* 129:1–4, 1981.

239. Schmidt K, et al: Oxidized low-density lipoprotein antagonizes the activation of purified soluble guanylate cyclase by endothelium-derived relaxing factor but does not interfere with its biosynthesis, *Cell Signal* 3:361, 1991.

240. Schneider J, et al: Metformin-induced changes in serum lipids, lipoproteins, and apoproteins in non-insulin-dependent diabetes mellitus, *Atherosclerosis* 82:97–103, 1990.

241. Schneider SL, Kohn RR: Glycosylation of human collagen in aging and diabetes mellitus, *J Clin Invest* 66:1179–1181, 1980.

242. Schneider SL, Kohn RR: Effects of age and diabetes mellitus on the solubility and non-enzymatic glucosylation of human skin collagen, *J Clin Invest* 67:1630–1635, 1981.

243. Schroeder H: *Hypertensive diseases*, Philadelphia, 1953, Lea & Febiger.

244. Seeger JM, et al: Lipid risk factors in patients requiring arterial reconstruction, *J Vasc Surg* 10:418–424, 1989.

245. Sell DR, Lapolla A, Monnier VM: Relationship between pentosidine and the complications of long-standing type 1 diabetes, *Diabetes* 40:302A. 1991.

246. Sell DR, Monnier VM: Structure elucidation of a senescence cross-link from human extracellular matrix: implication of pentoses in the aging process, *J Biol Chem* 264:21597–21602, 1989.

247. Sell DR, Monnier VM: End-stage renal disease and diabetes catalyze the formation of a pentose-derived crosslink from aging human collagen, *J Clin Invest* 85:380–384, 1990.

248. Semenkovich CF, Ostlund RE Jr, Schechtman KB: Plasma lipids in patients with type I diabetes mellitus: influence of race, gender, and plasma glucose control: lipids do not correlate with glucose control in black women, *Arch Intern Med* 149:51–56, 1989.

249. Shelburne F, et al: Effect of apoproteins on hepatic uptake of triglyceride emulsions in the rat, *J Clin Invest* 65:652, 1980.

250. Shimokawa H, Vanhoutte PM: Impaired endothelium-dependent relaxation to aggregating platelets and related substances in porcine coronary arteries in hypercholesterolemia and atherosclerosis, *Circ Res* 64:900, 1989.

251. Simon BC, Cunningham LD, Cohen RA: Oxidized low density lipoproteins cause contraction and inhibit endothelium-dependent relaxation in the pig coronary artery, *J Clin Invest* 86:75, 1990.

252. Simonson DC, Dzau VJ: Workshop IX—lipids, insulin, diabetes, *Am J Med* 90:85S–86S, 1991.

253. Sneddon JM, Vane JR: Endothelium-derived relaxing factor reduces platelet adhesion to bovine endothelial cells, *Proc Natl Acad Sci USA* 85:2800, 1988.

254. Sosenko JM, et al: Hyperglycemia and plasma lipid levels: a prospective study of young insulin-dependent diabetic patients, *N Engl J Med* 302:650, 1980.

255. Stamler J: Epidemiology, established major risk factors, and the primary prevention of coronary heart disease, in Parmley W, Chatterjee K, editors: *Cardiology*, Philadelphia, 1987, JB Lippincott, pp 1–41.

256. Standl E, Janka HV: High serum insulin concentrations in relation to other cardiovascular risk factors in macrovascular disease of type 2 diabetes, *Horm Metab Res* 17(suppl):46–51, 1985.

257. Steering Committee of the Physician's Health Study Research Group: Final report on the aspirin component of the ongoing physicians' health study, *N Engl J Med* 321:129–135, 1989.

258. Stein Y, et al: The removal of cholesterol from aortic smooth muscle cells in culture and Landschutz ascites cell fractions of human high density apoproteins, *Biochem Biophys Acta* 380:106, 1975.

259. Steinbrecher UP, Witztum JL: Glucosylation of low density lipoproteins to an extent comparable

to that seen in diabetes slows their catabolism, *Diabetes* 33:130–134, 1984.

260. Stiko-Rabrin A, et al: Secretion of plasminogen activator inhibitor 1 from cultured human umbilical vein endothelial cells is induced by very low density lipoprotein, *Arteriosclerosis* 10:1067–1073, 1990.

261. Stolar MW: Atherosclerosis in diabetes: the role of hyperinsulinemia, *Metabolism* 2(suppl 1):1–9, 1988.

262. Stout RW: Insulin and atheroma: an update, *Lancet* 1:1077, 1987.

263. Takahashi K, et al: Elevated plasma endothelin in patients with diabetes mellitus, *Diabetologia* 33:306, 1990.

264. Takahashi M, et al: Lipoproteins are inhibitors of endothelium-dependent relaxation of rabbit aorta, *Am J Physiol* 258:H1, 1990.

265. Takahashi K, et al: Endothelin-like immunoreactivity in rat models of diabetes mellitus, *J Endocrinol* 130:123, 1991.

266. Takeda Y, et al: Production of endothelin-1 from the mesenteric arteries of streptozotocin-induced diabetic rats, *Life Sci* 48:2553, 1991.

267. Tannenbaum SH, Gralnick HR: Gamma-interferon modulates von Willebrand factor release by cultured human endothelial cells, *Blood* 75:2177, 1990.

268. Tanner FC, et al: Oxidized low density lipoproteins inhibit relaxations of porcine coronary arteries: role of scavenger receptor and endothelium-derived nitric oxide, *Circulation* 83:2012, 1991.

269. Tesfamariam B, Jakubowski JA, Cohen RA: Contraction of diabetic rabbit aorta due to endothelium-derived $PGH_2/TXA_2$, *Am J Physiol* 257:H1327, 1989.

270. Tesfamariam B, et al: Elevated glucose promotes generation of endothelium-derived vasoconstrictor prostanoids in rabbit aorta, *J Clin Invest* 85:929, 1990.

271. Tomita T, et al: Rapid and reversible inhibition by low density lipoprotein of the endothelium-dependent relaxation to hemostatic substances in porcine coronary arteries: heat and acid labile factors in low density lipoprotein mediate the inhibition, *Circ Res* 66:18, 1990.

272. Tonnensen MG, et al: Adherence of neutrophils to cultured human microvascular endothelial cells, *J Clin Invest* 83:637, 1989.

273. Umeda F, Inoguchi T, Nawata H: Reduced stimulatory activity on prostacyclin production by cultured endothelial cells in serum from aged and diabetic patients, *Atherosclerosis* 75:61, 1989.

274. Uusitupa M, et al: The relationship of cardiovascular risk factors to the prevalence of coronary heart disease in newly diagnosed type 2 (non-insulin-dependent) diabetes, *Diabetologia* 28:653–659, 1985.

275. Uusitupa MIJ, et al: Serum lipids and lipoproteins in newly diagnosed non-insulin-dependent (type II) diabetic patients, with special reference to factors influencing HDL-cholesterol and triglyceride levels, *Diabetes Care* 9:17–22, 1986.

276. Uusitupa MIJ, et al: 5-year incidence of atherosclerotic vascular disease in relation of general risk factors, insulin level, and abnormalities in lipoprotein composition in non-insulin-dependent diabetic and nondiabetic subjects, *Circulation* 82:27–36, 1990.

277. VA Cooperative Study Group in Diabetes Mellitus (CSDM): A feasibility trial of glycemic control and complications in type II diabetes, *Diabetes* 40(suppl 1):467A, 1991.

278. Vague P: Insulin and the fibrinolytic system, *IDF Bull* 36:15–17, 1991.

279. Vague P, Juhan-Vague I, Aillaud MF, et al: Correlation between blood fibrinolytic activity, plasminogen activator inhibitor level, plasma insulin level and relative body weight in normal and obese subjects, *Metabolism* 2:250–253, 1986.

280. Vague P, et al: Fat distribution and plasminogen activator inhibitor activity in nondiabetic obese women, *Metabolism* 38:913–915, 1989.

281. Verbeuren TJ, et al: Release and vascular activity of endothelium-derived relaxing factor in atherosclerotic rabbit aorta, *Eur J Pharmacol* 191:173, 1990.

282. Villanueva GB, Allen N: Demonstration of altered antithrombin III activity due to nonenzymatic glycosylation at glucose concentration expected to be encountered in severely diabetic patients, *Diabetes* 37:1103–1107, 1988.

283. Vishwanath V, et al: Glycosylation of skin collagen in type I diabetes mellitus: correlations with long-term complications, *Diabetes* 35:916–921, 1986.

284. Vlassara H, Brownlee M, Cerami A: Novel macrophage receptor for glucose-modified proteins is distinct from previously described scavenger receptors, *J Exp Med* 164:1301–1309, 1986.

285. Vlassara H, et al: Advanced glycosylation end products on erythrocyte cell surface induce receptor-mediated phagocytosis by macrophages: a model for turnover of aging cells, *J Exp Med* 166:539–549, 1987.

286. Vlassara H, et al: Cachectin/TNF and IL-1 induced by glucose-modified proteins: role in normal tissue remodeling, *Science* 240:1546–1548, 1988.

287. Vogt BW, Schleicher ED, Wieland OH: ε-Amino-lysine-bound glucose in human tissues obtained at autopsy, *Diabetes* 31:1123–1127, 1982.

288. Vukovich TC, Schernthaner G: Decreased protein C levels in patients with insulin-dependent

type I diabetes mellitus, *Diabetes* 35:617–619, 1986.

289. Walmsley D, Hampton KK, Grant PJ: Contrasting fibrinolytic responses in type I (insulin-dependent) and type 2 (non-insulin-dependent) diabetes, *Diabetic Med* 8:954–959, 1991.

290. Wang-Iverson P, et al: Apo E–mediated uptake and degradation of normal very low density lipoproteins by human monocyte/macrophages: a saturable pathway distinct from the LDL receptor, *Biochem Biophys Res Commun* 126:578, 1985.

291. Warner SJC, Auger KR, Libby P: Interleukin-1 induces interleukin-1: II, recombinant human interleukin-1 induces interleukin-1 production by adult human vascular endothelial cells, *J Immunol* 139:1911–1917, 1987.

292. Watanabe J, et al: Enhancement of platelet aggregation by low density lipoproteins from IDDM patients, *Diabetes* 37:1652–1657, 1988.

293. Weisweiler P, Dransner M, Schwandt P: Dietary effects on very low density lipoproteins in type II (non-insulin dependent) diabetes mellitus, *Diabetologia* 23:101, 1982.

294. Welborne TA, Wearne K: Coronary heart disease incidence and cardiovascular mortality in Busselton with reference to glucose and insulin concentrations, *Diabetes Care* 2:154–160, 1979.

295. West KM, et al: The role of circulating glucose and triglyceride concentrations and their interactions with other "risk factors" as determinants of arterial disease in nine diabetic population samples from the WHO multinational study, *Diabetes Care* 6:361, 1983.

296. Wheelock FC, Marble A: Surgery and diabetes, in Marble A, White P, Bradley RF, et al, editors: *Joslin's diabetes mellitus*, ed 11, Philadelphia, 1971, Lea & Febiger, pp 599–620.

297. Wilhelmsen L, Svardsudd K, Korsan-Bengtsen K, et al: Fibrinogen as a risk factor for stroke and myocardial infarction, *N Engl J Med* 311:501–505, 1984.

298. Witztum JL, et al: Nonenzymatic glucosylation of high-density lipoprotein accelerates its catabolism in guinea pigs, *Diabetes* 31:1029–1032, 1982.

299. Witztum JL, et al: Nonenzymatic glucosylation of low-density lipoprotein alters its biologic activity, *Diabetes* 31:283–291, 1982.

300. Witztum JL, et al: Nonenzymatic glucosylation of homologous low density lipoprotein and albumin renders them immunogenic in the guinea pig, *Proc Natl Acad Sci USA* 80:2757–2761, 1983.

301. Witztum JL, et al: Autoantibodies to glucosylated proteins in the plasma of patients with diabetes mellitus, *Proc Natl Acad Sci USA* 81:3204–3208, 1984.

302. Wolff SP, Dean RT: Glucose autoxidation and protein modification: the potential role of "autoxidative glycosylation" in diabetes mellitus, *Biochem J* 245:243–250, 1987.

303. Wu MS, et al: Effect of metformin on carbohydrate and lipoprotein metabolism in NIDDM patients, *Diabetes Care* 13:1–8, 1990.

304. Yue DK, et al: The thermal stability of collagen in diabetic rats: correlation with severity of diabetes and non-enzymatic glycosylation, *Diabetologia* 24:282–285, 1983.

305. Zavoico GB, et al: IL-1 and related cytokines enhance thrombin stimulated $PGI_2$ production in cultured endothelial cells without affecting thrombin-stimulated von Willebrand factor secretion or platelet-activating factor biosynthesis, *J Immunol* 142:3993, 1989.

# CHAPTER 5

# Hemorheology

## Donald E. McMillan, M.D.

The foot needs blood to function. Blood is a fluid that is distributed through the body by the pumping action of the heart. Fluids are a broad class of materials that behave by flowing when acted on by any overall force. Fluids differ from solids because solids resist continuing movement by generating a force through the magnitude of their internal deformation (Fig 5–1). Fluids continue to move because their resistance to motion is generated by the motion itself. Even solids will flow (or break) when they are placed under sufficient force.

The systematic examination of flow is the scope of the scientific discipline called rheology, taken from rheos, the Greek word for flow. The study of blood's flow properties is called hemorheology. Blood has physical flow properties that are unique, and these unique properties are affected by disease states such as diabetes. In this chapter we review the features of blood flow and its control that are of potential use in understanding and managing foot problems in diabetes.

## CONCEPT OF BLOOD FLOW

Many fluids, including air and water, behave in a very regular way when acted on by force. They are referred to as newtonian because their response is analyzable using Newton's laws. In addition to formulating three basic laws for planetary motion (Book I, "The Motion of Bodies"), Newton experimented with movement of fluids, specifically water (Book II, "The Motion of Bodies In Resisting Mediums"). He found a simple and direct relation between applied force and responsive motion, like that expected from his second law of motion. The ratio of such a fluid's resistive force, $\sigma$, to its responsive motion or shear rate, $\dot{\gamma}$ (see the discussion of blood as a shear thinning fluid),

$$\eta = \frac{\sigma}{\dot{\gamma}}$$

where $\eta$ is the fluid's viscosity. Blood does not respond so simply and hence is said to be nonnewtonian. Nonnewtonian fluids make up a broad class. We have day-to-day contact with many of them, principally foods, inks, and cosmetics. None of the other nonnewtonian materials behaves exactly like blood.

Blood has unique cellular and plasma components. Its dominant cells are erythrocytes. They typically form 40% of blood's volume. Leukocytes form less than 1% of the volume but become very important in the microcirculation. Electrolytes and glucose are osmotically important, affecting red blood cell size, but they make only a very small direct contribution to blood's flow properties. Proteins in blood have effects on blood flow linked to both their shape and their concentration. This happens because they interact with red blood cells based on their shape. The protein–red blood cell mixture in blood generates different flow responses depending on vessel size and flow rate.

Blood is designed to flow and to deliver oxygen to the tissues, but it must also stop flowing when necessary. This happens regu-

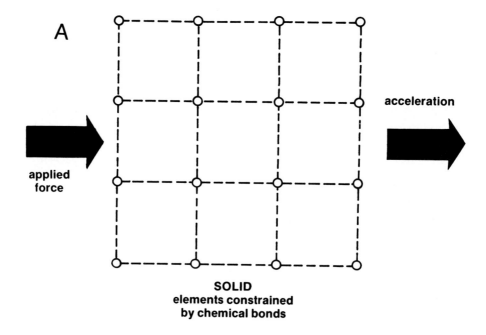

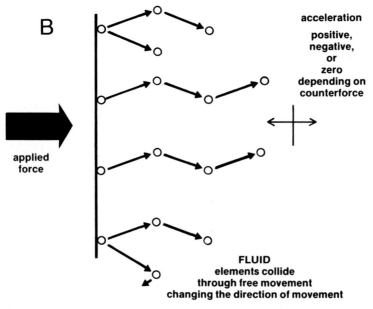

**FIG 5–1.**
Difference between solid **(A)** and fluid **(B)** deformation is diagrammed. In solid deformation, the elements of the material are held in place by interactions with their neighbors and resist movement more and more with greater displacement until the solid is disrupted. If no disruption occurs, the solid returns to its original shape by elastic recovery. A fluid resists deformation in proportion to the rate of displacement of its constituents relative to each other as long as there is time for the random motion of the elements relative to each other to dissipate the original momentum.

larly after trauma, during menstruation, and after parturition. To do this, blood contains platelets to plug small defects in the vessel walls, such as venipuncture sites and shaving nicks. Larger defects require local blood vessel constriction and the coagulation of the blood. A feature that helps slow local blood flow is the marked rise in blood flow resistance (viscosity; see Fig 5–5) when flow is slowed. This feature of blood is conferred to it by the plasma proteins, especially fibrinogen. Fibrinogen is also responsible for clot formation. In disease states such as diabetes and in pregnancy, fibrinogen levels rise and blood viscosity at low flow (shear) rates becomes elevated.[60] Fibrinogen and some closely related proteins have been associated cross-sectionally with diabetic complications.[69] Fibrinogen is also now well documented as a risk factor for cardiovascular disease in nondiabetics.[16, 109] One report shows it to have a similarly predictive role in diabetes.[82]

## INERTIAL VERSUS VISCOUS FLOW

Different blood flow properties are either more or less important in specific flow situations, particularly those seen in blood flow in the leg and foot. A review of both non-newtonian fluid and circulatory flow concepts is needed to understand which blood flow properties are most affected by diabetes. Fluid flow is commonly influenced by inertia, a property linked to mass. Fluids, like all materials in motion, try to continue movement in a straight line.

In the circulation there are few long straight paths, so that blood usually cannot maintain a straight line. It changes direction by using its motion energy and blood vessel walls to generate pressure gradients. These pressure gradients help blood to change in direction. Pressure waves and gradients are seen principally in the arteries and veins. In capillaries, the change in flow direction is controlled mainly by viscous drag generated by flow near the inner wall of a turn.

The relative importance of inertia and viscous drag to the flow of newtonian fluids was systematized by the work of Sir Osborne Reynolds, who studied liquid flow in straight tubes.[81] He showed that three factors controlled the relative importance of viscosity and inertia in linear flow. They are the velocity of the fluid, u, the diameter of the tube, d, and the kinematic viscosity of the fluid, $\nu$. Kinematic viscosity is the resistive viscosity divided by the fluid's density. The relation is usually represented by an equation as the flow's Reynolds' number, Re:

$$Re = \frac{u\ d}{\nu}$$

The ratio of the product of velocity and tube diameter to the kinematic viscosity has no dimension if the units used are the same and the fluid is newtonian. The result is called a Reynolds number. It portrays the relative importance of inertia and viscosity to flow in tubes and in structures roughly similar to tubes, the blood vessels (Table 5–1).

A flow at a Reynolds number that is less than 0.01 is characterized by a nearly uniform shearing motion in the fluid. Direction change is mediated by the resistive force generated by local differences in rate of shearing. In contrast, flows with a Reynolds number of 100 or more change direction through inertia-generated pressure gradients.

Two important effects are generated by the contrast between high Reynolds flow ($>$100) seen in arteries and low Reynolds flow ($<$0.01) seen in capillaries and small veins. Flow eddies are limited to larger vessels. Eddying has two effects. It causes the flow at the vessel wall to be uneven, increasing the local pressure drop, and it mixes blood locally, an important need in blood's oxygen delivery and other transport functions. In venules and small veins, mixing is absent. The flow is layered, as easily seen in fluorescein studies of the retina. Injected dye returns more rapidly after it passes through shorter and more direct vessel loops. The outer layers of the retinal venules fill with dye first, and almost no mixing occurs.[68]

Nonmixing of blood can be expected in most small vessels of the foot, but capillary

## TABLE 5–1.

Blood Vessel Reynolds' Numbers*

| Size of Vessel | Reynolds Number (Range) |
| --- | --- |
| Intracardiac | 400–1,500 |
| Aorta, large arteries | 500–5,800 |
| Muscular arteries | 100–1,000 |
| Primary arterioles | 0.05–1.0 |
| Small arterioles | 0.07–0.7 |
| Capillaries | Approx. 0.001 |
| Small venules | 0.05–0.5 |
| Moderate-sized veins | 50–500 |
| Large veins | 200–900 |

*Large Reynolds number flows (>100) are subject to much more inertial influence than lower Reynolds flows, whereas Reynolds number flows <0.01 are dominated by viscous drag. Reynolds number flows >2,000 are capable of generating turbulent patterns if tube length is long enough. Reynolds number flows around 1 (0.1–10) are mixtures of viscous and inertial behavior.

flow is a little more complex. Red blood cells pass through capillaries one at a time. They are greater in diameter (8 μm) than true capillaries (usually 4–6 μm). The erythrocytes must deform to pass through a capillary. They tend to fill it completely. Their movement disturbs the layered flow of the local plasma. The result is a flow that acts to mix plasma between red blood cells, called bolus flow.[43] This mixing effect enhances oxygen's passage into tissues. By this means, blood is uniquely well designed to defeat the lack of fluid mixing at low Reynolds flow by using cells to force the needed mixing. This helps to explain why blood can be more viscous than hemoglobin solutions made from it simply by destroying red blood cell membranes and still supply oxygen more effectively than oxygen-binding macromolecules.

Blood flow in arterioles and small veins falls between the two extremes discussed (see Table 5–1). Both inertial and viscous effects are important. Changes in local flow rate can affect mixing efficiency, but slowing always reduces mixing and causes the average tangential wall force caused by viscous drag to decline.

## ARTERIES TO LEG AND FOOT

Foot blood flow supplies three major tissue components: skin, muscle, and bone.

Little is known specifically about blood flow to bones of the foot; it is often assumed to be modest and stable. On the other hand, muscle flow is closely related to contractile activity, rising strikingly in parallel with oxygen consumption during intrinsic foot muscle contraction. Skin blood flow is strikingly affected by body core and environmental temperature, rising with the need to dissipate heat. It changes at least as strikingly as the flow associated with intrinsic muscle activity in the foot. A several-fold rise in foot flow is generated by vigorous walking or running.

It is useful to review the circulation to the foot with blood flow and flow properties in mind. Blood passes to the foot through the arteries. The aorta gives rise to the common iliac and then the external iliac and femoral arteries. The superficial femoral branch passes medially and posteriorly through the adductor canal to become the popliteal artery. Below the knee, the popliteal gives rise to three arteries (Fig 5–2). All three supply the foot, but two normally carry most of the flow. The anterior tibial artery changes direction abruptly as it passes forward and then through the anterolateral muscles of the leg. It passes then to the front of the ankle, where it becomes the dorsalis pedis artery, supplying the dorsal and even the plantar area of the foot. The posterior tibial and peroneal arteries arise more directly as medial and lateral branches of the popliteal artery. The posterior tibial artery (medial in Fig 5–2) is normally considerably larger. It passes behind the ankle medial malleolus to supply the plantar foot. The peroneal artery (lateral in Fig 5–2) passes behind the lateral malleolus to supply the less muscular lateral foot. The upper leg artery anatomy is responsible for some features of arterial pressure around the ankle. The pressure is highest in the large and direct posterior tibial artery. A somewhat lower pressure is commonly found in the dorsalis pedis artery. Intraluminal pressure is not infrequently low or the flow rate ultrasonically undetectable in the peroneal arteries at the ankle.

Two leg artery problems develop in diabetes. The more common is atherosclerotic occlusion. It is disproportionately distal, affecting the branches of the popliteal more

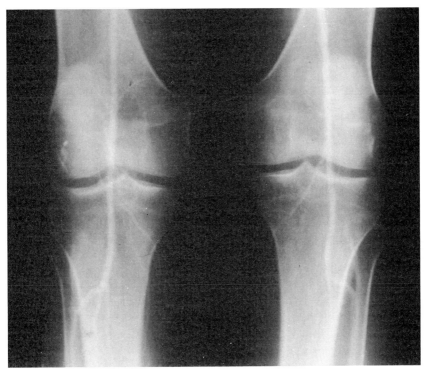

**FIG 5–2.**
Arteriogram of both knee areas shows how the popliteal artery gives rise to three branches after it passes behind the knee. The forklike configuration on the left deserves the name trifurcation. On the right the early takeoff of the anterior tibial and size disparity between the smaller posterior tibial and larger peroneal artery destroy the appropriateness of the name, also illustrating the variability of the arterial anatomy.

heavily than the iliac and femoral arteries.[49] The development of occlusive disease below the knee stimulates the collateral arteries around the knee to enlarge. Only infrequently is disease at this level associated with symptoms of intermittent claudication.[49] Two reasons exist for this absence. The low site of occlusion impairs calf flow less than higher blockages, and reduced pain appreciation caused by diabetic neuropathy can hide any remaining symptoms. Trouble is commonly associated with ankle artery pressures less than 80 mm Hg. At lower arterial perfusion pressure, injury- or infection-mediated gangrene is sometimes the initially recognized event. Several features of diabetic blood flow contribute to the low pressure and to gangrene development. Their identification can lead to new treatment modes (see Tables 5–3 to 5–5).

The second diabetes-associated problem is arterial wall calcification. This abnormality develops in the middle rather than the inner layer of the vessel wall. It interferes with leg blood pressure evaluation. Leg artery calcification also alters the distal arterial flow pattern and limits maximum blood flow to the foot.[15] Expansion of the artery wall during local systole is prevented so that larger rises in systolic pressure and greater systolic flow acceleration are transmitted to the microvessels of the foot. Arterial calcification interacts with gravity-mediated rises in intraluminal pressure to set the stage for atherosclerotic plaque development at the branches of the popliteal artery. Local flow-mediated force is enhanced in magnitude and distribution by stiffening of the arteries.

The plantar forefoot has a deep arterial arch connecting the posterior tibial and dorsalis pedis terminal branches like the one in the palm of the hand that connects radial and ulnar arteries. This arch may be thrombosed by local infection. Blood flow problems in diabetes appear to add to this likelihood. Distal thrombosis can result in digital artery occlusion and toe gangrene even when more proximal arteries are completely patent, but a leg artery occlusive cause for gangrene is far more common.

## BLOOD FLOW IN LEG VEINS

Venous return in the leg has some unusual features linked in part to the dependent position normally occupied by the lower extremities. The saphenous veins have valves, an anatomic feature shared with the superficial forearm veins. The anatomic situation of the deep leg veins below the trifurcation is more unique. They not only are valved but are paired and ensheathed in common with their associated arteries (venae comitantes). This allows the arterial pulse to act to propel deep leg vein blood toward the heart. Arterial stiffening interferes with this mechanism. The result is a rise in intraluminal leg vein pressure. Walking also acts to assist deep vein blood to return to the heart. Loss of muscle from diabetic neuropathy therefore further reduces blood return. Subcutaneous tissue pressure has been measured and found normally to be less than 3 mm Hg,[105] a value well below the oncotic pressure of the plasma. With a higher venous pressure in the ankle and foot, more fluid passes into the tissues and the efficiency of the lymphatic system is put to the test. This system is also equipped with valves and in health has the ability to contract and pump the lymph.

## EFFECTS OF AUTONOMIC NEUROPATHY ON FLOW

Diabetes is commonly followed by damage to the sympathetic nerves that control blood flow to the feet. A reduced vasoconstrictive response to standing has recently been found (Fig 5–3).[99] When the nondiabetic person stands up, skin blood flow to the feet drops to about 20% of resting supine flow. Reduced autonomic activity in diabetes interferes with this degree of vasoconstriction so that flow to the skin of the feet while standing remains high.[75, 99] This means that leg artery flow in the standing position is unusually high in diabetes at the same time

that gravity raises intraluminal leg artery pressure by more than 100 mm Hg. The unusually high intraluminal pressure stretches the arterial wall and reduces its degree of expansion with systole. Persistently high flow acts with reduced wall motion favor atherosclerotic plaque formation[52] that can develop in leg arteries that would otherwise be protected by reduced flow.

This reflex loss may explain why atherosclerotic plaques cause more blockage in leg than thigh arteries in diabetes and why leg artery atherosclerosis, in contrast with coronary disease, is commonly related in diabetes to disease duration, as well as to age.[12] The autonomic neuropathy that allows persistently high foot blood flow in the standing posture[99] is probably also responsible for lowering nutritional relative to shunt microvessel flow in the foot in long-standing diabetes.[26]

## ROLE OF LEUKOCYTES IN BLOOD FLOW

The leukocytes have unusual importance in the microcirculation. In the well-mixed flow present in large arteries and veins, white blood cells are kept in the main stream. But in smaller vessels, leukocytes tend to make contact with the vessel wall and roll along if flow is sufficiently rapid or to rest against the wall where flow is slow (in modest-sized venules). The tendency for leukocytes to be near the wall of small vessels is enhanced by plasma fibrinogen elevation,[24] so that leukocytes resting in small venules should be more numerous in diabetes.

Adherence of leukocytes to venule walls places them in the path of returning red blood cells, forcing the small aggregates of erythrocytes that have just passed through capillaries or shunt vessels and clumped together (Fig 5–4) to disaggregate again in order to pass the resting leukocytes.[84]

The leukocyte's microcirculatory role as an impeder of movement of red blood cells as they begin their return to the heart is furthered by fibrinogen. Fibrinogen promotes red blood cell aggregation. Two other agents that directly influence the leukocyte's role as

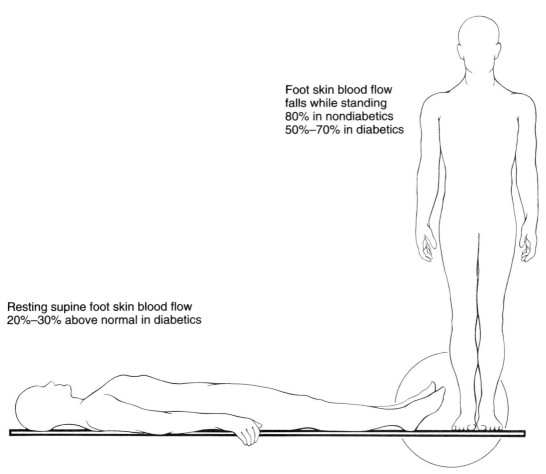

Foot skin blood flow
falls while standing
80% in nondiabetics
50%–70% in diabetics

Resting supine foot skin blood flow
20%–30% above normal in diabetics

**FIG 5–3.**
Figures portray two features of leg and foot blood flow in diabetes that may contribute to development of leg artery disease in diabetes. Resting (not maximal) skin blood flow is usually high in diabetes, but on standing the normal approximately 80% fall in skin blood flow fails to develop, favoring substantially higher leg artery flow in diabetes when the subject is standing.

a microcirculation obstructionist are adrenalin and leukocyte activating peptides. Adrenalin acts to alter microcirculatory flow and pressure. Both injected and endogenous epinephrine disgorge white blood cells resident in venules, reducing local flow resistance and raising the white blood cell count. Leukocyte activation by peptides such as f-Met·Leu·Phe that act to signal their increased responsiveness to chemoattractant chemicals and their ability to synthesize strong oxidants also increases their adherence to vessel walls. Their activation may even result in permanent occlusion of tissue if arterial pressure is insufficient to dislodge leukocytes that lodge in arterioles and capillaries,[83] an attractive mechanism to explain the development of toe gangrene in ad-

vanced diabetic occlusive leg artery disease. It has recently been shown that both activated monocytes and granulocytes may contribute to capillary nonperfusion in diabetic retinopathy.[86] Pharmacologic agents that can reverse the leukocyte's activation state and thereby improve microvascular flow may find a role in management of advanced diabetic leg artery disease.

## BLOOD AS SHEAR THINNING FLUID

With these physical, physiologic, and anatomic components of the diabetic foot's circulation, we can now point out more specific features of blood flow and the effects of diabetes on them. As already mentioned, blood

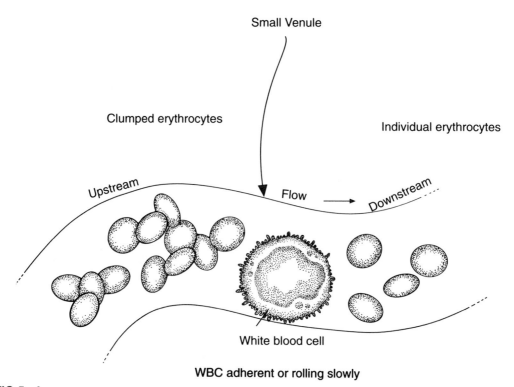

**FIG 5–4.**
Leukocytes tend to stay longest in small venules where they generate small clusters of erythrocytes by slowing their passage. The erythrocytes are forced to disaggregate to pass the standing or slowly moving white blood cell.

is much more resistant to flow at low than at high shear rates. This property is called shear thinning. Shear is a word used to describe that component of motion within a material that distorts its planes rather than simply changing the relative positions of two points. The rate of distortion of local surfaces during fluid motion is referred to as shear rate. Movement of a small fluid area relative to an adjacent area occurs at 1 inverse second (the unit of shear rate) if the two areas move relative to each other in both position and rotation the same distance as the distance between them. If a similar amount of motion takes only 10 msec, the local shear rate is 100 inverse seconds (100 $sec^{-1}$). For a newtonian fluid, the viscosity or ratio of resistive force generated locally by internal fluid motion is constant, so that 100 times as much force resisting flow develops at 100 $sec^{-1}$ as at 1 $sec^{-1}$ Blood is shear thinning (Fig 5–5), and the flow resistance ratio is only about 20 because its viscosity has fallen fivefold from 1 to 100 $sec^{-1}$ Overall, blood is typically at least 25 times as

thick or viscous at very low shear rate (0.01 $sec^{-1}$) as at high shear rate (500 $sec^{-1}$).

The basis for blood's shear thinning behavior is the interaction during flow of its red blood cells. At hematocrits less than 10%, blood shows little shear thinning, and a 40% to 55% suspension of erythrocytes in saline solution is also almost newtonian. But when either the concentration of red blood cells rises to more than 60% or plasma globulins are added, red blood cell suspensions become progressively more shear thinning, their low shear rate viscosity rising higher and higher. The basis for the rise is increasing contact between erythrocytes during flow. In the absence of globulins, each erythrocyte's negative surface charge actively reduces its contact with neighbors unless crowding by a hematocrit greater than 60% forces contact. Plasma globulins overcome the negative red blood cell charge, whereas albumin has little effect other than to stabilize red blood cell shape. Other large molecules that similarly enhance red blood cell contact during flow at low shear rate include

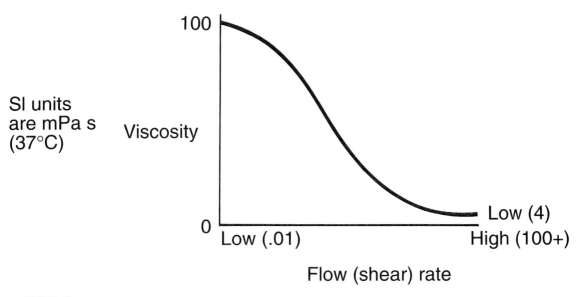

**FIG 5–5.**
Blood's nonnewtonian property of shear thinning is diagrammed. At high flow rates, blood is only five or six times as thick as water, but its flow resistance grows 20-fold as its internal motion slows. This property is useful in blood's need to flow easily and yet stop flowing after injury. Newtonian fluid would produce a horizontal line.

dextran (a large carbohydrate) and polyvinylpyrrolidinone (a pyrrole polymer). The plasma globulins share large size and substantial flow eccentricity with dextran and polyvinylpyrrolidinone. This physical property lets them enhance the attractiveness of red blood cell membranes for each other.

## PLASMA PROTEINS AND SHEAR THINNING

Molecular size and elongation affect the protein concentration required to produce red blood cell aggregation in flow. Fibrinogen is the most potent plasma globulin. Polyvinylpyrrolidinone (360,000 daltons) is ten times as potent as the dextran (150,000 daltons) commonly used in studies. Fibrinogen and other globulins generate blood's shear thinning properties. Haptoglobin is the most important of the globulins that remain in serum after clotting. In diabetes, all three plasma components favoring increased erythrocyte contact during low shear rate flow (fibrinogen, haptoglobin, and total globulin) are elevated. Total globulin elevation reflects, at least in part, a reduction in plasma albumin. Therefore, diabetic blood

typically shows more shear thinning (higher viscosity at low shear rate) than nondiabetic blood.

Increased low shear rate blood viscosity alters blood flow by reducing the shearing motion near the center of steady flow. This effect is in itself very modest. Increased shear thinning burdens flow at normal rates less than 2%. The increased pressure required to overcome this resistance increase is also less than 2%. This means that variations in plasma protein composition with age, gender, individual genetic predisposition, diabetes, and pregnancy have only this level of direct linkage to blood pressure and do not directly generate measurable changes in cardiac output.

## FLOW DESTABILIZATION

Blood has another continuously present nonnewtonian flow property of interest in addition to shear thinning (Table 5–2). Many nonnewtonian fluids lower fluid drag. Drag is a word used to describe the increased pressure drop generated by newtonian fluids during tube flow at high Reynolds' numbers. At Reynolds' numbers greater than 2,000, flow becomes unstable,

**TABLE 5-2.**

Types of Nonnewtonian Blood Flow Properties

A. Time independent (always present during flow)
   1. *Shear thinning* (lower viscosity at higher flow rate)
      Red blood cells interact with plasma globulins to try to aggregate blood at low flow rates, raising its viscosity. Red blood cells stretch progressively as flow rate rises, becoming more streamlined and continuing to lower blood viscosity.
   2. *Flow destabilization* (favors or opposes kinetically mediated change)
      Fluids fail to flow smoothly at high rates of absolute motion, developing irregular patterns with greater pressure drops. Substances that make the fluid nonnewtonian can affect this property, altering the fluid's ability to flow smoothly in curvilinear vessels, a major feature of artery and vein blood flow.
B. Time dependent (present as flow changes and shortly thereafter)
   1. *Viscoelasticity* (elastic strain energy stored as flow increases)
      Elastic erythrocytes (or stretchable molecules in other fluids) are deformed by the initiation or increase of flow rate. Red blood cell shape change reduces blood's initial resistance to flow but causes a persistence of internal force as a result of cell motion after the fluid's overall motion has ceased.
   2. *Transient resistance* (increased resistance to flow onset or restoration)
      Nonspherical elements in a fluid (erythrocytes in blood) become oriented to the flow as it is initiated or restored. Red blood cell orientation takes less time but more energy as blood's flow rate increases. Rapid red blood cell relaxation from flow orientation in blood causes its resistance to restarting flow to rise much more rapidly than that of other thixotropic fluids, an important feature of arterial flow.

with local eddies forming and dissipating much of the flow energy. This causes flow resistance to rise roughly as the 1.4 power of flow velocity.[81] Some substances that make the fluid nonnewtonian also lower this turbulence-related drag when added to the system.[47, 89] Red blood cells might reduce blood's drag in arteries by damping eddies; but the Reynolds number never achieves a value sufficiently high to make drag clearly important. On the other hand, early destabilization in curved flow (as opposed to straight flows) is seen in many nonnewtonian flows. Fortunately, blood is as stable as new-tonian fluids during curvilinear flow, and diabetes has no measurable effect on this non-time-based flow property.[53]

## TIME-BASED FLOW PROPERTIES OF BLOOD

Blood also has two time-based flow properties, viscoelasticity and transient resistance (see Table 5-2). Both are affected by diabetes. Time-based flow properties are seen for only brief periods when flow conditions change. They are not detectable during steady flow but affect blood flow only when it is pulsatile rather than steady. The pulsatility of blood flow in arteries gives these flow properties special importance.

### Blood Viscoelasticity

Viscoelasticity is responsible for blood's unusually low initial resistance to flow at low shear rate.[55] Because elastic behavior is characteristically reversible, blood's low initial flow resistance is associated with an essentially symmetric dissipation of resistive force when flow stops. Although visible mainly at low shear rate, viscoelastic behavior is a feature of flow initiation at all flow rates. To understand what is happening, we return to the concept of fluid deformation as principally the motion of one fluid area relative to another. Blood contains red cells and plasma, but only plasma can continue to move in this manner. Red cells begin to deform, but their solid shape causes them to resist further deformation. They simply achieve a new average shape while flowing that is lost as flow ceases. Erythrocyte shape change is easier to accomplish than plasma deformation at flow onset so that the flow resistance of blood is initially low, but the saving in early resistance shows up as a shear stress tail when flow stops.

Although commonly represented as individual red cell deformation, blood's viscoelastic deformation initially involves red cell rouleaux. Red cells are normally found in rouleaux when flow has stopped. Red cell suspensions that do not form rouleaux show

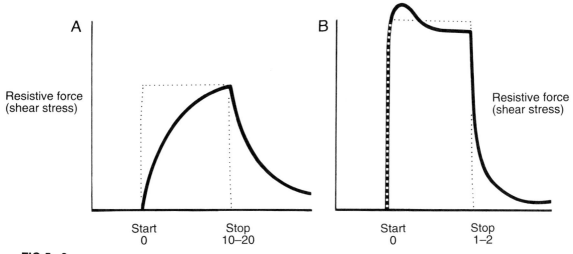

**FIG 5–6.**
Blood viscoelasticity **(A)** and transient resistance **(B)**. *Thicker lines* show blood's behavior, and *thinner broken lines* a newtonian fluid of similar viscosity to show the normal response. At slow onset of flow (shear rate 0.01–0.1 $\sec^{-1}$), red blood cell (RBC) bending dominates the fluid's interior motion, reducing its early resistance to deformation. But as flow ceases, the RBCs restore their shape and orient more randomly, accounting for the slow decline in internal force seen. At faster onset of flow (shear rate 0.2–30 $\sec^{-1}$), RBC bending is dominated by the need to orient the cells to rapidly developing flow. This need is directly linked to the rotation of the cells into line and therefore peaks sharply as shown. The slow red blood cell–based relaxation seen at the end of flow is proportionately smaller but still reflects blood's viscoelastic character.

much less viscoelasticity. At low shear rate ($<5$ seconds$^{-1}$), diabetic blood forms rouleaux more vigorously and is more viscoelastic than nondiabetic blood, but this difference becomes less evident as shear rate rises. The total elastic strain energy stored at flow initiation rises continuously up to at least 30 sec$^{-1}$ but less rapidly as this rate is approached.

## Transient Resistance of Blood (Fig 5–6)

A number of fluids that have solid components or that gel easily manifest a property called thixotropy,[64] a word coined from Greek to describe fluids and suspensions that fall in flow resistance after they initially undergo shear deformation. Good examples are found around the kitchen. One such material is mustard. When stirred or shaken, mustard will thin for a few minutes and pour or spread more easily. Blood was found to be thixotropic a number of years ago, but it does something that no other thixotropic fluid can do. It recovers its increased flow resistance very quickly, literally between heartbeats. For that reason, this property has been renamed transient flow resistance.[54] It has been shown to be caused by the extra work needed to align red cells into the plane of flow as flow begins or restarts. Transient resistance is recovered rapidly because elastic red blood cells move out of the plane of flow elastically as flow slows or stops. A large part of blood's transient resistance is mediated by growing contact between red cells as they move out of the orientation they maintained during flow.

Transient resistance is the blood flow property most strikingly affected by diabetes. It is elevated about 30%.[57] Its major direct effects are in the arterial system, where flow is clearly burdened more by increased transient resistance than by increased shear thinning because of diabetes. But it also has effects whose magnitude has not yet been assessed in local flow situations in which flow velocity suddenly changes at arterial and arteriolar branch sites. In these flow areas, inertial and transient resistance effects are additive. The largest macrovascular hemorheologic effects of diabetes should be in arterial areas where flow is suddenly accelerated.

## REDUCED ERYTHROCYTE DEFORMABILITY IN DIABETES

One of the truly unique features of diabetic blood is the reduced ability of diabetic red blood cells to pass through capillary-sized glass tubes[58] and filters.[8, 37, 44, 104] This defect is associated with two other red cell abnormalities. Diabetic red cells also manifest greater flow resistance at low shear rate when resuspended in an artificial medium.[56, 77] Most interesting of all is a slowing and reduced ability to form doublets,[59] the first stage of rouleau formation. This kind of motion is most susceptible to thermodynamic analysis. It indicates that diabetic erythrocyte membranes resist rate of bending about twice normally.[59] This means that diabetic red cells are slow to change shape as they enter capillaries, explaining the higher pressure at the arteriolar end of the capillaries seen in diabetic extremities even before mural sclerosis has developed.[98]

The basis for the abnormal behavior of diabetic red cells remains unclear. There is evidence that diabetic red cells are more glycated than normal red cells.[53] But rapid reversibility by insulin administration[7, 37, 44] and the uniformity of reduced red cell deformability in 4-μm glass tube flow[58] argue that glycosylation may not be the basis for the observed reduced deformability. The mechanism has importance because most studies have shown that the erythrocyte deformability problem is reduced when glucose control is better. If a mechanism other than glycation is responsible, a management strategy other than tight glucose control becomes possible.

## LEUKOCYTE DEFORMABILITY IN DIABETES

Filtration studies were susceptible to leukocyte plugging artifacts, suggesting initially that increased numbers of leukocytes in diabetes might be responsible for slowing filtration of diabetic blood.[96] But changes in technique to deal with this have still allowed the red cell deformability problem to be demonstrated.[18, 48, 95] In the meantime, studies of leukocytes showed that their passage through capillary-sized (5-μm) filters was impaired in diabetes.[21] Recent advances in leukocyte rheology have shown that the situation is quite complex. Activation alters leukocyte behavior,[86] further burdening clinical analysis.

Leukocytes normally pass through small arteriolovenular shunt vessels rather than true capillaries. This is in part because both red cells and white cells tend to be directed into the shunt vessels by the higher flow that these vessels experience while tissues are at rest. With less arterial pressure from leg artery disease in diabetes, leukocyte shunting loses efficiency, raising leukocyte residency frequency and duration in true capillaries,[83] a phenomenon that can lead to permanent tissue damage.[83] This becomes particularly important in the foot. The cutaneous vessels responsible for heat loss are mainly shunt vessels, whereas the nutritional vessels are true capillaries.[23] Foot skin nutrition is disproportionately compromised by diabetic leg artery disease.[23] Activation of leukocytes by infection can turn marginal blood flow into toe gangrene. This result illustrates how problems can add to each other to lead to amputation.

## TREATMENT CONSIDERATIONS

As described earlier, many hemorheologic changes in diabetes have been linked in severity to poor glucose control, but few randomized tests of the effects of improved glucose control on hemorheologic parameters have been carried out. Although weakened by the lack of an interventional trial, the cross-sectional and prospective data already cited[16, 82] make an argument that close control of blood glucose should reduce or prevent rheologically mediated vascular complications of diabetes.

Exercise (Table 5–3)[31, 85, 103, 106] is reported to lower blood viscosity through plasma protein changes. Both fibrinogen[31, 85, 103] and haptoglobin[106] fall. Haptoglobin's fall is thought to involve the feet; red cells are damaged as they pass through plantar capillaries when the feet hit the

**TABLE 5–3.**

Nonpharmacologic Hemorheologic Management

1. *Exercise.*
   Generalized hemoconcentration and intravascular hemolysis in the feet occur during activity, but fibrinolysis increases as physical condition improves with training[31, 85, 103, 106]
2. *Diet.*
   Diabetes control and an appropriately low-fat diet decreases VLDL (triglyceride) and its stimulated endothelial PAI-1 synthesis[92]
3. *Protein intake.*
   When adequate and timely, high-quality protein allows a normal albumin synthesis rate when combined with insulin[32, 36]
4. *Garlic/onion oil* (allyl propyl disulfide).
   When consumed in diet, acts to lower plasma free fatty acid levels and increase fibrinolysis[70]
5. *Trans-unsaturated fatty acids.*
   Present in margarine and other foods, have been shown to lower plasma fibrinogen levels in rats[70]
6. *Fish oil and supplements.*
   Act to lower blood viscosity,[13, 39, 108] fibrinogen levels,[74] red blood cell flow resistance[72] and membrane fluidity[38]
7. *Smoking cessation.*
   Fibrinogen and haptoglobin levels fall slowly after smoking stops in parallel with declining cardiovascular risk[63]
8. *Vitamins and nutrients* (often considered food supplements)
   See Table 5–5

VLDL = very low-density lipoprotein; PAI-1 = plasminogen activator inhibitor 1.

ground. Hemoglobin released binds to haptoglobin, and both are cleared from the bloodstream by the reticuloendothelial system.

Nutritional options are also thought to affect blood viscosity. Lowering the traditional U.S. dietary fat results in lower serum triglyceride levels.[11] Lowering of very low-density lipoprotein (VLDL) triglyceride levels leads in turn to reduced levels of plasminogen activator inhibitor 1 (PAI-1) the major opponent of plasmin-mediated clot dissolution and fibrinogenolysis because VLDL is a direct stimulator of PAI-1 formation by endothelial cells.[92] Adequate protein intake is necessary for normal serum albumin levels.[32, 36] Consumption of large amounts of fish[39] or its associated omega-3 unsaturated fatty acids[13, 74, 108] is reported to lower blood viscosity, but effects of the levels of dietary intake achieved by most Americans have not been studied. The fish oil effect appears to be mediated by lowering of triglyceride levels[90] and erythrocyte membrane lipid changes.[38, 72]

A number of parenteral regimes are used to manage serious hemorheologic problems (Table 5–4). Low molecular weight dextran, available as 40,000-dalton average Rheomacrodex, has been used in Europe to expand plasma volume as red blood cells are

**TABLE 5–4.**

Parenteral Agent Hemorheologic Management

1. *Hemodilution*
   A therapy designed to reduce blood viscosity by lowering hematocrit without decreasing blood volume and oxygen delivery. It is normally accomplished by removal of blood and replacement of plasma by an excess of low molecular weight dextran (40,000 daltons) or another oncotically active material. This is done to expand the plasma volume without raising blood viscosity. This management has been used in stroke,[93] peripheral arterial disease[110] and retinal vein thrombosis[30] with varying degrees of success. Its ultimate methodology and role in disease management are still being explored.[45]
2. *Plasmapheresis*
   Undesirable plasma components, usually proteins, are removed by phlebotomy. Red blood cells are separated by centrifugation and returned to the patient during the procedure; the plasma is either processed to remove specific substances and returned to the patient or replaced by salt-poor albumin. Treatment effectiveness depends on the half-life of the material being removed and the benefit derived from the feasible amount of lowering. The technique has been used to remove immune proteins[87] and lipoproteins,[88] and acts to lower plasma fibrinogen,[107] but it is both costly and inconvenient for the patient.
3. *Enzyme administration*
   a. Streptokinase, used in treating early acute myocardial infarction,[33] causes fibrinogen to fall to very low levels, altering blood flow properties.[4, 34]
   b. Urokinase, also used in acute myocardial infarction, has less antibody interference and less drop in fibrinogen levels[50] and blood viscosity[4] than streptokinase.
   c. Alteplase (tissue plasminogen activator), also used in acute myocardial infarction, has much less effect on fibrinogen levels and blood flow properties than streptokinase.[34]
   d. Ancrod (Arvin) has been used in treating peripheral artery disease.[46]

**TABLE 5–5.**

Oral Medication Hemorheologic Management

Aldose reductase inhibitors
  Sorbinil—lowers fibrinogen levels, improves RBC filterability[78]
  Ponairestat (statil)—improves RBC suspension viscosity[76]
Anabolic corticosteroids
  Furazabol—activates fibrinolytic system, lowers fibrinogen levels[1]
  Stanozolol—activates fibrinolytic system, lowers fibrinogen levels[16]
Anionic amphophiles
  Aspirin—suppresses fibrinogen synthesis,[70] reduces RBC aggregation[61]
  Calcium dobesilate—lowers fibrinogen levels,[102] blood viscosity,[10, 102]
    reduces RBC aggregation[61]
Anticlaudicants
  Buflomedil—lowers fibrinogen levels, WBV[101]
  Defibrotide—produces a fall in fibrinogen levels in claudication patients[16]
  Dipyridamole—improves filterability of processed RBCs in vitro[80]
  Pentoxifylline—lowers fibrinogen levels[6, 26] by a mechanism other than
    activating fibrinolysis,[70] opposes WBC activation[67]
  Suloctidil—lowers fibrinogen, mechanism not clear[79]
  Ticlopidine—lowers fibrinogen levels in claudication, transient ischemic
    attack[16]
Anticonvulsants
  Valproic acid—acts on liver, probably stops fibrinogen synthesis[97]
Antihypertensives
  β-Blockers
    Celiprolol—lowers fibrinogen levels in hypertension management[16]
    Propanolol—lowers fibrinogen levels and increases fibrinolysis in parallel[16]
  Calcium inhibitors
    Diltiazem—reported to lower blood viscosity, basis not clear[22]
    Flunarizine—reported to lower blood viscosity, basis not clear[17]
    Nimodipine—WBV falls without fall in plasma viscosity or fibrinogen
      levels[28]
  Central agents
    Clonidine—lowers fibrinogen levels modestly, basis not clear[70]
Antioxidants
  Idebenone—improves RBC filterability, aggregability, lowers plasma
    viscosity[66]
  Probucol—lowers fibrinogen and factor VIII in Watanabe rabbits[65]
Biguanides
  Buformin—increases fibrinolysis, decreases fibrinogen levels[29]
  Metformin—reported to increase fibrinolysis by lowering plasminogen
    activator inhibitor 1 levels[100]
  Phenformin—reported to increase fibrinolysis, not available in United States[25]
Fibric acid–derived triglyceride-lowering drugs
  Bezafibrate—lowers fibrinogen levels, more in hypertriglyceridemia[2]
  Ciprofibrate—lowers fibrinogen levels, more in hypertriglyceridemia[16]
  Clofibrate—lowers fibrinogen, more in hypertriglyceridemia[16, 71]
  Fenofibrate—lowers fibrinogen levels, more in hypertriglyceridemia[3, 16]
  Gemfibrozil—reported to raise fibrinogen level[94]
HMG-reductase inhibitors
  Lovastatin—raises fibrinogen levels while improving RBC filterability[9]; lowers
    plasma viscosity and RBC aggregation but does not change fibrinogen
    levels[41]; has its effect influenced by lipoprotein(a) level[40]
  Pravastatin—lowers fibrinogen level, plasma viscosity[35]; produces no
    change[5]
  Simvastatin—does not change fibrinogen level[51]
Vitamins-nutrients
  Ligustrazine (herb component)—lowers whole blood viscosity, cause not
    clear[111]
  Niceritrol (nicotinic acid + PETN)—lowers fibrinogen levels in diabetes[16]
  Nicotinic acid—lowers fibrinogen level in parallel with triglyceride levels[70, 91]
  Troxerutin—reduces RBC clumping in diabetic retinopathy[42]

*WBV = whole blood viscosity.*

removed to lower the hematocrit and reduce blood's flow resistance. Alternative plasma expanders based on starch and other large molecules are also being examined.[45]

Plasmapheresis is used when the level of a particular plasma protein needs to be lowered. Fibrinogen levels remain subnormal for 2 to 3 days, while plasma complement and other clotting components are restored in 1 day.[107]

The use of plasmin-activating enzymes to dissolve intravascular clots has become commonplace. Most of these agents also lower blood and plasma viscosity in parallel with their clot dissolving action, an effect considered to improve microcirculatory flow.[4] Streptokinase, acting throughout the plasma volume, produces a more striking change than urokinase and tissue-type plasminogen activator (t-PA) (alteplase) because the latter have a strong tendency to bind to thrombi.[34]

Information about oral pharmacologic agent effects on blood flow properties and fibrinogen levels is shown in Table 5–5. It has been growing steadily but remains far from complete. I have unpublished data that show that sulfonylurea drugs improve blood viscosity at the same time that they improve glucose control. Hypoglycemia mediates some additional changes in the flow properties of blood that are less desirable. They include increased blood and plasma viscosity, rising von Willebrand factor and t-PA levels, and falling PAI levels without change in fibrinogen level.[27]

Table 5–5 lists aldose reductase inhibitors, used in diabetic neuropathy management in some countries, anabolic corticosteroids, benzoic acid derivatives, and a series of agents used principally in Europe to treat intermittent claudication. They are also commonly described as vasodilators. A number of antihypertensive drugs used in diabetes have been reported to affect blood flow properties. Some of their therapeutic effects may ultimately be explained by this mechanism, but their major hypotensive effects appear to be from their influence on vascular smooth muscle. The biguanide drugs, used in diabetes management outside the United States, all have been shown to lower plasma fibrinogen levels as they increase fibrinolysis.[25, 29, 100] Agents used in controlling hyperlipidemias, also commonly used in diabetes management, make up a large fraction of the table.

The agent in Table 5–5 that is used most frequently in leg and foot disease in diabetes in the United States is pentoxifylline, a xanthine derivative with adenosine agonist effects. It has been shown to improve intermittent claudication.[73] Its effect was initially thought to be generated by improved red cell deformability,[20] but more recent work has suggested that the agent's adenosine action reverses leukocyte activation.[67] Such an inactivation could also help explain its ability to lower fibrinogen levels.[6, 26]

The major feature of Table 5–5 is the effect of many drugs on plasma fibrinogen levels. The mechanism for drug action in lowering or raising plasma fibrinogen levels is of interest. It is hinted at by an analysis of the cited reports. Fibrinogen is synthesized by the liver and after introduction into the plasma volume has a half-life of 2 to 4 days, a short period for plasma proteins. Valproic acid's effect in lowering fibrinogen levels is likely to be by direct suppression of hepatic synthesis, because it has been reported to disrupt liver metabolism and structure in idiosyncratic hepatotoxic reactions through generation of toxic metabolites.[19] Cytokines, especially interleukin 6 (IL-6), interact with surface receptors on hepatocytes to increase both fibrinogen levels and haptoglobin synthesis.[14] Pentoxifylline may act by reducing leukocyte-mediated signaling[67] by IL-6 and its resultant fibrinogen and haptoglobin synthesis.

The mechanism for the effect of many other drugs listed appears more complex. The relatively short half-life of fibrinogen and associations between hypertriglyceridemia and the coagulation process[90] argue that plasma fibrinogen is lost early in good part because the coagulation process is initiated or the enzyme plasmin has been activated. Either mechanism can lead to a fall in plasma fibrinogen level. Plasmin's activation is usually accomplished by t-PA, an enzyme whose two kringles encourage its attachment to coagulated fibrin. This enzyme is efficiently opposed by PAI-1. Both enzymes are principally products of the endothelium that lines the vascular space. Evidence that PAI-1 is directly stimulated from endothelial cells in culture by VLDL[92] creates a potential explanation for the effect of many of the drugs in Table 5–5. But a past report indicting suppression of hepatic synthesis in clofibrate's fibrinogen-lowering action[71] and the ability of gemfibrozil to lower triglyceride levels while raising fibrinogen levels[94] suggest that the situation is going to be more complex.

Fibrinogen is a well-documented risk factor predicting future cardiovascular disease[16, 109] that both alters blood's flow properties and accelerates its coagulability. Drug effects on its blood level should have at least as much interest as drug effects on serum cholesterol levels, a now widely known pharmacologic side effect. The current state of hemorheologic treatment is about a decade behind management of hyperlipidemia. The interaction of lipid lowering agents with blood fibrinogen levels should assist us in speeding our assimilation of information that will allow us to understand how better to restore the health of the feet and the other parts of the body through which blood passes in the diabetic patient.

## REFERENCES

1. Abiko Y, Kumada T: Enhancement of fibrinolytic and thrombolytic potential in the rat by an anabolic steroid, furazabol, *Thromb Res* 8:107–114, 1976.

2. Almer LO, Kjellstrom T: The fibrinolytic system and coagulation during bezafibrate treatment of hypertriglyceridemia, *Atherosclerosis* 61:81–85, 1986.

3. Arntz HR, et al: Influence of fenofibrate on blood rheology in type II hyperlipoproteinemia, *Clin Hemorheol* 10:297–307, 1990.

4. Arntz HR et al: The effects of different thrombolytic agents on blood rheology in acute myocardial infarction, *Clin Hemorheol* 11:63–78, 1991.

5. Arntz HR et al: Influence of pravastatin on blood rheology in type II hypercholesterolemia, *Clin Hemorheol* 11:785, 1991.

6. Bachet P, Lancrenon S, Chassoux G: Fibrinogen and pentoxifylline, *Thromb Res* 55:161–163, 1989.

7. Baldini P et al: Insulin effects on human red blood cells, *Mol Cell Endocrinol* 46:93–102, 1986.

8. Barnes AJ, et al: Is hyperviscosity a treatable component of diabetic microcirculatory disease? *Lancet* 2:789–791, 1977.

9. Beigel Y, et al: Lovastatin therapy in heterozygous familial hypercholesterolaemic patients: effect on blood rheology and fibrinogen levels, *J Intern Med* 230:23–27, 1991.

10. Benarroch IS, et al: Treatment of blood hyperviscosity with calcium dobesilate in patients with diabetic retinopathy, *Ophthalmic Res* 17:131–138, 1985.

11. Bierman EL, Brunzell JD: Diet low in saturated fat and cholesterol for diabetes, *Diabetes Care* 12:162–163, 1989.

12. Bild DE, et al: Lower-extremity amputation in people with diabetes epidemiology and prevention, *Diabetes Care* 12:24–31, 1989.

13. Cartwright IJ et al: The effects of dietary ω-3 polyunsaturated fatty acids on erythrocyte membrane phospholipids, erythrocyte deformability and blood viscosity in healthy volunteers, *Atherosclerosis* 55:267–281, 1985.

14. Castell JV et al: Recombinant human interleukin-6 (IL-6/BSF-2/HSF) regulates the synthesis of acute phase proteins in human hepatocytes, *FEBS Lett* 232:347–350, 1988.

15. Christensen NJ: Muscle blood flow, measured by xenon-133 and vascular calcifications in diabetics, *Acta Med Scand* 183:449–454, 1968

16. Cook NS, Ubben D: Fibrinogen as a major risk factor in cardiovascular disease, *Trends Pharmacol Sci* 11:444–451, 1990.

17. De Cree J, et al: The rheological effects of cinnarizine and flunarizine in normal and pathologic conditions, *Angiology* 30:505–515, 1979.

18. Diamantopoulos EJ, Raptis SA, Moulopoulos SD: Red blood cell deformability index in diabetic retinopathy, *Horm Metabol Res* 19:569–573, 1987.

19. Eadie MJ, Hooper WD, Dickinson RG: Valproate-associated hepatotoxicity and its biochemical mechanisms, *Med Toxicol* 3:85–106, 1988.

20. Ehrly AM: The effect of pentoxifylline on the deformability of erythrocytes and on the muscular oxygen pressure in patients with chronic arterial disease, *J Med* 10:331–338, 1979.

21. Ernst E, Matrai A: Altered red and white blood cell rheology in type II diabetes, *Diabetes* 35:1412–1415, 1986.

22. Ernst E, Matrai A: Diltiazem alters blood rheology, *Pharmatherapeutica* 5:213–216, 1988.

23. Fagrell B, et al: Vital capillary microscopy for assessment of skin viability and microangiopathy in patients with diabetes mellitus, *Acta Med Scand* 687(suppl):25–28, 1984.

24. Fahraeus R: The suspension-stability of the blood, *Acta Med Scand* 55:1–228, 1921.

25. Fearnley GR, Chakrabarti R: Fibrinolytic treatment of rheumatoid arthritis with phenformin plus ethyloestrenol, *Lancet* 2:757–761, 1966.

26. Ferrari E, et al: Effects of long-term treatment (4 years) with pentoxifylline on haemorheological changes and vascular complications in diabetic patients, *Pharmatherapeutica* 5:26–39, 1987.

27. Fisher BM, et al: Effects of acute insulin-induced hypoglycemia on haemostasis, fibrinolysis and haemorheology in insulin-dependent diabetic patients and control subjects, *Clin Sci* 80:525–553, 1990.

28. Forconi S, et al: Effect of treatment with the calcium-entry blocker nimodipine on cerebral blood flow (spect) and blood viscosity of patients affected by cerebral chronic vascular insufficiency, *Clin Hemorheol* 11:787, 1991.

29. Ghanem MH, Guirgis FK, El-Sawy M: Effect of buformin on fibrinolytic activity in rheumatoid arthritis, *Arzneimittelforschung* 22:1487–1489, 1972.

30. Hansen LL, Wiek J, Wiederholt M: A randomized prospective study of treatment of non-ischaemic central vein occlusion by isovolaemic haemodilution, *Br J Ophthalmol* 73:895–899, 1989.

31. Hornsby G, et al: Exercise conditioning reduces plasma fibrinogen in noninsulin-dependent diabetes mellitus, *Diabetes* 37(suppl 1):240a, 1988.

32. Hutson SM, et al: Regulation of albumin synthesis by hormones and amino acids in primary cultures of rat hepatocytes, *Am J Physiol* 252:E291–298, 1987.

33. I.S.A.M. Study Group: A prospective trial of intravenous streptokinase in acute myocardial infarction (I.S.A.M.), *N Engl J Med* 314:1465–1471, 1986.

34. Jan KM, et al: Altered rheological properties of blood following administrations of tissue plasminogen activator and streptokinase in patients with acute myocardial infarction, *Circulation* 72:417, 1985.

35. Jay RH, Rampling MW, Betteridge DJ: Abnormalities of blood rheology in familial hypercholesterolaemia: effects of treatment, *Atherosclerosis* 85:249–256, 1990.

36. Jeejeebhoy KN, et al: The comparative effects of nutritional and hormonal factors on the synthesis of albumin, fibrinogen and transferrin, *Clin Symp* 9:217–247, 1973.

37. Juhan I, et al: Effects of insulin on erythrocyte deformability in diabetics-relationship between erythrocyte deformability and platelet aggregation, *Scand J Clin Lab Invest* 41:159–164, 1981.

38. Kamada T, et al: Dietary sardine oil increases erythrocyte membrane fluidity in diabetic patients, *Diabetes* 35:604–611, 1986.

39. Kobayashi S, et al: Epidemiological and clinical studies of the effect of eicosapentaenoic acid (epa c20:5 ω-3) on blood viscosity, *Clin Hemorheol* 5:493–505, 1985.

40. Koenig W, et al: The effects of lovastatin on blood rheology, *Clin Hemorheol* 11:785, 1991.

41. Koppensteiner R, Minar E, Ehringer H: Effect of lovastatin on hemorheology in type II hyperlipoproteinemia, *Atherosclerosis* 83:53–58, 1990.

42. Ledevehat C, Vimeux M, Bondoux G: Hemorheological effects of oral troxerutin treatment versus placebo in venous insufficiency of the lower limbs, *Clin Hemorheol* 9:543, 1989.

43. Lew HS, Fung YC: The motion of the plasma between the red cells in the bolus flow, *Biorheology* 6:109–119, 1969.

44. Lipovac V, et al: Influence of lactate on the insulin action on red blood cell filterability, *Clin Hemorheol* 5:421–428, 1985.

45. Lowe GDO: Drugs in cerebral and peripheral arterial disease, *Br Med J* 300:524–528, 1990.

46. Lowe GDO, et al: Subcutaneous Ancrod therapy in peripheral arterial disease: improvement in blood viscosity and nutritional blood flow, *Angiology* 30:594–599, 1979.

47. Lumley JL, Kubo I: Turbulent drag reduction by polymer additives: a survey in Gampert B: *The influence of polymer additives on velocity and temperature fields*, New York, 1984, Springer-Verlag New York, pp 3–21.

48. MacRury SM, et al: Evaluation of red cell deformability by a filtration method in type 1 and type 2 diabetes mellitus with and without vascular complications, *Diabetes Res* 13:61–65, 1990.

49. Marinelli MR, et al: Noninvasive testing vs clinical evaluation of arterial disease, *JAMA* 241:2031–2034, 1979.

50. Mathey DG, et al: Intravenous urokinase in acute myocardial infarction, *Am J Cardiol* 55:878–882, 1985.

51. McDowell IFW, et al: Simvastatin in severe hypercholesterolaemia: a placebo controlled trial, *Br J Clin Pharmacol* 31:340–343, 1991.

52. McMillan DE: Blood flow and the localization of atherosclerotic plaques, *Stroke* 16:582–587, 1985.

53. McMillan DE, Brooks SM: Erythrocyte spectrin glucosylation in diabetes, *Diabetes* 31:64–69, 1982.

54. McMillan DE, Strigberger J, Utterback NG: Rapidly recovered transient flow resistance: a newly discovered property of blood, *Am J Physiol* 253:H919–H926, 1987.

55. McMillan DE, Utterback NG: Maxwell fluid behavior of blood at low shear rate, *Biorheology* 17:343–354, 1980.

56. McMillan DE, Utterback NG: Impaired flow properties of diabetic erythrocytes, *Clin Hemorheol* 1:147–152, 1981.

57. McMillan DE, Utterback NG: Viscoelasticity and thixotropy of diabetic blood measured at low shear rate, *Clin Hemorheol* 1:361–372, 1981.

58. McMillan DE, Utterback NG, La Puma J: Reduced erythrocyte deformability in diabetes, *Diabetes* 27:895–901, 1978.

59. McMillan DE, Utterback NG, Mitchell TP: Doublet formation of diabetic erythrocytes as a model of impaired membrane viscous deformation, *Microvasc Res* 26:205–220, 1983.

60. McMillan DE, Utterback NG, Stocki J: Low shear rate blood viscosity in diabetes, *Biorheology* 17:355–362, 1980.

61. McMillan DE, Utterback NG, Wujek JJ: Effect of anionic amphophiles on erythrocyte properties, *Ann NY Acad Sci* 416:633–641, 1983.

62. McMillan DE, et al: Taylor-Couette flow stability of diabetic blood, *Clin Hemorheol* 9:989–998, 1989.

63. Meade TW, Imeson J, Stirling Y: Effects of changes in smoking and other characteristics on clotting factors and the risk of ischaemic heart disease, *Lancet* 2:986–988, 1987.

64. Mewis J: Thixotropy—a general review, *J Non-Newtonian Fluid Mech* 6:1–20, 1979.

65. Mori Y, et al: Hypercoagulable state in the Watanabe heritable hyperlipidemic rabbit, an animal model for the progression of atherosclerosis, *Thromb Haemost* 61:140–143, 1989.

66. Nagakawa Y, et al: Effect of idebenone on hemorheologic variables in geriatric patients with cerebral infarction, *Clin Hemorheol* 11:351, 1991.

67. Nash GB, et al: Effects of acute trental infusion on white blood cell rheology in patients with critical leg ischaemia, *Clin Hemorheol* 11:309, 1991.

68. Nielsen NV: The normal fundus fluorescein angiogram and the normal fundus photograph, *Acta Ophthalmologica* 64(suppl 180):1–30, 1986.

69. Ostermann H, Van De Loo J: Factors of the hemostatic system in diabetic patients, *Haemostasis* 16:386–416, 1986.

70. Pickart L: Fat metabolism the fibrinogen/fibrinolytic system and blood flow: new potentials for the pharmacological treatment of coronary heart disease, *Pharmacology* 23:271–280, 1981.

71. Pickart L: Suppression of acute-phase synthesis of fibrinogen by a hypolipidemic drug (clofibrate), *Int J Tissue React* 3:65–72, 1981.

72. Popp-Snijders C, et al: Fatty fish-induced changes in membrane lipid composition and viscosity of human erythrocyte suspensions, *Scand J Clin Lab Invest* 46:253–258, 1986.

73. Porter JM, et al: Pentoxifylline efficacy in the treatment of intermittent claudication: multicenter controlled double-blind trial with objective assessment of chronic occlusive arterial disease patients, *Am Heart J* 104:66–72, 1982.

74. Radack K, Deck C, Huster G: Dietary supplementation with low-dose fish oils lowers fibrinogen levels: a randomized, double-blind controlled study, *Ann Intern Med* 111:757–758, 1989.

75. Rayman G, Hassan A, Tooke JE: Blood flow in the skin of the foot related to posture in diabetes mellitus, *Br Med J* 292:87–90, 1986.

76. Rillaerts EG, Vertommen JJ, De Leeuw IH: Effect of statil (ICI 128436) on erythrocyte viscosity in vitro, *Diabetes* 37:471–475, 1988.

77. Rillaerts E, et al: Increased low shear rate erythrocyte viscosity in insulin dependent diabetes mellitus, *Clin Hemorheol* 8:73–80, 1988.

78. Robey A, et al: Sorbinil partially prevents decreased erythrocyte deformability in experimental diabetes mellitus, *Diabetes* 36:1010–1013, 1987.

79. Roncucci R, et al: Effects of long-term treatment with suloctidil on blood viscosity, erythrocyte deformability and total fibrinogen plasma levels in diabetic patients, *Arzneim-Forsch Drug Res* 29:682–684, 1979.

80. Saniabadi AR, Fisher TC, Rimmer AR, et al: A study of the effect of dipyridamole on erythrocyte deformability using an improved filtration technique, *Clin Hemorheol* 10:263, 1990.

81. Schlichting H: *Boundary layer theory*, New York, 1979, McGraw-Hill.

82. Schmechel VH, Beikufner P, Panzram G: Langsschnittuntersuchungen zur progrenstischen bedeutung des plasmafibrinogens beim diabetes mellitus, *Z Gesamte Inn Med Jahrg* 39:453–457, 1984.

83. Schmid-Schonbein GW: Capillary plugging by granulocytes and the no-reflow phenomenon in the microcirculation, *Fed Proc* 46:2397–2401, 1987.

84. Schmid-Schonbein GW, et al: The interaction of leukocytes and erythrocytes in capillary and post-capillary vessels, *Microvasc Res* 19:45–70, 1980.

85. Schneider SH, et al: Impaired fibrinolytic response to exercise in type II diabetes: effects of exercise and physical training, *Metabolism* 37:924–929, 1988.

86. Schroder S, Palinski W, Schmid-Schonbein GW: Activated monocytes and granulocytes, capillary nonperfusion, and neovascularization in diabetic retinopathy, *Am J Pathol* 139:81–100, 1991.

87. Schwab PJ, Okun E, Fahey JL: Reversal of retinopathy in Waldenstrom's macroglobulinemia by plasmapheresis, *Arch Ophthalmol* 64:515–521, 1960.

88. Seidel D, et al: The HELP-LDL-apheresis multi-centre study, an angiographically assessed trial on the role of LDL-apheresis in the secondary prevention of coronary heart disease: part I, *Eur J Clin Invest* 21:375–383, 1991.

89. Sellin RHJ, Hoyt JW, Scrivener O: The effect of drag reducing additives on fluid flows and their industrial applications: part 1, basic aspects, *J Hydraulic Res* 20:29–68, 1982.

90. Simpson HCR, et al: Hypertriglyceridaemia and hypercoagulability, *Lancet* 1:786–790, 1983.

91. Sirs JA, Boroda C: Variations of blood rheology in diabetic patients on nicofuranose, *Clin Hemorheol* 11:191, 1991.

92. Stiko-Rahm A, et al: Secretion of plasminogen activator inhibitor 1 from cultured human umbilical vein endothelial cells is induced by very low density lipoprotein, *Arteriosclerosis* 10:1067–1073, 1990.

93. Strand T, et al: A randomized controlled trial of hemodilution therapy in acute ischemic stroke, *Stroke* 15:980–989, 1984.

94. Stringer MD, Rampling MW, Kakkar VV: Rheological effects of gemfibrozil in occlusive arterial disease, *Clin Hemorheol* 10:339, 1990.

95. Stuart J, Juhan-Vague I: Erythrocyte rheology in diabetes mellitus, *Clin Hemorheol* 7:239–245, 1987.

96. Stuart J, et al: Filtration of washed erythrocytes in atherosclerosis and diabetes mellitus, *Clin Hemorheol* 3:23–30, 1983.

97. Sussman NM, McLain LW Jr: A direct hepatotoxic effect of valproic acid, *JAMA* 242:1173–1177, 1979.

98. Tooke JE: Microvascular dynamics in diabetes mellitus, *Diabete Metab* 14:530–534, 1988.

99. Tooke JE, Rayman G, Boolell M: Blood flow abnormalities in the diabetic foot: diagnostic aid or research tool? in Connor H, Boulton AJ, Ward JD, editors: *The foot in diabetes*, Chichester, J Wiley, 1987, pp 23–31.

100. Vague P, et al: Metformin decreases the high plasminogen activator inhibition capacity, plasma insulin and triglyceride levels in nondiabetic obese subjects, *Thromb Haemost* 57:326–328, 1987.

101. Van Acker K, Rillaerts E, De Leeuw I: The influence of buflomedil on blood viscosity parameters in insulin-dependent diabetic patients: a preliminary study, *Biomed Pharmacother* 43:219–222, 1989.

102. Vinazzer H, Hachen HJ: Influence of calcium dobesilate (Doxium) on blood viscosity and coagulation parameters in diabetic retinopathy, *VASA* 16:190–192, 1987.

103. Volger E, Pfafferott C: Effects of acute physical effort versus endurance training on blood rheology in coronary heart disease patients, *Clin Hemorheol* 10:423, 1990.

104. Volger E, Schmid-Schonbein H: Mikrorheologisches verhalten des blutes beim diabetes mellitus, *Dtsch Gesellshaft Inner Med* 80:963–966, 1974.

105. Wiederhielm CA, Weston BV: Microvascular, lymphatic, and tissue pressures in the unanesthetized mammal, *Am J Physiol* 225:992–996, 1973.

106. Wolf PL, et al: Changes in serum enzymes, lactate, and haptoglobin following acute physical stress in international-class athletes, *Clin Biochem* 20:73–77, 1987.

107. Wood L, Jacobs P: The effect of serial therapeutic plasmapheresis on platelet count, coagulation factors, plasma immunoglobulin, and complement levels, *J Clin Apheresis* 3:124–128, 1986.

108. Woodcock BE, et al: Beneficial effect of fish oil on blood viscosity in peripheral vascular disease, *Br Med J* 288:592–594, 1984.

109. Yarnell JWG, et al: Fibrinogen, viscosity, and white blood cell count are major risk factors for ischemic heart disease, *Circulation* 83:836–844, 1991.

110. Yates CJP, et al: Increase in leg blood-flow by normovolaemic haemodilution in intermittent claudication, *Lancet* 2:166–168, 1979.

111. Zhao C, et al: The hemorheological study of ligustrazine treatment in diabetic subjects, *Clin Hemorheol* 9:615, 1989.

# CHAPTER 6

# Neuropathy in the Diabetic Foot: New Concepts in Etiology and Treatment

**Douglas A. Greene, M.D.**

**Eva L. Feldman, M.D., Ph.D.**

**Martin Stevens, M.D.**

Peripheral neuropathy is a common chronic complication of diabetes. It frequently is the initiating cause of foot lesions and ultimately leads to foot and leg amputations. Its incidence parallels the duration and severity of hyperglycemia in both type I (insulin-dependent) and type II (non-insulin-dependent) diabetes. It rarely occurs before the fifth year of diabetes except in type II patients with preexisting asymptomatic hyperglycemia. Diabetic neuropathy also complicates other forms of diabetes resulting from pancreatectomy, nonalcoholic pancreatitis, and hemachromatosis. Histologically, loss of both large and small myelinated nerve fibers accompanies paranodal and segmental demyelination, connective tissue proliferation, and thickening and reduplication of capillary basement membrane with capillary closure.[9]

## CLASSIFICATION

Diabetic neuropathy is classified into discrete clinical syndromes, each having a characteristic appearance and clinical course (Table 6–1). Clinical overlap often precludes rigid classification of individual cases.[10] Because identical neurologic syndromes occur in other diseases, diabetic neuropathy is a diagnosis of exclusion[14, 15] (Table 6–2).

## DISTAL SYMMETRIC POLYNEUROPATHY

Distal symmetric polyneuropathy is the most commonly recognized form of diabetic neuropathy.[19] Sensory deficits and symptoms, which generally predominate over motor involvement, appear first in the most distal portions of the extremities and progress proximally in a "stocking-glove" distribution.[27] In the most advanced cases, vertical bands of sensory deficit develop on the chest as the tips of the shorter truncal nerves become involved.[27] The signs, symptoms, and neurologic deficits of distal symmetric sensorimotor polyneuropathy vary, depending on the classes of nerve fibers involved.[14] Loss of large sensory and motor fibers diminishes light touch and proprioception, the latter resulting in ataxic gait and unsteadiness, as well as weakness of intrinsic muscles of the hands and feet. Involvement of small fibers diminishes pain and temperature perception, resulting in repeated injury especially to the feet. Typical neuropathic paresthesias (spontaneously occurring uncomfortable sensa-

**TABLE 6–1.**

Syndromes of Diabetic Neuropathy

1. Diffuse neuropathies (common, insidious onset, usually progressive)
   a. Distal symmetric sensorimotor polyneuropathy
   b. Autonomic neuropathy
2. Focal neuropathies (rare, sudden onset, usually transient)
   a. Cranial neuropathy
   b. Radiculopathy
   c. Plexopathy
   d. Mononeuropathy/mononeuropathy multiplex
      (1) Entrapment neuropathy
      (2) Other mononeuropathies

tions) or dysesthesias (contact paresthesias) may accompany both large- or small-fiber involvement.[14] A few patients complain of exquisite cutaneous contact hypersensitivity to light touch, unbearable superficial burning or stabbing pain, or severe bone-deep aching or tearing pain that can become disabling. Both neuropathic pain and paresthesias are speculated to reflect spontaneous depolarization of newly regenerating nerve fibers.[14, 15]

Many patients with distal symmetric polyneuropathy remain free of seriously troubling subjective symptoms, but subtle feelings of "numbness," "cold," or "dead" feet are elicited during careful questioning.

Inspection of the diabetic foot can give important clues as to whether significant neuropathy is present. Peripheral autonomic neuropathy is often found in association with somatic polyneuropathy and may occur at an earlier stage resulting in smooth atrophic skin, loss of nails and sweating abnormalities of the feet. Plantar callus formation, particularly over the areas of the foot subject to high pressure, predates ulceration and may be a sensitive indicator of the presence of neuropathy. Loss of sudomotor function may also precipitate cracking of the skin and fissure formation, which may become secondarily infected. More advanced neuropathy may cause structural changes of the foot resulting from ligamentous laxity and muscular weakness; prominence of the metatarsal heads, crowding of the toes, and subluxation of the tarsal and metatarsal bones all may indicate advanced neuropathy.

Testing of vibration perception at the great toe is a reliable and sensitive indicator of the presence of diabetic neuropathy. This can be adequately performed using a 128-Hz tuning fork or using a hand-held biothesiometer. For documenting the progress of neuropathy, however, a more sophisticated device, such as the Vibratron, is required. This instrument allows quantitative assessment of peripheral large afferent fiber function, and deficits in vibration perception have been found to correlate well with other tests of neurologic function. Deficits of cold perception, which is conveyed by the small myelinated A δ fibers that also convey pain, can be a sensitive and reproducible assessment of peripheral small fiber function. However an inexpensive and reproducible

**TABLE 6–2.**

Common Conditions Resembling Diabetic Neuropathy

1. Distal symmetric neuropathy
   a. Inflammatory neuropathies (vasculitic, such as systemic lupus erythematosis, polyarteritis, and other connective tissue diseases; sarcoidosis; leprosy)
   b. Metabolic neuropathies (hypothyroidism, uremia, nutritional, acute intermittent porphyria)
   c. Toxic neuropathies (alcohol; drugs; heavy metals, such as lead, mercury, arsenic; industrial hydrocarbons)
   d. Other neuropathies (paraneoplastic, dysproteinemic, amyloid, hereditary)
2. Autonomic neuropathy
   a. Loss of perspiration
   b. Idiopathic orthostatic hypotension
   c. Shy-Drager syndrome (progressive autonomic failure)
3. Cranial neuropathy
   a. Carotid aneurysm
   b. Intracranial mass
   c. Elevated intracranial pressure
4. Radiculopathy
   a. Spinal cord/root compression
   b. Transverse myelitis
   c. Coagulopathies
   d. Shingles
5. Plexopathy
   a. Mass lesions
   b. Coagulopathies
   c. Cauda equina lesions (femoral neuropathy)
6. Mononeuropathy/mononeuropathy multiplex
   a. Compression neuropathies
   b. Inflammatory (vasculitic) neuropathies
   c. Hypothyroidism, acromegaly

method of assessment is not yet readily available. This is disappointing, because small fiber defects may occur early in diabetes and may be the first sign of the development of neuropathy. Defects of peripheral thermal sensation may occur independently of vibration perception and may reflect similar defects in the small peripheral autonomic fibers. The Neurometer has been a recent introduction in the assessment of distal symmetric neuropathy. It uses a variable constant current sine wave, which at differing frequencies may allow assessment of both small and large fiber function. Its usefulness in the routine assessment of the diabetic patient awaits evaluation. Light touch perception, which is a large fiber modality, can be accurately assessed using a set of graduated nylon filaments. These filaments, when applied to the areas of the foot at maximal risk of ulceration, may allow the at-risk patient to be identified. This examination need not take substantially longer than using a cotton wisp, particularly if only a 10-g filament is used, because this is probably the pressure threshold required to protect the foot from ulceration.

It is desirable to perform at least an annual complete neurologic history and physical examination to detect evidence of early peripheral neuropathy. Patient education about the risks of neuropathy and foot care at this stage may make a substantial impact in reducing sepsis, ulceration, and neuroarthropathy by permitting an appropriate management strategy to be instigated. Electrophysiologic testing assists in quantifying the degree of peripheral nerve damage and may be required to exclude other causes of neuropathy if the history (e.g., rapid progression) or the clinical findings (predominantly unilateral) are unusual. A complete examination consists of motor and sensory nerve conduction studies and needle electromyography (Table 6–3).

## Late Complications

Undetected asymptomatic neuropathy may first appear with complications such as foot ulceration, embedded foreign bodies, unrecognized trauma to the extremities, or neuroarthropathy (Charcot's joints).[14] Acute foot ulcerations result from ill-fitting shoes or a nonpainful foreign body that penetrates, abrades, or becomes embedded under the skin of the foot. Diminished or absent pain sensation also predisposes to accidental injury during nail trimming. Plantar ulcers, which always form at the calloused sites of maximum walking pressure, result from a combination of motor, cutaneous sensory, and proprioceptive deficits. Patients with long-standing diabetes and neuropathy are also predisposed to chronic venous stasis ulcers, vascular ulcers as a result of macrovascular insufficiency, and ischemic gangrene. Neuroarthropathy refers to the joint erosions, unrecognized fractures, demineralization, and devitalization of the bones of the foot resulting from routine daily weight-bearing activities when normal protective proprioceptive and nociceptive functions are impaired by neuropathy. In the early stages the foot is swollen and red but not necessarily painful, and a distal symmetric sensory deficit with loss of pain is clearly demonstrable. The patient may report recent relatively painless trauma, and radiographic examination may be unrevealing or show healed fractures; however, a follow-up x-ray examination a few days or weeks later reveal clear traumatic changes. The initial clinical appearance may be misdiagnosed as cellulitis despite a normal white blood cell count and differential and the absence of fever. In more advanced cases, demineralization and devitalization of bone may mimic osteomyelitis, but fever and leukocytosis are absent. With progression, shortening and widening of the foot is evident, and in the most advanced stages the foot may appear to be a "bag of bones," with numerous fractures and extensive demineralization and resorption of bone.

Finally, the combination of decreased sensation, unintentional self-inflicted trauma, ulceration, osteomyelitis, vascular insufficiency, diminished leukocyte function, and increased tissue glucose all predispose to se-

**TABLE 6–3.**

Polyneuropathy Protocol

---

I. Conduction studies*
   A. General
      1. Test most involved site if mild or moderate, least involved if severe.
      2. Warm limb if temperature is < 32°C; monitor and maintain temperature throughout study.
      3. Use reproducible recording and stimulation sites (either fixed distances or standard landmarks).
      4. Use supramaximal percutaneous stimulation.
   B. Motor studies
      1. Peroneal motor (extensor digitorum brevis); stimulate at ankle and knee. Record F response latency following distal antidromic stimulation.
      2. If abnormal, tibial motor (abductor hallucis); stimulate at ankle; record F response latency.
      3. If no responses: peroneal motor (anterior tibial); stimulate at fibula.
      4. Ulnar motor (hypothenar); stimulate below wrist and elbow. Record F response latency.
      5. Median motor (thenar); stimulate wrist and anticubital fossa. Record F response latency.
   C. Sensory studies
      1. Sural sensory (ankle); may occasionally require:
         a. Needle recording.
         b. Response averaging.
      2. Median sensory (index); stimulate wrist and elbow. If antidromic response absent or focal entrapment suspected, record (wrist) stimulating palm.
      3. Ulnar sensory (fifth digit); stimulate wrist. If antidromic response absent or superimposed on motor artifact, perform orthodromic study.
   D. Autonomic studies
      1. Skin potential responses (palmar and plantar surfaces of hand and foot, respectively); stimulate contralateral median nerve.
   E. Additional
      1. Additional motor or sensory nerves can be evaluated if findings are equivocal. Definite abnormalities should result in:
         a. Evaluation of opposite extremity.
         b. Proceed to evaluation of specific suspected abnormality.
II. Needle examination
   A. Representative muscles
      1. Anterior tibial, medial gastrocnemius, first dorsal interosseous (hand), and lumbar paraspinal muscles.
      2. If normal, intrinsic foot muscles should be examined.
      3. Any abnormalities should be confirmed by examination of at least one contralateral muscle.
   B. Grading
      1. Abnormal spontaneous activity should be graded subjectively (0 to >4+) using conventional criteria.
      2. Motor unit action potential amplitude, duration, configuration, and recruitment graded subjectively.

*Recording sites indicated by parentheses.*
*(From Rifkin H, Porte D, editors: Diabetes mellitus: Theory and practice, ed 4, New York, 1990, Elsevier Scientific, p 734. Used by permission.)*

---

rious and rapidly progressive foot infections, often involving combinations of aerobic and anaerobic organisms that are not only limb threatening but also life threatening.

# AUTONOMIC NEUROPATHY

Autonomic neuropathy can impair virtually any function modulated by the autonomic nervous system in diabetic patients.[11]

While neuropathy produces diffuse subclinical autonomic nervous system dysfunction, symptoms are usually confined to one or two organ systems, producing the discrete syndromes listed in Table 6–4.

## Cardiovascular Autonomic Neuropathy

Asymptomatic cardiovascular autonomic neuropathy often initially manifests as an absence of the normal sleep bradycardia in hospitalized patients or as a diminished pulse rate variation with inspiration-expiration during physical examination or electrocardiography (reduced sinus arrhythmia), both the result of early vagal involvement.[4, 26] Sympathetic cardiac denervation interferes with normal cardiovascular reactivity, thus diminishing exercise tolerance and hypersensitizing the heart to circulating catecholamines, predisposing to tachyarrhythmias and sudden death.[4, 26] Autonomic neuropathy is also believed to be responsible for increased frequency of painless myocardial infarctions in patients with longstanding diabetes.[8] Severe central and peripheral cardiovascular sympathetic insufficiency produces orthostatic hypotension, especially when uncontrolled hyperglycemia produces concomitant hypovolemia.[4, 26] Treatment of hypotension should be aimed toward the underlying cause (Fig 6–1). Elastic stockings, increased salt intake, mineralocorticoids, vasoconstrictors, a military antigravity suit, or atrial pacing all have been effective in carefully evaluated patients.[14]

## Gastrointestinal Autonomic Neuropathy

Nonspecific gastrointestinal (GI) symptoms occur with great frequency in diabetic patients, reflecting diffuse but subtle GI autonomic dysfunction.[14, 15] Dysphagia, retrosternal discomfort, and "heartburn" often reflect disordered esophageal motility that also occurs in many patients without any referable symptoms. Gastric autonomic nervous system dysfunction decreases vagus-mediated gastric acid secretion believed to be responsible for the decreased incidence of peptic ulcers in diabetic patients and delays gastric emptying. The latter defect produces major clinical symptoms such as anorexia, nausea, vomiting that may become uncontrollable, early satiety, and postprandial bloating and fullness. Undigested food may be vomited days after it was consumed. Delayed nutrient absorption resulting from gastric hypomotility complicates glycemic control with otherwise unexplained swings of plasma glucose levels ranging from severe hyperglycemia to hypoglycemia. Diagnosis requires solid-phase radionuclide gastric emptying studies. Dopamine antagonists or parasympathetic agonists are initiated when the gastric emptying time is prolonged (Fig 6–2). Small frequent feedings, with a major portion of calories administered in liquid form (e.g., "liquid breakfasts") allow gastric emptying that is gravity dependent rather than motility dependent.[14] High-fiber diets should be avoided because they delay gastric emptying.[14]

Diabetic enteropathy encompasses the clinical syndromes of diabetic constipation, diabetic diarrhea, and fecal incontinence, all of which reflect widespread abnormalities

**TABLE 6–4.**
Autonomic Neuropathy Syndromes

1. Cardiovascular autonomic neuropathy
   a. Resting sinus tachycardia without sinus arrhythmia (fixed heart rate)
   b. Exercise intolerance
   c. Painless myocardial infarction
   d. Orthostatic hypotension
   e. (?) Sudden death
2. Gastrointestinal autonomic neuropathy
   a. Esophageal dysfunction
   b. Autonomic gastropathy and delayed gastric emptying
   c. Diabetic diarrhea
   d. Constipation
   e. Fecal incontinence
3. Genitourinary autonomic neuropathy
   a. Erectile impotence
   b. Retrograde ejaculation with infertility
   c. Bladder dysfunction
4. Hypoglycemic unawareness
5. Sudomotor neuropathy
   a. Facial sweating
   b. Heat intolerance
   c. "Gustatory" sweating
   d. Distal anhydrosis

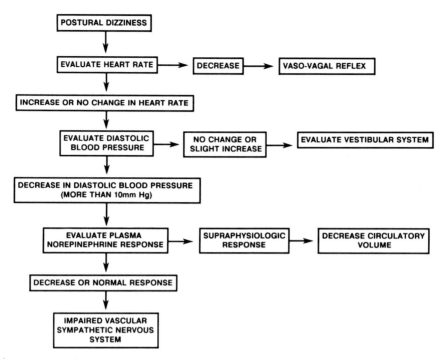

**FIG 6–1.**
Evaluation of postural dizziness in diabetic patients. *(From Rifkin H, Porte D, editors:* Diabetes mellitus, theory and practice, *ed 4, New York, 1990, Elsevier Scientific, p 751. Used by permission.)*

in the intestinal autonomic nervous system. Constipation is the most frequent GI complaint, occurring in 60% of diabetic patients. Stool softeners and judicious use of laxatives or cathartics are usually effective, although occasionally dopamine antagonists are indicated. Other patients suffer from diarrhea, often alternating with bouts of constipation. Diabetic diarrhea is painless, nocturnal, and associated with fecal incontinence.[14] The symptoms vary, depending on the various operative pathogenetic factors, which may include intestinal hypermotility because of diminished sympathetic inhibition, hypomotility with bacterial overgrowth, pancreatic exocrine insufficiency (particularly in type I diabetes), bile salt malabsorption, or "diabetic sprue" in which steatorrhea accompanies a mucosal pattern resembling that of gluten sensitivity. Diagnostic tests to define the contributing pathogenetic factors determine appropriate treatment; a positive hydrogen breath test supports a therapeutic trial of broad-spectrum antibiotics like ampicillin, tetracycline, and metronidazole, whereas evidence of bile salt

malabsorption suggests the use of bile salt sequestering agents (e.g., cholestyramine), both of which are effective in properly selected patients. Hypermotility is managed with loperamide. Finally, clonidine may be considered if all other treatments are unsuccessful (Fig 6–3).[14] These intestinal disorders and their treatment (which together may affect caloric absorption) can affect glycemic control, which should be monitored closely. Fecal incontinence, which is also usually nocturnal, reflects impaired sensation of rectal distention, and has been managed effectively with biofeedback techniques in a small series of patients.[14]

## Genitourinary Autonomic Neuropathy

Retrograde ejaculation, erectile impotence, and diabetic cystopathy all represent impaired autonomic nervous system function of the genitourinary tract. About 50% of diabetics report some degree of sexual dysfunction, but the problem in women has never been well studied.[14] Retrograde ejaculation reflects loss of the coordinated closure

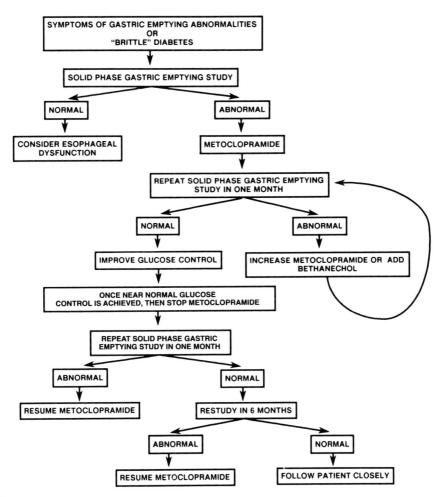

**FIG 6–2.**
Evaluation and treatment of gastric atony. *(From Rifkin H, Porte D, editors:* Diabetes mellitus, theory and practice, *ed 4, New York, 1990, Elsevier Scientific, p 749. Used by permission.)*

of the internal sphincter and relaxation of the external vesicle sphincter during ejaculation. Retrograde ejaculation appears as infertility, and the diagnosis is confirmed by documenting ejaculate azoospermia and the presence of motile sperm in the postcoital urine, which have been successfully employed for artificial insemination.

Erectile impotence may be psychogenic, endocrine, vascular, drug related, or neuropathic, and an appropriate diagnosis is essential for effective treatment. Psychogenic impotence and organic impotence are differentiated by lack of partner specificity, the absence of morning erections with organic causes, and diagnostic sleep studies. Sex steroid imbalances, hypogonadotrophism, and

hyperprolactinemia should be investigated by appropriate endocrine studies. Vascular insufficiency is usually seen in the form of femoral bruits, although localized obstruction of the penile artery has been reported and can be excluded only by measurements of the brachial/penile blood pressure ratio using Doppler-flow studies. Drugs known to produce impotence include various antihypertensives, anticholinergics, antipsychotics, antidepressants, narcotics, barbiturates, alcohol, and amphetamines. Neuropathic impotence is generally but not always accompanied by other manifestations of diabetic neuropathy. Proximal or localized vascular obstruction is managed by vascular surgical techniques. Drug-induced impotence is man-

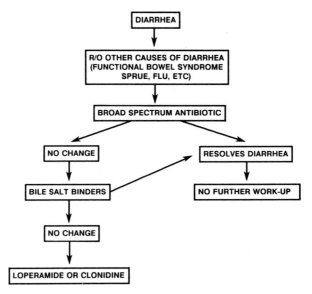

**FIG 6–3.**
Evaluation and treatment of diabetic diarrhea. *(From Rifkin H, Porte D, editors:* Diabetes mellitus, theory and practice, *ed 4, New York, 1990, Elsevier Scientific, p 750. Used by permission.)*

aged by altering the treatment regimen whenever possible. Neuropathic impotence is presently managed by appropriate counseling and the use of penile prostheses when indicated (Fig 6–4).[14]

Autonomic neuropathy of the bladder begins with the selective involvement of autonomic afferent nerves, resulting in diminished sensation of bladder fullness and a resultant reduction in urinary frequency.

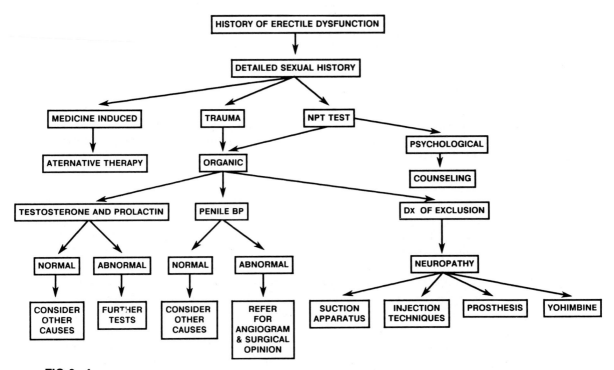

**FIG 6–4.**
Evaluation and treatment of erectile dysfunction in diabetic patients. *(From Rifkin H, Porte D, editors:* Diabetes mellitus, theory and practice, *ed 4, New York, 1990, Elsevier Scientific, p 746. Used by permission.)*

With efferent involvement, urination is incomplete, leading to poor stream, dribbling, and overflow incontinence. Residual urine predisposes the patient to urinary tract infections. Management involves scheduled voluntary urination, with or without the Crude maneuver, followed by cholinergic-stimulating drugs such as bethanecol, periodic catheterization, and bladder-neck resection of the internal sphincter in more advanced cases (Fig 6–5).[14]

## Hypoglycemic Unawareness

The diminished epinephrine response to hypoglycemia in chronic diabetes is generally believed to be the result of autonomic neuropathy of the adrenal medulla, which can blunt the usual adrenergic warning signs of impending hypoglycemia.[14] This "hypoglycemic unawareness" predisposes to severe hypoglycemic reactions and is generally conceded to be a major contraindication to intensive insulin treatment.[14]

## Sudomotor Neuropathy

Diabetic autonomic sudomotor dysfunction produces an asymptomatic distal anhydrosis in a stocking-glove distribution similar to that of distal symmetric polyneuropathy. This diminishes the thermoregulatory reserve, predisposing to heatstroke and hyperthermia, and produces a compensatory central hyperhidrosis that is often bothersome to the patient. Management is confined to avoidance of heat stress. An uncommon autonomic sudomotor syndrome is gustatory sweating, which consists of profuse sweating of the face during eating, often elicited by large meals, or, less commonly, specific foods such as cheese. Management consists of avoiding specific offending foods.[14]

## FOCAL NEUROPATHIES

Neural deficits corresponding to the distribution of single or multiple peripheral nerves (mononeuropathy and mononeuropathy multiplex), cranial nerves, areas of the brachial or lumbosacral plexuses (plexopathy), or the nerve roots (radiculopathy) are relatively uncommon, of sudden onset, and generally but not always self-limiting in diabetic patients.[1] Commonly the third cranial nerve is affected, accompanied by unilateral pain, diplopia, and ptosis but with pupillary sparing, in a syndrome that is termed *diabetic ophthalmoplegia*.[1] The differential diagnosis includes an aneurysm of the internal carotid artery and myasthenia gravis. Radiculopathy appears as a bandlike thoracic or abdominal pain that is often misdiagnosed as an acute intrathoracic or intra-abdominal emergency. Femoral neuropathy in diabetic patients often involves motor and sensory deficits at the level of the sacral plexus and the femoral nerve, with the relative excess of motor versus sensory involvement differentiating diabetic femoral neuropathy from that seen in other conditions.[1] Autopsy studies

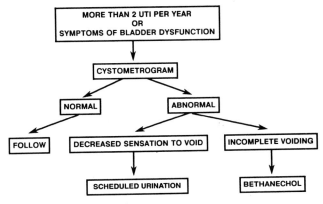

**FIG 6–5.**
Evaluation of diabetic autonomic dysfunction. *(From Rifkin H, Porte D, editors:* Diabetes mellitus, theory and practice, *ed 4, New York, 1990, Elsevier Scientific, p 745. Used by permission.)*

suggest that both diabetic femoral neuropathy and third nerve palsy constitute focal ischemic insults to the peripheral nervous system, presumably from diabetic vasculopathy.[1] Other mononeuropathies mimicking the compression neuropathies seen in nondiabetic individuals, such as carpal tunnel syndrome,[10] probably represent an increased susceptibility of the nerves of diabetics to mechanical or ischemic injury. Tarsal tunnel syndrome, secondary to compression of the posterior tibial nerve at the tarsal tunnel, manifests as unilateral pain and paresthesias in the medial aspect of the ankle and foot. Electrodiagnostic testing can assist in the diagnosis (Fig 6–6). Management of focal neuropathies involves excluding other causes, such as nerve entrapment or compression, and symptomatic palliation pending possible spontaneous resolution.[1]

## PATHOGENESIS OF DIABETIC NEUROPATHY

Both vascular and metabolic factors are implicated in the pathogenesis of diabetic neuropathy. In both the focal and diffuse diabetic neuropathies, the most important lesion is loss of myelinated and unmyelinated nerve fibers.[9] As mentioned previously, fragmentary but somewhat compelling evidence suggests that femoral and some cranial neuropathies constitute ischemic injury to diabetic nerves.[9] Recent autopsy studies show that nerve fiber loss exhibits a somewhat nonhomogeneous or focal distribution even in diffuse diabetic neuropathy and are interpreted to indicate that ischemia may play a prominent role in distal symmetric neuropathy as well.[9] Furthermore, animal studies have suggested that regulation of the microcirculation and oxygen delivery are faulty in diabetic peripheral nerves.[16, 17] In addition, extraneural arteriovenous shunting may be characteristic of diabetic patients with neuropathy, further contributing to impaired oxygen delivery to peripheral nerves.[30] A recently reported study of nerve biopsies from patients with diabetic neuropathy suggests that focal nerve fiber loss and by inference ischemic injury is more prominent in type II diabetes than in type I diabetes.[22] The ischemia and hypoxia hypothesis may also be related to other pathogenic mechanisms (Fig 6–7). It has been known for more than a decade that diabetic neuropathy is more common in patients who have poor metabolic control and that improved

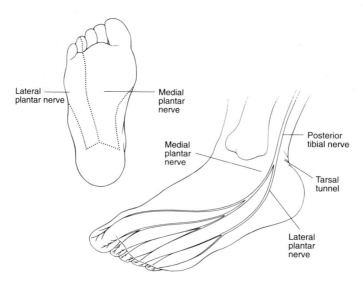

**FIG 6–6.**
Compression of posterior tibial nerve at tarsal tunnel or of plantar nerves causes sensory impairment in sole of foot and weakness of intrinsic pedal musculature. *(Modified from Aguayo AJ: Neuropathy due to compression and entrapment, in Dyck PJ, Thomas PK, Lambert EH, editors:* Peripheral neuropathy, *Philadelphia, 1975, WB Saunders. Used by permission.)*

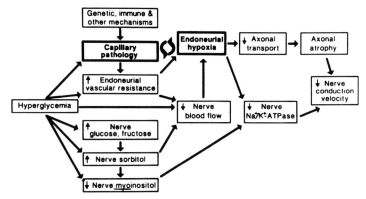

**FIG 6–7.**
Suggested pathogenesis of diabetic neuropathy. *(From Low PA, Tuck RR, Takeuchi M: Nerve microenvironment due to diabetic neuropathy, in Dyck PJ, Thomas PK, Asbury A, et al, editors:* Diabetic neuropathy, *Philadelphia, 1987, WB Saunders. Used by permission.)*

diabetic control improves nerve function in diabetic patients and animals.[12] Recent studies in animals and humans have demonstrated a cascade of metabolic abnormalities in diabetic peripheral nerves initiated by hyperglycemia and involving nerve sorbitol, *myo*-inositol, and sodium-potassium–adenosine triphosphatase, which explains the acutely reversible component of nerve conduction slowing and contributes to the development of highly characteristic neu-roanatomic lesions in both diabetic animals and patients (Fig 6–8).[13, 14] Furthermore, correction of these metabolic defects with al-dose reductase inhibitors, which prevents the initial conversion of excess neural glucose to sorbitol and improves nerve function,[13] also reverses many of these characteristic structural abnormalities and promotes nerve fiber regeneration.[18] Other metabolic abnormalities that may be instrumental in the pathogenesis of diabetic neuropathy include

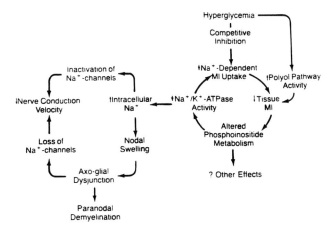

**FIG 6–8.**
Postulated relationship between hyperglycemia, polyol pathway, *myo*-inositol *(MI)*, Na$^+$-K$^+$-ATPase, and nerve conduction in diabetes. Hyperglycemia reduces nerve MI by competitively inhibiting its uptake and increasing polyol pathway activity by an indirect and yet unexplained mechanism related to the increased conversion of glucose to sorbitol by the enzyme aldose reductase. The reduction in nerve MI leads to a decrease in Na$^+$-K$^+$-ATPase activity, possibly through an alteration in phosphoinositide metabolism. Because MI uptake in nerve is sodium dependent, a self-reinforcing metabolic cycle involving MI is likely. Acute reduction in nerve conduction velocity in diabetes is ascribed in part to impaired Na$^+$-K$^+$-ATPase activity. A further consequence of impaired Na$^+$-K$^+$-ATPase activity is a reduction in sodium-dependent amino acid uptake; interference with other sodium-linked processes is probable but as yet unproved. Defects resulting from reduced nerve MI levels other than those mediated by changes in Na$^+$-K$^+$-ATPase await further investigation. *(From Rifkin H, Porte D, editors:* Diabetes mellitus, theory and practice, *ed 4, New York, 1990, Elsevier Scientific, p 715. Used by permission.)*

superoxide radical formation, abnormalities in lipid or amino acid metabolism, protein glycation, or blunting of neurotrophic action.[14]

## MANAGEMENT OF DIABETIC NEUROPATHY

The present treatment for diabetic neuropathy is symptomatic, palliative, and supportive, with primary emphasis on prophylactic measures to prevent late complications of neuropathy. In most cases of distal symmetric polyneuropathy, symptoms are generally mild unless complications ensue. Early diagnosis of asymptomatic neuropathy is essential for effective prophylaxis. In the neuropathic patient, reinforcement of good foot care and recognition of the exquisite vulnerability of their feet is paramount.[2, 3] Self-examination of the feet should be performed on a routine basis and with increased frequency during periods of unusual ambulation or when wearing new shoes. Areas of erythema that persist more than several minutes after removing footwear are cause for concern. Cushioned footwear should be worn, and neuropathic patients should never walk barefoot. New shoes should be broken in gradually. Toenails should be trimmed by a podiatrist. Callus formation over weight-bearing areas indicates the need for corrective footwear to redistribute weight bearing. Plantar ulcers should be managed by eliminating weight bearing with special walking casts or bed rest. Refractory or recurrent ulcers may be managed by surgical removal of the offending metatarsal bone. Neuroarthropathy is managed by reduced ambulation and weight bearing and cushioned footwear. Infection must be treated aggressively with appropriate consultation from infectious disease specialists. Antibiotics effective against anaerobic organisms should be included in the treatment regimen. Vascular bypass surgery or percutaneous angioplasty should be considered if arterial insufficiency is a major contributing factor.[2, 3, 14]

Mildly or intermittently painful or pares-thetic symptoms may signify neural repair (at times these symptoms are exacerbated when poorly controlled diabetes is brought under tighter control) or worsening neuropathy. Even severely painful symptoms, however, generally remit spontaneously within a few months, although they persist in a sizable minority of patients.[28]

The management of various autonomic syndromes is dictated by the respective pathophysiology, as alluded to previously, and involves various maneuvers to compensate for autonomic nervous system dysfunction, such as small frequent feedings and liquid meals for delayed gastric emptying, or mineralocorticoids for orthostatic hypotension. Focal neuropathies of vascular origin are generally self-limited, although rehabilitation improves the return of function in some cases. Focal neuropathies as compression sites respond to conventional protective measures, such as compression-limiting splints and pads, or surgical release procedures.[14]

A role for intensified hyperglycemia control is proposed by some investigators in the management or prevention of neuropathy, without conclusive substantiating evidence in the form of controlled clinical trials.[12] Dietary supplements of *myo*-inositol have been suggested on the basis of animal studies, but fragmentary clinical experience has been inconclusive.[12] Aldose reductase inhibitors, which block the accumulation of sorbitol and loss of *myo*-inositol from nerves and improve conduction in diabetic animals and patients, are still undergoing clinical trials in symptomatic neuropathy and are therefore not presently available.[12, 18, 23] Painful neuropathy has been treated with transcutaneous stimulation[29] and various drugs, including standard analgesics and drugs normally used to treat pain in other conditions. Although not substantiated by controlled clinical trials, phenytoin,[6] carbamazepine,[21, 31] and mexiletine[8] have been used, based on their membrane-stabilizing properties. Tricylic antidepressants, either alone[24] or in combination with fluphenazine, have also been reported but without supporting controlled clinical trials.[15] Use of the selective serotonin reuptake inhibitor paroxetine has been recommended, although it may not be as effective as imipramine.[24] Topical capsaicin cream was recently proved effective in a multicenter, double-blind trial,[5] validating earlier claims of its utility in treating painful diabetic neuropathy.[20, 22] In contrast, a controlled study of pentoxifylline revealed it was no more effective than placebo in the treatment of diabetic neuropathy.[7]

## REFERENCES

1. Asbury AK: Focal and multifocal neuropathies of diabetes, in Dyck PJ, Thomas PK, Ashbury AK, et al, editors: *Diabetic neuropathy*, Philadelphia, 1987, WB Saunders.

2. Boulton AJM: The diabetic foot: neuropathic in aetiology? *Diabetic Med* 7:852–858, 1990.

3. Boulton AJM: Clinical presentation and management of diabetic neuropathy and foot ulceration, *Diabetic Med* 8:S52–S57, 1991.

4. Broadstone VL, Roy T, Self M, et al: Cardiovascular autonomic dysfunction: diagnosis and prognosis, *Diabetic Med* 8:S88–S93, 1991.

5. Capsaicin Study Group: Treatment of painful diabetic neuropathy with topical capsaicin: a multicenter, double-blind, vehicle-controlled study, *Arch Intern Med* 151:2225–2229, 1991.

6. Chadda VS, Mathur MS: Double-blind study of the effects of diphenylhydantoin sodium on diabetic neuropathy, *J Assoc Phys India* 26:403, 1978.

7. Cohen SM, Matthews T: Pentoxifylline in the treatment of distal diabetic neuropathy, *Angiology* 42:741–746, 1991.

8. Dejgard A, Petersen P, Kastrup J: Mexilitine for treatment of chronic painful diabetic neuropathy, *Lancet* 2:9–11, 1985.

9. Dyck PJ: Pathology, in Dyck PJ, Thomas PK, Asbury AK, et al, editors: *Diabetic neuropathy*, Philadelphia, 1987, WB Saunders.

10. Dyck PJ, Karnes J, O'Brien PC: Diagnosis, staging, and classification of diabetic neuropathy and associations with other complications, in Dyck PJ, Thomas PK, Asbury AK, et al, editors: *Diabetic neuropathy*, Philadelphia, 1987, WB Saunders.

11. Fagius J: Aspects of autonomic neurophysiology in diabetic polyneuropathy: a brief review, *Diabetic Med* 10:S58–S62, 1991.

12. Greene DA: Glycemic control, in Dyck PJ, Thomas PK, Asbury AK, et al, editors: *Diabetic neuropathy*, Philadelphia, 1987, WB Saunders.

13. Greene DA, Lattimer SA, Sima AAF: Sorbitol, phosphoinositides, and sodium-potassium-ATPase in the pathogenesis of diabetic complications, *N Engl J Med* 316:599, 1987.

14. Greene DA, Sima AAF, Albers J, et al: Diabetic neuropathy, in Rifkin H, Porte D, editors, *Diabetes mellitus, theory and practice*, ed 4, 1990, St Louis, Mosby-Year Book.

15. Greene DA, Sima AAF, Pfeifer MA, et al: Diabetic neuropathy, *Annu Rev Med* 41:303–317, 1990.

16. Low PA, Lagerlund TD, McManis PG: Nerve blood flow and oxygen delivery in normal, diabetic, and ischemic neuropathy, *Int Rev Neurobiol* 31:355–429, 1989.

17. Low PA, Tuck RR, Takeuchi M: Nerve microenvironment in diabetic neuropathy, in Dyck PJ, Thomas PK, Asbury AK, et al: editors: *Diabetic neuropathy*, Philadelphia, 1987, WB Saunders.

18. Masson EA, Boulton AJM: Aldose reductase inhibitors in the treatment of diabetic neuropathy: a review of the rationale and clinical evidence, *Drugs* 39:190–202, 1990.

19. Melton LJ, Dyck PJ: Epidemiology, in Dyck PJ, Thomas PK, Asbury AK, et al, editors: *Diabetic neuropathy*, Philadelphia, 1987, WB Saunders.

20. Ross DR, Varipapa RJ: Treatment of painful diabetic neuropathy with topical capsaicin, *N Engl J Med* 321:474–475, 1989.

21. Rull JA, Quibrera R, Gonzalez-Millan H, et al: Symptomatic treatment of peripheral diabetic neuropathy with carbamazepine (Tegretol): double-blind crossover trial, *Diabetologia* 5:215–218, 1969.

22. Scheffler NM, Sheitel PL, Lipton MN: Treatment of painful diabetic neuropathy with capsaicin 0.075%, *J Am Podiatr Med Assoc* 81:288–293, 1991.

23. Sima AA, Nathaniel V, Greene DA: Peripheral nerve repair following ARI treatment, *Adv Exp Med Biol* 291:265–270, 1991.

24. Sindrup SH, Gram LF, Brosen K, et al: The selective serotonin reuptake inhibitor paroxetine is effective in the treatment of diabetic neuropathy symptoms, *Pain* 42:135–144, 1990.

25. Sindrup SH, Gram LF, Skjold T, et al: Clomipramine vs desipramine vs placebo in the treatment of diabetic neuropathy symptoms: a double-blind cross-over study, *Br J Clin Pharmacol* 30:683–691, 1990.

26. Stevens MJ, Watkins PJ: Diabetic autonomic neuropathy, *Acta Diabetol Lat* 28:105–112, 1991.

27. Thomas PK, Brown PJ: Diabetic polyneuropathy, in Dyck PJ, Thomas PK, Asbury AK, et al, editors: *Diabetic neuropathy*, Philadelphia, 1987, WB Saunders.

28. Thomas PK, Scadding JW: Treatment of pain in diabetic neuropathy, in Dyck PJ, Thomas PK,

Asbury AK, et al, editors: *Diabetic neuropathy*, Philadelphia, 1987, WB Saunders.

29. Thorsteinsson G, Stonnington HH, Stillwell GK, et al: Transcutaneous electrical stimulation: a double-blind trial of its efficacy for pain, *Arch Phys Med Rehabil* 58:8–14, 1977.

30. Ward JD, Boulton AJM: Peripheral vascular abnormalities and diabetic neuropathy, in Dyck PJ, Thomas PK, Asbury AK, et al, editors: *Diabetic neuropathy*, Philadelphia, 1987, WB Saunders.

31. Wilton TD: Tegretol in the treatment of diabetic neuropathy, *S Afr Med J* 48:869–873, 1974.

# CHAPTER 7

# Charcot Foot

**Lee J. Sanders, D.P.M.**
**Robert G. Frykberg, D.P.M.**

The Charcot foot is a poorly understood and frequently overlooked complication of diabetes mellitus that poses a formidable diagnostic and treatment challenge for all members of the health care team. The probability of successful management is greatly increased with heightened awareness and thorough understanding of the pathogenesis, natural history, and anatomic patterns of neuropathic osteoarthropathy. Identification of high-risk individuals facilitates early implementation of management strategies directed toward prevention and minimization of foot deformity, joint instability, ulceration, disability, and surgery.

Early recognition and timely treatment will often result in a more satisfactory outcome. The key to treatment is prevention, with avoidance of further trauma until the bone and soft tissues heal. The aim of treatment should be to obtain stability of the foot and to avoid excessive pressure on the skin from a bony prominence.

Since William Reily Jordan's linkage of neuropathic arthropathy of the foot and ankle with diabetes mellitus in 1936, the number of case reports has steadily increased.[21-24, 38, 53, 93] The growing number of cases reflects the seriousness of this disorder, as well as increased recognition of Charcot's joints.

## CHARCOT'S PERSPECTIVE

During the last third of the 19th century, Jean-Martin Charcot's clinicoanatomic studies of patients with tabes dorsalis at the Salpêtrière enabled him to describe a distinct pathologic entity, the arthropathy of ataxia. He[18, 19, 20] noted that "among the diverse conditions that may develop in the extremities as a result of certain traumatic or spontaneous lesions of the peripheral nerves, some as we know, have a predilection for the joints. This group of arthropathies . . . is frequently discussed today as an example of various nutritional disturbances that sometimes affect the distribution of nerve trunks affected by some alteration of a greater or lesser degree . . . To begin with, we shall note one more time the absence of any external cause, traumatic or otherwise . . . As for the site, the arthropathy . . . showed no preference to one side . . . It always started unexpectedly, rather suddenly, without precipitating cause."

Charcot[18-20] believed that lesions of the spinal cord, particularly of the gray matter, were responsible for disorders of the skin, the muscles, and the bones and joints commonly associated with the tabetic arthropathies.[46] "The irritative lesions of the spinal cord . . . react sometimes on the periphery, and determine various *nutritive* disorders . . . The bones and articulations do not appear to escape this law. It follows that the arthropathies of locomotor ataxia would be . . .one of the forms of these articular affections, developed under the more or less direct influence of the spinal centre."[19] His concept of a *nutritive* trophic regulation of bones and joints, mediated by the spinal cord, became the basis of the *French theory*, for the etiology of arthropathy seen in ataxic patients.[11-13, 18-20, 46] Charcot's theory was vehemently opposed by the German surgeons Volkmann and Virchow, who believed that the arthropathy of ataxia was nothing more than a "traumatic arthritis caused by the manner of locomotion peculiar to these patients."[19] Their concept became known as the *German*, mechanical or neurotraumatic theory.[11-13, 27]

Charcot described his observations of a sudden and unexpected arthropathy, which often began without apparent cause. Lancinating pains in the limbs often preceded the joint affection. He described a sudden onset of generalized tumefaction of the limb with rapid changes in the articular surfaces of the joint. Crepitations in the joint would occur within a few days after the onset and would normally precede the development of the characteristic motor incoordination of tabes. He argued that these arthropathies did not result exclusively from the distention of the ligaments and capsules of the joints or from the awkward gaits of these patients. "Anatomically the enormous wear and tear shown by the heads of the bones, the extensive looseness of the ligaments of the joints, and the frequent occurrence of luxations seem to distinguish these arthropathies from the ordinary type of osteoarthritis."[19]

Charcot's contribution to the understanding of spinal arthropathies was recognized in the *Rapport du Congrès* (Transactions of Congress) published in London in 1882, where it was written that "these bone changes constitute a distinct pathological entity. They deserve the name of 'Charcot's joint.' "[46] Accordingly, this term has been perpetuated to describe the bone and joint changes associated with all of the neuropathic arthropathies.

Charcot reasoned that "behind the dis-

ease of the joint there was a disease far more important in character, which in reality dominated the situation."[19] This reasoning applies equally well to diabetes mellitus with its neuropathic influence and ravaging effects on the bones and joints of the foot and ankle.

## DISORDERS PRODUCING CHARCOT JOINT

A variety of disorders affecting the spinal cord and peripheral nerves have been reported to destroy the protective mechanisms of joints and interfere with the "nutritive" trophic regulation of bone.[11-13, 18-20, 27, 46, 94, 99] The mechanisms of destruction may be precipitated by a single injury or by repetitive moderate stress applied to the bones and joints of an insensate foot and ankle. The results are fractures, effusions, and ligamentous laxity, followed by erosion of articular cartilage, fragmentation, luxation, disintegration, and collapse of the foot. The presence of peripheral neuropathy and the clinical and laboratory evidence of diabetes mellitus,[41-44, 69, 74] tabes dorsalis,[15, 77, 95] leprosy,[13, 44, 47, 100] syringomyelia,[15, 44, 52, 77, 78] spina bifida,[13, 77, 78] meningomyelcoele,[77] congenital insensitivity to pain,[44, 77] chronic alcoholism,[7, 77] spinal cord injury and compression,[18-20, 44, 46, 52] and peripheral nerve injuries[57, 77] complete the picture of neuroarthropathy, or bona fide Charcot joint. The key characteristic that all of these disorders have in common is the absence or decrease of pain sensation in the presence of uninterrupted physical activity.

As the number of cases of tabes dorsalis has declined, diabetes mellitus has emerged as the leading cause of neuropathic arthropathy today.[41-44, 69, 72] The importance of the diabetic form of neuropathic arthropathy was established in 1955 in a report by Miller and Lichtman[69] at the Cook County Hospital and Chicago Medical School. They[69] noted that "whereas tabes of syphilitic origin was formerly the usual cause of these painless deformities of the feet, with complicating soft tissue infections, ulcers and osteomyelitis, the diabetic neuropathic foot is now showing the higher incidence. Perhaps there is greater alertness in recognition."

## PREVALENCE AND PATIENT CHARACTERISTICS

The prevalence of diagnosed neuropathic bone and joint disease associated with diabetes mellitus has been reported to be from 0.08% to 7.5%.[4, 38, 75, 93] Pogonowska et al.[75] reported on a clinical and radiologic survey of 242 patients in Houston, Texas. They noted 6.8% of the cases had bone abnormalities classified as "diabetic osteopathy." Forgács in a comprehensive literature review of data on 237 patients estimated that diabetic neuropathic osteoarthropathy (DNOAP) occurs in 0.3% to 0.5% of all diabetic patients.[38] Radiographic evidence of lower limb bone and joint changes was found in 29% of 333 diabetics with peripheral neuropathy, reported by Cofield et al.[24] It is very likely that there are many more cases of DNOAP that go undetected or misdiagnosed.[41-44]

The average age reported for the onset of DNOAP is approximately 57 years, with the majority of patients in their fifth and sixth decades.[4, 22-24, 38, 69, 84, 93] Of greater significance, the average duration of diabetes at the time of diagnosis of neuropathic bone changes is approximately 15 years, with 80% of the patients being diabetic for more than 10 years and 60% more than 15 years.[4, 22-24, 38, 84, 93] Clohisy and Thompson[22] reported on a homogeneous group of 18 adult juvenile-onset diabetics with neuropathic arthropathy, an average age of 33.5 years, and a 20-year history of diabetes mellitus. Age therefore does not appear to be as important a factor in the development of DNOAP as the duration of diabetes mellitus (Table 7-1).

Bilateral involvement has been reported to occur in 5.9% to 39.3% of the heterogeneous cases.[23, 69, 84, 93] Seventy-five percent of the cases reported by Clohisy and Thompson[22] had bilateral involvement, with a very

## TABLE 7-1.

Reported Characteristics of Diabetics With Neuropathic Osteoarthropathy*

| Reference | No. of Cases Reported | Age (yr) (range) | Duration DM[†] (yr) (range) | % Bilateral Involvement |
|---|---|---|---|---|
| Bailey and Root[4] | 17 | 56 (30-69) | 11.5 | 23.5 4/17 |
| Miller and Lichtman[69] | 17 | 53 | | 5.9 1/17 |
| Sinha et al.[93] | 101 | 2/3s 50s-60s (20-79) | 83% > 10 65% > 15 | 23.8 24/101 |
| Clouse et al.[23] | 90 | 55 (25-78) | 18 (1.5-43) | 18 |
| Forgács[38] | 23 | 63 (48-79) | 14.8 (2-32) | |
| Cofield et al.[24] | 96 | 56 (27-79) | 81% > 10 16 (1-40) | 21 20/96 |
| Clohisy and Thompson[22] | 18 | 33.5 (25-52) | 20 | 75 14/18 |
| Sanders and Mrdjenovich[84] | 28 | 79% 50s-60s 57.2 (36-70) | 78% > 10 59% > 15 15.1 (1-27) | 39.3 11/28 |

*Modified from Sanders LJ, Frykberg R: Diabetic neuropathic osteoarthropathy: the Charcot foot, in The high risk foot in diabetes mellitus, New York, 1991, Churchill Livingstone.
[†]DM = diabetes mellitus.

high incidence of serious fractures of the ankle and the tarsal bones. There does not appear to be a significant difference in sex distribution, with men and women affected
equally.

## NATURAL HISTORY OF CHARCOT FOOT

Various descriptions of the course of
bone and joint changes associated with neuropathic arthropathies have appeared in the
literature over the last century. The terms
atrophic, destructive, and hyperemic have
been used to describe acute or early radiographic findings. Hypertrophic, reparative,
proliferative, sclerotic, and quiescent all are
terms used to describe chronic or late
findings.[41–44, 59, 90, 95] These descriptions
are based on clinical, radiologic, and histologic observations, as well as the chronicity
of disease. Norman et al.[74] suggested that

neuropathic joints be classified as acute or
chronic, on the basis of the suddenness of
their onset and speed of development.
They[74] believed that "since both reaction to
injury and repair occur simultaneously in
the joint two separate phases of development
do not take place." What seems to link these
opposite states is the process of bony resorption and repair, as determined by the balance of osteoclastic and osteoblastic activity
(Fig 7–1).

The acute phase of neuroarthropathy is
often precipitated by minor trauma and is
characterized by swelling, local heat,
erythema, laxity of ligaments, joint effusion,
and bone resorption. Early findings may be
indistinguishable from those of osteoarthritis
and infection. Nearly all reports confirm the
role of trauma in initiating the evolution of
neuropathic osteoarthropathy in patients
with an underlying neurologic deficit.

Newman[71] suggested that the earliest
changes in the evolution of neuropathic

**MINOR TRAUMA**   STAGE OF DEVELOPMENT

**REST AND IMMOBIL-IZATION**   STAGES OF COALESCENCE AND RECONSTRUCTION

Swelling and Joint Effusion
Local Elevation in Skin Temperature
Bone Resorption & Softening from Hyperemia
Osteolysis  and Osteopenia
Ligaments Weakened by Hyperemic Resorption
Abnormal Joint Alignment (subluxation)
Increased Joint Mobility
Erosion of Cartilage & Subchondral Bone
Dislocation and  Fragmentation of Bone
Bone and Cartilage Debris (detritus)
Hemorrhage into Periarticular Tissues

Absorption of Fine Debris
Periosteal New Bone Formation
Fusion and Rounding of
Large Fragments
Exuberant (metaplastic) Bone
Decreased Joint Mobility
*** Increased Stabilization ***
Increased Bone Density and Sclerosis
Deformity

RESORPTION OF BONE

REPAIR

ATROPHIC PHASE
(DESTRUCTIVE OR HYPEREMIC CHANGES)
ACUTE (EARLY) FINDINGS
ACTIVE

HYPERTROPHIC PHASE
(REPARATIVE OR SCLEROTIC CHANGES)
CHRONIC (LATE) FINDINGS
QUIESCENT

*LJS '92*

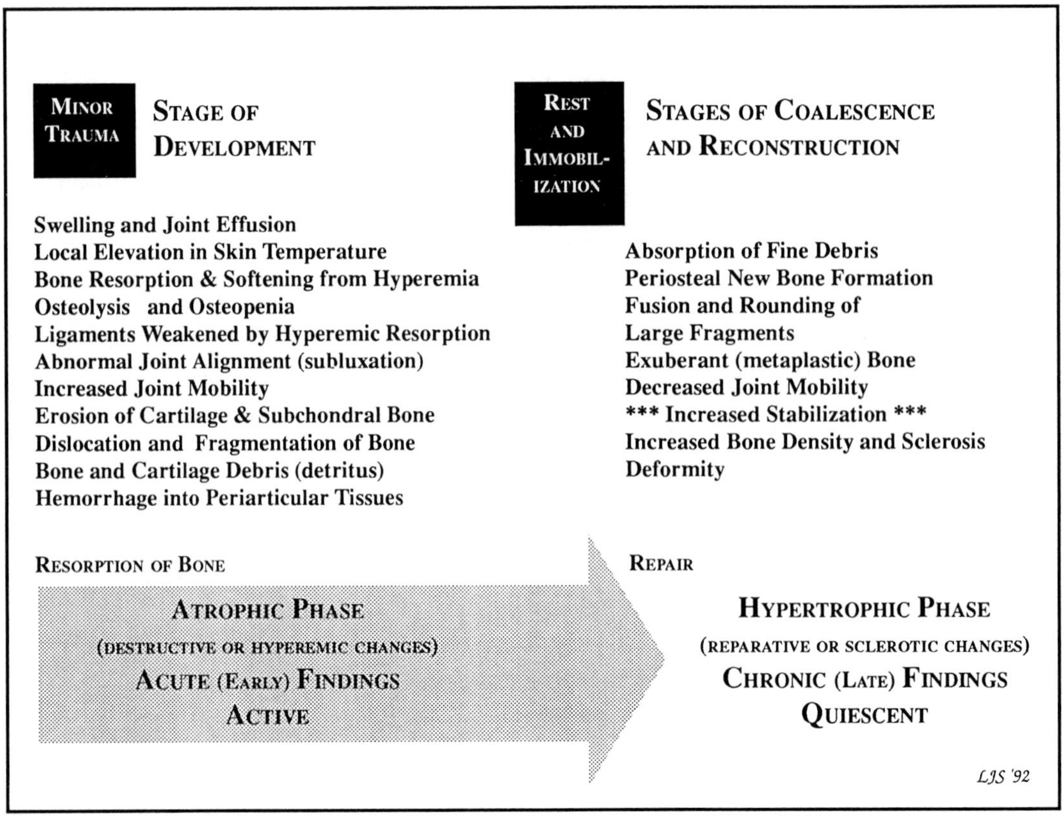

**FIG 7–1.**
Natural history of Charcot foot.

joints involve the soft tissues. He postulated that gross neuropathic changes in the ligaments were responsible for spontaneous dislocation of the foot, which he observed in five cases occurring without bone destruction. In those cases of neuropathic osteoarthropathy that do not begin with spontaneous fractures, ligamentous lesions may be of paramount importance, leading to spontaneous dislocation of the foot. Ligaments and joint capsule are thought to be stretched by the abnormal stresses applied to the joints, allowing them to go beyond their normal range of motion. They may be further weakened at their insertions into bone by hyperemic resorption allowing complete dislocation to take place.[52]

Eichenholtz[34] divided the disease process into three radiographically distinct stages: development, coalescence, and reconstruction. The *stage of development* represents the acute, destructive period, which is distinguished by joint effusions, soft tissue edema, subluxation, formation of bone and cartilage debris (detritus), intra-articular fractures, and fragmentation of bone. This phase of bone and joint destruction is induced by minor trauma and aggravated by persistent ambulation on an insensitive foot. The consequence of trauma is a hyperemic response, which promotes additional resorption of bone and increases the susceptibility to further injury and progressive deterioration. Non–weight bearing must be initiated during this acute phase of the disease process.

The *stage of coalescence* is noted by a lessening of edema, absorption of fine debris, and healing of fractures. Clinical and radiographic evidence of coalescence indicates that the reparative phase of healing has begun. The final phase of bone healing is the *stage of reconstruction*, wherein further repair and remodeling of bone take place in an attempt to restore stability and homeostasis (see Fig 7–1). Neuropathic osteoarthropathy can be arrested during the stage of development if diagnosed before the disease has had a chance to mature. Early identification and treatment will ideally result in minimal joint destruction and deformity.

Late neuropathic bone and joint changes are an exaggeration of those seen in osteoarthritis: cartilage fibrillation, loose body formation, subchondral sclerosis, and marginal osteophytes.[44] These lesions often heal with the formation of hyperplastic dense bone, especially in the midfoot. The early phase of healing is distinguished by the gradual absorption of fine debris and hematoma, with callus formation and the coalescence and reattachment of loose fragments of bone or cartilage. Proliferative changes are characteristic of this phase, with usual findings being intra-articular and extra-articular osteophytes, exostoses, ossification of ligaments and joint cartilage and marginal lipping at contact points.[27] Proliferation of new bone is often evidenced by exuberant overgrowth, "florid ossification" with decreased joint mobility and increased stabilization of the foot. Fusion and rounding of large fragments are late findings.

## PATHOGENESIS OF CHARCOT FOOT

Multiple factors appear to contribute to the development of bone and joint destruction in diabetics. Peripheral neuropathy with loss of protective sensation, mechanical stress, ankle equinus, autonomic neuropathy with increased blood flow to bone, and trauma have emerged as the most important determinants. Diabetic neuropathic osteoarthropathy may also be caused by metabolic factors, renal disease, renal transplantation, corticosteroid-induced osteoporosis, decreased cartilage growth activity, and possibly to nonenzymatic glycosylation of bone proteins and extra-articular soft tissues (Fig 7–2). Notwithstanding, the mechanism for development of neuropathic bone and joint lesions is not completely understood.

Two mechanisms have been described for the development of bony resorption (osteolysis); one mechanism is mediated by increased blood flow to bone and the other through osteoclastic activity.[1] Infection may cause increased blood flow to bone through granulation tissue as is often the case with a mal perforans ulcer. The resultant radiographic changes in bone are usually nonspe-

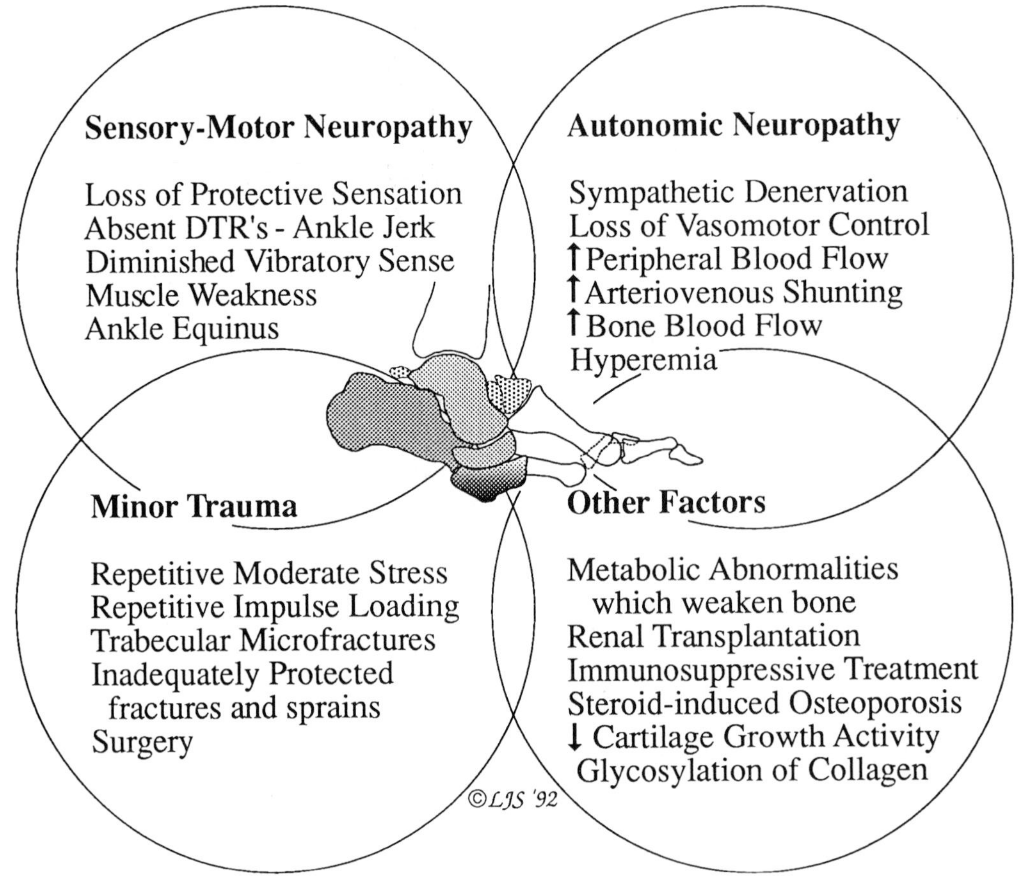

**FIG 7–2.**
Pathogenesis of Charcot foot. *(Modified from Sanders LJ, Frykberg RG: Diabetic neuropathic osteoarthropathy: the Charcot foot, in Frykberg RG, editor:* The high risk foot in diabetes mellitus, *New York, 1991, Churchill Livingstone. Used by permission.)*

cific. What initially appears to be bone destruction consistent with osteomyelitis may not be caused by direct extension of infection to the bone but may instead represent osteolysis secondary to increased peripheral blood flow, inflammatory hyperemia, granulation tissue, or soft tissue infection.

Bone resorption and joint deformity, especially in the metatarsophalangeal joints, may be exaggerated by the presence of trophic ulceration and infection.[56, 98] The diagnostic dilemma in these cases is which came first, the osteoarthropathy or the infection. Because the presenting symptoms of ulceration and infection often precede radiographic evaluation of the foot, it is invariably construed that pathologic bone and joint changes must have occurred secondary to infection. In their discussion of the role of infection in the pathogenesis of the Charcot

foot and ankle, Lippman et al.[64] determined that in 4 of their 12 patients, collapse preceded infection. In four other cases it seemed likely that ulceration and bacterial invasion occurred after the Charcot lesion had been established for some time.[64] Other authors[66, 67] have reported similar observations. The role of infection in many of these patients should be viewed as a complication and not an etiologic factor.[75]

The relationship that exists between certain lesions of the spinal cord and the peripheral nerves and the subsequent development of neuropathic joints has been well documented.* The presence of peripheral sensory-motor neuropathy characterized by loss of protective sensation, absent deep ten-

*References 10–12, 15, 18–20, 46, 52, 53, 57, 59, 67, 91, 95.

don reflexes, diminished vibratory perception, and muscle weakness sets into motion a series of events that eventually result in the development of Charcot's joint. The following discussion is directed at understanding the neurovascular etiology of DNOAP, as well as the possible roles of other important factors, that may be less well known.

## Increased Peripheral Blood Flow

Autonomic nervous system dysfunction has been noted as an associated finding in patients with neuropathic osteoarthropathy.* Support for the hypothesis that increased blood flow and active bone resorption are responsible for the development of Charcot's joint is evidenced by several case reports and experimental data.† Schwarz et al.[90] described the case of a 61-year-old diabetic who developed severe whittling down of the metatarsal bones and proximal phalanges of the left foot after a left lumbar sympathectomy 22 years earlier. Edelman et al.[29] reported three cases where neuropathic osteoarthropathy developed within 2 to 5 years after successful lower limb revascularization. Lippman et al.[64] suggested that excess local arterial flow can be a contributing factor to osseous breakdown under stress.

A neurally initiated vascular reflex leading to increased blood flow and active bone resorption has been proposed as an important etiologic factor in the development of bone and joint destruction in neuropathic patients.[11-13, 29, 99] Wartenberg[99] noted a possible role of the sympathetic nervous system in the manifestations of tabes dorsalis and in the production of tabetic joints. He observed local disturbances in sympathetic vessel innervation in unilateral tabetic arthropathies, in proximity to the affected joints. "The following pathologic disturbances were found: elevation of the local temperature, rise in the arterial and venous blood pressure, increase in the oscillometric index, anomalies of the sweat secretion and disturbances in the pilomotor reflex."[99]

Normal circulation with palpable pedal pulses have consistently been reported in diabetic patients with neuropathic osteoarthropathy.[4, 39, 53, 93] "Pedal pulses in most of our patients were accentuated. The feet were warm with bounding dorsalis pedis and posterior tibial pulses."[93] The existence of autonomic neuropathy in patients with diabetic neuropathic arthropathies has likewise been reported with regularity.[39, 67, 69, 90]

Evidence exists that autonomic neuropathy with sympathetic denervation resulting in high peripheral blood flow is common in patients with diabetes mellitus.‡ Archer et al.,[2] at the King's College Hospital, measured resting foot blood flow in 22 diabetic patients with severe sensory neuropathy using mercury strain gauge plethysmography and Doppler sonogram techniques. They found blood flow to be increased on the average five times greater than normal at 20° C to 22° C. They noted that foot skin temperature was also elevated, reflecting the increased circulation.

Edmonds et al.,[31] also from King's College Hospital, studied the uptake of methylene diphosphonate labeled with technetium 99m in 13 neuropathic diabetics and 8 nondiabetic controls. Bone scans were performed, and uptake of radiopharmaceutical was monitored in three phases. Uptake in all three phases (2 minutes after injection, at 4 minutes, and at 4 hours) was markedly elevated and confined to the feet in all neuropathic subjects. Increased uptake at 2 and 4 minutes indicated increased blood flow. These investigators concluded that the most likely explanation for their findings was increased bony blood flow secondary to sympathetic denervation. Edmonds et al.[31] noted that severely abnormal autonomic function occurs in association with neuropathic ulceration. High blood flow, vasodilatation, and arteriovenous shunting, which result from sympathetic denervation, could lead to abnormal venous pooling.[101]

Mean venous $P_{O_2}$ in the feet of neuropathic subjects with ulcers was found to be significantly higher than in controls.[8] Boul-

---

*References 2, 18, 29, 33, 39, 65, 69, 99.

†References 11–13, 29, 31, 32, 64, 66, 67, 90, 99, 101.

‡References 2, 8, 10, 26, 31, 33, 101.

ton et al.[8] frequently observed the presence of prominent pedal arteries and distended dorsal foot veins in their diabetic patients who had noninfected neuropathic foot ulcers. These observations led them to believe that arteriovenous (AV) shunting with increased venous oxygenation was important in the pathogenesis of ulceration.[8]

## Mechanical Stress

Mechanical elements have long been recognized in the etiology of osteoarthritis. Situations that impose chronically increased stress on articular cartilage can act as the inciting primary cause. The repetitive mechanical stress of ambulation with impulsive loading of bone, applied to a foot that has lost protective sensation, results in soft tissue injury (ulcers) and tensile fatigue of cartilage and bone. Trabecular microfractures in the subchondral cancellous bone are the earliest ultrastructural evidence of cartilage damage.[76] The result of healing of these microfractures and remodeling is an increase in the stiffness of the subchondral bone,[78] which reduces the bones' normal resilience and ability to absorb shock. Total collapse of the neuropathic foot can occur over a very short period and may be evidenced clinically by depression of the medial longitudinal arch and complaints by the patient that "my arch has fallen."[85]

Any disturbance of the bones and joints of the neuropathic foot resulting in a change of shape, bony deformity, or alteration of foot mechanics has the potential for causing skeletal and soft tissue lesions. The consequence of increased vertical force and shear stress directed on the soft tissues overlying prominent bone is ulceration, followed by infection and further collapse of the foot. The degree of injury is determined by the extent of sensory loss, amount of stress on the joint, duration of the inflammatory process, and the patient's persistent ambulation in spite of the swelling, redness, and deformity.

## Fractures

Fractures of significant magnitude were responsible for initiating or increasing joint changes in the majority of the 118 cases of neuroarthropathy reported by Johnson.[52] He concluded that "the behaviour of the bones and joints in neuroarthropathy can be explained on the basis of the usual responses of these tissues to trauma modified by the presence of decreased protective sensation." Lack of attentive recognition and a cavalier attitude with regard to protection of fractures, sprains, and effusions sustain the atrophic phase and result in bone and joint destruction. As long as resorption outpaces new bone formation, this destructive cycle continues.

Eleven percent of the cases reported by Newman[72] had spontaneous fractures and dislocations. These cases presented the greatest therapeutic problems compared with other noninfective diseases of bone. Newman[72] stressed the importance of recognizing these conditions and distinguishing them from osteomyelitis.

Autonomic neuropathy with loss of vasomotor control and increased peripheral blood flow to bone, coupled with an inflammatory hyperemia of the soft tissues, results in resorption of bone with further weakening. Atrophic bone is easily fractured or fragmented. Frequent spontaneous fractures in neuropathic patients has led some authors[35] to believe that intrinsic bone disease may be an etiologic factor.

## Equinus Deformity

Weakness of the anterior group muscles of the leg (ankle dorsiflexors) may result in a compensatory contracture of the gastrocnemius-soleus muscles, with equinus deformity.[5, 82, 88] Although there are no data confirming a direct causal relationship between equinus deformity and the development of neuroarthropathy, intuitively this appears to be a reasonable assumption, especially at the tarsometatarsal and midtarsal joints. Weight bearing on a neuropathic foot with weak ankle dorsiflexors causes the achilles tendon to forcefully plantarflex the foot, resulting in increased pressure over the metatarsophalangeal joints, a slapping gait, and stress at the tarsometatarsal, naviculo-cuneiform, and midtarsal joints once calf contracture occurs.

## Renal Transplantation

Isolated reports have shown an association between renal transplantation with long-term corticosteroid or other immunosuppressive treatment and the subsequent development of neuropathic osteoarthropathy.[22] These reviews show that after renal transplantation, diabetics have a much higher incidence of neurotrophic joint disease than the nontransplanted diabetic population. Clohisy and Thompson[22] reported on 18 patients with juvenile-onset diabetes and severe neuropathic arthropathy of the ankle and tarsus. Fourteen of these patients had received a renal transplant before the fracture was diagnosed, and none had a history of major trauma.

It remains unclear whether corticosteroid-induced osteoporosis or some other metabolic abnormality, which tends to weaken bone, was the underlying factor responsible for the development of bone and joint destruction in these patients. Further discussion of this subject follows in the section on anatomic patterns of bone and joint destruction, pattern V.

## Glycosylation of Collagen

The synthesis of abnormal collagen types not usually found in cartilage, bone, ligaments, or other soft tissues may be another possible factor in the development of DNOAP. Nonenzymatic glycosylation of proteins associated with chronic hyperglycemia, in particular hemaglobin and dermal collagen, has been reported in several publications.[9, 14, 16, 70] Digital sclerosis and joint contractures were found affecting the hands in 18% of children with insulin-dependent diabetes mellitus.[16] Biopsies of patients with limited joint mobility have shown increased cross-linking and glycosylation of collagen.[9] Limited subtalar joint mobility has been observed in neuropathic diabetics compared with an age-matched nondiabetic control group. Routine lateral view radiographs did not reveal remarkable subtalar joint abnormalities in the diabetic subjects (Sanders LJ, unpublished data).

Abnormal (type 1) collagen has been found by immunohistochemical assays in the immediate vicinity of chondrocytes in osteoarthritic cartilage.[50] Diminution of chondroitin sulfate content relative to the collagen matrix is a feature common to osteoarthritic alteration of joint cartilage. Hough and Sokoloff[50] suggest that this change might alter the material properties of cartilage with respect to wear and tear.

## Decreased Cartilage Growth Activity

Skeletal integrity may be affected by insulin deficiency through its effect on insulin-like growth factor 1 (IGF-1). Insulin growth factor 1, also known as somatomedin C, is synthesized in response to growth hormone influence and acts directly to produce cartilage proliferation and skeletal growth. Data suggest that IGF-1 serves as a mitogenic signal to cause mitosis of newly differentiated chondrocytes.[89] The induction of streptozotocin-induced diabetes in rats has been shown to result in a significant decrease in serum somatomedin and cartilage growth activity.[63]

## PATTERNS OF BONE AND JOINT DESTRUCTION

Five characteristic anatomic patterns of bone and joint destruction have been observed to occur in diabetics with neuropathic osteoarthropathy (DNOAP) or osteopathy.[83, 84] Sanders and Frykberg compiled information on the distribution of bone and joint involvement in neuropathic diabetics, reported in the English literature, as well as his own cases from a Veterans Administration retrospective study, and developed the following anatomic classification: pattern I, forefoot; pattern II, tarsometatarsal joints; pattern III, naviculocuneiform, talonavicular, and calcaneocuboid joints; pattern IV, ankle joint; and pattern V, calcaneus. Two of these patterns, I and II, are frequently associated with bony deformity and ulceration. The most frequent joint involvement is seen in patterns I, II, and III, with the most severe structural deformity and functional instability seen in patterns II and IV. Pattern V osteopathy is the least common and may be seen as an isolated fracture of the calcaneus or in association with involvement of other tarsal bones. These anatomic patterns may be seen singly or in combination in any given individual (Fig 7–3).

## Pattern I: The Forefoot

This commonly occurring pattern of osteoarthropathy is characterized by involvement of the forefoot, in other words, the interphalangeal joints, phalanges, metatarsophalangeal joints, or distal metatarsal bones. Radiographic findings in this location are typically atrophic and destructive in nature, characterized by osteopenia, osteolysis, juxta-articular cortical bone defects, subluxation, and destruction. Pattern I involvement has been reported to occur in from 26% to 67% of all affected sites.[24, 69, 84, 93] Of the affected joints (10/21) in Miller and Lichtman's[69] study, 47.6% in-

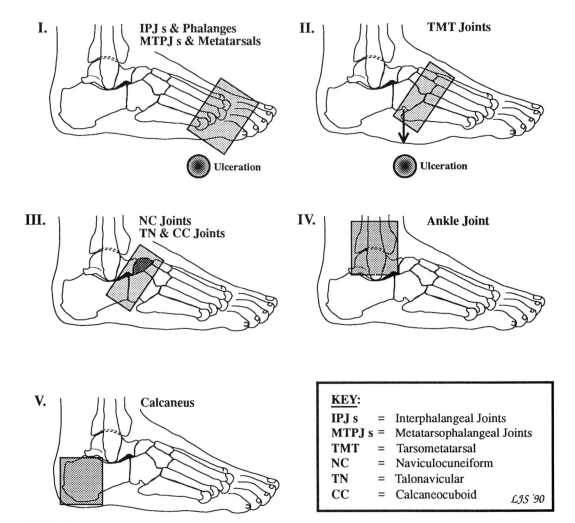

**FIG 7–3.**
Anatomic patterns of bone and joint destruction reported in diabetics with neuropathic osteoarthropathy of the foot and ankle. Patterns I and II are frequently associated with bony deformity and ulceration. The most frequent joint involvement is seen in patterns I, II, and III, with the most severe structural deformity and functional instability associated with patterns II and IV. *(From Sanders LJ, Frykberg RG: Diabetic neuropathic osteoarthropathy: the Charcot foot, in Frykberg RG, editor:* The high risk foot in diabetes mellitus, *New York, 1991, Churchill Livingstone, Used by permission.)*

volved the metatarsophalangeal and interphalangeal joints. Sanders and Mrdjenovich[84] found pattern I involvement in 30% of affected sites (20/66); Cofield et al.[24] reported metatarsophalangeal and interphalangeal joint involvement in 67% of 116 affected limbs. Sinha et al.[93] reported metatarsophalangeal joint involvement in 26.8% (34/127) of all affected sites.

Plantar ulceration is a common finding associated with osteopathy of the forefoot. Cofield et al.[24] reported that 91% of their patients with radiographic evidence of metatarsophalangeal joint involvement had underlying ulcers. It may not be readily apparent whether the bone and joint changes preceded or developed as a result of the ulceration. The presence of neuropathic plantar ulceration should be considered a serious finding, which may lead to major disability. This finding may, in fact, be a cutaneous marker for neuropathic arthropathy of the forefoot. Newman et al.[73] assessed the prevalence of osteomyelitis in 35 diabetic patients with 41 foot ulcers (38 classic mal perforans ulcers). As determined by bone biopsy and culture, these investigators found osteomyelitis to underlie 68% of the foot ulcers. All patients with ulcers exposed to bone had osteomyelitis.

Digital findings include concentric resorption of bone that may be seen to affect the phalangeal diaphyses with a characteristic *hourglass* appearance. Broadening of the bases of the proximal phalanges occurs, with the formation of a *cup* around the metatarsal head (Fig 7–4).[60, 90]

Resorption of the distal metatarsal bones and phalanges is characteristic of atrophic, destructive diabetic osteopathy. This is evidenced, on anteroposterior radiographs, as a pencil-like tapering of the metatarsal bones with a *licked peppermint stick*, or sucked candy, appearance (Fig 7–5). The histopathologic picture reveals erosion of articular cartilage, periarticular fibrosis, increased vascularity, synchronous resorption of bone, and new bone formation. There is disorganization of subchondral bone, with bony resorption and a fatty marrow. Chronic ulceration and infection may be associated with these changes.

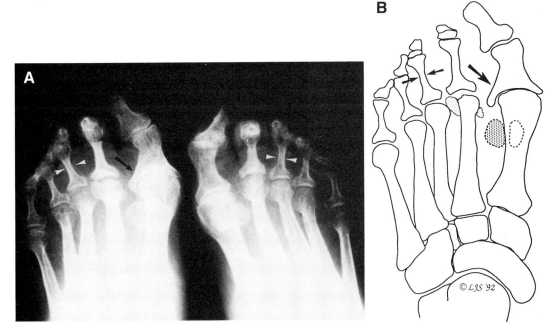

**FIG 7–4.**
**A,** concentric resorption of bone involving proximal phalangeal shafts of the lesser toes *(arrowheads).* Note hourglass appearance of the phalanges. Note also, broadening of the phalangeal base of the hallux and cupping of the first metatarsal head *(arrow).* Proliferative changes of the second metatarsal head are also noted. **B,** graphic illustration of radiographic findings.

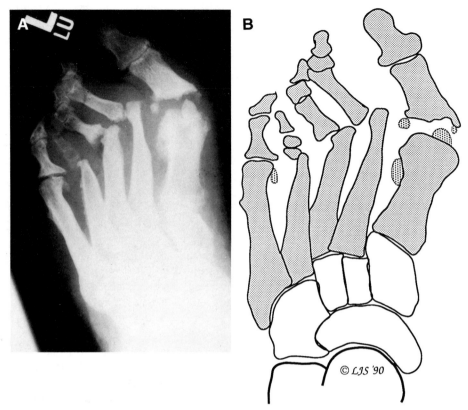

**FIG 7–5.**
**A,** anteroposterior radiograph reveals osteolytic destruction of all metatarsophalangeal joints, with pencil-like tapering of the metatarsal shafts resembling "sucked candy" or "licked peppermint stick." **B,** graphic representation of radiographic findings. *(From Sanders LJ, Frykberg RG: Diabetic neuropathic osteoarthropathy: the Charcot foot, in Frykberg RG, editor:* The high risk foot in diabetes mellitus, *New York, 1991, Churchill Livingstone, Used by permission.)*

## Pattern II: Tarsometatarsal Joints

Pattern II osteoarthropathy is distinguished by affection of the tarsometatarsal (Lisfranc's) joints and is often associated with plantar ulceration at the apex of the collapsed cuneiforms or cuboid. Tarsometatarsal involvement has been reported to occur in 15% to 43% of the cases of DNOAP.[24, 69, 77, 93] This pattern of osteoarthropathy occurs spontaneously and with greater frequency in diabetics than in patients with leprosy (Hansen's disease). Unlike the cuneiform-metatarsal base pattern associated with Hansen's disease, this pattern is rarely caused by "definite violence."[47]

The normal anatomic relationships of the tarsometatarsal joints are illustrated in Figure 7–6. The second metatarsal base is securely recessed in the intercuneiform mortise. This tenon-in-mortise relationship creates a very stable keystone for the midfoot. Disturbance of this relationship weakens the foot and allows for dorsolateral displacement of the metatarsal bones on the lesser tarsus, followed by architectural collapse of the cuneiforms and cuboid.

Early changes in the tarsometatarsal joints may be subtle and consistent with incipient osteoarthritis; there may be slight dorsal prominence of the metatarsal bases with local swelling and increased skin temperature on the dorsum of the foot. Late changes reveal degenerative arthritis with fragmentation and subluxation of the cuneiform bones and the metatarsal bases. The metatarsal bases often override the cuneiforms. There may be evidence of total disintegration of the cuneiforms, with collapse of the midfoot and a resultant *rocker bottom* foot deformity.

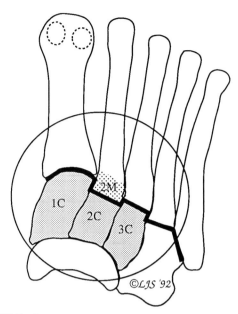

**FIG 7–6.**
Normal anatomy of the tarsometatarsal (Lisfranc's) joints. Note recessed position of the second metatarsal base *(stippled area)* in the intercuneiform mortise. *M* = metatarsal, *C* = cuneiform.

A fracture at the base of the second metatarsal, in the absence of major trauma, may precede collapse of the tarsometatarsal joints, as seen in the following case. A 66-year-old neuropathic diabetic man had mild swelling and erythema on the dorsum of his right foot after a fall in his kitchen. Radiographs revealed a laterally displaced fracture of the second metatarsal base (Fig 7–7). The patient was placed in a plaster cast, non–weight bearing, with crutches for 6 weeks. During this time he was poorly compliant and refused further treatment. Within 8 months the patient's midfoot collapsed.

Diabetics may have an erythematous, hot, painful, swollen foot, with no history of trauma. The clinical picture may be nonspecific, resembling an acute gouty arthritis, septic arthritis, or cellulitis. Patients are usually afebrile with no clinical or laboratory evidence of infection. There may, however, be a mildly elevated erythrocyte sedimentation rate (ESR) with normal white blood cell (WBC) count. Sanders and Mrdjenovich[84] reported a mean ESR of 32 ± 6.7 mm/hour (range 22–41) in a group of 13 neuropathic diabetics with bone and joint

changes and normal WBC counts. The radiographic picture, however, is quite remarkable, revealing subluxation or fracture dislocation of Lisfranc's joint. The base of the second metatarsal is laterally displaced from its normal recessed position in the intercuneiform mortise, and all of the metatarsals are shifted laterally on the lesser tarsus.

The following case represents an acute neuropathic osteoarthropathy affecting the tarsometatarsal articulations. The patient, a 63-year-old neuropathic diabetic man with a 15-year history of diabetes mellitus, poorly controlled with insulin, was admitted to the emergency room with acute erythema, swelling, increased skin temperature, and deformity of the right foot. He reported having mild pain and no history of trauma. The patient, a unilateral transtibial amputee, was afebrile with an elevated blood glucose level of 447 mg/dL. Radiographs revealed a tarsometatarsal joint dislocation, with all of the metatarsal bases shifted laterally on the lesser tarsus. The lateral radiograph re-

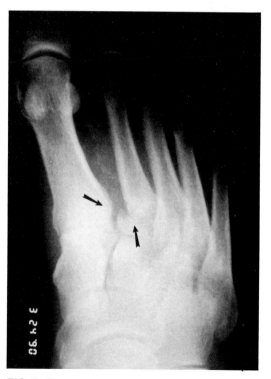

**FIG 7–7.**
Laterally displaced fracture of the second metatarsal base *(arrows).*

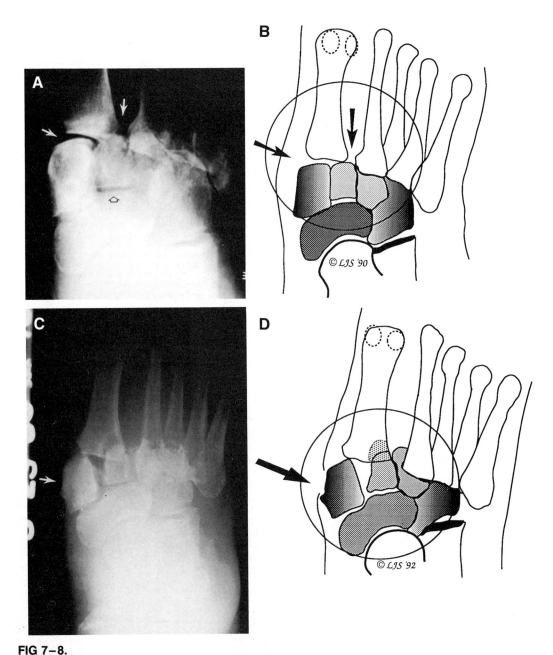

**FIG 7–8.**
**A,** anteroposterior radiograph reveals dislocation of the tarsometatarsal joints, with lateral displacement of the metatarsal bases on the cuneiforms and cuboid. Second metatarsal base is completely displaced from the inter-cuneiform mortise, with the first metatarsal base articulating with the medial half of the second cuneiform *(arrows)*. Note distal migration of the second cuneiform *(arrowhead)*. **B,** graphic illustration of radiographic findings in **A. C,** anteroposterior radiograph taken 6 months after initial presentation. There has been extensive deterioration of the tarsometatarsal, navicular cuneiform, and midtarsal joints. Note extrusion of the medial cuneiform *(arrow)*. The second cuneiform has eroded its way into the plantar-lateral aspect of the first metatarsal base. **D,** graphic illustration of radiographic findings in **C.** (From Sanders LJ, Frykberg RG: Diabetic neuropathic osteoarthropathy: the Charcot foot, in Frykberg RG, editor: *The high risk foot in diabetes mellitus,* New York, 1991, Churchill Livingstone, Used by permission.)

vealed plantar dislocation of the cuneiforms and navicular, with dorsal displacement of the metatarsal bases. The patient was admitted to the hospital for conservative management of the right foot, an unsuccessful attempt at closed reduction of the dislocation, and control of diabetes mellitus. In spite of efforts to immobilize the limb and to limit weight bearing, this unilateral amputee continued to walk on his right lower limb. Within 6 months total collapse of the foot occurred, along with extrusion of the medial cuneiform. Ulceration developed from shear stress over the prominent medial cuneiform (Fig 7–8).

## Pattern III: Naviculocuneiform, Talonavicular and Calcaneocuboid Joints

This pattern of osteoarthropathy involves the naviculocuneiform and midtarsal joints. Pattern III is frequently characterized by dislocation of the navicular or by disintegration of the naviculocuneiform joints. Sanders and Mrdjenovich[84] reported naviculocuneiform, talonavicular, or calcaneocuboid involvement in approximately 32% of the affected joints (21/66 sites) in 28 cases. Very early radiographic changes of impending Charcot's joint destruction may be evidenced by osteolysis of the naviculocuneiform joints. Typical fragmentation, osteolysis, and sharply defined osseous debris are

visible on the lateral radiograph (Fig 7–9). Observation of this finding signals the need for non–weight bearing cast immobilization of the foot. Ignoring this finding may result in progressive deterioration of the lesser tarsal bones and ultimately in collapse of the midfoot.

Isolated midtarsal joint dislocations associated with neuropathic diabetics have been reported by several authors.[52, 61, 71] Lesko and Maurer,[61] reported their experience with eight talonavicular dislocations, in which dislocations of the navicular were described as either inferomedial, mediodorsal, or medial. Fragmentation of bone frequently accompanies these dislocations. Talonavicular dislocation may be seen alone or in association with involvement of the naviculocuneiform joints, disintegration of the cuneiform bones, or with deterioration of the head and neck of the talus (Fig 7–10).

A combination of patterns II and III is represented in Figure 7–11. Note the dramatic collapse of the midfoot with a rocker bottom appearance. Ulceration of the skin occurred at the apex of the rocker. The tarsometatarsal, naviculocuneiform, talonavicular, and calcaneocuboid joints all are involved.

## Pattern IV: Ankle Joint

Ankle joint involvement accounts for only 3% to 10% of the reported cases,[24, 69, 84, 93]

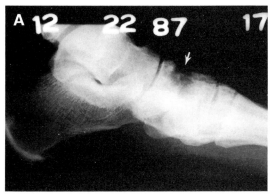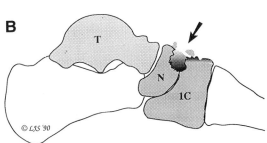

**FIG 7–9.**
**A,** osteolytic destruction of the naviculocuneiform joints *(arrow).* Fragmentation, osteolysis, and sharply defined osseous debris are noted. **B,** graphic illustration of radiographic findings. *1C* = first cuneiform bone, *N* = navicular bone, *T* = talus. *(From Sanders LJ, Frykberg RG: Diabetic neuropathic osteoarthropathy: the Charcot foot, in Frykberg RG, editor:* The high risk foot in diabetes mellitus, *New York, 1991, Churchill Livingstone. Used by permission.)*

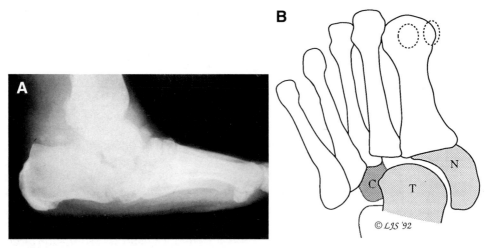

FIG 7–10.
**A,** disorganization of the talonavicular and calcaneocuboid joints. **B,** graphic illustration of talonavicular dislocation with inferomedial displacement of the navicular bone.

yet this pattern invariably results in severe structural deformity and functional instability of the ankle. Charcot's joint affecting the ankle may develop suddenly without any appreciable external cause, with spontaneous swelling and localized redness of the foot and ankle. Patients will initially notice swell-

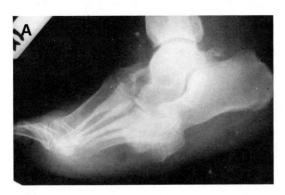

ing and deformity of the affected ankle, with little pain. They often continue to walk on the affected limb until the collateral ligaments stretch or tear, and there is erosion of bone and cartilage with collapse of the joint. Steindler's[95] observations of foot and ankle fractures in patients with tabetic joints

FIG 7–11.
**A,** lateral radiograph demonstrates collapse of the tarsometatarsal, naviculocuneiform, talonavicular, and calcaneocuboid joints (combination of patterns II and III). **B** and **C,** graphic illustrations of radiographic findings, with identification of involved structures. *C* = cuboid; *N* = navicular; *T* = talus; *OC* = calcaneus; *1C* = medial cuneiform; *M* = metatarsal. (**A** *and* **B** *from Sanders LJ, Frykberg RG: Diabetic neuropathic osteoarthropathy: the Charcot foot, in Frykberg RG, editor:* The high risk foot in diabetes mellitus, *New York, 1991, Churchill Livingstone. Used by permission.)*

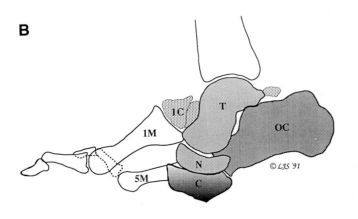

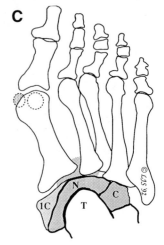

caused him to conclude that "the greatest pathological changes correspond to the maximum of mechanical stress. . .in the direction of the greatest weight-bearing." He noted two types of destruction: one in the direction of the long axis of the leg, breaking down the talus and calcaneus; the other evidenced by collapse of the forefoot and tarsus. Free bodies were seen in the ankle joint in 8 of 21 cases.

Harris and Brand[47] noted that if during weight bearing "the posture of the foot is disturbed by external forces or paralysis an abnormal position results, and the new weight stream will cross the trabecular lines so that minor fractures occur more readily and ligaments may rupture." They[47] described "a relatively rapid and catastrophic disintegration of the proximal tarsal bones allowing the tibia to grind its way through the foot to the ground."

Even trivial trauma associated with an ankle sprain or a relatively minor fracture may result in instability of the ankle joint, with resultant collapse and disintegration.[47, 52, 69] Miller and Lichtman[69] described a case in which total destruction of the ankle joint resulted after surgical intervention for a fractured medial malleolus. Johnson[52] reported the case of a 55-year-old woman who 8 weeks after a sprained left ankle developed complete displacement of the medial malleolus with grinding away of one half of the talus and part of the distal end of the tibia.

Rapid disintegration of the ankle joint occurred in a 59-year-old neuropathic woman with a 15-year history of diabetes mellitus. Her chief complaints were pain, redness, and swelling of her left foot and ankle of 1 week's duration. There was no history of trauma; however, she had recently been treated by her family physician for "an infected blister" on her left fifth toe. Infection resolved promptly, but shortly thereafter pain and swelling developed over the lateral aspect of her foot and ankle. The patient had bounding pedal pulses and a dense peripheral neuropathy. Radiographs revealed osteopenia of the tarsal bones, with evidence of osteoarthritis of the tarsometatarsal joints. Radionucleotide scan with methylene

diphosphonate labeled with $^{99m}$Tc revealed very high uptake in the left ankle and tarsal bones, as well as marked uptake in the asymptomatic right ankle. Blood cultures and ankle joint aspirate obtained on admission grew *Staphylococcus aureus*. The opinion of an infectious disease consultant was that a septic arthritis was overlying a diabetic neuropathic arthropathy.[80] In spite of appropriate treatment with parenteral antibiotics, bed rest, elevation of the limb, and non−weight bearing casts, progressive deformity of the left ankle ensued. The clinical picture was characterized by lateral bulging and instability of the ankle, with medial displacement of the foot and fragmentation of bone. Radiographs and clinical photographs revealed extensive joint destruction with dislocation of the foot to the medial side of the leg (Fig 7–12).

## Pattern V: Calcaneus

### Calcaneal Insufficiency Avulsion Fractures

Pattern V osteopathy involves fractures of the calcaneus, characterized by avulsion of the posterior tubercle, and until just recently has been the least frequently reported pattern of bone destruction seen in neuropathic diabetics.[22, 25, 35, 54] Kathol et al.[54] reported on 21 diabetic patients with calcaneal fractures, of which 18 fractures were nontraumatic and 14 were limited to the posterior third of the calcaneus. This fracture pattern occurs in the same plane as a fatigue-type calcaneal fracture, with displacement and rotation of the posterior tuberosity. The term calcaneal insufficiency avulsion fracture was coined by Kathol's group to describe this specific pattern.[54]

Harris and Brand[47] attributed increased vulnerability of the calcaneus in an insensitive foot to (1) increased force on the heel caused by the patient's landing more heavily on an insensitive foot, (2) continued walking on a fractured bone, and (3) previous or concurrent ulceration "which may have weakened the bone by hyperaemic decalcification or may allow infection and osteomyelitis to complicate the fracture."

A bilateral calcaneal fracture was re-

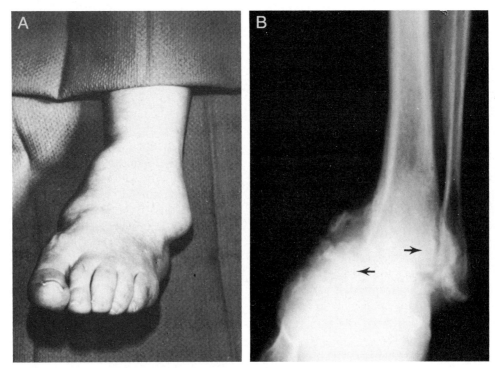

**FIG 7–12.**
**A,** unstable neuropathic left ankle, with lateral bulging. **B,** anteroposterior radiograph reveals extensive joint destruction with fragmentation of bone. Note dislocation of the joint *(arrows),* with the foot displaced medially. *(From Sanders LJ, Frykberg RG: Diabetic neuropathic osteoarthropathy: the Charcot foot, in Frykberg RG, editor: The high risk foot in diabetes mellitus, New York, 1991, Churchill Livingstone. Used by permission.)*

ported by Coventry and Rothacker[25] in a 45-year-old neuropathic woman with juvenile-onset diabetes. El-Khoury and Kathol[35] reported on four patients with spontaneous, unusual avulsion fractures of the posterior tubercle of the calcaneus, "where the avulsed fragment migrated superiorly due to the constant pull of the achilles tendon." These patients had diminished pain and vibratory perception. Clohisy and Thompson[22] reported 19 calcaneal fractures in 18 neuropathic juvenile-onset diabetics who had no history of major trauma to their limbs. Five of these patients had bilateral calcaneal fractures. In 17 limbs the calcaneal fractures were seen together with fractures of more than 1 other tarsal bone. Fourteen of the patients in this study underwent renal transplant surgery before the fracture was diagnosed.[22]

Thompson et al.,[97] in a retrospective review of 55 neuropathic kidney transplant patients, found a 20% incidence of skeletal disease among diabetic patients, with the highest incidence occurring in the third and fourth years after transplantation. They reported seeing three calcaneal fractures in 11 patients with neurotrophic joint disease. The initial manifestation in all patients was a pathologic fracture, usually in a metaphyseal area near a joint. Only later did they see actual joint destruction that seemed to result from the subchondral collapse associated with the initial fracture.

A calcaneal insufficiency avulsion fracture of the posterior tubercle of the right calcaneus occurred spontaneously in an active 53-year-old neuropathic diabetic woman with a 5-year history of diabetes mellitus. She reported hearing a loud crack and feeling a sharp pain in the back of her right heel while walking in the hallway at work. Lateral radiographs revealed posterior and superior displacement of the posterior process of the calcaneus (Fig 7–13). In addition to the calcaneal insufficiency avulsion fracture, radiographs of the asymptomatic left foot revealed concentric resorption of the proximal

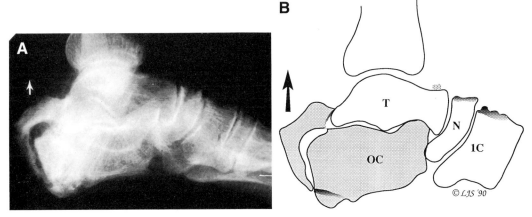

**FIG 7–13.**
**A,** lateral radiograph demonstrates an avulsion fracture of the posterior tubercle of the calcaneus. *Arrow* points in the direction of pull of the Achilles tendon. Early osteolytic changes are seen to affect the naviculocuneiform joint. **B,** graphic illustration of radiographic findings. *(From Sanders LJ, Frykberg RG: Diabetic neuropathic osteoarthropathy: the Charcot foot, in Frykberg RG, editor:* The high risk foot in diabetes mellitus, *New York, 1991, Churchill Livingstone. Used by permission.)*

phalanges, a cup-shaped proximal phalangeal base of the hallux, and fragmentation of the second metatarsal head.

## Diagnostic Studies

The diagnosis of DNOAP depends primarily on the physician's clinical suspicion of the disease. Medical history, clinical manifestation, and radiographic findings should help to narrow down the differential diagnosis. This disorder should be suspected when bone and joint pathologic conditions are found in a diabetic patient with loss of protective sensation, absent deep tendon reflexes, and diminished vibratory sense.

The most specific diagnostic tools for distinguishing between DNOAP and osteomyelitis in the diabetic foot are careful clinical, radiographic, and magnetic resonance imaging (MRI) examinations, followed by bone biopsy, bone cultures and histopathologic examination. Bone biopsy should be reserved for those cases that are equivocal, when there has been a chronic nonhealing wound or soft tissue infection contiguous to bone. Radiographs may occasionally be unremarkable during the early manifestation of the Charcot foot. At this time, the clinical picture may be very subtle, with only mild inflammation of the soft tissues and radiographic findings consistent with incipient os-

teoarthritis or osteolysis. In cases where there is a clear history of injury but the initial plain films are negative, radiographic studies should be repeated within 2 to 3 weeks to rule out stress fractures, fragmentation of bone, and periosteal new bone formation. During this time a cautious approach to treatment should be taken with a high index of suspicion. Neuropathic individuals should be immobilized and kept non–weight bearing. Serial radiographs are beneficial in following the course of this disease through the stage of reconstruction.

Computed tomography (CT) and MRI are valuable adjuncts in the evaluation of the diabetic Charcot foot. Williamson et al.,[102] at the University of Virginia Medical School, reported CT scans correctly predicted the presence or absence of osteomyelitis in all of a series of seven patients. Nuclide bone scans had one false positive and one false negative result. Beltran et al.[6] found MRI to be particularly helpful in differentiating neuroarthropathy from osteomyelitis. They identified a distinctive pattern for Charcot's joints consisting of low signal intensity on $T_1$- and $T_2$-weighted images within the bone marrow space adjacent to the involved joint. The following example demonstrates the use of MRI for evaluation of a 54-year-old woman with collapsed midfoot and associated plantar ulcer. The sagittal image clearly demonstrates the talus and calcaneus with no alteration of signal intensity to suggest edema or active osteomyelitis. The MRI scan allows clear visualization of the soft tissue structures demonstrating ulceration penetrating through the plantar aponeurosis (Fig 7–14).

Positive technetium and gallium bone scans may be seen with osteomyelitis, but they may also be false positive because of neuropathic bone disease.[85] Diffuse and focal uptake of technetium has been reported in neuropathic feet by several authors in areas of active bone turnover and increased bony blood flow, as seen in patients with osteoarthropathy.[31, 32, 37, 48] Positive scans have been reported to sometimes precede radiographic changes.[37] Gallium 67 citrate, which accumulates in sites of infection, has also been reported to localize in noninfected neuropathic bone.[45, 49]

Leukocyte scanning with indium 111 has been shown to have a high specificity and a very high negative predictive value for osteomyelitis.[55, 68, 79, 86, 87, 103] Newman et al.[73] from the Mount Sinai Medical Center in New York compared the results of radiographs, leukocyte scans with [111]In oxyquinolone, and bone scans with bone biopsy and culture results. Of all imaging tests, the leukocyte scan had the highest sensitivity, 89%.[73] The specificity for osteomyelitis with [111]In has been reported to be from 78% to 89%[55, 68, 86] compared with 38% to 75% for three-phase bone scans.[55, 79] Schauwecker et al.[86, 87] found that in the absence of infection, [111]In-labeled leukocytes do not accumulate in neuropathic bone.[68]

## MANAGEMENT STRATEGIES

Management of the Charcot foot should be based on the acuteness of symptoms, the anatomic pattern of bone and joint destruction, the degree of involvement (e.g., deformity, fractures, bone fragmentation, and instability) and presence of infection. Surgery should be contemplated only when attempts at conservative care have failed to establish a stable, plantigrade foot. An objective rationale of treatment based on the chronicity of injury, anatomic alignment, and associated degree of deformity has been outlined

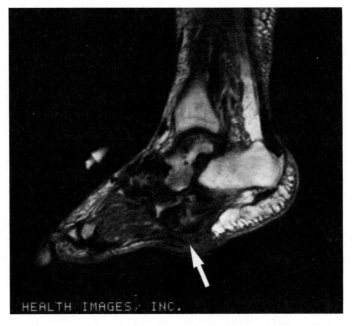

**FIG 7–14.**
MRI scan in a 54-year-old diabetic woman with collapsed midfoot and associated plantar ulcer. Note defect in the plantar aponeurosis *(arrow)* secondary to chronic ulceration. There is no alteration in signal intensity of the bones to suggest edema or active osteomyelitis. *(Courtesy of Health Images, Inc., Atlanta Magnetic Imaging, and John A. Ruch, D.P.M.)*

by Lesko and Maurer[58] at the University of California, San Francisco. For acute injuries with acceptable alignment, they suggest immobilization and protective weight bearing to prevent further progression of neuropathic joint destruction. For acute dislocation with marked deformity and little bone fragmentation, reduction and surgical arthrodesis may be indicated. For chronic dislocation with severe deformity and bone fragmentation, surgical treatment is recommended only as a last resort if soft tissue breakdown cannot be prevented by therapeutic footwear and bracing. Lesko and Maurer[61] emphasized that surgical reduction and arthrodesis should be reserved for the acute dislocation and for correction of deformities so severe that soft tissue breakdown cannot be prevented by footwear and bracing alone.

Diabetics with acute symptoms of neuropathic osteoarthropathy, as evidenced by erythema, swelling and bone and joint destruction, may be best treated by early hospitalization, bed rest, non–weight bearing, and cast immobilization. Hospitalization, although not always necessary, may be required to establish the diagnosis of the Charcot foot or to facilitate the treatment of poorly compliant or high-risk individuals. Compliant patients with supportive family members or friends may be efficiently managed on an outpatient basis.

Surgical intervention during the atrophic phase should be avoided, because it may accelerate the destructive process. If the acute injury goes unnoticed and unprotected, luxation, fragmentation, architectural collapse, hypertrophic bone formation, and deformity will follow. The aim of treatment should be to *obtain stability* of the foot with no excessive pressure on the skin from a bony prominence.[52, 71, 74] The key to treatment is *prevention*, with avoidance of further trauma and inflammation until the soft tissues heal.

Progressive destruction of the neuropathic foot can be halted if recognized early enough.[47, 64, 83] The appropriate way to treat the Charcot foot is first to prevent its occurrence. Careful history and physical examination directed toward risk assessment and stratification will help to identify individuals at greatest risk. Patients in their fifth and sixth decade, who have been diabetic for more than 10 years, and who demonstrate peripheral neuropathy with loss of protective sensation are prime candidates for the development of neuropathic osteoarthropathy. Added risk factors include the presence of nephropathy and retinopathy.[22, 93]

Early recognition of DNOAP with a *high index of suspicion* is vitally important. The physician and patient must look for areas of mild swelling, increased skin temperature, deformity, or instability of the foot and ankle. *Local temperature assessment* is valuable for monitoring tissue damage in the insensitive foot. Areas of increased warmth correspond to areas of inflammation in the insensitive limb that are at risk for bony resorption and ulceration. A hand-held infrared digital thermometer is a useful tool for the physician to monitor the inflammatory response in insensate patients. Any increase in skin temperature greater than 2°C should be considered a significant finding indicating impending osteoarthropathy or preulcerative inflammation.[85] Degenerative changes in any foot with proved peripheral sensory impairment are indicative of neuropathic arthropathy.[56]

In contrast to Charcot's description of a painless arthropathy, *pain* is often an associated feature but appears to be less severe than would normally be expected in view of the pathologic changes present. Elevation of the limb to reduce edema, cessation of weight bearing, prolonged cast immobilization, and comprehensive patient education are basic components of effective treatment.

## Immobilization

A general rule of thumb to follow in managing patients with neuropathic osteoarthropathy is that at least 3 months of non–weight-bearing cast immobilization is required before the resumption of partial weight bearing in a therapeutic shoe or walking brace. The duration of immobilization should be determined by assessment of skin temperature, as well as by radiographic evidence of consolidation of fractures and fragmented bone. Warmth of the skin indicates persistent inflammation, which requires continued immobilization. This period may be as short as 2 to 3 months or perhaps as long as 4 to 6 months, depending on the anatomic pattern and extent of involvement. Attention should be directed to the "asymptomatic" limb with respect to the development of bilateral osteoarthropathy. Clohisy and Thompson[22] observed that when an affected limb was prevented from weight bearing, involvement of the contralateral limb became evident after an average of 4.5 months. They therefore recommend prophylactic immobilization of the contralateral limb with a protective cast or orthosis.

### Orthoses and Shoes

A patella tendon–bearing (PTB) orthosis used together with therapeutic shoes may effectively decrease load on the foot.[22, 61, 81] Clohisy and Thompson[22] suggest short-term prophylactic protection of the "uninvolved" limb with a PTB cast or orthosis during the period of cast immobilization of the involved limb. For long-term protection of the affected limb they institute a calf-containment PTB orthosis.[22] Saltzman et al.[81] at the Mayo Clinic measured mean peak force transmitted to the foot in six diabetics with neurotrophic arthropathy. They found that use of a properly fitted standard PTB orthosis with a free ankle and an extradepth shoe reduced mean peak force to the entire foot by 15%. The addition of extra padding to the orthosis decreased the force by 32%. Interestingly, these investigators found that although load transmission was reduced in the hindfoot, it was not reduced in the midfoot or forefoot.

Prescription footwear and foot orthoses should be considered essential for the management of diabetics with loss of protective sensation. Cavanagh et al.[17] reported a significant reduction in the incidence of plantar lesions after the provision of special footwear to a group of high-risk neuropathic patients. Extra-depth, super-extra-depth, and thermal moldable shoes with soft leather uppers and well-molded insoles

are a cost-effective approach to management of patients with mild to moderate deformity. Shoes should be employed only after adequate medical or surgical management with crutch or walker assisted non–weight bearing immobilization of the limb. Ulcers should be healed or very shallow before ambulation is allowed. An interim healing shoe can be fabricated using a custom-molded orthosis in a surgical shoe. More comprehensive coverage of this subject follows in the chapters on footwear (Chapters 24 and 25).

## SURGICAL MANAGEMENT

Once the acute inflammatory stage has subsided, unstable joints and deformities that predispose to shearing stress and ulceration should be corrected. When surgery is attempted during the early stages of Charcot's joint development, the operative trauma further contributes to the process and is destined to fail.[34, 44, 58] Most reports advise surgical intervention only if the deformity is severe, the foot or ankle is unstable, or weight bearing is difficult.[34, 52, 58, 69] In Johnson's[52] series, surgery on the feet was limited to excision of bony prominences, except in one patient in whom two unsuccessful attempts at midtarsal fusion were made. In Newman's[71] series, it was found that there was always an adequate blood supply to allow simple operations to be undertaken. He[71] recommends prolonged immobilization during the active phase of the disease, followed by "removing of the lump," ensuring that there is no excessive pressure on the overlying skin.

### Indications and Criteria

Instability, deformity, chronic ulceration, and progressive joint destruction, despite rest and immobilization, are the primary indications for surgical intervention in diabetic individuals with neuropathic osteoarthropathy[5, 32, 52, 83] (Table 7–2).

Age, physical condition, patient compli-

**TABLE 7–2.**

Criteria for Surgery on the Charcot Foot

1. Instability
2. Deformity
3. Recurrent ulceration
4. Refractory to conservative treatment
5. Must be quiescent
6. Circulation intact
7. No active infection
8. Medically stable

ance, and comorbidities must also be considered in the surgical decision-making process. The benefits of surgery must be weighed carefully against the possible risks of lengthy operative procedures. A simple ostectomy or limited arthrodesis might be preferable in high-risk patients rather than subjecting them to extensive reconstructive surgery. Regional ankle block anesthesia, continuous epidural, or long spinal are preferable to general anesthesia.

Contraindications to surgical management of the Charcot foot include infection, ischemia, active bone disease, poorly controlled diabetes mellitus, a medically unstable patient, and a history of noncompliance.

## Surgical Techniques

Regardless of the surgical procedure employed the patient's condition should be optimized before surgery. Patients should be admitted to the hospital for thorough evaluation, bed rest, medical management, local wound care, and non–weight bearing several days before surgery. The initial approach to treatment should be directed at metabolic control, reduction of peripheral edema, and treatment of possible infection. Appropriate wound cultures should be performed with Gram's stain to assist in the selection of antibiotics. Daily debridement of ulcers and saline solution wet-to-dry dressing changes will help to maximize the condition of the wound before surgery.

### Ostectomy

The most commonly employed procedure for the treatment of chronic neuropathic ul-

ceration involves excision of bony prominences through either a plantar, medial, or lateral approach (Fig 7–15). Decompression of the ulcer in some cases may be sufficient to prevent recurrence even when there is residual deformity of the foot. The surgeon should consider excision of the ulcer, resection of underlying bony prominence, and primary closure of the wound as a reasonable method of treatment associated with minimal morbidity.[62, 83] For coverage of large plantar wounds ($> 3$ cm in diameter), consideration should be given to plastic surgical repair.

Fusiform excision of plantar ulcers with resection and saucerization of bone appears to provide prompt resolution of chronic plantar ulceration (Fig 7–16).[62, 83] Long-term results of this procedure have not been published. In a series of seven cases (Sanders LJ, unpublished data), five patients developed new ulcers within 2 years, adjacent to the site of the original lesion. Two patients underwent a second operation, and three healed with local wound care and shoe modifications.

Excision of the medial cuneiform was performed on a 65-year-old man with triopathy after 15 weeks of cast immobilization for an acute pattern II osteoarthropathy. At the time of surgery the foot was stable, skin temperature was normal, and radiographs revealed consolidation of bone. The skin overlying the convex medial border of the foot was believed to be at risk for shearing stress and development of ulceration. Postoperative photographs and radiographs reveal improved appearance of the foot, with resolution of the medial prominence. The anteroposterior radiograph reveals satisfactory alignment, with the first metatarsal base articulating with the intermediate cuneiform (Fig 7–17).

### Arthrodesis

Arthrodesis of neuropathic joints has been reported by some authors as uniformly poor despite the use of acceptable surgical and technical operative procedures.[25, 34, 52, 71] Attempts at open reduction and rigid in-

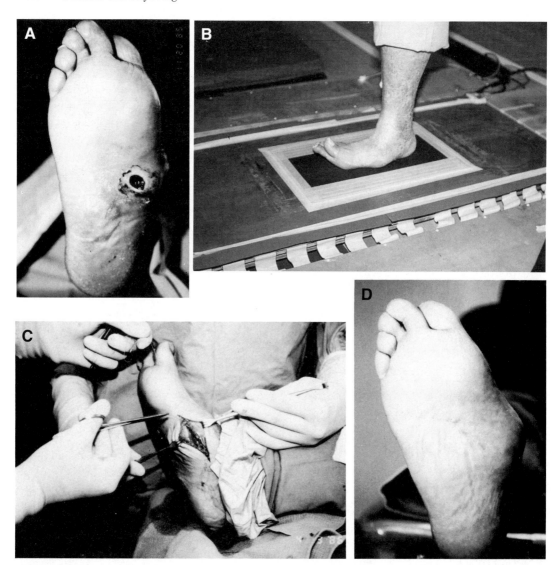

**FIG 7–15.**
**A,** neuropathic plantar ulceration beneath the medial cuneiform–first metatarsal base. **B,** weight-bearing view of the right foot. Note rocker bottom appearance. **C,** medial surgical approach for removal of prominent bone with an osteotome. **D,** postoperative photograph taken almost 3 years after surgery. The patient has remained lesion free. (**A, C,** and **D** from Sanders LJ, Frykberg RG: Diabetic neuropathic osteoarthropathy: the Charcot foot, in Frykberg RG, editor: The high risk foot in diabetes mellitus, New York, 1991, Churchill Livingstone. Used by permission.)

ternal fixation of subluxed and dislocated joints, especially the tarsometatarsal joints and ankle joint, should be approached with caution. This is often met with failure, as evidenced by increased destruction of bone, redislocation, nonunion, and altered foot mechanics that result in subluxation or disintegration of more proximal articulations.[52, 71]

Contrary to these reports, Banks and McGlamry,[5] at the Northlake Regional Medical Center in Tucker, Georgia, and Downey at the Pennsylvania College of Podiatric Medicine in Philadelphia (personal communication), report satisfactory preliminary results with arthrodesis in the Charcot patient. Stabilization of the medial column of the foot appears to be crucial to the success of this surgery (Fig 7–18). Surgical complication rates, long term results, patient char-

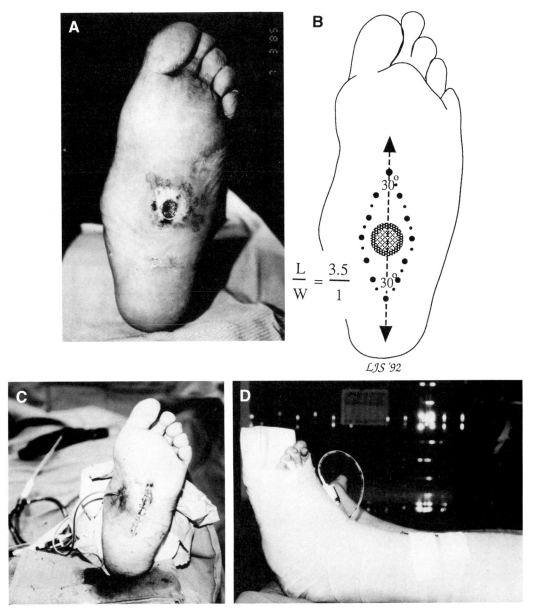

**FIG 7–16.**
**A,** plantar ulcer, left foot, overlying the cuboid. **B,** graphic illustration of surgical technique using a fusiform excision of the ulcer and saucerization of underlying bone. Length of the skin ellipse is three and one-half times the width. **C,** primary wound closure over a tube low suction drain. **D,** postoperative immobilization in a posterior splint.

acteristics and incidence of progressive joint involvement have not as yet been published by these podiatric surgeons. Until such essential data are available for evaluation, these procedures must be considered developmental.

Important factors leading to successful arthrodesis in Hansen's disease include pre-

operative condition of the foot, operative technique, and postoperative management.[92] Generally speaking, no patient should be considered for surgery without converting an active Charcot joint to its quiescent stage. Regardless of which joints are fused, basic surgical techniques remain the same. Technique for successful arthrodesis should

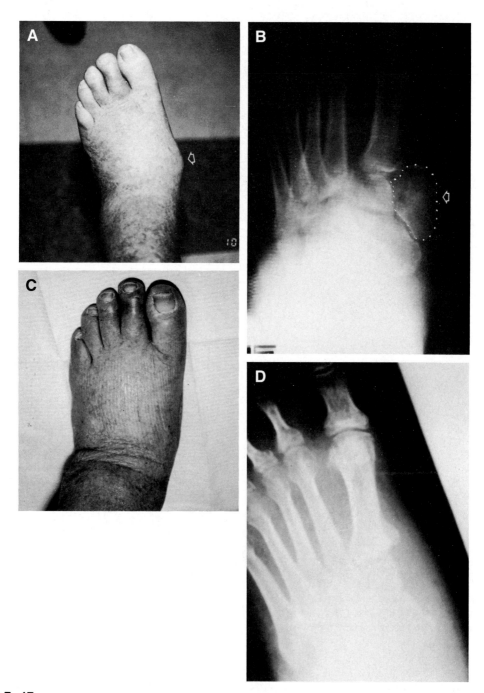

**FIG 7–17.**
Excision of the medial cuneiform in a 65-year-old diabetic man after 15 weeks of cast immobilization to treat acute pattern II osteoarthropathy. **A,** preoperative clinical photograph reveals a prominent convexity *(arrow)* along the medial aspect of the foot. **B,** preoperative radiograph reveals medial dislocation of the first cuneiform *(arrow)*. **C,** postoperative photograph demonstrates absent medial convexity with improved alignment of the foot. **D,** postoperative anteroposterior radiograph reveals absence of the medial cuneiform, and the first metatarsal base articulating with the intermediate cuneiform.

include (1) thorough removal of all cartilage and detritus, with debridement of synovial and scarred capsular tissues; (2) careful removal of sclerotic bone down to healthy bleeding bone; (3) meticulous fashioning of congruent bone surfaces for apposition; (4) firm fixation of bone with appropriate use of Kirschner wires, intramedullary nails, staples, plates, and screws which is extremely important. This has been found to greatly increase the chances for successful outcome.[5, 28, 52, 82, 92] Of equal importance is the necessity for prolonged postoperative immobilization, non–weight bearing, and a gradual return to protected weight bearing.

The following case is an example of major Charcot foot reconstruction, performed by Downey, on a 52-year-old diabetic woman with collapse of the right foot and chronic recurrent plantar ulceration. Conservative methods of treatment were unsuccessful, and the patient was told that a transtibial amputation was necessary. Preoperative radiographs revealed extensive disruption of the tarsometatarsal, naviculocuneiform, calcaneocuboid, and talonavicular joints. Open re-

duction with rigid internal fixation of fractures and dislocations was performed. The surgery included lengthening of the Achilles tendon and arthrodesis of Lisfranc's, naviculocuneiform, and midtarsal joints. The patient was immobilized in a short leg non–weight bearing cast for 3 months, followed by a weight-bearing short leg cast for 1 month. Clinical photographs and radiographs taken 1 year after surgery reveal complete healing of the plantar ulcer, with improved structural alignment and foot posture. There was a solid fusion of the medial column of the foot. The patient is currently ambulatory in custom-molded shoes and a PTB orthosis (Fig 7–19).

Achieving anatomic reduction of isolated tarsometatarsal dislocations in neuropathic diabetics may not be as critical as it is in nonneuropathic individuals who sustain trauma to the foot. In the latter case, incomplete reduction of the fracture or dislocation will often result in permanent disability in the form of chronic pain, deformity, and difficulty wearing shoes.[3] Painful arthritis is generally not a problem for neuropathic pa-

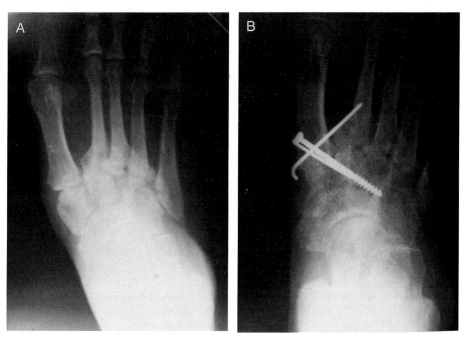

**FIG 7–18.**
**A,** anteroposterior radiograph reveals pattern II osteoarthropathy. There was instability of the medial column of the right foot. **B,** postoperative radiograph after open reduction and internal fixation of the first metatarsal–cuneiform and intercuneiform joints.

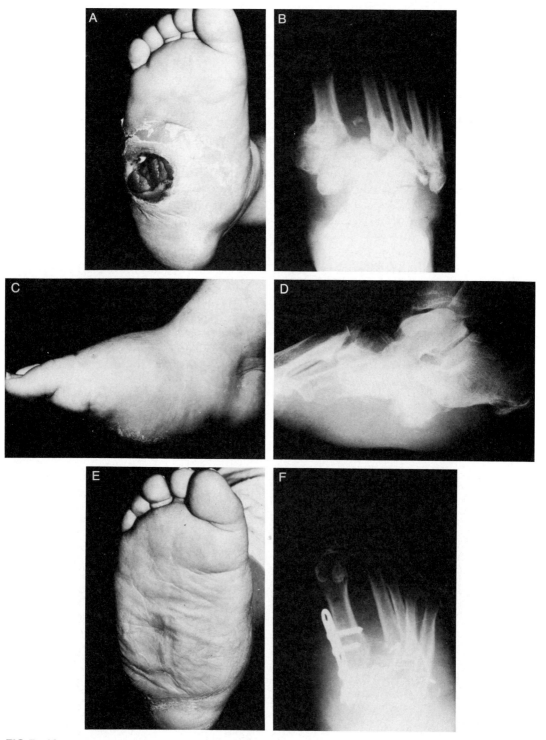

## FIG 7–19.

Charcot foot reconstruction in a 52-year-old woman with collapse of the right midfoot and history of chronic plantar ulceration. **A,** preoperative photograph reveals a large full-thickness ulcer on the sole of the right foot. **B,** anteroposterior radiograph reveals fracture dislocation of the tarsometatarsal, naviculocuneiform, and midtarsal joints. **C,** preoperative lateral photograph of the right foot demonstrates plantar bulging of the midfoot. **D,** lateral radiograph reveals exensive collapse of the midfoot with patterns II and III involvement. **E,** postoperative photograph of the right foot reveals complete healing of the plantar ulcer. **F,** anteroposterior radiograph demonstrates functional reduction of fractures and dislocations with internal fixation devices in place. Note improved alignment of the foot. **G,** postopoerative lateral photograph demonstrates improved structure and alignment of the foot. **H,** postoperative lateral radiograph reveals restoration of skeletal alignment with internal fixation devices in place.
*(Courtesy of Michael S. Downey, D.P.M.)*

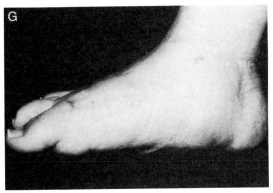

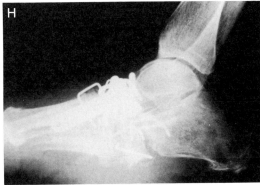

**FIG 7–19 (cont.).**

tients, and a reasonable amount of deformity can be accommodated with a therapeutic shoe.

### Ankle Arthrodesis

Ankle arthrodesis has been reported to have the greatest incidence of nonunion and pseudoarthrosis in patients with neuroarthropathy. Johnson[52] achieved successful fusion in only 33% of his series but was pleased enough with the position and stability of his failures to consider them as clinically successful. Stuart and Morrey[96] recently reported a 78% complication rate with neuropathic ankle fusions, achieving a satisfactory result in only 38% of their patients. Shibata et al.[92] reported on 24 patients with leprotic neuroarthropathy, who were followed for an average of 9 years. They achieved solid ankle fusion in 19 of 26 ankles (73%). Fusion was not obtained because of postoperative infection in four patients, deficiency of the arthrodesis site in one patient, and refracture through the site of fusion in two patients.[92] Others report satisfactory treatment of unstable ankles by simply repositioning the foot under the tibia and driving two heavy, threaded pins up through the heel into the distal tibia, followed by prolonged cast immobilization.[51] This alternative to solid ankle fusion provides a stable, fibrous ankylosis with satisfactory alignment. Jacobs[51] notes that immobilization may need to be two to three times longer than that required for a patient without neuropathic bone disease. This can be 4 to 6 months or longer.

### Complications of Surgery

Infection, nonunion, pseudoarthrosis, progressive bone and joint destruction, and pathologic fractures all have been reported after surgery on Charcot feet. Attention to detail, appropriate antibiotic coverage, meticulous surgical technique, and postoperative non–weight bearing immobilization will help to minimize these complications.

Postoperative infection is perhaps the greatest hazard after surgery on any neuropathic joint[52] and can result in further destruction of bone, followed by total collapse of the foot and ankle, and ultimately in loss of limb. Preoperative condition of the patient, metabolic and nutritional status, surgical technique, extent of dissection, length of operation, and use of internal fixation devices may affect postoperative morbidity.

### Acknowledgments

We thank Barbara E. Deaven, medical librarian, and Roxanne Felli, library technician, Medical Library Service, VA Medical Center, Lebanon, Pennsylvania, for assistance in searching the medical literature; and Patricia Whitehead and the Lebanon VA Medical Center podiatry staff for support during preparation of this chapter.

### REFERENCES

1. Aegerter E, Kirkpatrick JA: Metabolic diseases of bone, in Aegerter E, Kirkpatrick JA, editors: *Orthopedic diseases*, Philadelphia, 1983, WB Saunders, p 33.

2. Archer AG, Roberts VC, Watkins PJ: Blood flow patterns in diabetic neuropathy, *Diabetologia* 27:563, 1984.

3. Arntz CT, Veith RG, Hansen ST: Fractures and fracture-dislocations of the tarsometatarsal joint, *J Bone Joint Surg* 70A:173, 1988.

4. Bailey CC, Root HF: Neuropathic foot lesions in diabetes mellitus, *N Engl J Med* 236:397, 1947.

5. Banks AS, McGlamry ED: Charcot foot, *J Am Podiatr Med Assoc* 79:213, 1989.

6. Beltran J, Campanini S, Knight C, et al: The diabetic foot: magnetic resonance imaging evaluation, *Skeletal Radiol* 19:37, 1990.

7. Bjorkengren AG, Weisman M, Pathria MN, et al: Neuroarthropathy associated with chronic alcoholism, *Am J Radiol* 151:743, 1988.

8. Boulton AJM, Scarpello JHB, Ward JD: Venous oxygenation in the diabetic neuropathic foot: evidence of arteriovenous shunting? *Diabetologia* 22:6, 1982.

9. Brink SJ: Limited joint mobility as a risk factor for diabetes complications, *Clin Diabetes* 5:122, 1987.

10. Brooks AP: The neuropathic foot in diabetes: part II, Charcot's neuroarthropathy, *Diabetic Med* 3:116, 1986.

11. Brower AC, Allman RM: The neuropathic joint: a neurovascular bone disorder, *Radiol Clin North Am* 19:571, 1981.

12. Brower AC, Allman RM: Pathogenesis of the neurotrophic joint: neurotraumatic vs. neurovascular, *Radiology* 139:349, 1981.

13. Brower AC, Allman RM: Neuropathic osteoarthropathy in the adult, in Taveras JM, Ferrucci JT, editors: *Radiology: diagnosis—imaging—intervention*, Philadelphia, 1989, JB Lippincott, vol 5, p 1.

14. Brownlee M, Cerami A, Vlassara H: Advanced glycosylation end products in tissue and the biochemical basis of diabetic complications, *N Engl J Med* 318:1315, 1988.

15. Bruckner FE, Howell A: Neuropathic joints, *Semin Arthritis Rheum* 2:47, 1972.

16. Buckinham BA, Uitto J, Sanborg C, et al: Scleroderma-like changes in insulin-dependent diabetes mellitus: clinical and biochemical studies, *Diabetes Care* 7:163, 1984.

17. Cavanagh PR, Sanders LJ, Sims DS: The role of pressure distribution measurement in diabetic foot care: rehabilitation R&D progress reports 1987, *J Rehabil Res Dev* 25:53, 1988.

18. Charcot JM: Sur quelques arthropathies qui paraissent dépendre d'une lésion du cerveau ou de la moelle épinière, *Arch Physiol Norm Pathol* 1:161, 1868.

19. Charcot JM: Lectures on the diseases of the ner-

vous system: lecture IV, on some visceral derangements in locomotor ataxia, arthropathies of ataxic patients, edited and translated by Sigerson G, London, 1881, New Sydenham Society.

20. Charcot JM: On some arthropathies apparently related to a lesion of the brain or spinal cord [by Charcot JM, January 1868; translated and edited by Hoché G, Sanders LJ], *J Hist Neurosci* 1:75–87, 1992.

21. Classen JN: Neuropathic arthropathy with ulceration, *Ann Surg* 159:891, 1964.

22. Clohisy DR, Thompson RC: Fractures associated with neuropathic arthropathy in adults who have juvenile-onset diabetes, *J Bone Joint Surg* 70A:1192, 1988.

23. Clouse ME, Gramm HF, Legg M, et al: Diabetic osteoarthropathy: clinical and roentgenographic observations in 90 cases, *AJR* 121:22, 1974.

24. Cofield RH, Morison MJ, Beabout JW: Diabetic neuroarthropathy in the foot: patient characteristics and patterns of radiographic change, *Foot Ankle* 4:15, 1983.

25. Coventry MB, Rothacker GW: Bilateral calcaneal fracture in a diabetic patient, *J Bone Joint Surg* 61A:462, 1979.

26. Cundy TF, Edmonds ME, Watkins PJ: Osteopenia and metatarsal fractures in diabetic neuropathy, *Diabetic Med* 2:461, 1985.

27. Delano PJ: The pathogenesis of Charcot's joint, *AJR* 56:189, 1946.

28. Drennan DB, Fahey JJ, Maylahn DJ: Important factors in achieving arthrodesis of the Charcot knee, *J Bone Joint Surg* 53A:1180, 1971.

29. Edelman SV, Kosofsky EM, et al: Neuro-osteoarthropathy (Charcot's joints) in diabetes mellitus following revascularization surgery: three case reports and a review of the literature, *Arch Intern Med* 147:1504, 1987.

30. Edmonds, ME: The neuropathic foot in diabetes: part I, blood flow, *Diabetic Med* 3:111, 1986.

31. Edmonds ME, Clarke MB, Newton S, et al: Increased uptake of bone radiopharmaceutical in diabetic neuropathy, *Q J Med (New Ser)* 57:843, 1985.

32. Edmonds ME, Morrison N, Laws JW, et al: Medial arterial calcification and diabetic neuropathy, *Br Med J* 284:938, 1982.

33. Edmonds ME, Nicolaides KH, Watkins PJ: Autonomic neuropathy and diabetic foot ulceration, *Diabetic Med* 3:56, 1986.

34. Eichenholtz SN: *Charcot joints*, Springfield, Ill, 1966, Charles C Thomas.

35. El-Khoury GY, Kathol MH: Neuropathic fractures in patients with diabetes mellitus, *Radiology* 134:313, 1980.

36. Ellman MH: Neuropathic joint disease (Charcot

joints), in McCarty DJ, editor: *Arthritis and allied conditions: a textbook of rheumatology*, Philadelphia, 1989, Lea & Febiger, p 1255.

37. Eymont MJ, Alavi A, Dalinka MK, et al: Bone scintigraphy in diabetic osteoarthropathy, *Radiology* 140:475, 1981.

38. Forgács S: Clinical picture of diabetic osteoarthropathy, *Acta Diabetol Lat* 13:111, 1976.

39. Foster DB, Bassett RC: Neurogenic arthropathy (Charcot joint) associated with diabetic neuropathy: report of two cases, *Arch Neurol Psychiatry* 57:173, 1947.

40. Friedman SA, Rakow RB: Osseous lesions of the foot in diabetic neuropathy, *Diabetes* 20:302, 1971.

41. Frykberg RG: The diabetic Charcot foot, *Arch Podiatr Med Foot Surg* 4:15, 1978.

42. Frykberg RG: Diabetic osteoarthropathy, in Brenner MA, editor: *Management of the diabetic foot*, Baltimore, 1987, Williams & Wilkins, p 75.

43. Frykberg RG: Osteoarthropathy, *Clin Podiatr Med Surg* 4:351, 1987.

44. Frykberg RG, Kozak GP: Neuropathic arthropathy in the diabetic foot, *Am Fam Phys* 17:105, 1978.

45. Glynn TP: Marked gallium accumulation in neuropathic arthropathy, *J Nucl Med* 22:1016, 1981.

46. Guillain G: *J.M. Charcot 1825–1893 his life—his work* [edited and translated by Pearce Bailey], New York, 1959, Paul B. Hoeber.

47. Harris JR, Brand PW: Patterns of disintegration of the tarsus in the anaesthetic foot, *J Bone Joint Surg* 48B:4, 1966.

48. Hart TJ, Healey K: Diabetic osteoarthropathy versus diabetic osteomyelitis, *J Foot Surg* 25:464, 1986.

49. Hartshorne MF, Peters V: Nuclear medicine applications for the diabetic foot, *Clin Podiatr Med Surg* 4:361, 1987

50. Hough AJ, Sokoloff L: Pathology of osteoarthritis, in McCarty DJ, editor: *Arthritis and allied conditions: a textbook of rheumatology*, Philadelphia, 1989, Lea & Febiger, p 1571.

51. Jacobs RL: Charcot foot, in Jahss MH, editor: *Disorders of the foot and ankle: medical and surgical management*, ed 2, Philadelphia, 1991, WB Saunders, p 2156.

52. Johnson JTH: Neuropathic fractures and joint injuries: pathogenesis and rationale of prevention and treatment, *J Bone Joint Surg* 49A:1, 1967.

53. Jordan WR: Neuritic manifestations in diabetes mellitus, *Arch Intern Med* 57:307, 1936.

54. Kathol MH, El-Koury GY, Moore TE: Calcaneal insufficiency avulsion fractures in patients with diabetes mellitus, *Radiology* 180:725–729, 1991.

55. Keenan AM, Tindel NL, Alavi A: Diagnosis of pedal osteomyelitis in diabetic patients using current scintigraphic techniques, *Arch Intern Med* 149:2262, 1989.

56. Kelly PJ, Coventry MB: Neurotrophic ulcers of the feet: review of forty-seven cases, *JAMA* 168:388, 1958.

57. Kernwein G, Lyon WF: Neuropathic arthropathy of the ankle joint resulting from complete severance of the sciatic nerve, *Ann Surg* 115:267, 1942.

58. Kidd JG: The Charcot joint: some pathologic and pathogenetic considerations, *South Med J* 67:597, 1974.

59. Knaggs LR: Charcot joints, in Knaggs RL: *Inflammatory and toxic diseases of bone*, Bristol, 1926, John Wright and Sons, p 105.

60. Kraft E, Spyropoulos E, Finby N: Neurogenic disorders of the foot in diabetes mellitus, *AJR* 124:17, 1975.

61. Lesko P, Maurer RC: Talonavicular dislocations and midfoot arthropathy in neuropathic diabetic feet: natural course and principles of treatment, *Clin Orthop* 240:226, 1989.

62. Leventen EO: Charcot foot—a technique for treatment of chronic plantar ulcer by saucerization and primary closure, *Foot Ankle* 6:295, 1986.

63. Levin ME: Diabetes and bone, *Compr Ther* 4:63, 1978.

64. Lippman HI, Perotto A, Farrar R: The neuropathic foot of the diabetic, *Bull NY Acad Med* 52:1159, 1976.

65. Lister J, Maudsley RH: Charcot joints in diabetic neuropathy, *Lancet* 2:1110, 1951

66. Martin MM: Charcot joints in diabetes mellitus, *Proc R Soc Med* 45:503, 1952.

67. Martin MM: Diabetic neuropathy: a clinical study of 150 cases, *Brain* 76:594, 1953.

68. Maurer AH, Millmond SH, Knight LC, et al: Infection in diabetic osteoarthropathy: use of indium-111 labeled leukocytes for diagnosis, *Radiology* 161:221, 1986.

69. Miller DS, Lichtman WF: Diabetic neuropathic arthropathy of feet, *Arch Surg* 70:513, 1955.

70. Monnier VM, Vishwanath V, Frank KE, et al: Relation between complications of type I diabetes mellitus and collagen-linked fluorescence, *N Engl J Med* 314:403, 1986.

71. Newman JH: Spontaneous dislocation in diabetic neuropathy. *J Bone Joint Surg* 61B:484–488, 1979.

72. Newman JH: Non-infective disease of the diabetic foot, *J Bone Joint Surg* 63B:593, 1981.

73. Newman LG, Waller J, Palestro CJ, et al: Unsuspected osteomyelitis in diabetic foot ulcers: diag-

nosis and monitoring by leukocyte scanning with indium In 111 oxyquinoline, *JAMA* 266:1246, 1991.

74. Norman A, Robbins H, Milgram JE: The acute neuropathic arthropathy—a rapid, severely disorganizing form of arthritis, *Radiology* 90:1159, 1968

75. Pogonowska MJ, Collins LC, Dobson HL: Diabetic osteopathy, *Radiology* 89:265, 1967.

76. Radin EL: Mechanical aspects of osteoarthrosis, *Bull Rheum Dis* 26:862, 1976

77. Resnick D: Neuroarthropathy, in Resnick D, Niwayama G, editors: *Diagnosis of bone and joint disorders with emphasis on articular abnormalities*, Philadelphia, 1981, WB Saunders, vol 3, p 2422.

78. Rodnan GP: Neuropathic joint disease (Charcot joints), in Hollander JL, et al, editors: *Arthritis and Allied Conditions*, Philadelphia, 1985, Lea & Febiger, p 1095.

79. Rosenblatt S: Principles of evaluation and treatment of osteomyelitis in the diabetic foot, *Clin Diabetes* 7:85, 1989.

80. Rubinow A, Spark EC, Canoso JJ: Septic arthritis in a Charcot joint, *Clin Orthop* 147:203, 1980.

81. Saltzman CL, Johnson KA, Goldstein RH, et al: The patellar tendon-bearing brace as treatment for neurotrophic arthropathy: a dynamic force monitoring study, *Foot Ankle* 13:14, 1992.

82. Sammarco GJ: Diabetic arthropathy, in Sammarco GJ, editor: *The foot in diabetes*, Philadelphia, 1991, Lea & Febiger.

83. Sanders LJ, Frykberg RG: Diabetic neuropathic osteoarthropathy: the Charcot foot, in Frykberg RG, editor: *The high risk foot in diabetes mellitus*, New York, 1991, Churchill Livingstone.

84. Sanders LJ, Mrdjenovich D: Anatomical patterns of bone and joint destruction in neuropathic diabetics, *Diabetes* 40(suppl 1):529A, 1991.

85. Sanders LJ, Murray-Leisure K: Infections of the diabetic foot, in Abramson C, McCarthy DJ, Rupp M, editors: *Infectious diseases of the lower extremity*, Baltimore, 1991, Williams & Wilkins.

86. Schauwecker DS: Osteomyelitis: diagnosis with in-111-labeled leukocytes, *Radiology* 171:141, 1989.

87. Schauwecker DS, Park HM, Burt RW, et al: Combined bone scintigraphy and indium-111 leukocyte scans in neuropathic foot disease, *J Nucl Med* 29:1651, 1988.

88. Schoenhaus HD, Wernick E, Cohen R: Biomechanics of the diabetic foot, in Frykberg RG, editor: *The high risk foot in diabetes mellitus*. New York, 1991, Churchill Livingstone.

89. Schwartz ER: Chondrocyte structure and function, in McCarty DJ, editor: *Arthritis and allied conditions: a textbook of rheumatology*, Philadelphia, 1989, Lea & Febiger, p 289.

90. Schwarz GS, Berenyi MR, Siegel MW: Atrophic arthropathy and diabetic neuritis, *AJR* 106:523, 1969.

91. Shands AR: Neuropathies of the bones and joints: report of a case of an arthropathy of the ankle due to a peripheral nerve lesion, *Arch Surg* 20:614, 1930.

92. Shibata T, Tada K, Hashizume C: The results of arthrodesis of the ankle for leprotic neuroarthropathy, *J Bone Joint Surg* 72A:749, 1990.

93. Sinha S, Munichoodappa C, Kozak GP: Neuroarthropathy (Charcot joints) in diabetes mellitus: clinical study of 101 cases, *Medicine (Baltimore)* 52:191, 1972.

94. Soto-Hall R, Haldeman KO: The diagnosis of neuropathic joint disease (Charcot joint): an analysis of 40 cases, *JAMA* 114:2076, 1940.

95. Steindler A: The tabetic arthropathies, *JAMA* 96:250, 1931.

96. Stuart MJ, Morrey BF: Arthrodesis of the diabetic neuropathic ankle joint, *Clin Orthop* 253:209, 1990.

97. Thompson RC, Havel P, Goetz F: Presumed neurotrophic skeletal disease in diabetic kidney transplant recipients, *JAMA* 249:1317, 1983.

98. Treves F: Treatment of perforating ulcer of the foot, *Lancet* 2:949, 1884.

99. Wartenberg R: Neuropathic joint disease, *JAMA* 111:2044, 1938.

100. Wastie ML: Radiological changes in serial x-rays of the foot and tarsus in leprosy, *Clin Radiol* 26:285, 1975.

101. Watkins PJ, Edmonds ME: Sympathetic nerve failure in diabetes, *Diabetologia* 25:73–77, 1983.

102. Williamson B, Treates CD, Phillips CD, et al: Computed tomography as a diagnostic aid in diabetic and other problem feet, *Clin Imag* 13:159, 1989.

103. Zeiger LS, Fox IM: Use of indium-111 labeled white blood cells in the diagnosis of diabetic foot infections, *J Foot Surg* 29:46, 1990.

104. Zlatkin MB, Pathria M, Sartoris DJ, et al: The diabetic foot, *Radiol Clin North Am* 25:1095, 1987.

# CHAPTER 8

# Infection of the Diabetic Foot

**J. Russell Little, M.D.**

**George S. Kobayashi, Ph.D.**

**Thomas C. Bailey, M.D.**

Infections are a frequent problem in patients with diabetes mellitus, and foot infections are a major cause of limb loss and other morbidity.[46] Many diabetic foot ulcers are neglected because they may produce few symptoms and because their importance is not appreciated by the patient, leading to potentially serious complications. Determining which pathogens are involved is problematic, and culture results can even be misleading. Further, the diagnosis of osteomyelitis associated with a foot ulcer can be a formidable challenge. We consider these and several other areas that contribute to our understanding of the pathogenesis and treatment of these important infections.

## MICROBIOLOGY OF SKIN

Microbiologic studies of human skin have revealed that different areas are populated by a complex and changing bacterial and fungal flora. Various environments predispose to different types of microbial colonization.[60, 70] On the drier portions of the lower leg, the flora is restricted (about 1,000 bacteria/cm$^2$) because of the physical and chemical conditions on the skin surface. Strong, selective pressures against microbial growth on the lower leg and foot are exerted by (1) skin temperature, which is much lower than optimum for many human pathogens; (2) the presence of metabolic products of the skin that have direct antimicrobial chemical effects (e.g., fatty acids) to lower the pH or increase the ionicity on the skin surface; (3) the relatively arid surface of the dorsum of the foot and lower leg, making survival dependent on the ability of various microbes to resist drying; and (4) the stratum corneum of the sole, which is thicker than anywhere else on the body and less permeable to ingress and egress of nutrients and fluids than other skin surfaces.[70]

However, a number of local conditions on the foot favor the growth of certain microbial flora. Although the feet of diabetics with impaired sweating because of peripheral neuropathy are colonized with flora similar to nondiabetic patients,[52] the importance of moisture in promoting bacterial and fungal growth is suggested by the density and variety of organisms in the toe webs, which are even greater than in the axilla (where > 1 million bacteria/cm$^2$ can be recovered).[30, 45, 60] The presence of *Corynebacterium minutissimum* (the causative agent of erythrasma); lipophilic and nonlipophilic diphtheroids; enterobacteraciae; and *Pseudomonas, Acinetobacter,* and *Candida* organisms in the toe webs differs greatly from the coccal and lipophilic diphtheroid flora of the drier and, therefore, less hospitable lower calf. In addition, the higher microbial density of intertriginous areas is supported by a higher surface pH, a result of the metabolism of nitrogenous substances and the low availability of carbohydrate substrates reducing acid production. Further, although the low temperature of the distal lower extremity has a significant selective effect against many common bacteria and fungi, *Mycobacterium marinum* and the dermatophytes flourish in areas where the temperature seldom exceeds 30° to 31° C.[44]

Colonization of the foot by dermatophyte fungi occurs in healthy individuals, facilitated by the necessity of wearing shoes in our society, which leads to retention of skin products, especially water. The amount of fatty acids secreted by sebaceous glands of the covered foot is also diminished, predisposing to ringworm (dermatophyte) infection.[61] In one study of 124 recruits without clinical evidence of skin disease, 23 (18.6%) yielded one or more of three fungal species (*Trichophyton mentagrophytes, Trichophyton rubrum,* or *Epidermophyton floccosum*) from foot scrapings.[40] However, the diabetic patient may be at increased risk of colonization by these fungi. In Greenwood and Rockwood's study[28] of 100 patients with generally well-controlled diabetes, 70 were found to have dermatophytosis of the interdigital areas of the feet.

Interdigital dermatophytosis is a major factor in predisposing the diabetic patient to serious infection, because the resultant epidermal fissures and erosions create portals of entry for pyogenic bacteria, leading to cellulitis and "infectious" gangrene of the digits.[20] The importance of interacting flora is exemplified on the moist skin of the toe webs, where combined colonization by dermatophyte fungi, *Staphylococcus aureus* and *Candida albicans*, intensifies itching, aggravating the inflammatory response and providing a greater opportunity for invasion.[43] The diabetic patient may also suffer adverse effects from ill-fitting shoes, resulting in repeated minor trauma and leading directly to stasis and ulceration, followed by penetration of potentially pathogenic skin fungi and bacteria and, ultimately, overt infection. The problem of minor trauma by ill-fitting shoes, followed by infection at these sites, can be exacerbated by neuropathic changes, producing hypoesthesia and unawareness by the patient of the usual symptoms of local inflammation.

## DIABETES MELLITUS AND INFECTION

Although it is commonly stated that patients with diabetes mellitus are more susceptible to infection than normal individuals, epidemiologic studies have produced conflicting results.[11] It may be that awareness of the hazard of infection in diabetics has given rise to the impression of higher infection rates. There is no convincing evidence that immunologic competence is impaired in patients with diabetes mellitus,[30, 42, 64, 75] nor is there any significant difference in antibody responses in murine models of diabetes.[5, 13]

However, experiments with induced diabetes in rabbits and rats have provided some support for the concept that diabetes does increase susceptibility to bacterial and fungal infections.[8, 14, 67] Also, Robbins and Tucker[62] found an increased frequency of infection of the extremities and of pyelonephritis in an autopsy comparison of 307 adult diabetics with 2,800 nondiabetics. Much interest has centered around possible abnormalities in the diabetic host phagocytic cells. Brayton et al.[4] found evidence for reduced leukocyte mobilization in patients with diabetes mellitus. Perillie et al.[57] found reduced leukocyte mobilization only when ketoacidosis was present, whereas Mowat and Baum[49] and Fortes et al.[19] have provided additional evidence of defective chemotaxis in diabetic leukocytes.

Tan et al.,[71] Dziatkowiak et al.,[16] and Sima et al.[68] have independently found neutrophil bactericidal defects in phagocytes from diabetic animals and patients. Studies have shown that neutrophil respiratory burst activity is subnormal in diabetics, prompting the speculation that host resistance is impaired because of a defect in the formation of reactive oxygen metabolites.[59, 65] Cruickshank and Payne[8] have shown that the whole blood of animals with alloxan-induced diabetes (regardless of glucose content) had a weaker bactericidal activity than blood from normal animals. Nolan et al.[53] studied a similar defect in granulocyte bactericidal function in peripheral blood leukocytes from poorly controlled diabetics. Others have claimed that the bactericidal and phagocytic activities of the diabetic's polymorphonuclear leukocytes are normal,[6, 7, 32] although phagocytosis was decreased during ketoacidosis.[6]

Of all the infections seen in diabetic patients, none is more common than bacterial and fungal infections of the skin. Greenwood[27] has suggested that 25% of patients with diabetes have a history of significant cutaneous infection, and 10% show active infections at any one time. Authors disagree about an increased susceptibility to staphylococcal skin infections, but there is general accord that once an infection of the foot or lower leg has become established, it is generally more severe and refractory in the diabetic patient.

The exact mechanisms of increased frequency and severity of infections of the feet are nearly as obscure as the relationship of diabetes and infection in general. Hyperglycemia per se does not generally increase the growth rate of the common bacterial pathogens. Despite disagreement about the existence of a greater susceptibility to or severity of infection, it has been proposed that effective antibiotic therapy for infection is second only to the availability of insulin in significantly increasing the life span of diabetic patients.[7, 72] Although the experimental data are lacking to explain an increased susceptibility of diabetics to infection at the cellular level, it is likely that peripheral neuropathy and vascular insufficiency are the major pathobiologic contributors to the predisposition of diabetic feet to serious infections (see later discussion).

## INFECTIONS OF NAILS

Infections of the toenails, nail beds, and adjacent structures comprise an important and frequently encountered group of problems in diabetic patients. The general, and perhaps mistaken, consensus is that nail infections are almost always caused by fungi. In fact, even though species of dermatophytes belonging to the genus *Trichophyton*, particularly *T. rubrum*, have been accepted as etiologic agents in tinea unguium (invasion of the nail plate by dermatophytes), attempts to prove them pathogens according to Koch's postulates have failed.[73] The latter failure may reflect experimental deficiencies, but clinical series have provided evidence that bacterial infections,[80] congenital abnormalities, viral infections, traumatic injury, and various other dermatologic diseases (e.g., lichen planus and psoriasis) of toenails also occur commonly and may be clinically indistinguishable from disease caused by dermatophytes. A heterogeneous group of other ubiquitous fungi, including *C. albicans*, *Scopulariopsis brevicalis*, and various species of *Aspergillus*, have been isolated and identified in nail infections, frequently in association with dystrophic nail changes.[80] The clinical term employed to describe fungal infection of the nail is onychomycosis.[73]

The clinical appearance of tinea unguium (any dermatophyte infection of the nail plate) and onychomycosis caused by any one species of fungus is indistinguishable from that caused by any other species. The fungal infection per se is asymptomatic. Often most of the fingernails and toenails are involved, although sparing of one or more digits is fairly common. Subungual keratosis is the most reliable and most commonly seen clinical sign (distal subungual onychomycosis). The fungus gains access to the nail from under the distal free edge or from the lateral nail folds. The nail plate appears normal during the early phase of infection, but later the normal nail plate–nail bed attachment is disrupted, permitting air to collect under the nail, which produces the white appearance termed onycholysis. (The latter is often seen in other nail conditions as well.) As the process progresses, the offending organism advances proximally, growing on the stratum corneum of the nail bed and invading the undersurface of the nail plate. The excessive horn produced by the diseased nail bed epidermis usually elevates the nail plate, giving the appearance of a dramatically thickened nail. Subsequently, the nail plate loses its usual transparency and its quality of hardness, becoming crumbly and dough-like. In the advanced stages of onychomycosis, coexisting bacterial flora usually abound; *Pseudomonas aeruginosa* and *Proteus* species are the most common. In the final stages of the process, the abnormal nail plate crumbles or is traumatically removed. The process can arrest itself and remain unchanged at any of its stages or may progress rapidly through all of them.

The diagnosis of onychomycosis is usually verified by microscopic examination and culture. The nails are scraped vigorously, and the material removed from infected areas is digested with 10% potassium hydroxide and examined microscopically for hyphae or pseudohyphae (*Candida* species).[80] Gentle heating over a flame will hasten the hydrolytic process. The coverslip should be firmly pressed down, producing a thin film of material for examination. Cultures are grown on Mycosel agar (Sabouraud's dextrose agar with chloramphenicol and cycloheximide) for 4 weeks before being discarded as negative. Because many "nonpathogens" (e.g., *Aspergillus* and *Scopulariopsis* organisms) have been implicated in clinical infections, cultures should also be seeded on Sabouraud's medium containing chloramphenicol alone, because these latter organisms may be sensitive to cycloheximide.

Difficulties are occasionally encountered in collecting adequate clinical material because of the greater pain sensitivity of the affected nail plate. In such cases the patient can collect clippings from the affected area on a sheet of paper, place it in an envelope, and submit them on a subsequent visit to the physician for microscopic examination and culture. In general, the dermatophytes withstand short periods of desiccation and remain viable.

In the treatment of dermatophytic onychomycosis, it is clear that oral griseofulvin in adequate amounts results in high response rates. However, in many patients, fungal toenail disease promptly recurs after the cessation of therapy. Griseofulvin is absorbed well with food, and dietary fat promotes greater absorption. The drug is incorporated into the cells of the epidermis in concentrations sufficient to inhibit but not kill the dermatophyte fungi.

Microsize griseofulvin 0.5–1.0 g/day orally is administered in a single dose or in two divided doses. Griseofulvin is remarkably nontoxic, but gastrointestinal complaints such as eructations or diarrhea may occur, and skin eruptions have occasionally required discontinuation of the drug. Headache occurs in approximately 15% of those treated, but it is usually mild. Reversible leukopenia occasionally occurs. Symptomatic relief of dermatophyte skin infections generally occurs after 48 to 96 hours of griseofulvin therapy, but therapy should generally be continued for 4 to 6 months, although the dosage can usually be reduced by one half after the initial 6 weeks of treatment.

It is important to recognize that griseofulvin is useless in noninfectious dermatoses and even in skin infections caused by the nondermatophyte fungi *C. albicans* and *Pityrosporum obiculare*. The imidazole and azole compounds such as ketoconazole, fluconazole, and the currently experimental agent itraconazole represent an advance in the treatment of systemic fungal infections.[12] However, they are also effective in the treatment of superficial fungal infections such as paronychia caused by *C. albicans* and the dermatophytoses (e.g., tinea infections). For some patients, oral antifungal therapy may prove to be more convenient, but topical azoles (butoconazole, clotrimazole, ketoconazole, miconazole, and econazole) are widely used and comparably effective. Of the oral agents, ketoconazole is the least expensive. It is administered in daily doses of one or two 200-mg tablets taken with a meal or with orange juice. Gastric acidity is needed to dissolve the drug and promote absorption from the gastrointestinal contents. At the beginning of treatment, a blood ketoconazole level should always be obtained (90 minutes after the daily dose) to document the adequacy of absorption. Itraconazole (soon to be approved by the Food and Drug Administration [FDA]) is similar to ketoconazole in its dependence on acid for intestinal absorption, and antacids (including $H_2$-antagonists) interfere with the absorption of both agents. Fluconazole has advantages of acid-independent absorption and five to ten times greater activity against *C. albicans* than ketoconazole.[22] Adverse effects of these newer azoles appear to be remarkably few. Pruritis, mild nausea, and occasional vomiting are more likely to occur at higher doses such as 400 to 600 mg/day. Results of renal function tests, urinalysis, and blood counts have shown few abnormalities, but hepatic toxicity, usually mild and reversible, has been an idiosyncratic serious problem in some patients taking ketoconazole. Azoles may be administered for prolonged periods to establish or maintain clinical remission or to prevent reinfection. Efficacy has often been dramatic in the acute dermatophytoses and in chronic mucocutaneous candidiasis. Ketoconazole is also effective in chronic dermatophyte infections, including those resistant to griseofulvin.[23, 29, 34] Skin lesions clear much more quickly than nail lesions, which may require many months of therapy.

## PARONYCHIA

Paronychia is an important problem in diabetic foot care, although it is less common on the feet than on the hands. In either location the infection is often related to initial trauma and to the predisposing influence of moist or macerated skin. Either bacteria or fungi are common infectious agents found in paronychia. *Candida albicans* is the most common mycotic agent, and *S. aureus* is frequently a secondary invader. The differential diagnosis includes herpes simplex infection (whitlow), but this is uncommon, quite painful, and almost always occurs on the hands, usually in health care workers. In chronic paronychia there is usually only slight erythema and little swelling or pain, but tenderness on pressure is common.

Paronychial involvement by *C. albicans* can be effectively managed by nystatin ointment (100,000 units/g) or with oral ketoconazole or fluconazole. Secondary infections with *S. aureus* may be treated with oral dicloxacillin, 250 to 500 mg four times daily. Several weeks of continuous therapy are usually necessary to cure chronic paronychia. The patient must be warned that the injudicious use of hot compresses in the treatment of paronychia or other infections of the leg or feet may contribute to the development of gangrene if the blood supply is marginal. Keeping the area clean, elevating the leg, and avoiding trauma do more to aid in localization of infection than do most other steps, and early surgical drainage is also encouraged.

## NEUROPATHY AND VASCULAR INSUFFICIENCY AS RISK FACTORS FOR FOOT INFECTIONS

The pathophysiology of the development of infected foot ulcers in diabetic patients relates principally to neuropathy and ischemia. Peripheral sensory neuropathy predisposes to foot injuries, which often go unnoticed because of reduced pain sensation,[55] and motor neuropathy affecting the foot can cause alterations in pressure distribution that predispose to traumatic skin ulceration.[9] A common scenario is that motor neuropathy causes weakness of the intrinsic muscles of the foot. The development of weak foot muscles creates an imbalance, with the stronger muscles of the calf pulling up on the foot and resulting in clawing of the toes. This claw foot deformity changes the mechanics of the foot and even the patient's gait, so that more weight is placed on the metatarsal heads, resulting in callus formation in the overlying skin. Inflammatory changes tend to occur underneath the callus, leading to tissue autolysis, hemorrhage, necrosis, and ulcer formation over the metatarsal heads (mal perforans ulcer). Patients often fail to note discomfort from pressure points, callus formation, or even ulceration because of the associated sensory neuropathy. These considerations are discussed in greater detail in Chapters 2 and 6.

Although it is unproved, it seems probable that a second major etiologic factor in infection is vascular insufficiency. Tissue ischemia resulting from poor blood supply probably contributes significantly to infection in the foot and lower leg. In the normal individual, the blood supply is increased at the site of inflammation, whereas patients with diabetes respond to inflammation in regions with inadequate blood supply by developing vascular thrombosis and resulting tissue necrosis. The importance of microvascular occlusive changes[1] in the etiology of diabetic foot disease has been seriously questioned and the evidence reviewed critically by LoGerfo and Coffman.[38] These and other authors maintain that diabetic neuropathy, not microvascular disease, is the primary cause of foot lesions in the presence of a normal arterial system.

## CLINICAL AND BACTERIOLOGIC CHARACTERISTICS OF DIABETIC FOOT INFECTIONS

The relationship between infection and gangrene (see Chapters 4 and 17) is a critical consideration in understanding the pathogenesis and optimum therapy of foot infections in the diabetic. The two central processes that determine the occurrence and distribution of gangrene in the affected limb are (1) preexisting major arterial insufficiency (see discussion on vascular disease in Chapters 17 and 18), and (2) the regional increased tissue turgor and metabolic rate that result from edema, the local inflammatory reaction, or both.

The finding of gas in infected tissues in diabetic patients has been a recognized phenomenon for many years. The soft tissue gas produced during bacterial infections is principally hydrogen and carbon dioxide. The capacity for gas formation is shown not only by *Clostridium* spp. but also by aerobic and anaerobic gram-negative bacilli and anaerobic gram-positive cocci. It was once believed that crepitus in a gangrenous extremity was certain evidence of clostridial infection. However, most of these infections in diabetic patients are caused by anaerobic streptococci and enterobacteriaceae and do not represent classical "gas gangrene."[78] A typical example of cellulitis with soft tissue gas is shown in Figure 8–1.

Arterial insufficiency and locally increased tissue pressure and metabolism act synergistically to increase the tissue demand for oxygen while reducing its delivery. Increased extravascular tissue tension and the local production of tissue-destructive en-

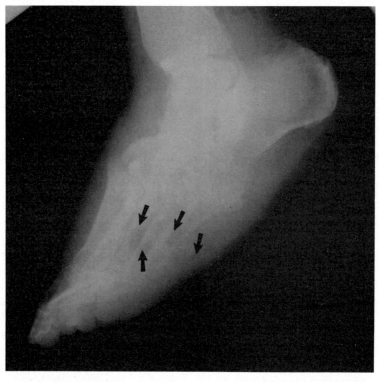

**FIG 8–1.**
Radiograph of foot with bacterial cellulitis. Lateral view shows accentuated soft tissues and diffuse soft tissue swelling. Numerous air collections *(arrows)* throughout soft tissue are consistent with cellulitis.

zymes, derived mainly from phagocyte lysosomes, lead to local thrombosis and small-vessel occlusion. Bacterial endotoxins liberated from infecting microbes and acting on mononuclear phagocytes may also play a role in the initiation of local thrombosis. With certain infections, the vascular compression resulting from increased tissue tension may partly result from bacterial gas formation by *Clostridium* species, *Bacteroides* species, or *Escherichia coli* organisms or the anaerobic streptococci. The anatomic progression of tissue infection may be alarmingly swift if the extremity was previously edematous or, alternatively, if *Streptococcus pyogenes* or clostridia are the predominant pathogens. These microorganisms secrete an array of biologically potent toxins and enzymes, some of which cause increased capillary permeability with severe swelling and edema formation. In such a setting, the application of a tight bandage or a tightly fitting shoe often leads to pressure necrosis and the initiation of gangrenous process.

The choice of appropriate therapy for foot infections, like infections elsewhere, depends on clinical judgments regarding severity, duration, rate of progression, and the probable pathogenic flora. Clearly the most satisfactory form of treatment is preventive and depends on the patient's motivation and understanding of the rules of hygiene and meticulous care outlined in Chapter 2. Important therapeutic generalizations that relate to an already established infection are (1) to provide for immobilization and elevation of the extremity and (2) to incise surgically and drain early if there is any perceived fluctuance or partially drained abscess. Surgical drainage is an important part of the therapy, as well as providing material for culture and antibiotic susceptibility testing.

The question of whether diabetic foot infections should be routinely cultured is complex and controversial. Recent successful results with empirical antibiotic therapy, taken together with our knowledge that specimens are often contaminated with colonizing organisms, make it difficult to provide a simple answer. If only superficial cultures can be obtained, they may be of very little value or even misleading. If a deep curettage specimen or pus aspirated through unbroken skin is cultured, the relevant bacteriology is more likely to be revealed. One argument for routine culturing is that occasionally less common pathogens may be identified (e.g., methicillin-oxacillin-resistant *S. aureus* [MRSA], group B streptococci, *Clostridium* spp.), providing important clues for management. Because about 70% of foot infections involve mixed bacterial flora, anaerobic as well as aerobic culture methods should be employed. In interpreting the culture results, it should be borne in mind that the pathogenic roles of weakly virulent bacteria such as coagulase-negative staphylococci, enterococci, viridans streptococci, corynebacteria, and certain anaerobes are unknown. Treatment directed specifically at each and every isolated agent is difficult and usually unnecessary.

Obligate anaerobes are often present in neurotrophic foot ulcers whether or not they show signs of infection. These ulcers usually contain mixed bacterial flora, including facultative and obligate anaerobes, and they have certain clinical characteristics that distinguish them from infections caused by staphylococci or other aerobes.[17] Specifically, these mixed anaerobe infections are frequently foul smelling and associated with soft tissue gas. Figure 8–2 shows the typical appearance of a diabetic neurotrophic ulcer.

If a diabetic patient with an infected foot appears nontoxic and is afebrile without recent mental status changes, a decision may be made regarding possible outpatient management.[37] Improvement of the patient's metabolic regulation may dictate the need for inpatient therapy, but after careful consideration, some patients may still be suitable candidates for outpatient management. Generally this will include patients whose infections lack evidence of deep soft tissue involvement, osteomyelitis, or gangrene. Outpatient management requires a supportive home environment where the patient may be inactive with the foot elevated and, in most patients, will involve the use of oral antibiotics (Table 8–1). One recently published study by Lipsky et al.[37] involved 56 assessable patients randomly assigned to outpa-

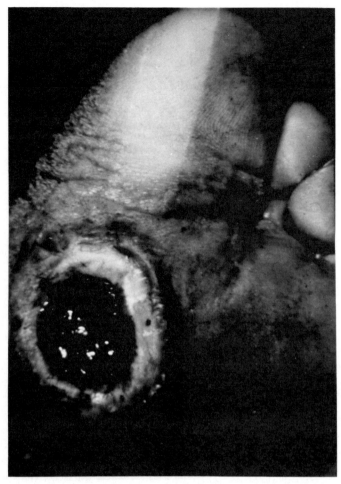

**FIG 8–2.**
Neurotrophic (mal perforans) ulcers *(arrows)* appear over areas of pressure and trauma in anesthetic skin. Why such changes follow cutaneous denervation is not completely understood, but any clinical disorder resulting in loss of sensation can produce them. Most common sites are at pressure points, particularly on sole of foot over base of first metatarsal head. *(Courtesy of Dr. Howard C. Welgus, St. Louis.)*

tient treatment with oral clindamycin (Cleocin, 300 mg qid) or cephalexin (Keflex, 500 mg qid) for 2 weeks. Ninety-one percent of these patients were regarded as cured, requiring no further antibiotic treatment after a mean follow-up interval of 15 months. This is surprising, because the two antibiotics are not ideal, especially when used as monotherapy. Clearly these encouraging data are crucially dependent on patient selection. Notably, the authors state that patients whose infections failed to improve or worsened initially were withdrawn from the study and hospitalized for parenteral antibiotic therapy. Although the study design makes it virtually impossible to interpret the

authors' very high success rate, it is true that the newer oral antibiotics, particularly the fluoroquinolones[50, 56] and extended spectrum β-lactams,[25] along with oral clindamycin (Cleocin) or metronidazole (Flagyl), have reduced the number of patients requiring hospitalization for treatment of their foot infections. For example, a combination of oral ciprofloxacin (Cipro) and clindamycin (Cleocin) provides broad antibacterial action (vs. *S. aureus*, aerobic gram-negative bacilli and anaerobes).

However, hospitalization and parenteral antibiotics will still be required for initial therapy of patients with complicated infections (e.g., gangrene or osteomyelitis), for

**TABLE 8-1.**

Guide to Useful Antimicrobial Agents for Diabetic Foot Infections

| Antibiotic | Route and Dosage | Major Targeted Bacteria | Comments |
|---|---|---|---|
| Ciprofloxacin | PO 750 mg bid<br>IV 400 mg, q12h | Aerobic gram-negative rods (bacilli), *Staphylococcus aureus* | Good bone penetration; useful against *Pseudomonas aeruginosa.* |
| Ofloxacin | PO 400 mg bid | Aerobic and modest anaerobic spectrum | New agent. Less active vs. *P. aeruginosa* than ciprofloxacin |
| Ticarcillin-clavulanate | IV 3.1 g q4–8h | Aerobic gram-negative rods, *S. aureus,* anaerobes | Timentin; expensive |
| Ampicillin-clavulanate | PO 500 mg tid | Aerobic gram-negative rods, *S. aureus,* anaerobes | Augmentin; causes diarrhea in ∼ 10% |
| Ampicillin-sulbactam | IV 3 g q6h | *S. aureus,* aerobic gram-negative rods, anaerobes, enterococci | Unasyn; expensive |
| Cefoxitin | IV 2 g q4–8h | Aerobic gram-negative rods, anaerobes | Not active vs. *P. aeruginosa, Enterobacter* sp. |
| Cefotetan | IV 1–3 g q12h | Aerobic gram-negative rods, anaerobes | Long half-life |
| Ceftazidime | IV 1–2 g q8h | Aerobic gram-negative rods, gram-positive cocci, anaerobes | Potent vs. *P. aeruginosa* and other aerobic gnr |
| Ceftriaxione | IV 1 g q24h<br>IM 1 g q24h | Aerobic gram-negative rods, gram-positive cocci | Long half-life; expensive |
| Imipenem-cilastatin | IV 0.5 g q6h<br>IM 0.5–0.75 g q12h | Aerobic gram-negative rods, gram-positive cocci, anaerobes | Combination of Primaxin; Expensive; very broad spectrum |
| Clindamycin | PO 300 mg qid<br>IV 600 mg q8h | Anaerobes and common gram-positive cocci | Good bone penetration; not active vs. aerobic gnr |
| Metronidazole | PO 500 mg tid<br>IV 500 mg q8h | Obligate anaerobes only | Used along with other antibiotics |
| Vancomycin | IV 1 g q12h | Methicillin-resistant *S. aureus,* enterococci, coagulase-negative *Staphylococcus* | Drug of choice for methicillin-resistant *S. aureus,* most coagulase-negative *Staphylococcus* |

patients who appear toxic or acutely ill, and for those who may have failed to respond to oral antibiotics. In such patients there are at least five different parenteral antibiotic regimens that provide empirical therapy directed at infections, including aerobic gram-negative bacilli, mixed anaerobic bacteria, and most isolates of *S. aureus.* These are, in order of increasing cost, (1) cefazolin (Ancef or Kefzol) plus clindamycin (Cleocin) or metronidazole (Flagyl), (2) cefotetan (Cefotan) or cefoxitin (Mefoxin), (3) ampicillin-sulbactam (Unasyn), (4) ticarcillin-clavulanate (Timentin), and (5) imipenem-cilastatin (Primaxin). Only Unasyn, Timentin, and Primaxin are active against *Enterococcus* spp. Only Timentin and Primaxin provide coverage for *Pseudomonas aeruginosa;* cefotetan (Cefotan) and cefoxitin (Mefoxin) have the weakest coverage for staphylococci, and none of these is active against methicillin-resistant coagulase-negative staphylococci or MRSA, for which vancomycin is the drug of choice. If the patient has had a previous penicillin allergy, aztreonam (Azactam) may be substituted for cefazolin (Ancef or Kefzol) in regimen 1 (with clindamycin [Cleocin]).

Blood culture results and, in some cases, the results of local wound cultures may dictate changes in antibiotics from the empirical choices cited earlier (e.g., *Enterococcus* spp., MRSA, or highly resistant aerobic gram-negative bacilli), but it is desirable in most diabetic patients to avoid the use of aminoglycosides (e.g., gentamicin [Garamycin]) because of their potential nephrotoxicity and ototoxicity. Patients with known or suspected gram-negative sepsis are exceptions to this rule in which a loading dose of aminoglycoside (e.g., 1.5–2.0 mg/kg gentamicin) should be added to a β-lactam (e.g., ceftazidime [Fortaz or Tazidime]) and clindamycin (Cleocin) or metronidazole (Flagyl). Once the patient's condition is stabilized and the culture and susceptibility data are known, a reevaluation of the need for continued aminoglycoside therapy is encouraged.

Synergistic gangrene has been observed repeatedly in patients with mixed anaerobic infections of the foot. Synergy implies that two or more bacteria can produce a pathologic process that cannot be produced by a simple microbe in pure culture. The synergy concept underlies an attractive hypothesis to explain the pathophysiology of mixed anaerobic infections in general. One well-studied synergistic bacterial pair is anaerobic streptococci, occurring with *S. aureus* to produce a burrowing, undermining ulcer.[69] *Staphylococcus aureus* produces a hyaluronidase that permits the streptococcus to invade at the inflammatory front.[47] When these infections are seen in patients who have been treated previously for diabetic foot ulcers, the assumption is often made erroneously that they are monomicrobial infections caused by staphylococci and may be treated with semisynthetic penicillins, perhaps even on an outpatient basis. This may involve a great risk because most anaerobes fail to respond to the usual semisynthetic antistaphylococcal agents, and the soft tissue infection may spread rapidly to involve the entire leg.

## OSTEOMYELITIS

Osteomyelitis is one of the most serious problems of foot care in diabetic patients. In a review by Waldvogel et al.,[74] approximately one third of 247 patients with osteomyelitis were diabetic. Most diabetic patients with osteomyelitis are between 50 and 70 years of age, and almost all infections involve the toes or small bones of the feet. Few have systemic manifestations of infection (fever, malaise, leukocytosis), but most patients have long-standing indolent ulcers with swelling and erythema. Mixed infections are common; staphylococci are usually associated with anaerobic or aerobic streptococci (not group A) or with one of the enterobacteriaceae (*E. coli, Klebsiella, Proteus, Enterobacter,* etc.). Conservative treatment with antimicrobial drugs, incision, and drainage is frequently unsuccessful, especially in the presence of vascular insufficiency; amputation may be required for cure.

It should be emphasized that neither clinical, radiographic, nor radionuclide evaluations can distinguish consistently between osteomyelitis and the lesions of diabetic osteopathy (Figs 8–3 to 8–5) or neuropathic joint disease (Charcot joints) that occur in severe peripheral neuropathy.[21] Osteopathy related to denervation does not require surgical intervention even if the bone changes are demonstrably progressive. A useful radiographic sign of neuropathic disease in the feet is the presence of a characteristically pointed distal metatarsal called the "peppermint stick sign." The multifocal and bilateral distribution of diabetic neuropathic osteopathy is helpful, if present, in differentiating it from osteomyelitis. In addition, patients with neuropathic bone dissolution will usually have normal total leukocyte counts and erythrocyte sedimentation rates (ESRs). Clearly, the presence of an overlying ulcer strongly suggests that underlying bone lesion or lesions may be osteomyelitis. Ultimately the distinction between osteomyelitis and diabetic osteopathy is a clinical one; it can best be made by careful sequential observations.

Most cases of osteomyelitis of the foot or lower leg in diabetics begin as chronic perfo-

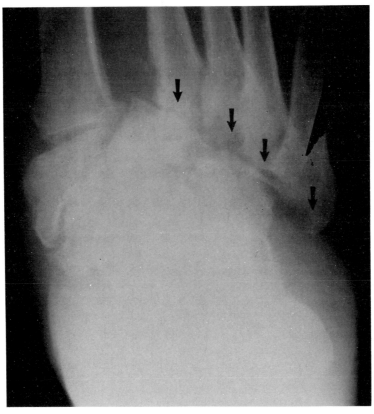

**FIG 8–3.**
Radiograph of diabetic neurotrophic arthropathy. Anteroposterior view of foot to show tarsometatarsal joints. Note disorganization of joints and lateral dislocation of second to fifth metatarsal bases *(arrows)* with respect to tarsal bones (Lisfranc's fracture dislocation). Note destruction of metatarsal bases and bones of distal tarsal row. *(Courtesy of Dr. William F. Conway, St. Louis.)*

rating ulcers. These may heal and recur repeatedly over long periods, because the predisposing factors of poor tissue nutrition and decreased antimicrobial defenses remain unchanged. Generally, chronic skin and subcutaneous ulcers ultimately become populated with mixed bacterial species. If the ulcer is neglected or improperly cared for, bacteria may invade the base of the lesion and spread along fascial planes or may penetrate fascia and soft tissues to reach the periosteum. Puncture wounds of the foot may result in a similar sequence, and diabetic patients with neuropathic hypoesthesia are particularly susceptible to puncture trauma.[48] Punctures through a tennis shoe often become infected with *P. aeruginosa*.[18] Retained foreign bodies in the soft tissue should always be considered in cases of perforating trauma. The patient must be made

aware that draining lesions require prompt treatment even when there is relatively little pain, redness, or local swelling.

The well-known problems in evaluating conventional bone x-ray films or tomograms in osteomyelitis have been offset somewhat by the progress achieved with newer imaging techniques, such as radionuclide scanning and magnetic resonance imaging (MRI). It should be emphasized, however, that plain x-ray films of the feet are the logical first step in the imaging of foot infections, because they may reveal air in the tissues or the presence of foreign bodies, and sometimes they may provide convincing evidence of osteomyelitis. However, negative x-ray films cannot exclude bone infection, and other imaging studies are often recommended by radiologists. Generally bone scans or gallium scans, although much more sensitive than plain x-ray films, are too non-specific.[31, 33, 41, 79] Twenty-four-hour indium 111–labeled white blood cell scanning has been employed by Newman et al.,[51] who found that the majority of diabetic foot ulcers had underlying osteomyelitis (confirmed by bone biopsy) that was clinically unsuspected. These authors also concluded that the [111]In-labeled leukocyte scan was the most useful of the noninvasive techniques (89% sensitivity) and that it was also valuable for monitoring the response to antibiot-ics. Drawbacks in the use of [111]In-labeled leukocyte scanning are high cost, the long time required (48–72 hours), and relatively high radiation dose to the spleen.[81] It has also been found less sensitive in the detection of chronic than in acute infections, and false positive scans have been observed in noninfected closed fractures. In one recent series,[33] poor spatial resolution and poor uptake by necrotic bone were cited as possible causes of lower sensitivity (79%) than had been reported by other authors. Taken together, these results suggest that [111]In-labeled leukocyte scanning shares many of the same limitations of other radionuclide scanning procedures, and while generally quite sensitive, they are costly, lacking in specificity and spatial resolution, and cannot be recommended for routine use.

Magnetic resonance imaging is the newest of the radiographic techniques for evaluating musculoskeletal infections. A small but rapidly growing literature suggests that this costly but powerful imaging technique can be quite useful in the diagnosis of osteomyelitis and in the detection and precise localization of abscesses that complicate severe diabetic foot infections. Bone marrow images with *decreased* signal intensity of $T_1$-weighted images and *increased* intensity of $T_2$-weighted and STIR (short tau inversion recovery) images (Fig 8–6) are highly consistent findings in osteomyelitis, but similar changes may be produced by fracture, Charcot joint, or other bony disease.[2, 76] Septic arthritis and tenosynovitis are not easily confirmed by MRI, but unsuspected or poorly localized abscess cavities can be readily differentiated from cellulitis and pinpointed for surgical drainage or needle aspiration.[15] Expense is a major drawback of MRI, and it should probably be reserved for cases such as treatment failures where there may be unsuspected abscess or as an adjunct in the planning of amputation or drainage procedures. Although it is very useful in the diagnosis of osteomyelitis, a strong clinical suspicion that bone infection is probable will often be sufficient (without MRI) to justify a 6- to 8-week course of antibiotics.

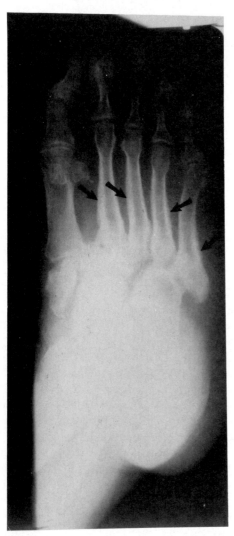

**FIG 8–4.**
Radiographic appearance of hypertrophic form of neurotrophic arthropathy. Anteroposterior view demonstrates findings noted in Figure 8–2. Note periosteal reaction of second to fifth metatarsal shafts *(arrows)*. *(Courtesy of Dr. William F. Conway, St. Louis.)*

A          B

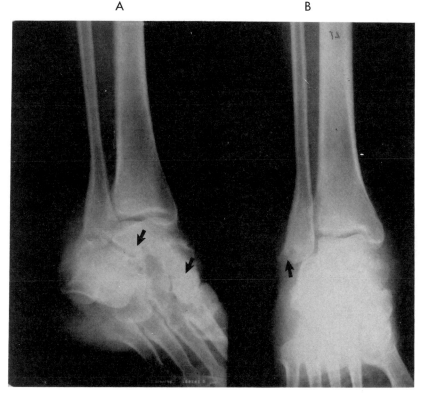

**FIG 8–5.**
Hypertrophic neurotrophic arthropathy. **A,** oblique radiographic view of ankle and hindfoot. Note destructive changes in sinus tarsus *(left arrow)* and sclerosis of tarsal navicular *(right arrow).* **B,** mortise view of ankle. Note hypertrophic changes of lateral malleolus *(arrow). (Courtesy of Dr. William F. Conway, St. Louis.)*

Surgery often plays a role in the successful treatment of osteomyelitis of the foot in diabetic patients. Bone necrosis is a crucial problem. If cure is a realistic therapeutic goal, all dead bone must be surgically excised. When surgery is not feasible, long-term antibiotic suppressive therapy may control the infection and prevent bacteremia. In general, surgery and antibiotic therapy are complementary. Because osteomyelitis in bones of the feet is most often related to a chronic perforating ulcer, most cases must be regarded as chronic bone infection requiring 6 weeks or more of antibiotic therapy, as well as debridement. In many cases, treatment failure and recurrence may dictate amputation. A very reasonable therapeutic approach to suspected osteomyelitis in diabetic foot infections has been recently proposed by Levin.[35] According to this algorithm, if the patient has bone exposure by inspection or by probe (100% osteomyelitis), has an ulcer wider than 2 cm (94% osteomyelitis), has ulcer inflammation (77% osteomyelitis), or has a sedimentation rate greater than 70 mm/hour with a noninflamed ulcer (100% osteomyelitis), then why not just treat the patient for osteomyelitis? Treatment for 6 to 8 weeks would include a fluoroquinolone[24, 54] and possibly a second antibiotic to cover anaerobes (metronidazole [Flagyl] or clindamycin [Cleocin]).

The use of antibiotic-impregnated polymethylmethacrylate (cement) beads for the treatment of localized osteomyelitis has achieved wider popularity in Europe than in the United States.[58] Most of the published experience with this strategy is difficult to evaluate, because it is provided as case reports rather than controlled comparative trials. Gentamicin- (Garamycin)–impregnated beads of uniform size and composition are

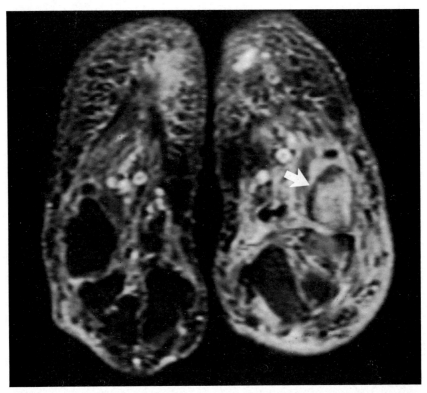

**FIG 8–6.**
STIR image from MRI scan of infected *(right)* and uninfected *(left)* feet after resection of distal right toes for osteomyelitis. Right foot shows extensive soft tissue swelling, as well as increased signal intensity of the cuboid *(white arrow)* and second and third cuneiform bones. This increased signal intensity reflects increased water content of the bone marrow and is indicative of osteomyelitis. Note that the corresponding bones of the left foot show *decreased* signal intensity compared with surrounding soft tissue. *(Courtesy of Dr. Scott Mirowitz, St. Louis.)*

commercially available in some European countries, but use in the United States requires extemporaneous preparation and lacks FDA approval.[26] There is a theoretical but generally unsubstantiated appeal in achieving locally high concentrations of antibiotics as they elute from surgically implanted beads. However, the availability of broad-spectrum β-lactams and fluoroquinolones has more than offset the lack of systemic aminoglycoside toxicity associated with gentamicin- or tobramycin-impregnated beads.

## LABORATORY DIAGNOSIS

Aerobic and anaerobic bacterial cultures, as well as Gram stains, should be obtained from almost all suspected foot infections. If the drainage is foul smelling, suggesting an anaerobic bacterial infection, anaerobic sampling equipment and transport medium should be brought to the bedside (Fig 8–7), unless prompt plating of the specimen under anaerobic conditions can be otherwise assured.

The importance of various anaerobic bacteria and the generally polymicrobial nature of diabetic foot infections have led to considerable uncertainty as to the optimal techniques for obtaining clinical samples for bacteriological testing. Sapico et al.[63] have carefully compared the bacterial isolates obtained from the same foot lesions before and immediately after amputation. None of the specimen collection methods showed good concordance with deep tissue cultures obtained from the surgical specimen. However, of the methods tested, curettage of the base of the ulcer as described by Louie et al.[39] showed the best correspondence, and surface swabs were the least reliable method of collection. Wheat[77] and Lipsky et al.[36] have also emphasized the unreliability of superficial swab cultures or of culture specimens obtained from openly draining lesions. Such samples often give poor correspondence with needle aspiration, curettage, or surgical biopsy specimens. Figure 8–7 shows a typical anaerobic sampling kit with a syringe and oxygen-free transport medium. Ideally, suitable anaerobic specimens should be obtained at the bedside by deep inoculation of an anaerobic transport swab into the transport medium or by injecting the sample through the diaphragm in the tube cap. The studies of Sapico et al.[63] confirm the numer-

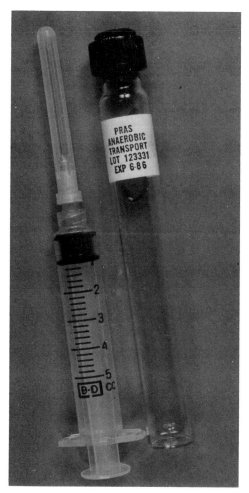

**FIG 8–7.**
Bedside kit for collection of bacteriologic samples likely to contain strict anaerobes. Samples should be aspirated carefully to avoid drawing air into syringe or injecting it with sample into oxygen-free transport medium.

ical dominance of anaerobes in many infected diabetic foot lesions, especially in chronic ulcers and in the presence of tissue necrosis. Fever and foul-smelling ulcers correlate with the presence of polymicrobial infections containing anaerobic bacteria, the so-called fetid foot of diabetes.[17] However, strictly anaerobic bacteria seldom comprise the only organism.[66]

Gram stains of the specimen provide a guide for the selection of empirical antibiotic therapy, but broad initial coverage is the rule, and the results of stained smears should not lead to restricted coverage (e.g., based on a single type of organism seen on Gram stain), especially in a seriously ill patient. Gram stain is also helpful in determining the presence or absence of inflammatory cells. The lack of an inflammatory response (few or no white blood cells) in the presence of gram-positive bacilli (*Clostridia* species) indicates the possibility of a histotoxic clostridial infection. The absence of leukocytes is attributed to the effects of clostridial exotoxins, whereas a substantial leukocyte response in the wound exudate is usually associated with nonclostridial soft tissue infections.[10] Although foot infections caused by mixed flora are common, *S. aureus* or streptococci, but rarely aerobic gram-negative bacilli, may cause monomicrobial foot or leg infections (e.g., common bacterial cellulitis).

Antibiotic susceptibility testing may reveal that an isolated *Staphylococcus* species is penicillin sensitive and does not require the use of one of the β-lactamase-resistant agents. For penicillin-resistant *S. aureus* or organisms of intermediate sensitivity, the use of intravenous oxacillin (Prostaphlin) or nafcillin (Unipen) or oral dicloxacillin (Dynapen or Pathocil) is optimal, but for *S. aureus* resistant to these drugs (MRSA), vancomycin is the drug of choice. Less often, susceptibility testing may give an impression of microbial susceptibility when factors of poor blood supply, abscess formation, or unsuspected mixed infection may lead to a poor clinical response to the antimicrobial agents.

Diabetic foot infections continue to require individualized diagnostic and therapeutic strategies that rely heavily on clinical judgment. The three interrelated complications—neuropathy, vascular insufficiency, and infection—create a formidable complexity. These foot infections are usually polymicrobial, but the methods for obtaining and identifying the relevant pathogens are seriously flawed. Osteomyelitis is common, but a secure diagnosis of bone infection is often difficult, and a plethora of radiographic imaging techniques often seem to contribute more to the expense of diagnosis than to its competent management. Antibiotics such as the fluoroquinolones (e.g., ciprofloxacin [Cipro], ofloxacin [Floxin]), and extended spectrum β-lactams (e.g., amoxacillin-clavulanate [Augmentin]) have provided new therapeutic options. These may help to reduce reliance on IV antimicrobials, reduce the length of hospital stay, or even permit entirely outpatient management. Meanwhile, the importance of clinical judgment is underscored by the epidemiology of lower-extremity amputations.[3, 46] In the United States, about one half of the nontraumatic lower extremity amputations occur in individuals with diabetes. Many, perhaps as much as one half of these are preventable, whereas the 3-year survival rate for diabetic patients who have undergone such amputations is only 50%.

# REFERENCES

1. Beaumont P, et al: Growth hormone, sorbital, and diabetic capillary disease, *Lancet* 1:579–581, 1971.

2. Beltran J, et al: The diabetic foot: magnetic resonance imaging evaluation, *Skeletal Radiol* 19:37–41, 1990.

3. Bild DE, et al: Lower-extremity amputation in people with diabetes, *Diabetes Care* 12:24–31, 1989.

4. Brayton RG, et al: Effect of alcohol and various diseases on leukocyte mobilization, phagocytosis, and intracellular bacterial killing, *N Engl J Med* 282:123–128, 1970.

5. Briscoe HF, Allison F Jr: Diabetes and host resistance: I, effect of alloxan diabetes upon the phagocytic and bactericidal efficiency of rat leukocytes for *Pneumococcus*, *J Bacteriol* 90:1537–1541, 1965.

6. Bybee JD, Rogers DE: The phagocytic activity of polymorphonuclear leukocytes obtained from patients with diabetes mellitus, *J Lab Clin Med* 64:1–13, 1964.

7. Crosby B, Allison F Jr: Phagocytic and bactericidal capacity of polymorphonuclear leukocytes recovered from venous blood of human beings, *Proc Soc Exp Biol Med* 123:660–664, 1966.

8. Cruickshank AH, Payne TPB: Anti-pneumococcal powers of the blood in alloxan diabetes in the rabbit, *Bull Johns Hopkins Hosp* 84:334–343, 1949.

9. Delbridge L, et al: The aetiology of diabetic neuropathic ulceration of the foot, *Br J Surg* 72:1–6, 1985.

10. Dellinger EP: Severe necrotizing soft-tissue infections, *JAMA* 246:1717–1721, 1981.

11. Diabetes mellitus and pyelonephritis [editorial], *N Engl J Med* 261:1247–1248, 1959.

12. Dismukes WE: Azole antifungal drugs: old and new [editorial], *Ann Intern Med* 109:177–179, 1988.

13. Dolkart RE, Halpern B, Perlman J: Comparison of antibody responses in normal and alloxan diabetic mice, *Diabetes* 20:162–167, 1971.

14. Drachman RH, Root RK, Wood WB Jr: Studies on the effect of experimental nonketotic diabetes mellitus on antibacterial defense: I, demonstration of a defect in phagocytosis, *J Exp Med* 124:227–240, 1966.

15. Durham JR, et al: Impact of magnetic resonance imaging on the management of diabetic foot infections, *Am J Surg* 162:150–154, 1991.

16. Dziatkowiak H, Kowalska M, Denys A: Phagocytic and bactericidal activity of granulocytes in diabetic children, *Diabetes* 31:1041–1043, 1982.

17. Fierer J, Daniel D, Davis C: The fetid foot: Lower extremity infections in patients with diabetes mellitus, *Rev Infect Dis* 1:210–217, 1979.

18. Fisher WC, Goldsmith JF, Gilligan PH: Sneakers as a source of *Pseudomonas aeruginosa* in children with osteomyelitis following puncture wounds, *J Pediatr* 106:608–609, 1985.

19. Fortes ZB, et al: Direct vital microscopic study of defective leukocyte-endothelial interaction in diabetes mellitus, *Diabetes* 40:1267–1273, 1991.

20. Freinkel RK, Freinkel N: Cutaneous manifestations of endocrine disorders, in Fitzpatrick TB, Eisen AZ, Wolff K, et al, editors: *Dermatology in general medicine*, ed 3, New York, 1987, McGraw-Hill.

21. Friedman SA, Rakow RB: Osseous lesions of the foot in diabetic neuropathy, *Diabetes* 20:302–307, 1971.

22. Fromtling RA: Overview of medically important antifungal azole derivatives, *Clin Microbiol Rev* 1:187–217, 1988.

23. Galimberti R, et al: The activity of ketoconazole in the treatment of onychomycosis, *Rev Infect Dis* 2:596–598, 1980.

24. Gentry LO: Oral quinolone therapy for difficult-to-treat skin and soft-tissue infections, *Postgrad Med* April 12, 48–54, 1991.

25. Gentry LO: Therapy with newer oral β-lactam and quinolone agents for infections of the skin and skin structures: a review, *Clin Infect Dis* 14:285–297, 1992.

26. Goodell JA, et al: Preparation and release characteristics of tobramycin-impregnated polymethylmethacrylate beads, *Am J Hosp Pharm* 43:1454–1461, 1986.

27. Greenwood AM: A study of the skin in five hundred cases of diabetes, *JAMA* 89:774–776, 1927.

28. Greenwood AM, Rockwood EM: The skin in diabetic patients: further studies, *Arch Dermatol Syphilol* 21:96–107, 1930.

29. Hay RJ, Clayton YM: Treatment of chronic dermatophyte infections: the use of ketoconazole in griseofulvin treatment failures, *Clin Exp Dermatol* 7:611–617, 1982.

30. Kass EH: Hormones and host resistance to infection, *Bacteriol Rev* 24:177–185, 1960.

31. Keenan AM, Tindel NL, Alavi A: Diagnosis of pedal osteomyelitis in diabetic patients using current scintigraphic techniques, *Arch Intern Med* 149:2262–2266, 1989.

32. Kontras SB, Bodenbender JG: Studies of the inflammatory cycle in juvenile diabetes, *Am J Dis Child* 116:130–134, 1968.

33. Larcos G, Brown ML, Sutton RT: Diagnosis of osteomyelitis of the foot in diabetic patients: Value of $^{111}$In-leukocyte scintigraphy, *Am J Roentgenol* 157:527–531, 1991.

34. Legendre R, Steltz M: A multicenter, double-blind comparison of ketoconazole and griseofulvin in the treatment of infections due to dermatophytes, *Rev Infect Dis* 2:586–591, 1980.

35. Levin S: Digest of current literature, *Infect Dis Clin Pract* 1:49–50, 1992.

36. Lipsky BA, Pecoraro RE, Wheat LJ: The diabetic foot: soft tissue and bone infection, *Infect Dis Clin North Am* 4:409–432, 1990.

37. Lipsky BA, et al: Outpatient management of uncomplicated lower-extremity infections in diabetic patients, *Arch Intern Med* 150:790–797, 1990.

38. LoGerfo FW, Coffman JD: Vascular and microvascular disease of the foot in diabetes, *N Engl J Med* 311:1615–1619, 1984.

39. Louie TJ, et al: Aerobic and anaerobic bacteria in diabetic foot ulcers, *Ann Intern Med* 85:461–463, 1976.

40. Maibach HI, Hildick-Smith G: *Skin bacteria and their role in infection*, New York, 1965, McGraw-Hill.

41. Majd M: Radionuclide imaging in early detection of childhood osteomyelitis and its differentiation from cellulitis and bone infarction, *Ann Radiol (Paris)* 20:9–18, 1977.

42. Marble A, White HJ, Fernald AT: The nature of the lowered resistance to infection in diabetes mellitus, *J Clin Invest* 17:423–430, 1938.

43. Marples MJ, Bailey MJ: A search for the presence of pathogenic bacteria and fungi in the interdigital space of the foot, *Br J Dermatol* 69:379–388, 1957.

44. Marples RR: *The ecology of the human skin*, Springfield, Ill, 1965, Charles C Thomas.

45. Marples RR: Diphtheroids of normal human skin, *Br J Dermatol* 81 (suppl 1):47–54, 1969.

46. Massachusetts Medical Society: Lower extremity amputations among persons with diabetes mellitus—Washington, 1988. *MMWR* 40:737–739, 1991.

47. Mergenhagen SE, Thonard JC, Scherp HW: Studies on synergistic infections: I, experimental infections with anaerobic streptococci, *J Infect Dis* 103:33–44, 1958.

48. Miller EH, Semian DW: Gram-negative osteomyelitis following puncture wounds of the foot, *J Bone Joint Surg* 57A:535–537, 1975.

49. Mowat AG, Baum J: Chemotaxis of polymorphonuclear leukocytes from patients with diabetes mellitus, *N Engl J Med* 284:621–627, 1971.

50. Neu HC: Use of fluoroquinolones, *Infect Dis Clin Pract* 1:1–10, 1992.

51. Newman LG, et al: Unsuspected osteomyelitis in diabetic foot ulcers: diagnosis and monitoring by leukocyte scanning with indium in 111 oxyquinoline, *JAMA* 266:1246–1251, 1991.

52. Newrick PG, et al: Impaired sweating in the diabetic neuropathic foot and its influence on skin flora, *Diabetes Res* 12:173–176, 1989.

53. Nolan CM, Beaty HN, Bagdade JD: Further characterization of the impaired bactericidal function of granulocytes in patients with poorly controlled diabetes, *Diabetes* 27:889–894, 1978.

54. Parish LC, Jungkind DL: Systemic antimicrobial therapy in skin and skin structure infections: comparison of temafloxacin and ciprofloxacin, *Am J Med* 91(suppl 6A):115S–119S, 1991.

55. Parkhouse N, Le Quesne PM: Impaired neurogenic vascular response in patients with diabetes and neuropathic foot lesions, *N Engl J Med* 318:1306–1309, 1988.

56. Peterson LR, et al: Therapy of lower extremity infections with ciprofloxacin in patients with diabetes mellitus, peripheral vascular disease, or both, *Am J Med* 86:801–808, 1989.

57. Perillie PE, Nolan JP, Finch SC: Studies of the resistance to infection in diabetes mellitus: local exudative cellular response, *J Lab Clin Med* 59:1008–1015, 1962.

58. Popham GJ, et al: Antibiotic-impregnated beads:

part II, factors in antibiotic selection, *Orthop Rev* 20:331–337, 1991.

59. Qvist R, Larkins RG: Diminished production of thromboxane B$_2$ and prostaglandin E by stimulated polymorphonuclear leukocytes from insulin-treated diabetic subjects, *Diabetes* 32:622–626, 1983.

60. Rebell G, et al: Factors affecting rapid disappearance of bacteria placed on the normal skin, *J Invest Dermatol* 14:247–264, 1950.

61. Richardson MD, Warnock DW: Mechanisms of resistance to fungal infection in the non-compromised host, in Warnock DW, Richardson MD, editors: *Fungal infection in the compromised patient*, New York, 1982, John Wiley & Sons.

62. Robbins SL, Tucker AW Jr: The cause of death in diabetes: a report of 307 autopsied cases, *N Engl J Med* 231:865–868, 1944.

63. Sapico FL, et al: The infected foot of the diabetic patient: quantitative microbiology and analysis of clinical features, *Rev Infect Dis* 6(suppl 1):S171–S176, 1984.

64. Savin JA: Bacterial infections in diabetes mellitus, *Br J Dermatol* 91:481–487, 1974.

65. Shah SV, Wallin JD, Eilen SD: Chemiluminescence and superoxide anion production by leukocytes from diabetic patients, *J Clin Endocrinol Metab* 57:402–409, 1983.

66. Sharp CS, et al: Microbiology of superficial and deep tissues in infected diabetic gangrene, *Surg Gynecol Obstet* 149:217–219, 1979.

67. Sheldon WH, Bauer H: The development of the acute inflammatory response to experimental cutaneous mucormycosis in normal and diabetic rabbits, *J Exp Med* 110:845–852, 1959.

68. Sima AAF, et al: Bacterial phagocytosis and intra-cellular killing by alveolar macrophages in BB rats, *Diabetes* 37:544–549, 1988.

69. Stone HH, Martin JD Jr: Synergistic necrotizing cellulitis, *Ann Surg* 175:702–711, 1972.

70. Tachibana DK: Microbiology of the foot, *Annu Rev Microbiol* 30:351–375, 1976.

71. Tan JS, et al: Neutrophil dysfunction in diabetes mellitus, *J Lab Clin Med* 85:26–33, 1975.

72. Thornton GF: Infections and diabetes, *Med Clin North Am* 55:931–938, 1971.

73. Vilanova X, Casanovas M, Francino J: Onychomycosis: an experimental study, *J Invest Dermatol* 27:77–101, 1956.

74. Waldvogel FA, Medoff G, Swartz MN: Osteomyelitis: a review of clinical features, therapeutic considerations and unusual aspects, *N Engl J Med* 282:198, 260, 316, 1970.

75. Wale RS, Madders K: Staphylococcal toxoid in the treatment of diabetes, *Br J Exp Pathol* 17:279–281, 1936.

76. Wang A, et al: MRI and diabetic foot infections, *Magn Reson Imaging* 8:805–809, 1990.

77. Wheat J: Diagnostic strategies in osteomyelitis, *Am J Med* 78(suppl 6B):218–224, 1985.

78. Wills MR, Reece MW: Non-clostridial gas infections in diabetes mellitus, *Br Med J* 2:566, 1960.

79. Yuh WTC, et al: Osteomyelitis of the foot in diabetic patients: evaluation with plain film, [99m]Tc-MDP bone scintigraphy, and MR imaging, *AJR* 152:795–800, 1989.

80. Zaias N, Oertel I, Elliott DF: Fungi in toenails, *J Invest Dermatol* 53:140–142, 1969.

81. Zeiger LS, Fox IM: Use of indium-111-labeled white blood cells in the diagnosis of diabetic foot infections, *J Foot Surg* 29:46–51, 1990.

# CHAPTER 9

# Biomechanics of the Foot in Diabetes Mellitus

**Peter R. Cavanagh, Ph.D.**

**Jan S. Ulbrecht, M.D.**

The aim of this chapter is to provide a biomechanical framework on which an understanding of the cause, treatment, and prevention of foot injury in patients with diabetes can be built. Although peripheral vascular disease long has been implicated in lower limb problems in the diabetic patient, it is now well-recognized that the majority of injuries to the plantar surface of the foot are a consequence of trauma not recognized by the patient.[47] Diabetes-related distal symmetric polyneuropathy results in a loss of protective sensation, and subsequently a number of biomechanical risk factors conspire to cause injury. Thus biomechanics has great relevance to neuropathic injury. In this chapter we attempt to describe how the forces that injure the foot are generated, how they may cause injury, and how they might be modified to achieve healing, and better still, to prevent injury.

Most of the skin injuries seen on the feet of patients with diabetic neuropathy occur on the plantar surface (Diabetes Foot Clinic, unpublished data, 1992), frequently at the sites of the highest pressure under the foot. Although this has been known for some time, recent developments make this a particularly exciting time for biomechanical studies of the foot in diabetes. Barefoot plantar pressure measurement is becoming less costly and more available, and, perhaps of most consequence, in-shoe pressure measurement is becoming available as a clinical decision-making tool.[31, 38] On average, patients with diabetes have higher pressures under their feet than persons without diabetes,[18] and there has been a rapid growth in the understanding of why this may be so.[40, 48, 89] The topic of shear stress as a possible mechanism of skin injury is being revisited,[58] and the biomechanical consequences of peripheral neuropathy for posture and gait are being explored.[29, 75, 76] Experimental determinations of tissue properties are expanding our knowledge of the effects of diabetes on the mechanical behavior of skin, collagen, and adipose tissue,[26, 45] and objective assessment of footwear designs is providing an understanding of how to best intervene to treat or prevent injury.[42]

Yet the field is still relatively young, and many areas remain where current diagnoses and approaches to treatment can be neither supported nor refuted by scientific evidence. This is also true of our understanding of pathogenesis; for example, it is likely that many Charcot fractures (see Chapter 7) have a partly mechanical etiology, although no experimental evidence for this exists at present.[71] We attempt to concentrate in this chapter on topics where evidence is available to support our assertions. However, by necessity, we also mention a number of areas in need of further biomechanical study and attempt to provide some hypotheses to guide such study. We also intend to keep this chapter firmly directed at clinical reality, because a frequent and usually valid criticism of biomechanical and bioengineering texts is their inaccessibility to clinicians.

After a brief discussion of the mechanics of gait, we turn to the mechanics of the plantar aspect of the foot and then to the mechanics of footwear. We also present an outline of a simple physical examination of the foot and lower limb, which, if performed on individual patients, should provide some insight into the issues addressed in this chapter even when some of the more sophisticated methodology is not available.

## GAIT: INTERNAL AND EXTERNAL MECHANICS

Most foot injuries occur while the patient is walking and are caused by the forces generated during gait. Thus, a natural place to begin the discussion of injury is with an overview of the mechanics of gait. When we watch a patient ambulate in the clinic, we are attempting to assess certain aspects of the external mechanics of the patient's gait. What we actually see are the limb movements in space, which bear little relationship to the most important quantities in the current context, the injurious stresses in the tissue, which could be labeled the internal mechanics. Yet it is worth dwelling briefly on the external mechanics of gait, because observation and, preferably, measurement can sometimes provide insight into the reasons for high forces and pressures during gait.

A number of techniques are available to track the spatial position of targets attached to segments of the lower limb during gait.[57, 59] Most commonly, reflective markers are used and tracked by high-speed video (Fig 9–1,A). This allows joint motion in the foot to be quantitatively measured during normal function rather than depending on inferences from a static examination. For example, the pattern of dorsiflexion and plantarflexion of the first metatarsophalangeal (MTP) joint in a diabetic patient during gait is shown in Figure 9–1,B. Very few such measurements of foot movement in diabetes have actually been performed to date, although the techniques are widely

used in orthopedic biomechanics for the study of conditions such as cerebral palsy and joint replacement.[4, 46]

The example just chosen is quite relevant to the current context, because plantar ulceration of the hallux is a common occurrence in patients with diabetic neuropathy.[10] Dorsiflexion at the first MTP joint is essential during the toe-off phase of gait. When the ability of that joint to dorsiflex is mechanically limited, very high pressure must be expected under the hallux during toe-off, a common finding in patients who ulcerate in this region. An understanding of the necessary range of dorsiflexion of the first MTP joint during gait, taken together with a static measurement of dorsiflexion at that joint, can provide insight into why high plantar pressure may occur at that particular site.

Although the likelihood of high pressure between a region of the foot and the floor can be inferred from an analysis of movement as described earlier, neither the eye nor the most sophisticated video analysis system can measure these forces and pressures, because it is only the *consequences* of force that can be actually "seen." The area of mechanics in which the forces that cause movement are studied is called *kinetics*, whereas the label *kinematics* is applied to studies (e.g., those described earlier) when the movement per se is measured. The forces that are most frequently measured and studied are the external forces between the foot and either the floor or the footwear. Less frequently, internal forces in tissues or forces between the articulating surfaces of joints can be measured, estimated, or modeled.

When the foot strikes the ground in gait, Newton's third law tells us that there will be equal forces experienced by both the foot and the floor. Because it is more convenient to measure the force with an instrument mounted on the floor than on the foot, a device called a "force platform" is frequently found in gait laboratories. As demonstrated in Figure 9–2, the force measured by a force platform during a single foot contact is usually expressed in three components: vertical (or *normal* to use the engineering term), anteroposterior shear, and mediolateral shear.

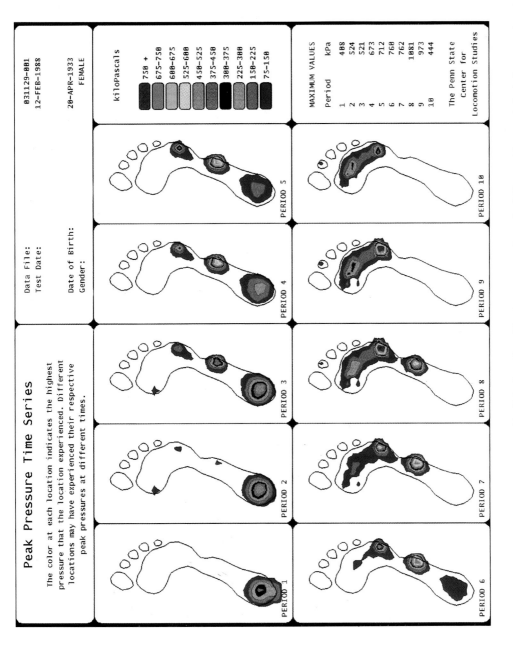

**Peak Pressure Time Series**

The color at each location indicates the highest pressure that the location experienced. Different locations may have experienced their respective peak pressures at different times.

Data File: 031129-001
Test Date: 12-FEB-1988

Date of Birth: 20-APR-1933
Gender: FEMALE

kiloPascals

750 +
675-750
600-675
525-600
450-525
375-450
300-375
225-300
150-225
75-150

| MAXIMUM VALUES | |
|---|---|
| Period | kPa |
| 1 | 408 |
| 2 | 524 |
| 3 | 521 |
| 4 | 673 |
| 5 | 712 |
| 6 | 768 |
| 7 | 762 |
| 8 | 1081 |
| 9 | 973 |
| 10 | 444 |

The Penn State
Center for
Locomotion Studies

PERIOD 1  PERIOD 2  PERIOD 3  PERIOD 4  PERIOD 5

PERIOD 6  PERIOD 7  PERIOD 8  PERIOD 9  PERIOD 10

## PLATE 9.
Plantar pressures measured during barefoot walking in a neuropathic diabetic patient. Plantar pressures in each of 10 equal time periods during ground contact of the right foot. The "cool" colors represent low pressures, and the "hot" colors high pressures (see bar scale). Note that after the initial heel strike there is a focus of pressure in the midfoot, which continues to be loaded during more than 60% of the ground contact. An area under the head of the fifth metatarsal also experiences extremely high pressures for 60% to 90% of the contact time. The toes are virtually unused throughout.

## PLATE 10.

Peak pressure plot, which on the right summarizes the data shown in Plate 10. Peak pressure plot for the left foot of the same patient also is shown, and demonstrates a fairly symmetric pattern of pressure distribution. In this summary plot the most pressure at each location under the foot from any point in the ground contact is shown in the diagram with the same scale and color key used in Plate 9. This display is a useful addition to the patient's chart.

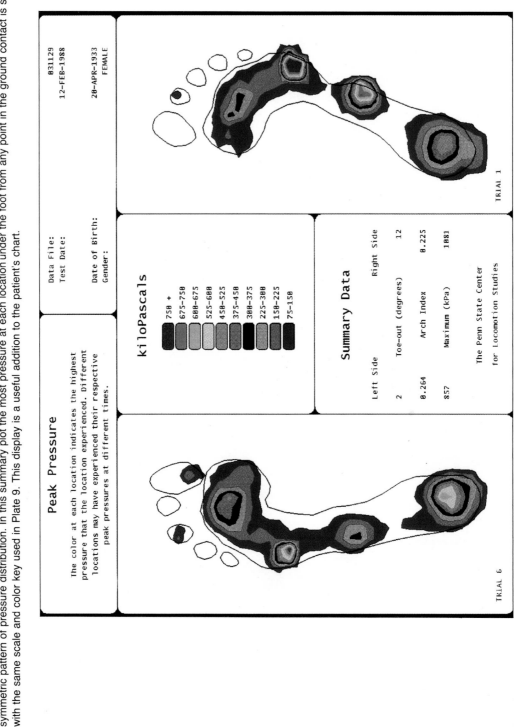

### Peak Pressure

The color at each location indicates the highest pressure that the location experienced. Different locations may have experienced their respective peak pressures at different times.

| Data File: | 031129 |
| Test Date: | 12-FEB-1988 |
| Date of Birth: | 20-APR-1933 |
| Gender: | FEMALE |

**kiloPascals**

- 750 +
- 675-750
- 600-675
- 525-600
- 450-525
- 375-450
- 300-375
- 225-300
- 150-225
- 75-150

### Summary Data

| Left Side | | Right Side |
|---|---|---|
| 2 | Toe-out (degrees) | 12 |
| 0.264 | Arch Index | 0.225 |
| 857 | Maximum (kPa) | 1001 |

The Penn State Center
for Locomotion Studies

TRIAL 1

TRIAL 6

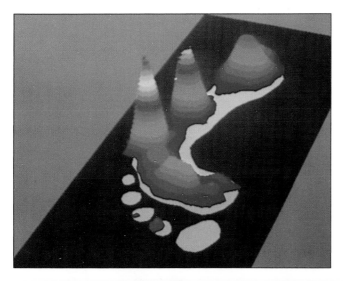

**PLATE 11.**
Three-dimensional view of the same peak pressure data shown in Plate 10. Representation of the pressure as colored "mountains" allows the magnitudes of the regions of elevated pressure to be appreciated better.

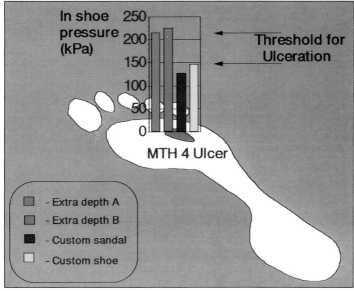

**PLATE 12.**
Peak pressure between the shoe and the head of the fourth metatarsal in the same patient in four different footwear conditions measured using a Mikro EMED insole. The patient had experienced a recurrent ulcer at this site after wearing shoes A and B, both of which were rigid rocker shoes with custom-molded insoles. The tissue did not break down when wearing a custom sandal with a deep Plastazote insole, which reduced the peak pressure at the ulcer site by more than 40%. A definitive shoe was built, similar to a sandal, and this reduced pressure by approximately 35% compared with the earlier devices. The patient remains ulcer free after 4 months of very active living in this shoe. These measurements therefore demonstrate that in this patient at this site the threshold for ulceration lies between approximately 150 and 215 kPa.

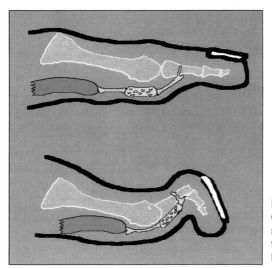

**PLATE 13.**
Cartoon cross section of the anatomy of the second ray shows displacement of the plantar fat pad *(yellow)* believed to occur with clawing of the toes. This mechanism needs to be confirmed by objective study.

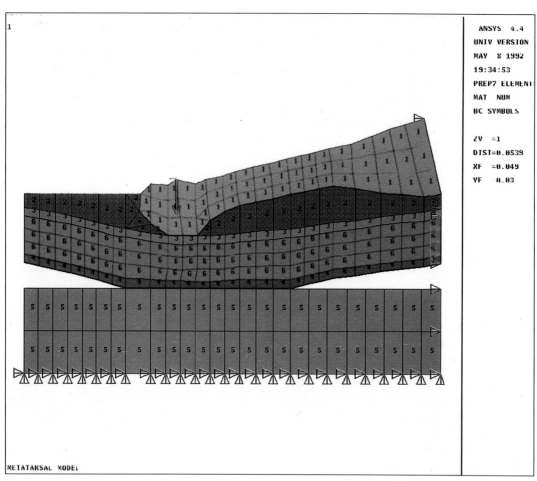

ANSYS 4.4
UNIV VERSION
MAY 8 1992
19:34:53
PREP7 ELEMENT
MAT NUM
BC SYMBOLS

ZV =1
DIST=0.0539
XF =0.049
YF =0.03

METATARSAL MODEL

**PLATE 14.**
Model of the second metatarsal and associated structures comprising a "mesh" of small geometric elements that can be given material properties, constraints, and to which external forces can be applied. Successive mathematical solution of resulting stress and strain in each small element of the model allows the behavior of the entire model to be defined. Without this technique, called finite element analysis, the problem would be too complex for solution.

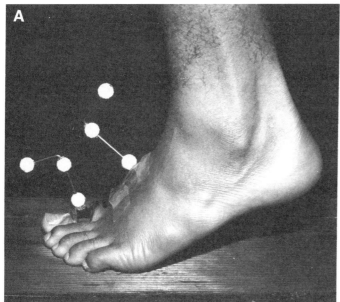

**FIG 9–1.**

**A,** foot with targets attached for automated video analysis of motion of the first metatarsophalangeal joint. At least three targets must be placed on each segment of interest (or on a base firmly attached to it). If the targets are visible in two or more video cameras, the three dimensional locations of the targets can be obtained automatically by computer analysis of the resulting videotape and the unique position of the segment in space determined. **B,** dynamic flexion-extension pattern of the first metatarsophalangeal joint during slow barefoot walking in a patient with diabetic neuropathy and limited joint mobility. Measurements were made using automated analysis of video, as described in **A.** *Dashed line* represents the maximum extension (37 degrees) measured statically during physical examination. Note that the maximum dynamic value is approximately 90% of the static value.

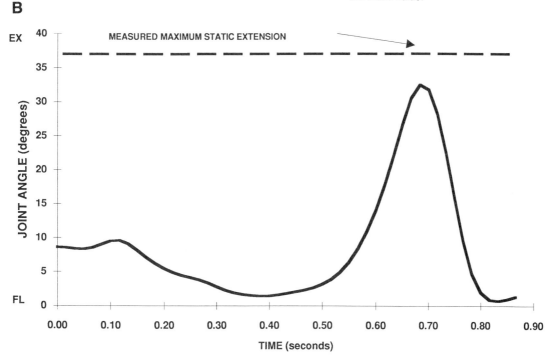

The forces shown in Figure 9–2 can be thought of as the mechanical input to the foot, yet their magnitude does not necessarily reflect the risk of injury. As Brand[20] has so aptly said, "Pressure is the critical quantity that determines the harm done by the force." The link between force and pressure is, of course, the area of force application. Much more damage can be done by a force transmitted through a few plantar prominences than by the same force distributed over a larger area of the plantar surface. Consequently, plantar pressure measurement is a topic of critical interest in the field of diabetes-related foot injury (see Chapter 10).

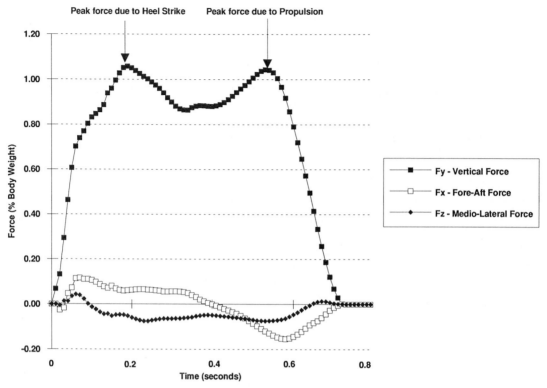

**FIG 9–2.**

Three components of ground reaction force underneath one foot during a single step. The step begins with heel-strike at time 0, and ends with toe off. The three components of the force are fore-aft shear component (*Fx*), vertical component (*Fy*), and mediolateral shear component (*Fz*). Note that the vertical component is six times larger than the anteroposterior shear, and 15 times larger that the mediolateral shear. *Left arrow* marks the peak vertical force after heel strike; *right arrow* marks the peak vertical force during the late part of the step cycle and is used for calculation of pressure in Figure 9–3.

Average pressure is calculated by dividing the applied force by the area over which it acts. What is widely called "plantar pressure" in the diabetes literature is known in mechanical terms as "normal stress"; "stress" because it is the result of force applied to a defined area and "normal" because it is measured at right angles to the supporting surface. Shear stress is calculated in the same manner but using the magnitude of the shear force and its area of application, which may be the same as that for the normal stress. For example, consider the effects of the peak ground reaction forces shown in Figure 9–2 on a "rocker bottom foot" with concentrated force application to a midfoot prominence. As shown in Figure 9–3, the calculation leads directly to estimates of large "normal" and "shear" stresses (Table 9–1). In practice, however,

the areas of application are rarely known, and as we[35] have previously shown, similar calculations of pressures based on body weight or ground reaction forces and total foot area are not valid, because "effective foot area" is much smaller than the area of the footprint. Plantar pressure must therefore be directly measured where possible rather than estimated. Although we measure plantar pressure routinely in all patients in our Diabetes Foot Clinic, we are still frequently surprised by the discrepancies between our preconceptions of how a particular foot functions and the evidence from direct plantar pressure measurement. Clinically apparent plantar bony prominence does not guarantee a high pressure in that region, and more important, the absence of any obvious bony deformity is not a guarantee of low pressure.

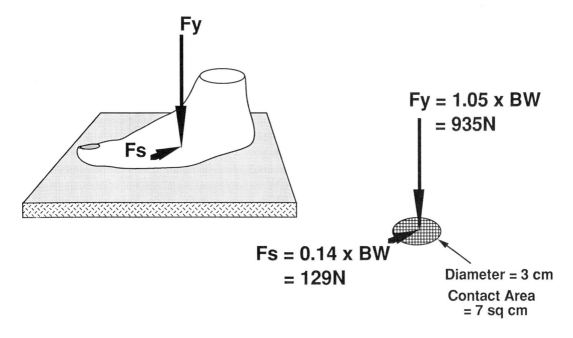

Normal Stress  = 935/ (7 x .0001) = 1340 kPa =1.34 MPa

Shear Stress    = 129/ (7 x .0001) =   184 kPa

**FIG 9–3.**
Schematic of a rocker bottom "Charcot" foot in contact with the ground during the late-support phase of gait at the instant shown by the *right arrow* in Figure 9–2. If the contact area is assumed to be circular with a diameter of 3 cm, the normal stress will be 1.34 MPa and the shear stress 184 kPa.

## PLANTAR PRESSURE MEASUREMENT

Methods for the measurement of plantar pressure have been discussed in detail by ourselves and others.[1, 9, 31, 36–38] Several devices for barefoot plantar pressure measurement are currently commercially available, and two insole devices for in-shoe pressure measurement have been recently introduced commercially.[31] Although several different principles of measurement of pressure are used in the manufacture of the sensors that make up the devices,[31] in the majority of the platform instruments for measurement of barefoot pressure a matrix of transducers is used. This is also the case with the two in-shoe instruments. For barefoot measurement, the patient walks onto the platform and keeps walking. In this situation, information from a single foot contact is collected. For in-shoe measurement the matrix of transducers is manufactured into a thin pliable "insole," which is placed in the shoe in direct contact with the foot. In this case, information from multiple steps can be obtained.[31]

When any of the instruments are used, attention must be given to several technical considerations: dynamic range, sampling rate, spatial resolution, frequency response, linearity, hysteresis, temperature sensitivity, reliability, and reproducibility; all of these have been reviewed elsewhere.[36, 37] Of particular importance is an understanding of the relevance of effective sensor size on the pressure measured. Generally speaking, the smaller the sensor, the larger the apparent pressure recorded in the same region of the same foot.[36–38] Thus, normative data must be developed for each instrument used and cannot be interchanged.

Also to be considered are several aspects of the data collection process that will impact the results. These include stride length

**TABLE 9–1.**

Clinical Biomechanics*

| Examination | Outcome | Treatment |
| --- | --- | --- |
| Deformity | Dorsal prominence | Rule out Charcot's fracture |
| | Clawed toes | Needs special footwear |
| | Bunions | Needs special footwear |
| | Wide forefoot | Needs special footwear |
| | Forefoot supination/ pronation | Possibly posted foot orthosis |
| | Unusual deformity | Radiograph for fracture |
| Soft tissue changes | Reduced plantar tissue | Consider more protection |
| | Altered plantar tissue | Consider more protection |
| | Scarring and adhesions | Teach scar mobilization |
| Limited joint mobility | Reduced hallux dorsiflexion | Consider a rockered shoe |
| Callus | Callus present | Teach or provide proper care |
| Weakness | Foot drop | Shoes to protect toes and an ankle foot orthosis to prevent tripping |

*This table assumes that an examination to determine loss of protective sensation[79] has already been performed. If sensation is adequate, further examination of the foot is not needed beyond noting major deformities and inappropriate footwear, both of which are likely to be problematic if sensation becomes impaired.*

(natural or mandated), speed of walking (natural or mandated), first step, or midgait.[80] In our daily clinical use, we choose not to standardize gait speed or stride length to make the step as "normal" for the subject as possible. We recognize that step length and speed will affect plantar pressure; however, we believe that, in a clinical setting, measuring the consequences of a "normal" step for that patient is more meaningful than attempting to make the subject conform to a set of conditions that may be unnatural for him or her.[31] In our barefoot studies we have chosen to look at the average of five "first steps,"[37] whereas for in-shoe testing we average many steps during normal gait.

Most published work with plantar pressure measurement has been with the platform devices, and these are discussed next in more detail. Although the pressure measured by any particular transducer during any instant of foot contact is accessible, we usually present the results either as a set of snapshots taken throughout the contact phase (Plate 10) or as a single contour plot of the peak pressure achieved at each site during that foot contact (so-called peak pressure plot; Plates 11 and 12). We also find it useful to present the data as the average peak pressure in standard anatomic regions during multiple steps. Such regional analysis from a group of nondiabetic pa-

**FIG 9–4.**
**A,** regional analysis of data from five walking trials in the same patient as in Plates 10 to 12. The foot has been divided into 10 anatomic regions based on a standard algorithm. Division also could be done on an individual basis by inspection on the computer screen. The regions shown are the medial and lateral rearfoot (regions 1 and 2); medial and lateral midfoot (regions 3 and 4); first, second, and lateral metatarsal heads (regions 5, 6, and 7, respectively); hallux (region 8); second toe (region 9), and lateral toes (region 10). Location of the peak pressure within each region from each trial is shown by the squares. Note that the location of peak pressure in the different trials is somewhat inconsistent in the forefoot; in particular, the fifth metatarsal head is not the most loaded region in the lateral forefoot in two of the five trials. Means and standard deviations from five trials are given; *asterisks* mark regions outside normal limits for the platform used. **B,** mean regional peak pressure values (±2 SD) in kilopascals in 14 nondiabetic subjects during first-step gait on a Novel EMED SF pressure distribution platform. Regions are numbered according to the scheme shown in **A,** Similar data in larger groups are needed to provide confidence limits for evaluation of pressure in a neuropathic diabetic population.

A

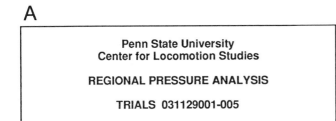

Penn State University
Center for Locomotion Studies

REGIONAL PRESSURE ANALYSIS

TRIALS 031129001-005

Subject Details:

| | |
|---|---|
| ID: | 031 |
| Gender: | Female |
| Height: | 166 cm |
| Weight: | 720 N |
| | |
| Footprint area: | 71.8 sq cm |
| Arch Index: | 22.5% |
| Mean Toe Out: | 9.2 degrees |
| sd | 2.7 degrees |

| REGION | PMAX (kPa) | sd (kPa) | CV % |
|---|---|---|---|
| 1. | 421.4 | 114.6 | 27.2 |
| 2. | 506.3 | 36.4 | 7.2 |
| 3. | 0.0 | 0.0 | 0.0 |
| *4. | 588.0 | 370.8 | 63.1 |
| 5. | 524.7 | 389.3 | 74.2 |
| 6. | 444.5 | 70.4 | 15.8 |
| *7. | 856.2 | 486.7 | 56.8 |
| 8. | 104.0 | 43.7 | 42.0 |
| 9. | 229.3 | 73.0 | 31.8 |
| 10. | 93.8 | 64.1 | 68.3 |

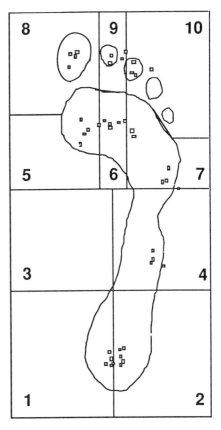

B

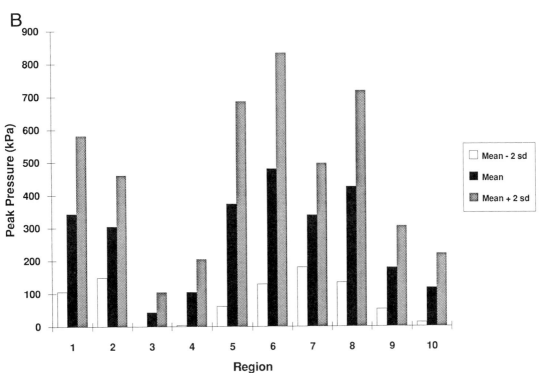

tients is shown in Figure 9–4. The considerable variability (and therefore range of these normal results) should be noted. This issue is addressed again later on in the context of reference or normative values.

We suspect that regional analysis may be important because areas of the foot normally involved in weight bearing may be better adapted for this function and may thus tolerate higher pressure before breakdown. Conversely, the pressure threshold for tissue breakdown may be lower in regions of the foot not normally involved in weight bearing; an example of this would be the midfoot exposed to weight bearing because of an underlying Charcot fracture deformity (see Fig 9–3). We have also found the appearance of elevated regional plantar pressure in the midfoot a very helpful tool in the early diagnosis of Charcot's fractures.[37]

Because most patients wear shoes and often sustain injury while wearing them, the ability to measure pressures inside the shoe is an important extension of investigative techniques. Bauman and Brand[8] and Brand and Ebner[22] used single in-shoe transducers almost 30 years ago; more recently, similar studies have been performed to investigate principles of footwear management.[42, 63, 65] Although these have been principally research studies, devices suitable for clinical use have recently become available,[31, 34] with the likelihood that this approach will revolutionize footwear prescription in the future. A case study from our own initial clinical use of an in-shoe matrix of transducers is shown in Plate 13. After several unsuccessful empirical attempts to prevent reulceration by different footwear designs, we prescribed further footwear for this patient on the basis of measured pressure reduction at the ulcer site. Low-pressure values were achieved by this method, with the patient remaining free of ulceration for a 3-month follow-up of very active living.

## PLANTAR PRESSURE AND ULCERATION

As already alluded to, plantar ulceration has been linked in several retrospective studies and in one recent prospective study[16, 18, 43, 81] to high plantar pressure. However, there is no clear agreement yet on the pressure threshold for ulceration. This may be a consequence of several factors. First, results obtained using one pressure platform cannot be extrapolated to other platforms because of the effect of element size. Second, different regions of the foot may have different pressure thresholds for breakdown. Third, the pressure threshold for tissue breakdown may vary, depending on the health of the tissue related to vascular supply, tissue perfusion,[84] degree of glycosylation of the tissues, and scarring. Fourth, shear, although not measured by any of the currently available platforms, may interact with normal forces in ways not yet understood. Fifth, time $\times$ pressure product, currently not often calculated, may be more relevant than simple peak pressure.[36, 37]

It is not possible to simply take the foot pressure distribution of a healthy population and consider similar values safe for patients with insensitive feet. Healthy individuals remain ulcer free not because they have lower plantar pressures but because they can feel injury. As mentioned earlier, the range of "normal" regional peak pressure values—defined as mean $\pm$ 2 standard deviations—is very wide (see Fig 9–4), with peak values approaching 1,000 kPa at several regions. Yet plantar ulcerations can and do occur in the feet of neuropathic patients at sites where peak pressure is as low as 500 kPa. Based on our experience with pressure measurement on more than 200 patients in our clinic using the EMED SF (Novel gmbh, Munich) pressure platform, we regard barefoot peak plantar pressure under the metatarsal heads and under the hallux greater than 500 kPa as possibly dangerous and pressure greater than 1,000 kPa as very dangerous. These values are not, however, based on a rigorous prospective analysis of the relationship between pressure and ulceration. Not all subjects with peak pressures in excess of these values will ulcerate; ulceration will still depend on care taken by the patient, activity level, and tissue characteristics.

It should also be remembered that in all the studies published to date, an association has been drawn between ulceration, which usually occurs in shoes, and barefoot plantar pressure. The whole premise of trying to provide patients at risk with appropriate footwear rests on the concept that footwear can lower pressure. Therefore, a patient theoretically "at risk" because of high barefoot plantar pressure will remain ulcer free if he or she wears footwear that distributes pressure adequately. Thus the most that barefoot pressure measurement can ever do is to suggest who is at risk. Particular threshold values for tissue breakdown can be approached only by measuring pressure in shoes in which an ulceration has occurred.

## WHAT CAUSES HIGH PRESSURE?

As noted earlier, pressures generated under apparently healthy feet (see Fig 9–4) can be high enough to cause ulceration in the presence of neuropathy. It is also true that diabetes, and particularly diabetes complicated by neuropathy, is associated with higher than normal plantar pressure.[15, 18] It is generally believed that diabetes mellitus may alter both the musculoskeletal and soft tissue mechanics in a manner that elevates plantar pressure and makes tissue damage more likely. Few of these effects have been observed in prospective studies, and thus evidence rests on retrospective analysis and cross-sectional studies.

As discussed by Boulton and colleagues (see Chapter 10), claw toes are a frequent clinical finding, and this phenomenon has been ascribed to atrophy of the intrinsic muscles that control the position of the proximal phalanges on the metatarsals.[62] In addition to the fact that claw toes increase the likelihood of dorsal ulceration from footwear, it is hypothesized that the soft tissue "metatarsal cushions"[52] are displaced distally, leaving the condyles of the metatarsal heads exposed (Plate 14). Gooding et al.[50, 51] have investigated tissue thickness under the metatarsal heads using ultrasound, but the results have been inconclusive.

More direct metabolic consequences of diabetes may also affect plantar soft tissue structure and function. Nonenzymatic glycosylation (NEG) of many proteins in the body has been demonstrated in patients with diabetes,[25, 26] and this process has been shown to affect the mechanical properties of tissue, usually reducing elasticity. The foot is no exception, and Delbridge et al.[45] have shown that keratin in the stratum corneum of the foot is glycosylated compared with nondiabetic skin. Although no direct mechanical measurements have been made on these tissues, it is possible that NEG will make plantar skin (and possibly deeper tissues) stiffer and thus less able to distribute pressure through deformation. Because the adipose tissues of the plantar aspect of the foot (particularly the heel) are tightly bound by connective tissue,[12, 14, 55] the possibility exists that changes in connective tissue stiffness will affect the overall intrinsic "cushioning" properties of the foot.

A further presumed by-product of NEG is the observed limitation of range of movement in many joints of the body in persons with diabetes. Although first demonstrated in the hand,[68] this has now been found in the joints of the foot and ankle.[10, 48] Anecdotally, limitation of motion in the first MTP joint is frequently associated with ulceration of the hallux in neuropathic patients (see earlier discussion and Fig 9–1,B). Decreased subtalar joint mobility has been associated with elevated plantar pressure,[48] although there are indications that protective sensation may allow compensation to occur such that pressure may not necessarily be elevated in the setting of subtalar limited joint mobility without neuropathy.[30]

It has been suggested that neuropathy predisposes patients to the production of excessive plantar keratoses.[70] Whether or not this is true, recent evidence has shown that the removal of callus from bony prominences in the forefoot reduces plantar pressure by an average of 29%.[89] The formation of callus has frequently been ascribed to elevated shear stress,[52] although experimental evidence for this view is lacking. It appears, however, that excessive callus acts to elevate pressure, and this may result in positive feedback for the production of further callus. This observation confirms the critical importance of callus care in the patient at risk for neuropathic ulceration.

We have recently examined the relationship between the bony structure of the foot and elevated plantar pressure.[40] A variety of angular and linear measurements was taken from standardized anteroposterior and lateral weight-bearing radiographs in a large group of patients. A multivariate statistical technique (stepwise multiple regression) was used to identify those structural variables associated with high pressure. Among the strongest predictors of high pressure under the first metatarsal head were soft tissue thickness between the sesamoids and ground, inclination of the metatarsal in a sagittal plane, and frontal plane splay of the first and fifth metatarsals. It is encouraging to find that static structural measurements of the foot are statistically related to dynamic functional characteristics. This suggests that it may be possible in the future to add such measurements as a component of a larger risk factor profile to predict risk of injury.

In the course of examining the radiographs just described, a number of clinical abnormalities were also noted.[39] In particular, there was a 12% prevalence of fractures (mostly metatarsal shaft) in neuropathic patients, and most of these had not been previously diagnosed. In addition, an 8% prevalence of Charcot joint fractures was found. Fractures can result in alteration of weight bearing and load sharing by regions of the foot not specialized for this purpose. Thus, unperceived injury to bone can be a risk factor for elevated plantar pressure and ulceration.

Previous ulceration is widely regarded as a leading risk factor for future ulceration. This is reasonable, because the initial ulceration represents tangible proof that the patient has the combination of other risk factors that together produce ulceration. Yet there may also be a direct risk linked to prior ulceration steming from altered mechanical properties of the new tissue generated during the wound repair process.[24] Although little is known about the mechanical properties of tissue generated during wound repair,[54] clinically one can feel the adhesion between different tissue layers and the lack of mobility of the skin overlying bony prominences. The exact role of adhesion and scar tissue in causing further tissue breakdown is not well known, but certainly stress concentration is a possible explanation. Thus, scar tissue may act in much the same way that callus appears to act—by transferring large, concentrated loads to the immediately underlying softer tissue.

The previous discussion is by no means an exhaustive coverage of those factors that contribute to elevated plantar pressure. A comprehensive risk factor model has yet to be developed, and until such time, the factors mentioned must be considered as at least part of the pathway to high plantar pressure and subsequent ulceration.

## SHEAR STRESS

Most of the previous discussion concerning the interaction of the foot with the shoe or ground has centered on the normal (vertical) pressures. But as shown in Figure 9–2, there are also forces during gait that tend to make the foot slip from its relatively fixed position on the ground, so-called shear forces. These forces generate shear stress in the tissues and in the shoe materials, which are considered on a theoretical basis in the following discussion. Little is known at present about the magnitude and direction of shear stress during everyday activities or its role in causing plantar injury. This is because there are only isolated examples in the literature of instrumentation to measure shear stress.[58, 65, 82]

Nevertheless, many authorities believe that shear stress is an important pathogenic factor in foot injury;[20, 52, 56] it should not be ignored simply because there is no satisfactory measurement device at present. Shear stress can probably be modulated by the fit of a shoe (see Fig 9–11), and it may emerge that the minimization of shear stress is an important criterion in defining appropriate fit. A number of groups (including our own) are actively engaged in development projects to refine methods of shear measurement with the anticipation of rapid developments in the near future.

## HOW DOES FOOT INJURY OCCUR?

Although elevated plantar pressure is now accepted as a major factor in the etiopathogenesis of plantar ulcers in diabetics, exactly how tissue damage occurs is not well known. Various mechanisms have been discussed by Brand and Coleman,[21] Delbridge et al.,[44] Pecoraro et al.,[64] and others.[89] Certainly the strong possibility exists that plantar soft tissue in regions of high pressure becomes ischemic when the foot is loaded. A systolic blood pressure of 120 mm Hg is only 15 kPa, and capillary pressure is less than half this value. Reference to Figure 9–4 shows that typical peak plantar pressures in the forefoot during gait are at least 30 times higher, implying that blood flow will be occluded during at least part of the gait cycle. Recovery from this ischemia may be affected by such factors as glycosylation or the state of the microcirculation, which has recently been shown to be abnormal even in early diabetes.[84]

Factors leading to tissue breakdown have been studied much more systematically by those interested in pressure ulcers of the buttocks than by scientists with an interest in the foot.[7] It is believed that pressures as small as 6 to 8 kPa can, when applied for periods of 15 minutes or more, affect the microcirculation, lymph flow and interstitial transport in the tissues over the ischial tuberosities. Although the loading pattern in this region is fundamentally different from that which occurs in the foot, the protocols used by Bader[6] to examine recovery of tissue transcutaneous oxygen pressure ($tcPo_2$) after repetitive loading would seem to have merit for application to the foot. Delayed recovery of normal tissue oxygenation was found in elderly and neuropathic patients, and this may have been because of the delayed elastic recovery of the aging tissue.

The ischemic injury hypothesis is only one of several possible options for the cause of tissue injury. For instance, it is also likely that the unperceived stresses in the plantar soft tissues are high enough to actually rupture the microanatomic and macroanatomic structures that are usually protected from damage by the exquisite sensitivity of the plantar aspect of a normal foot. In any case, there can be no doubt that the acute and chronic phases of foot injury deserve more study experimentally than they have received to date.

## BIOMECHANICS OF FOOT-INSOLE INTERFACE: TISSUE AND MATERIAL PROPERTIES

We have referred to studies that show a link between areas of high plantar pressure and plantar ulceration.[16, 18, 43, 81] We have also noted that diabetes is associated with plantar pressures higher than those found in a nondiabetic population[15, 18] and have discussed why this may be the case. Many of the presumed reasons for elevated plantar pressure in diabetes have to do with changes in the plantar soft tissues, whereas footwear is prescribed to redistribute plantar forces and thereby lower plantar pressure. Thus, a deeper understanding of the properties of footwear materials and the plantar tissues, in particular, how they respond to force, is key in providing further insight into why high pressure may occur and how it may be dealt with. The excellent chapter by Thompson[83] in the fourth edition of this book is recommended as a good primer on tissue mechanics, as is the more mathematical treatment by Wainwright et al.[87]

When a force is applied to an object, some deformation always occurs. If the material is very hard (e.g., bone), the deformation may not be visible to the naked eye, but if the material is soft (e.g., the heel pad), deformation is obvious. Because both the area over which the force is applied and the initial length of the material will affect the outcome of a given interaction, engineers have chosen to standardize the approach to these kinds of problems using the quantities *stress* and *strain*. As discussed earlier, stress is synonymous with pressure and is calculated by dividing force by the area over which it acts. Strain is simply fractional deformation, calculated by dividing the change in length by the original length. Thus, stress causes strain; it is important that these terms not be used interchangeably.

The field of solid mechanics examines the relationship between stress and strain in materials. In a biologic context, it is most developed in the area of tensile (elongation) testing of hard tissues; for example, both experimental and theoretical determination of the effects of stress on bone are well documented.[53] In contrast, soft tissues have received less attention, particularly in compression, and little is known about the mechanical properties of the tissues of the plantar surface of the foot. The same is true for the mechanical properties of the materials that are typically put in contact with the foot, such as polyethylene foam (e.g., Plastazote) and urethane foam (e.g., PPT). Both soft tissues and these materials are complex because they exhibit large deformation, non-linearity, and viscoelastic behavior, all properties that make theoretical approaches difficult.

Figure 9–5 shows theoretical examples of deformation (strain) under the action of stress. A normal (vertical) stress causes both compression in the direction of the stress and expansion at right angles to the stress. When a shear stress is applied (see Fig 9–5,C), the entire material "rotates," that is, it experiences the most absolute deflection at the free surface and possibly zero deflection at the opposite surface. In general, tissues in the foot will experience both shear and normal stress (Fig 9–5, D), with resultant compression along the line of normal stress, expansion at right angles to the stress, and "rotation" simultaneously. The same will be true of insole materials.

The mechanical properties of materials can be characterized by performing controlled tests on uniformly shaped samples such that the strain resulting from a known

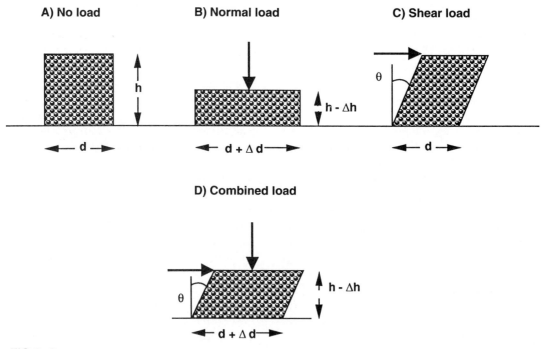

**FIG 9–5.**
Tissue deformation (strain) under the action of stress. From the unloaded position **(a),** normal stress applied to the top of the cube **(b),** causes compression in the direction of the stress by an amount Δh and expansion at right angles to the stress by an amount Δd. When a shear stress is applied **(c)** the entire material "rotates" and the deflection is measured by the angular change Θ. In the general case **(d),** tissue in the foot will express all consequences of stress; compression along the line of normal stress, expansion at right angles to the stress, and rotation will occur simultaneously.

stress can be measured. In the present application, compression and shear tests are most relevant, although these are less frequently conducted than tension tests. Tests can be done either in vitro or, in some cases, in vivo.

Examples of the results of compression tests for a perfect spring, an insole material (Plastazote I closed-cell polyethylene foam), and the human heel pad are shown in Figure 9–6. Note that the graphs for materials have a standard form. Stress is plotted on the Y axis (in units of force divided by area, kilopascals in the SI system), and strain on the X axis in dimensionless form (change in thickness divided by initial thickness).

The relationship between stress and strain in the working range of a perfect spring is linear (see Fig 9–6,A), and this curve can therefore be described by a single constant equal to the gradient of the curve, the so-called spring constant. Notice, however, that in this idealized spring a point is reached when further application of force causes no further change in thickness and the spring is said to be "bottomed out."

In almost all biologic tissues and in most insole applications, the materials are nonlinear in compression. The particular form of nonlinearity most often seen is the stiffening of materials as strain increases (see Fig 9–9,B and C). When stress is high enough to cause materials to reach that part of their range where they become extremely stiff (see Fig 9–6,B), this is the equivalent of the spring bottoming out. Although an objective in insole design is to avoid bottoming out, prolonged use causes degradation of material which may bring it closer to the bottoming out regions.[28]

The curve for Plastazote I shown in Figure 9–6,B is clearly nonlinear and thus cannot be described by a single "spring constant." As shown in this figure, a variety of slopes (equivalent to spring constants) can be used to characterize these curves, and their values describe the stiffness of the materials over different regions of their operating ranges. If we compare Plastazote I with another insole material (Pelite), we find that Pelite is three times stiffer than Plastazote I in the middle part of the range. Similar tests

can be performed with the materials being subjected to shear stress.

There are several points of interest about the heel pad data (Fig 9–6,C); note that the early part of the curve (phase 1) is quite flat. This indicates that very little stress is required to produce significant strain. The tissue then seems to "stiffen" first along one line (phase 2) and then along another steeper line (phase 3). The anatomic correlates of this behavior remain to be identified. A comparison of the heel pad data with the insole material is also of interest. Note that the initial stiffness of the heel pad is less than that of the insole material, the phase 2 slope is about equal, and the phase 3 slope is stiffer.

Another major departure from perfect spring behavior is that both the insole material and the heel pad follow different paths during loading and unloading. This feature, which is discussed later, is known as "hysteresis" and results in energy loss during repeated loading and unloading.

Although some data describing the mechanical properties of commonly used shoe materials are available,[23] most prescribers and fabricators follow an empirical approach to insole and shoe manufacture at the present time.[60] However, reference to such data will become vital as more quantitative methods of footwear design become possible. Similarly, investigation of the mechanical properties of the plantar soft tissues will be helpful in ascertaining the presumed role of soft tissue change in the increase in plantar pressure associated with diabetes. With better understanding of the relationship between these relatively simple material characteristics and cushioning, it should be possible to pick the correct material for a given situation.

## FOOTWEAR

That footwear is so central to injury prevention in diabetes is emphasized by the fact that three other chapters in this book (see Chapters 10, 24, and 25) deal with the various aspects of footwear design and prescrip-

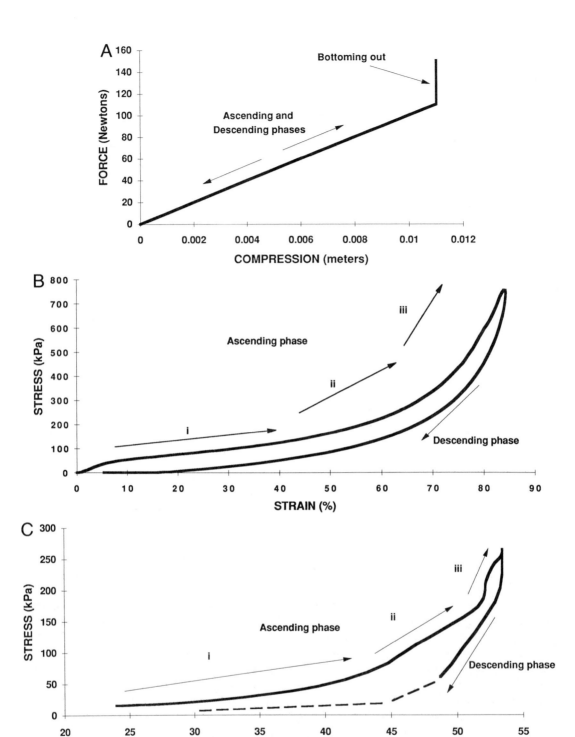

**FIG 9–6.**
Results of compression tests for a perfect spring **(A),** material used in insole construction (Plastazote I; **B**), and the human heel pad **(C).** Note that the idealized spring is linear and follows the same path during the ascending (loading) and descending (unloading) phases but that a "bottoming out" point is reached where force increases sharply with minor change in compression. Gradient of the spring (change in force divided by change in deformation) in its linear portion is known as spring "stiffness." Graphs for materials have a standard form: stress is plotted on the Y axis and strain on the X axis. No single value can be used to characterize the slopes of the curves for the Plastazote material and the human heel pad, because these curves get steeper in three phases (i.e., the materials become stiffer) as more compression occurs. Stiffness (or modulus) can be calculated for each of these phases. Both insole material and the heel show hysteresis, meaning that loading and unloading follow different paths.

tion. Footwear can be critical in preventing the first injury in patients with newly diagnosed neuropathy and becomes an issue of lifetime concern for a patient who has experienced a neuropathic ulcer. Given the emphasis on the practical aspects of footwear in other chapters, we describe some of the principles behind the action of footwear and explore ways in which some science may be applied to this area, which has been widely described as "an art form." We have already alluded to the use of in-shoe plantar pressure measurement in footwear design and in the next section explore four further important issues, cushioning, modeling, shoe fit, and the rocker bottom outsole modification.

## Cushioning

If asked to choose a single word to describe the objective of footwear for the neuropathic foot, many workers in the field would probably choose the term *cushioning*. Yet the definition of cushioning in a footwear context is elusive: it has no units, it is not easily measured, and it is often misinterpreted. Webster's dictionary[88] offers the definition "to protect against force or shock," and goes on to define a cushion as "an elastic body for reducing shock." This definition might be paraphrased in more mechanical terms as "controlling the energy of a collision." To understand the inadequacy of this definition and to seek a better one, it is helpful to divide the contact of the shoe and the floor into two distinct phases: a *dynamic phase*, which starts at heel strike and ends at foot flat; and a *quasistatic phase*, which includes the remainder of ground contact. It may come as a surprise that the late support and toe-off phases are considered quasistatic, but compared with the high impact forces of the landing phase,[66] the rather slowly changing forces of the second part of support have minimal dynamic components.

The major difference between these two phases is that the net or total force acting on the foot through the shoe can be reduced by the cushioning effect of footwear during the dynamic phase, but the net force during the quasistatic phase cannot be changed. However, during both phases, the net force can be distributed so that local pressures on the foot are reduced. By net force, we mean the total, at any instant in time, of all the forces acting on each part of the foot. For example, if there were forces of 300 N and 200 N on the forefoot and hindfoot, respectively, at 0.3 seconds after footstrike, a net force of 500 N would be acting, and this could be recorded by a force platform as shown in Fig 9–2.

To appreciate the difference between the dynamic and static phases, consider the two situations shown in Figure 9–7. In Figure 9–7,A an egg is dropped from the same height onto surfaces of successively softer characteristics. On the hard surface, it breaks, but on the foams the impact is "cushioned" and breakage does not occur. The appropriate models are of a mass with velocity $v$ and acceleration $g$, contacting first a rigid link and then springs of stiffness $k_1$ and $k_2$ (where $k_1 > k_2$). Hypothetical force-time curves show that the peak force at impact would be reduced and the time to peak force increased. Both of these effects are forms of cushioning that can occur in a dynamic situation.

In the static situation, a flat plate is shown standing on the same materials (see Figure 9–7,B). Despite the fact that the plate sinks more deeply into the softer foams, the net (or total) force acting on the plate is the same in each case and is equal to its weight.

In the case of a collision, as occurs at heel strike, Webster's definition is appropriate, because we are concerned with managing the energy of the collision to reduce the force on the foot. Certainly therapeutic shoes can be cushioned in this way, but we know that neuropathic ulceration rarely occurs in the heel regions, except for pressure ulcers, which have a different etiology. Thus, collision energy is not really what causes ulcers. Because the static example (see Fig 9–7,B) shows that net force cannot be reduced during the midsupport phase when forefoot plantar pressures are largest (see Plate 10), we must search elsewhere to find a definition

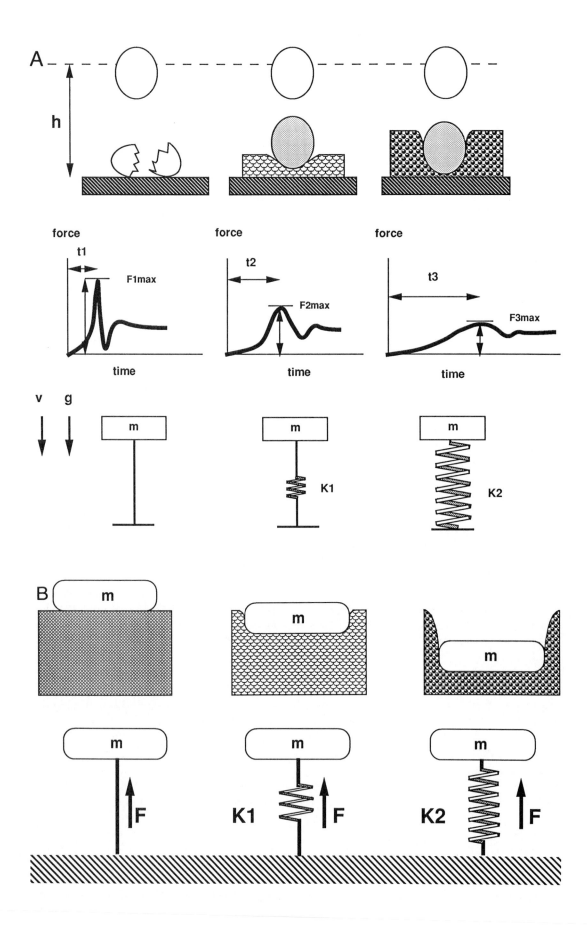

of cushioning that is relevant to the prevention of neuropathic foot injury.

This search leads to a definition of cushioning that is based on "distribution" of force rather than attenuation of net force. As mentioned earlier, the term "net" is key to understanding the action of footwear because, although the net or total force acting on the forefoot at any instant in time may remain the same, the local forces acting on individual anatomic structures, which, when totaled, must equal the net force, can be altered dramatically by footwear.

A further model of cushioning in the context of forefoot deformity is proposed in Figure 9–8. If a bony prominence such as the head of a plantar flexed metatarsal contacts a rigid surface, most of the ground reaction force will be applied to the small area of the bony prominence, with resultant large local pressures (see Fig 9–8,A). Patients are always encouraged to avoid walking barefoot for precisely this reason. The model of this foot in a conventional (nontherapeutic) shoe is shown in Figure 9–8,B. The uniform stiffness of the midsole material (i.e., its spring constant k) is so large that even though the shoe does deform slightly, the amount of deformation is not enough to engage the adjacent spring elements with the foot so that the load can be shared. Thus no pressure reduction occurs.

When a compliant material is placed in the shoe, the situation becomes much more favorable for the soft tissue. The appropriate model now consists of a series of springs with lower spring constants than before, arranged in parallel with each other (see Fig 9–8,C). Because the spring constant is smaller, more deformation will occur, allowing adjacent spring elements to begin to share the load as the material under the bony prominence is compressed. This action results in the so-called accommodative behavior of shoes for the neuropathic foot. The total force from all the spring elements at any instant will be the same as the force in Figure 9–8,A but the local pressure (force in each spring element divided by its area of application) will be reduced.

This situation in Figure 9–8,C clearly is not perfect, because the greater compression of the spring element under the prominence will still result in greater local pressure. The available options are to increase the length of the adjacent springs (see Fig 9–8,D) or to reduce both the stiffness and the length of the spring under the prominence (see Fig 9–8,E). In practice, the first of these options is easier to achieve, because the deformation range over which a less stiff spring could work is limited by the room in the shoe. Molding of the insole to the shape of foot is the practical embodiment of this theory. This process brings the insole up to meet those parts of the plantar aspect that would otherwise not share in the load-bearing process.

As long as the molding is "perfect" and the platform under the molded area does not deform, softness is not an essential requirement. This is apparent from the success that can be achieved healing neuropathic ulcers with a total contact cast[17, 61, 78] where the individual springs in the model are very stiff but there is an infinitely large number of

---

**FIG 9–7.**
Schematic illustrations on the effects of different types of "cushioning" during the dynamic phase and quasi-static phases of contact. **(A)**, dynamic phase. Egg falling from the same height onto surfaces of successively softer characteristics. The appropriate models are of a mass with velocity *v* and acceleration *g*, contacting first a rigid link, then springs of stiffness k1 and k2 (k1 > k2). Hypothetical force-time curves show that the peak impact force would be reduced and the time to peak force increased by the softer material; however, the area under each curve (which represents the change in momentum of the egg) is the same in each case. Thus, in the dynamic phase (as occurs during gait primarily only at foot strike) soft materials can change the peak force acting on the foot. **B**, static phase. Flat plate standing on materials of progressively increasing softness: rigid; stiffness, k1; stiffness k2 (k1 > k2). Note that despite the fact that the plate sinks more deeply into the softer material, the net (total) force acting on the plate is the same in each case and is equal to its weight. Therefore, in the static phase of foot contact with the ground (as occurs in the later phases of support) soft materials cannot change the total force acting on the foot, but can affect the distribution of the force (see also Fig 9–8).

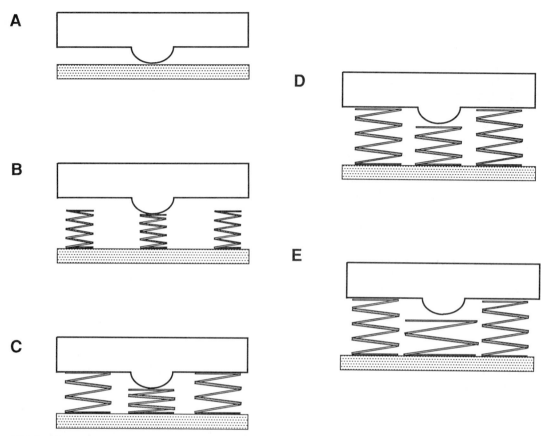

**FIG 9–8.**
Role of footwear during the quasi-static phase of ground contact in "cushioning" by distribution of load. **A,** schematic cross section of a foot with a plantar prominence resting on a flat rigid surface. **B,** conceptual model of the foot in contact with a rigid shoe. Spring elements are all the same, and extremely stiff. Even though slight deformation occurs under the prominence, this does not cause enough deflection to bring other regions of the foot-shoe interface into the load-bearing process. Thus the pressure under the prominence is as high as in **A,** because the total force still is transmitted through this region. **C,** when a more compliant material is placed in the shoe the appropriate model now consists of springs with lower spring stiffness than before in parallel with each other. Because the spring stiffness is smaller more deformation will occur, and as the material under the bony prominence is compressed, adjacent spring elements begin to share the load. This action results in the "accommodative" behavior of shoes for the neuropathic foot. The force transmitted through the prominence now will be less. **D,** alternative solution (shown for the almost unloaded foot) is to reduce the length of the spring under the prominence and/or increase the length of the springs away from this region, so that all springs will engage immediately on loading. This occurs with a molded insole, where load sharing begins as soon as the foot is loaded and peak pressures are reduced. **E,** better solution still is to make the spring under the prominence both shorter and less stiff. This reduces the loading on the prominence and increases loading on other structures. This occurs with a composite insole with different material under the bony prominence.

them, so that the individual tissue stresses are reduced.* In the case of an insole, however, molding of a rigid interface is rarely perfect, and there is some deformation in the supporting shoe, even with a rigid rocker. Nor can the foot be immobilized in a shoe the way it is in a cast to ensure that the

appropriately molded parts of the foot and insole stay in contact with each other. Relative movement between foot and footbed brings prominent parts of the foot into contact with raised parts of the rigid insole, leading to tissue damage. Thus, we depend on soft materials that modify their contour and keep the load shared between adjacent regions even when shearing movements occur. It has recently been shown that socks

*Load may also be shared by the sidewalls of the cast, which are tightly molded around the leg, although this hypothesis remains to be proved.

must be considered in this equation[85, 86] because socks alone can reduce barefoot peak pressures by approximately 30%. One can conceptualize the way they achieve this in the same manner as insoles have their effect, by providing a large number of short springs that can bring new, albeit small, regions of the foot surrounding bony prominences into a weight-bearing role.

Even with a well-molded insole (e.g., Plastazote backed with PPT), there will still be elevated pressures under bony prominences compared with the adjacent regions. This is because the molding results in a thin, compressed layer of material under the prominence, which probably acts as a stiffer spring and will give greater force for a given compression than the uncompressed material in surrounding areas. There are presently no data in the literature on the mechanical characteristics of moldable materials after they have been reduced in thickness.

From the point of view of equalizing the pressure in different areas of the foot, the ideal foot-shoe interface would be a hydrostatic cushion (a fluid-filled bag) that could adapt to local curvatures and apply equal loads to all regions of the foot. This principle has been implemented in the area of pressure ulcers of the buttocks.[72] Fluid-filled insoles have been proposed, but this design has no ability to resist movement of the foot in the anteroposterior or mediolateral directions, providing a very unstable platform for the foot. The depth would also have to be great enough to prevent bottoming out. These problems do not appear to be insurmountable, however, with an appropriate restraint applied through the upper and with the kind of depth that is already incorporated into a rocker shoe. The problem of excessive weight in fluid-filled insoles may prove more difficult to resolve.

The example of lack of control in the "fluid bag" brings us to the last additions to the conceptual model of the shoe-foot interface, and these are damping and spring stiffness in the anteroposterior and mediolateral directions. We note from the stress-strain experiments on shoe materials shown in Figure 9–6 that these materials exhibit hysteresis, showing that energy absorbing (damping) elements are present. Perfect springs store all of the available energy when they deform and return that energy during the rebound phase. If no damping were present in the earlier example of the falling egg (see Fig 9–7), the egg would rebound from the foam cushions up to its initial height.

Whereas springs store energy, dampers redirect it. The first law of thermodynamics tells us that energy cannot be created or destroyed; it can only be transformed. Energy used to deform a damper is converted to heat and thus cannot be usefully recovered as mechanical energy. When a viscous element is cyclically loaded, stress and strain are not in phase, and a characteristic loop is developed (see Fig 9–6). The area enclosed by the loop is a measure of how much energy has been lost. Practically speaking, the damping elements control the rate of compression of the spring and its tendency to oscillate or bounce. They are usually represented as "dashpots" (Fig 9–9,A), which in our model would be in parallel with the spring. Thus, each spring element in our cushioning models of Figures 9–7 and 9–8 should be replaced with the combined element shown in Figure 9–9,A.

Finally, we turn to the issue of stiffness and damping in shear directions. The potential role of shear stress in causing foot injury has been discussed earlier, and we consider here how footwear may affect shear stress. As long as there is sufficient friction between the insole and the foot or sock, points on the foot will tend to remain in contact with the same points on the surface of the insole when shear forces are applied, causing the insole material to experience shear strain. When there is not enough friction, the foot will, of course, slip. Exactly how much strain occurs for a given shear stress will be determined by the stiffness of the material in shear, and this can be added conceptually to our unit element by a spring in the horizontal plane as shown in Figure 9–9,B. In the examples discussed previously, the spring constant of the horizontal components in the hydrostatic cushion would be extremely small, that on a rigid surface extremely large, and that in traditional insole materials intermediate in value. The provision of a

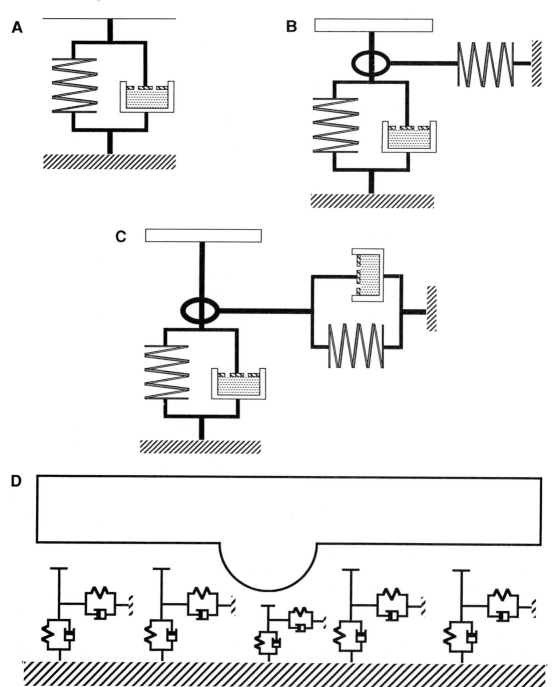

**FIG 9–9.**
Single-spring models cannot describe shear stress or the hysteresis noted in actual materials (see Fig 9–6,B). However, refinements to such simple models are possible. **A,** damping element is added in parallel with the spring. This controls the rate at which the spring compresses and controls the rebound. It also can model hysteresis in the materials. **B,** stiffness of the material in shear is modeled by a spring grounded at one end and attached to the vertical element at the other. Stiffness of the spring can be measured as the shear stiffness (or modulus) in actual shoe materials. **C,** final model element with both compliance and damping in both vertical and horizontal directions. (See text for further details.) **D,** refined large conceptual model of the foot in cross section. Load sharing will begin as soon as the foot is loaded in both horizontal and vertical directions. Damping is incorporated into each element, and the spring constants of the material under the prominence are smaller than those elsewhere.

material that allows an appropriate amount of shear strain to occur is a critically important factor in the specification of an insole. There will also be a damping action in the horizontal plane, and this is shown by the added horizontal dashpot in Figure 9–9,C, which represents the final configuration of a conceptual model that is appropriate for the consideration of cushioning in the shoe. The complete conceptual model, which incorporates different spring constants under the bony prominence, as well as compliance and damping in both vertical and horizontal directions, is shown in Figure 9–9,D.

Although the concept of individual springs and dampers is useful for conceptually discrete models, when the materials are continuous, the compression modulus and shear modulus are better quantities for the characterization of the vertical and horizontal spring stiffness. As mentioned earlier, although values for these quantities are not common knowledge at the present time,[23] it is expected that they will become the basis for a more quantitative approach to footwear design and manufacture in the future.

## Biomechanical Models

The models presented earlier are useful to help understand the concepts behind therapeutic footwear interventions in the diabetic patient. They do not, however, allow direct predictions of the efficacy of different approaches to be made, because they lack the quantitative detail and sufficient complexity to approximate the real situation. The two most accessible methods presently available to assess different types of footwear are (1) to use different materials in experiments with patients and measure plantar pressure at the foot shoe interface and (2) to try to predict plantar pressure from known forces, material properties, and tissue architecture by modeling. Most previous models have attempted to explore the effects of major structural or surgical changes,[2] but little has been done on the modeling of events leading to tissue breakdown in the normal foot with relatively normal gross structure but with important changes in the plantar adipose tissue, for example.

Although calculations of the effects of stress on uniform rigid solids (e.g., beams and plates) are routinely performed in engineering, the effects of stress on multiple layers of soft, irregular, nonlinear, viscoelastic tissues is more problematic. We have recently begun to explore a technique known as finite element analysis,[33, 74] and some of the preliminary results from this technique are shown in Figure 9–10 and Plate 15. The basic approach is to divide the problem into small geometric elements (in either two or three dimensions) that can be mathematically characterized one at a time by a sophisticated computer program. The geometry and mechanical properties of each element are first defined; the boundary conditions and external loads are then added, and the program is set in motion. The model allows the combined effects of all these factors to be used in the prediction of the resulting deformations and stresses at any point in the model.

The particular benefit of this approach is that any of the input parameters can be varied at will and a set of new predictions obtained. In the examples shown (see Fig 9–10), a two-dimensional model of a single weight-bearing metatarsal head has been formulated. Bone, muscle, tendon, adipose tissue, and skin all have been included, and the three different weight-bearing surfaces (a rigid floor, a stiff shoe, and a compliant shoe) have been modeled. Also, the effects of changes in the thickness of the adipose tissue layer have been explored.

Even these preliminary results provide considerable insight into mechanical conditions under the foot that could lead to tissue damage. The foot with adequate adipose tissue cushions under the metatarsal head is predicted to show low pressures that are distributed broadly under the area of study. The poor footwear yields values for plantar pressure that are virtually the same as barefoot while some reduction in pressure is seen in the compliant shoe condition. The model predictions for the foot without adipose tissue show focal pressures in the area of the metatarsal head that are over five times higher than those in the normal foot. Even the poor footwear causes a marked reduc-

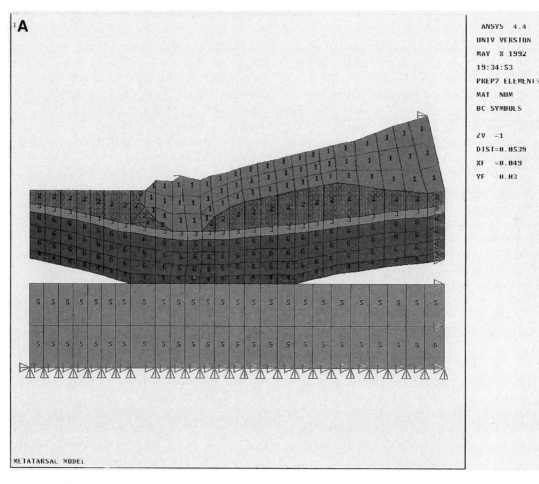

B

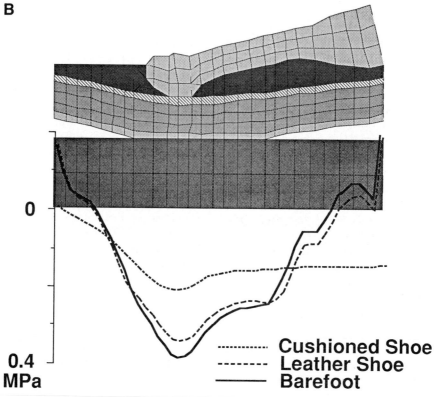

0

0.4
MPa

.......... Cushioned Shoe
- - - - Leather Shoe
——— Barefoot

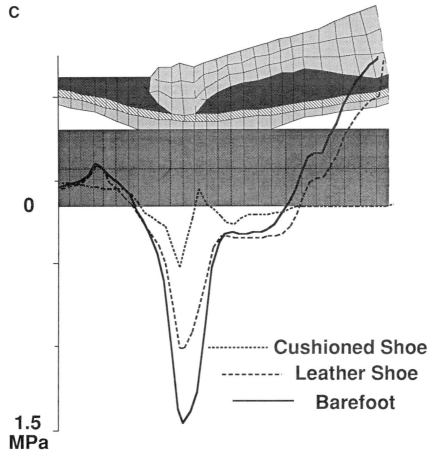

**C**

**0**

**1.5**
**MPa**

·········· **Cushioned Shoe**
·········· **Leather Shoe**
—————— **Barefoot**

**FIG 9–10.**
**A,** model of the second metatarsal and associated structures comprising a "mesh" of small geometric elements that can be given material properties, constraints, and to which external forces can be applied. Successive mathematical solution of resulting stress and strain in each small element of the model allows the behavior of the entire model to be defined. Without this technique, called finite element analysis, the problem would be too complex for solution. **B,** predicted pressure (normal stress) under the metatarsal head model shown in **A**, with "good" submetatarsal head tissue cushioning in three different footwear conditions. Cushioned shoe is predicted to reduce barefoot pressures by 45%. **C,** effects of loss or displacement of the submetatarsal cushion. Barefoot pressures are predicted to be almost four times greater than in the foot with intact tissue **(B)**, and footwear is predicted to have a much more dramatic effect on pressure reduction.

tion in pressure, but pressures in the compliant shoe are still more than twice as great as those predicted for the barefoot condition in the normal foot. These results highlight the importance of footwear intervention in a foot with bony prominences. We expect that further development of the modeling approach will yield significant insight into the etiology of elevated plantar pressures.

**Fit**

Shoe fit is a critical issue in the prevention of both dorsal and plantar ulcers. Despite its importance, it is usually left to the subjective opinion of the fitter and the wearer. When the fitter is inexperienced and the wearer has limited sensation, it is clear that this approach can lead to a less than perfect solution. A shoe with ideal fit would control the motion of the foot relative to the weight-bearing surface without applying any pressure whatsoever to the dorsum of the foot. This is not possible in practice, however, and thus a working definition of shoe fit might be "a covering for the dorsum of the foot that minimizes the application of pressures to the dorsum while controlling

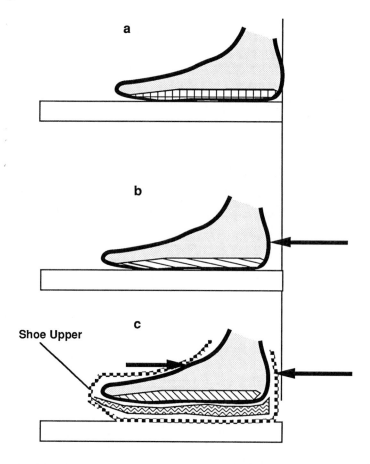

**FIG 9–11.**

Hypothesis for the role of the shoe upper and a soft insole in reducing the shear strain of the plantar tissues. Soft tissues on the plantar surface of the foot are shown with schematic shading to indicate the amount of shear stress experienced. From the resting position on a flat surface with minimum shear stress in the tissues **(a)**, an anteriorly directed shear force applied to a foot with no upper **(b)** causes forward movement of the foot about the fixed plantar surface, which will lead to high shear stress in the tissues. If the same force is applied to a foot in a shoe with an upper and a compliant insole **(c)** the resulting shear stress is reduced because the upper applies a re-straining force to the foot once the insole has allowed forward movement. Note that there would be no reduction in the shear of the plantar tissue without the restraint of the shoe upper. Thus the shoe and the insole together reduce the amount of shear stress in the plantar tissues, and possibly the risk of injury. This hypothesis can be investigated experimentally.

mediolateral and anteroposterior foot move-ment." The exact values for the pressures between the upper and the foot encountered in different types of footwear have not been quantitatively explored, although several of the available devices to measure in-shoe plantar pressure (mentioned earlier) could also be used for this purpose. It is expected that such measurements will become routine in footwear prescription for high-risk dia-betics in the near future.

In the absence of experimental data on shoe fit, the following represents a working hypothesis of the role of fit of the upper in providing a safe shoe. Although relief of pressure over bony prominences is an obvi-ous need, a less frequently expressed role of the upper may be to limit the amount of shear strain that the tissue on the plantar aspect of the foot experiences. As shown in Figure 9–11, in the presence of shear forces, the upper acts on the dorsum of the foot to generate opposing forces. This has the effect of reducing the forward movement of the foot on the shoe compared with what would occur with the shoe platform alone, consequently reducing the amount of shear strain in the plantar tissues. An insole that allows shear strain will facilitate this forward movement of the foot relative to the shoe and allow the upper to "engage" the dorsum at a lower value of shear strain. Because excessive shear strain in the tissue is likely to be damaging, the combination of an appropriate insole and a well-fitting upper has the potential to reduce plantar injury based on the principles described here rather than from a simple cushioning approach. If the upper does not fit correctly or the insole does not permit shear strain, this role could be lost; if the upper fits too tightly, direct injury could result.

In practice, the shoe fitter attempts, by palpation, to establish that any bony prominences have adequate pressure relief and to locate the position of the most distal toe. Once this latter position has been determined, there must be some attempt to determine how much relative movement between foot and shoe will occur with the given combination of insole materials, upper, gait, and physical characteristics of the patient. There are, at present, almost no quantitative tools available to assist with this extremely complex process.

## Rocker Bottom Shoes

The discussion of footwear so far has concentrated principally on the interface between the foot and shoe, and there is no doubt that this is the most important aspect of footwear for the neuropathic foot. However, a number of investigators have shown either clinically or through direct measurement that outsole modifications can also have an important effect on preventing injury.[41, 42, 63, 73, 77] The commonest of these is the rigid rocker bottom shoe, or a variant thereof, which has been advocated by Brand[19] for many years. The general principle behind this design (Fig 9–12) is that it allows the patient to walk with minimum motion of the joints of the foot. In particular, no extension of the MTP joints is required during the phase of forefoot weight bearing, and this appears to reduce forefoot pressures compared with walking in flexible shoes by up to 50%.[63, 73, 77] It is frequently said that the rigid sole, usually accompanied

by a molded insole, loads the entire foot throughout the contact phase. Pressure measurements have shown that this is not the case.[73] There are many design variables, including the location of the rocker axis, the anteroposterior curvature of the "roller," and the mediolateral position of the axis. In addition, a given shoe can actually increase the load under some parts of the foot while reducing it elsewhere.[73]

The uncertainty over the positioning of the rocker axis is a good example of why more objective research is needed in this field before footwear can be designed according to established principles rather than simply basing designs on clinical experience. Many of the ideas outlined in this section on footwear need to be confirmed by experimental investigations. The entire field of therapeutic footwear biomechanics is still in a primitive stage, where trial and error is the principal modus operandi. This is not a satisfactory situation for either patient or provider and frequently results in a long and frustrating search for a solution that will keep the patient healed. One can only hope that the continued application of technologies such as biomechanical modeling, pressure measurement, materials testing, and shape measurement will result in a more complete understanding of the principles of different approaches and faster convergence toward appropriate interventions.

## IMPLICATIONS FOR HEALING

Even in the presence of many of the presumed risk factors for injury mentioned earlier, it is clear that footwear can act as the final preventive or permissive link in the chain between elevated pressure and injury. There is little doubt that inappropriate footwear can be a major factor in the development of plantar ulcers, and because plantar injury is caused by mechanical stress, healing is likely to be impaired by continued mechanical insult. We believe that the term "nonhealing" plantar ulcer could frequently be replaced by the term "nontreated" ulcer. This view is based on the rapid healing of many long-standing plantar ulcers once a

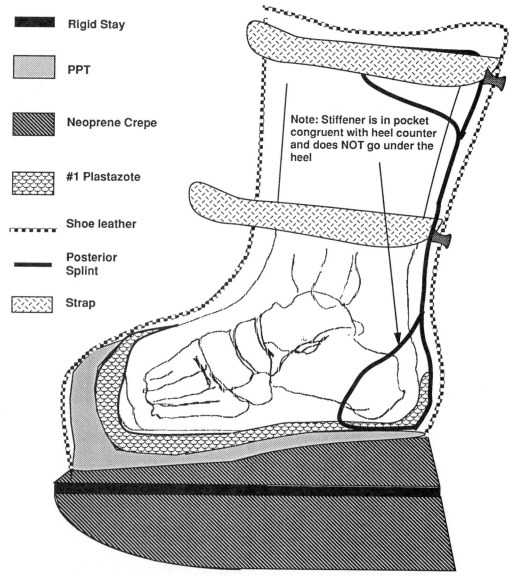

Rigid Stay

PPT

Neoprene Crepe

#1 Plastazote

Shoe leather

Posterior Splint

Strap

Note: Stiffener is in pocket congruent with heel counter and does NOT go under the heel

**FIG 9–12.**
Longitudinal section of a short rocker bottom shoe shown with the outline of the patient's foot taken from a lateral radiograph. This particular shoe has a rigid midsole and no single rocker axis but a "roller" outsole that permits the center of pressure to slowly move forward during support. Patient had ulceration of the distal tip of the foot with several full length shoes with toe fillers, but remained ulcer free in this shoe. We frequently make such a diagram as a means of communicating our footwear concepts to the prosthetist and shoe technician.

non-weight-bearing regimen has been instituted. The only exceptions to complete non–weight-bearing that appear to have some role in ulcer healing are the total contact cast[17, 78, 86] and the fiberglass cast boot.[27]

It must be stressed that the principles and examples of therapeutic footwear presented earlier are definitely not intended to be described as "healing shoes." In fact, we

would go so far as to say that the term healing shoe is an oxymoron, because continued ambulation in any kind of footwear other than the casts mentioned earlier for a patient with a neuropathic ulcer is incompatible with healing. If this single idea were better communicated to primary care physicians, who are often the first to see neuropathic ulcers, there can be little doubt that the morbidity associated with neuropathic ulceration would be dramatically reduced.

## CLINICAL BIOMECHANICS

So far we have discussed the biomechanics of gait, of the soft tissues of the foot, and of footwear in the context of understanding the cause and prevention of diabetic foot injury. At each point we have tried to draw clinical implications and either supported our assertions by reference to measurements or pointed out where no evidence exists. Often data produced from sophisticated and expensive equipment have been referred to. However desirable such an in-depth examination might be, we recognize that in many settings this kind of examination is simply not practical. Thus, the goal of the final section of this chapter to pull together the information provided so far into a coherent, usable clinical strategy when the facilities of a well-equipped gait laboratory are not available (see Table 9–1).

The key permissive factor in diabetic foot injury is loss of protective sensation because of the distal symmetric peripheral neuropathy that can result from diabetes (see Chapter 6). The degree of nerve damage can be assessed in many ways, and it has been recently proposed that to fully define the degree of neuropathy an objective assessment of symptoms, function and electrophysiologic tests should be performed.[5] However, in the context of defining the level of sensory loss that is permissive of unperceived injury, simple functional sensory tests appear to provide the best discrimination.[11, 18, 37, 79] Loss of protective sensation has been defined in terms of touch-pressure sensation using the Semmes-Weinstein monofilaments[11, 79] and in terms of vibration perception threshold using the Biosthesiometer[13, 18] and the Vibratron.[79] A calibrated tuning fork is in use in Switzerland.

We use primarily the Semmes-Weinstein monofilaments and believe that in clinical practice this simple tool provides the quickest and best method of defining loss of protective sensation. In several studies using a "method of limits" rather than a "forced choice" protocol,[11, 37] the 5.07 monofilament has been found to be discriminatory. We believe that this extremely simple and inexpensive tool should be in the office of all physicians who care for patients with diabetes. Just as an annual examination of the retina is viewed as essential to good care,[3] an annual assessment of sensory level in the feet should be seen as critical. If the patient can easily feel the 5.07 monofilament at multiple sites in the feet, he or she can be considered to require little or no additional special footcare. The only possible exception to this would be a patient who wears shoes that are inappropriate even for a healthy person, such as those with high heels and a cramped toe box. In that case, a discussion of reasonable footwear styles, as an "investment" for the future, might be appropriate.

Once the loss of protective sensation is identified, a detailed evaluation of foot structure and function and of gait and footwear is essential. The following section is designed to help the clinician determine what to look for.

### Foot Deformity

High pressure on both the dorsal and plantar surfaces is the immediate cause of skin injury. On the dorsal aspect of the foot, the problems encountered are usually the result of deformity, the most common from clawing of toes. On occasion the toes will actually become dorsally dislocated, and in that situation, off-the-shelf shoe fit is usually not possible. Although uncommon, bony prominences on the dorsal aspect of the midfoot are very troublesome because this region of the foot is likely to be particularly involved in the transfer of propulsive forces from the foot through footwear to the floor during gait. Such dorsal prominences are sometimes seen in patients with Charcot's fractures. Bunions, secondary to hallux valgus, are important deformities, particularly when associated with a wide forefoot. They are usually covered by very little soft tissue, making shoe fitting difficult.

Another important deformity is that of forefoot supination or pronation (rotation of the plane of the metatarsal heads so that they are no longer in the same plane as the hindfoot).[67] When the forefoot is in supination, the fifth metatarsal head tends to hit the ground first during gait with predictably higher plantar pressure in this region. Similarly, when the forefoot is in pronation, one could predict higher plantar pressure under the first metatarsal head. However, this is a good example of how very difficult it is to predict plantar pressure from a casual examination of the foot. The pressures just implied will, in fact, depend on whether the supination or pronation is fixed or flexible, in other words, on how difficult it is to bring all the metatarsal heads onto the ground during stance and gait. Thus, no firm conclusions about footwear modifications should be made in this situation without plantar pressure measurement although careful observation of barefoot stance and gait, preferably on video, might provide enough information in some cases. Plantar flexed metatarsals (particularly the first) also result in focal areas of pressure, and an attempt should always be made to identify potentially dangerous plantar prominences in the forefoot.

Unusual deformities or prominences usually imply underlying fractures. Often fractures are not noted by the patient,[39] and we therefore recommend that radiographs of the feet of patients with diabetic neuropathy be routinely obtained; radiographs of a patient with a major deformity is mandatory. Unusual prominences of the midfoot are of particular relevance because they are usually an indication of an underlying Charcot fracture. In the acute stages of a Charcot process, the foot is also erythematous, hot, and swollen, but in the "healed" stage of a Charcot fracture these findings are absent.

### Soft Tissue Changes

Bones can appear to be prominent either because of deformity or because of changes in the soft tissues overlying the bones. The plantar surface is usually well "padded," with soft tissue so that some attempt at an examination of the soft tissues there is important. Because most ulcers occur under the hallux and metatarsal heads, these are the regions that should be inspected most carefully.

Because there is an association between soft tissue thickness under a metatarsal head and peak plantar pressure in that region, an assessment of the quantity of the soft tissues under the metatarsal heads is relevant. In a healthy young foot, the metatarsal heads are not visible through the plantar skin nor palpable to a light stroking movement by the examiner's finger across them. As the toes becoming clawed as a consequence of intrinsic muscle atrophy, the plantar fat pad slides forward away from the metatarsal heads so that the tissue between the skin and the metatarsal heads becomes thinner. As discussed earlier, the quantity and quality of the plantar soft tissues may also be affected by glycosylation. Thus, in an extreme case, the metatarsal heads will be visible and directly palpable, seeming to be covered by skin only. On average, pressure under a metatarsal head covered by skin only will be much greater than when there is a good amount of healthy plantar tissue between the metatarsal head and the floor.

Scarring and adhesions of the soft tissues of the plantar surface can also be detected clinically; because of their possible consequences to plantar soft tissue function and thus to ulceration, we teach our patients to try to mobilize scar tissue by massage. It is also our impression that the quality of the "normal" soft tissues of the plantar surface of the foot changes in diabetes, but we have no data as yet to support this hypothesis. Healthy tissue between the skin and the metatarsal heads feels thick and resilient when compressed, whereas in some patients even reasonably thick plantar tissue seems to lose its resilience.

With experience, some useful information can be obtained from a clinical examination of the quality and quantity of plantar tissue. In a patient who has already had an ulceration, high pressure at that site can be inferred and appropriate footwear provided. The plantar tissue examination takes on most importance, however, in the initial evaluation of a patient with loss of protective sensation before any skin injuries have occurred. In that situation, direct measurement of plantar pressure is far preferable to any clinical examination.[38] As discussed earlier, areas that do not look prominent can be regions of high pressure (particularly in the midfoot), whereas prominent areas not actually involved in weight bearing will not have high pressure.

## Limited Joint Mobility

Limited joint mobility is statistically associated with higher plantar pressure.[48] The possible mechanisms for this association have been discussed. Although direct prediction of plantar pressure from measurement of the range of motion of a joint is not possible, there is nevertheless one measurement that is probably worthwhile: the measurement of hallux dorsiflexion. Normal range of hallux dorsiflexion is 70 degrees, measured with a simple goniometer,[49] with marked reductions of hallux dorsiflexion associated with high hallux pressure.[10] One would similarly predict that a reduction in ankle dorsiflexion would tend to increase forefoot plantar pressure. In general, however, this is not convincing on a patient by patient basis probably because many other factors contribute to forefoot pressure. For completeness, both ankle dorsiflexion, with the knee flexed and extended, and subtalar range of motion should be assessed. Since accuracy and inter-rater reliability are controversial topics in such measurements,[69] those made by a single examiner are preferable. Certain measurements (e.g., subtalar neutral position) may be almost worthless because of lack of appropriate landmarks.

## Callus

Even though the etiology of callus is not at all clear, the fact that callus contributes to high plantar pressure is clear.[89] It is therefore recommended that callus be looked for and that appropriate measures be taken to prevent, limit, and remove it. An extremely important sign in the evaluation of the neuropathic foot is hemorrhage into a callus, also called a preulcer. Although this may be quite subtle at times, it implies that enough trauma has occurred to cause tissue damage. Therefore, hematoma in a callus must be taken as seriously as an ulcer.

## Weakness

Although much emphasis in the evaluation and treatment of the diabetic patient is placed on sensory neuropathy, patients with a significant motor component to their neuropathy can also display major functional problems with the feet. A quick evaluation of the patient's ability to rise repeatedly on the toes from a neutral standing position is a worthwhile component of the clinical examination to reveal triceps surae weakness. Loss of strength of the ankle dorsiflexors will be apparent on gait, where foot drop, a steppage gait, or both will be seen. Patients with foot drop can injure their toes by dragging them on the floor; this can be prevented if good shoes are always worn. Falling because of the toes catching on the floor can be prevented using an ankle-foot orthosis.

## Gait

Additional information that might help predict risk of injury to the neuropathic foot can also be obtained from an assessment of gait. An important question to ask patients is how much they use their feet. It is important to ask about both the amount and type of use, because running, for example, leads to much greater forces being transmitted through the plantar tissues than walking.[32] A patient who is bed or chair bound will not need sophisticated footwear to protect the feet, whereas a very athletic patient who has significant foot problems may have to consider altering his or her behavior and footwear.

Instability during standing or walking can also result from more generalized lower limb muscle weakness or from proprioceptive deficits.[29] Instability leads to trips and falls and can also cause foot injury. The use of some form of an ankle-foot orthosis to deal with instability has already been alluded to. A number of patients feel more stable when their shoes are rockered or when they are provided with molded ankle-foot orthoses;

we have, as yet, no quantitative data to support either approach.

An important aspect of gait to observe before designing rocker bottom modifications of footwear is that of foot angle or toe-out during gait. This can be measured simply by putting ink on the sole of the shoes, one spot at mid forefoot and one at midheel. The patient can then walk down a runway on a roll of paper; the toe-out angle can be easily measured from the ink marks left on the paper. The rocker angle of the shoes can then be built to match the natural gait pattern of the patient. If this is not done for a patient with a marked degree of toe-out, the patient will be forced from his or her normal gait pattern, causing abnormal stresses and possible pain at the knees, hips, or both.

### Shoes

It is through shoes that the forces of gait that can potentially damage the foot are transmitted from the ground, and it is therefore in shoes that most injuries occur. Shoes can protect from injury, but they can also cause injury directly. Thus, a thorough examination of footwear must be considered to be an essential component of the clinical biomechanical examination of the patient at risk for neuropathic injury.

Concepts of fit must be applied to the clinical situation, with particular attention to dorsal deformities, clawed toes, and forefoot width. Construction of the insole will depend on what the clinical situation demands, but any insole already worn must be examined for excessive wear (bottoming out). This can provide insight into the location of high plantar pressure and will also suggest that a particular type of insole is not sufficient (e.g., if it bottoms out very quickly) or is simply too old.

Evaluation of the wear of both the uppers and outsoles of the shoes worn by a patient can also be helpful. Excessive wear of the outsole is probably a consequence of relative movement ("scuffing") during the early and late phases of foot contact and thus is probably not helpful in predicting where high plantar pressure occurs. Deformations of the upper, however, are often extremely useful, because they are evidence of shear forces tending to move the foot off the platform of the shoe. Significant uncompensated supination and pronation deformities of the forefoot can usually be inferred from deformations in the shoe upper.

## CONCLUDING REMARKS

It is our hope that the techniques and principles presented here will make the biomechanical aspects of etiology and prevention of foot injury more understandable, hence more accessible to those involved in the treatment of diabetic foot problems. There is little doubt that much remains to be learned, but the acceptance of quantitative approaches to what is frequently seen as a subjective field will eventually benefit both patient and clinician.

### Acknowledgments

We are grateful to the many patients from whom we have learned. They have been our untiring companions through frequently long searches for solutions to complex problems. Arleen Norkitis, P.T., has set consistently high standards of clinical care, and Mary Becker, R.N., M.S., has facilitated our experimental efforts. Tzyy-Yuang Shiang provided leadership on the finite element modeling efforts, and discussions with Don Streit, Ph.D., and Gerrit Jan van Ingen Schenau, Ph.D., were helpful. The contributions of the graduate students and staff of the Center for Locomotion Studies at Pennsylvania State University also are gratefully acknowledged.

Research supported by the American Diabetes Association, the National Institutes of Health, the Orthopedic Research and Education Foundation, and the Veterans Administration.

## REFERENCES

1. Alexander IJ, Chao EYS, Johnson KA: The assessment of dynamic foot-to-ground contact forces and plantar pressure distribution: A review of the evolution of current techniques and clinical applications, *Foot Ankle* 11:152–167; 1990.

2. Allard P, Stokes IAF, Salathe EP, et al: Modeling

of the foot and ankle, in Jahss MH, editor: *Disorders of the foot and ankle: medical and surgical management*, ed 2, Philadelphia, 1991, WB Saunders, vol I.

3. American College of Physicians, American Diabetes Association, and American Academy of Opthalmology: Screening for diabetic retinopathy [position statement], *Diabetes Care* 15:16–18, 1992.

4. Andriacchi TP: Biomechanics and gait analysis in total knee replacement, *Orthop Rev* 17:470–473, 1988.

5. Asbury AK, Porte D Jr: Report and recommendations of the San Antonio Conference on Diabetic Neuropathy, *Diabetes Care* 11:592–597, 1988.

6. Bader DL: Effects of compressive loading regimens on tissue viability, in Bader DL, editor: *Pressure sores—clinical practice and scientific approach*, New York, 1990, MacMillan.

7. Bader DL: *Pressure sores—clinical practice and scientific approach*, New York, 1990, MacMillan.

8. Bauman JH, Brand PW: Measurement of pressure between foot and shoe, *Lancet* 1:629–632, 1963.

9. Betts RP, Franks CI, Duckworth T: Foot pressure studies: normal and pathologic gait analyses, in Jahss MH, editor: *Disorders of the foot and ankle: medical and surgical management*, ed 2, Philadelphia, 1991, WB Saunders, vol I, pp 484–519.

10. Birke JA, Cornwall MA, Jackson M: Relationship between hallux limitus and ulceration of the great toe, *J Orthop Sports Phys Ther* 10:172–176, 1988.

11. Birke JA, Sims DS: Plantar sensory threshold in the ulcerative foot, *Leprosy Rev* 57:261–267, 1986.

12. Blechschmidt E: Die Architektur des Fersenpolsters, *Morphol Jahrb*, 72:60–68, 1933. (Reprinted as The structure of the calcaneal padding, *Foot Ankle* 2:260–283, 1982.)

13. Bloom S, Till S, Sonksen P, et al: Use of biothesiometer to measure individual vibration thresholds and their variation in 519 non-diabetic subjects, *Br Med J* 288:1793–1795, 1984.

14. Bojsen-Moller F: Anatomy of the forefoot, normal and pathologic, *Clin Orthop* 142:10–18, 1979.

15. Boulton AJM, Betts RP, Franks CI, et al: Abnormalities of foot pressure in early diabetic neuropathy, *Diabetic Med* 4: 1987.

16. Boulton AJM, Betts RP, Franks CI, et al: The natural history of foot pressure abnormalities in neuropathic diabetic subjects, *Diabetes Res* 5:73–77, 1987.

17. Boulton AJM, Bowker JH, Gadia M, et al: Use of plaster casts in the management of diabetic neuropathic foot ulcers, *Diabetes Care* 9:149–153, 1986.

18. Boulton AJM, Hardisty CA, Betts RP, et al: Dynamic foot pressure and other studies as diagnostic and management aids in diabetic neuropathy, *Diabetes Care* 6:26–33, 1983.

19. Brand PW: Management of the insensitive limb, *Phys Ther* 59:8–12, 1979.

20. Brand PW: Repetitive stress in the development of diabetic foot ulcers, in Levin ME, O'Neal LW, editors: *The diabetic foot*, ed 4, St Louis, 1988, Mosby-Year Book.

21. Brand PW, Coleman WC: The diabetic foot, in Rifkin H, Porte D, editors: *Ellenberg and Rifkin's diabetes mellitus: theory and practice*, ed 4, New York, 1990, Elsevier.

22. Brand PW, Ebner JD: Pressure sensitive devices for denervated hands and feet, *J Bone Joint Surg* 51A:109–116, 1969.

23. Brodsky JW, Kourosh S, Stills M, et al: Objective evaluation of insert material for diabetic and athletic footwear, *Foot Ankle* 9:111–116, 1988.

24. Brown GL, Curtsinger LJ, White M, et al: Acceleration of tensile strength of incisions treated with ECG and TGF-β, *Ann Surg* 208:788–794, 1988.

25. Brownlee M, Cerami A, Vlassara H: Advanced glycosylation end products in tissue and the biochemical basis of diabetic complications, *N Engl J Med* 318:1315–1321, 1988.

26. Brownlee M, Vlassara H, Cerami A: Nonenzymatic glycosylation and the pathogenesis of diabetic complications, *Ann Intern Med* 101:527–537, 1984.

27. Burden AC, Jones GR, Jones R, et al: Use of the "Scotchcast boot" in treating diabetic foot ulcers, *Br Med J* 286:1555–1557, 1983.

28. Campbell GJ, McLure M, Newell EN: Compressive behavior after simulated service conditions of some foamed materials intended as orthotic shoe insoles, *J Rehab Res Dev* 21:57–65, 1984.

29. Cavanagh PR, Derr JA, Ulbrecht JS, et al: Problems with gait and posture in neuropathic patients with insulin dependent diabetes mellitus, *Diabetic Med* 9:482–485, 1992.

30. Cavanagh PR, Fernando DJS, Masson EA, et al: Limited joint mobility (LJM) and loss of vibration sensation are predictors of elevated plantar pressure in diabetes [abstract] *Diabetes* 40:531A, 1991.

31. Cavanagh PR, Hewitt FG Jr, Perry JE: In-shoe plantar pressure measurement: a review, *Foot* (in press).

32. Cavanagh PR, Rodgers MM: Pressure distribution underneath the human foot, in Perren SM, Schneider E, editors: *Biomechanics: current interdisciplinary research*, Dordrecht, The Netherlands, 1985, Martinus Nijhoff.

33. Cavanagh PR, Shiang T-Y: Approaches to finite element analysis of the foot-shoe interface in diabetic patients [abstract], NACOB II: The Second North American Congress on Biomechanics, Aug 24–28, 1992, Chicago.

34. Cavanagh PR, Simoneau GG, Ulbrecht JS: Ulceration, unsteadiness, and uncertainty: the biomechanical consequences of diabetes mellitus, *J Biomech*, (in press).

35. Cavanagh PR, Sims DS Jr, Sanders LJ: Body mass is a poor predictor of peak plantar pressure in diabetic men, *Diabetes Care* 14:750–755, 1991.

36. Cavanagh PR, Ulbrecht JS: Plantar pressure in the diabetic foot, in Sammarco GJ, editor: *The foot in diabetes*, Philadelphia, 1991, Lea & Febiger.

37. Cavanagh PR, Ulbrecht JS: Biomechanics of the diabetic foot: a quantitative approach to the assessment of neuropathy, deformity, and plantar pressure, in Jahss MH, editor: *Disorders of the foot and ankle, medical and surgical management*, ed 2, Philadelphia, 1991, WB Saunders.

38. Cavanagh PR, Ulbrecht JS: Clinical plantar pressure measurement in diabetes: rationale and methodology, *Foot* (in press).

39. Cavanagh PR, Young MJ, Adams JE, et al: Bony abnormalities in the feet of neuropathic diabetic patients [abstract], Abstracts of the First International Symposium on the Diabetic Foot, Amsterdam, May 3–4, 1991.

40. Cavanagh PR, Young MJ, Adams JE, et al: Correlates of structure and function in neuropathic diabetic feet [abstract], *Diabetologia* 34:A39, 1991.

41. Chantelau E, Kushner T, Spraul M: How effective is cushioned therapeutic footwear in protecting diabetic feet? a clinical study, *Diabetic Med* 7:355–359, 1990.

42. Coleman WC: The relief of forefoot pressures using outer shoe sole modifications, in Mothiramipatil K, Srinivasa H, editors: *Proceedings of the International Conference on Biomechanics and Clinical Kinesiology of Hand and Foot*, Madras, India, 1985, Indian Institute of Technology.

43. Ctercteko GC, Dhanendran M, Hutton WC, et al: Vertical forces acting on the feet of diabetic patients with neuropathic ulceration, *Br J Surg* 68:608–614, 1981.

44. Delbridge L, Ctercteko G, Fowler C, et al: The aetiology of diabetic neuropathic ulceration of the foot, *Br J Surg* 72:1–6, 1985.

45. Delbridge L, Ellis CS, Robertson K: Nonenzymatic glycosylation of keratin from the stratum corneum of the diabetic foot, *Br J Dermatol* 112:547–554, 1985.

46. DeLuca PA: Gait analysis in the treatment of the ambulatory child with cerebral palsy, *Clin Orthop* 264:65–75, 1991.

47. Edmonds ME: Experience in a multidisciplinary diabetic foot clinic, in Connor H, Boulton AJM, Ward JD, editors: *The foot in diabetes*, New York, 1987, John Wiley & Sons.

48. Fernando DJS, Masson EA, Veves A, et al: Relationship of limited joint mobility to abnormal foot pressures and foot ulceration, *Diabetes Care* 14:8–11, 1991.

49. Fromherz WA: Examination, in Hunt GC, editor: *Physical therapy of the foot and ankle*, vol 15: *Clinics in physical therapy*, New York, 1988, Churchill Livingstone.

50. Gooding GAW, Stess RM, Graf PM: Sonography of the sole of the foot: evidence for loss of foot pad thickness in diabetes and its relationship to ulceration of the foot, *Invest Radiol* 21:45–48, 1986.

51. Gooding GAW, Stess RM, Graf PM, et al: Heel pad thickness: determination by high-resolution ultrasonography, *J Ultrasound Med* 4:173–174, 1985.

52. Habershaw G, Donovan JC: Biomechanical considerations of the diabetic foot, in Kozak GP, Hoar CS, Rowbotham JL, et al, editors: *Management of diabetic foot problems*, Philadelphia, 1984, WB Saunders.

53. Hayes WC: Biomechanics of cortical and trabecular bone: implications for assessment of fracture risk, in Mow VC, Hayes WC, editors: *Basic orthopaedic biomechanics*, New York, 1991, Raven Press.

54. Holm-Pederson P, Viidik A: Tensile properties of and morphology of healing wounds in young and old rats, *Scand J Plast Reconstr Surg* 6:24–35, 1972.

55. Jahss MH, Michelson JD, Desai P, et al: Investigations into the fat pads of the sole of the foot: anatomy and histology, *Foot Ankle* 13:233–242, 1992.

56. Jenkin WM, Palladino SNJ: Environmental stress and tissue breakdown, in Frykberg RG, editor: *The high risk foot in diabetes mellitus*, New York, 1991, Churchill Livingstone.

57. Krag MH: Quantitative techniques for analysis of gait, *Automedica* 6:85–97, 1985.

58. Laing P, Cogley D, Crerand S, et al: The Liverpool shear transducer [abstract], Abstracts of the First International Symposium on the Diabetic Foot. Amsterdam, May 3–4, 1991.

59. McBride ID, Wyss UP, Cooke TDV, et al: First metatarsophalangeal joint reaction forces during high-heel gait, *Foot Ankle* 11:282–288, 1991.

60. Miller J: Custom-made shoe therapy for the diabetic foot, in Brenner MA, editor: *Management of the diabetic foot*, Baltimore, 1987, Williams & Wilkins.

61. Myerson M: The total-contact cast for management of neuropathic plantar ulceration of the foot, *J Bone Joint Surg (Am)* 74:261–269, 1992.

62. Myerson MS, Shereff MJ: The pathological anatomy of claw and hammer toes, *J Bone Joint Surg [Am]* 71:45–49, 1989.

63. Nawoczenski DA, Birke JA, Coleman WC: Effect of rocker sole design on plantar forefoot pressures, *J Am Podiatr Med Assoc* 78:455–460, 1988.

64. Pecoraro RE, Reiber GE, Burgess EM: Pathways to diabetic limb amputation: basis for prevention, *Diabetes Care* 13:513–521, 1990.

65. Pollard JP, LeQuesne LP, Tappin JW: Forces under the foot, *J Biomed Eng* 5:37–40, 1983.

66. Radin EL, Yang KH, Riegger C, et al: Relationship between lower limb dynamics and knee joint pain, *J Orthop Res* 9:398–405, 1991.

67. Rose GK: Pes planus, in Jahss MH, editor: *Disorders of the Foot Ankle, medical and surgical management*, ed 2, Philadelphia, 1991, WB Saunders, vol I.

68. Rosenbloom AL, Silverstein JH, Lezotte DC, et al: Limited joint mobility in childhood diabetes mellitus indicates increased risk for microvascular disease, *N Engl J Med* 305:191–194, 1981.

69. Rothstein JM, Miller PJ, Roettger RF: Goniometric reliability in a clinical setting: elbow and knee measurements, *Phys Ther* 63:1611, 1983.

70. Sage RA: Diabetic ulcers: evaluation and management, in Harkless LB, Dennis KH, editors: *Clinics in podiatric medicine and surgery: the diabetic foot*, Philadelphia, 1987, WB Saunders.

71. Sanders LJ, Frykberg RG: Diabetic neuropathic osteoarthropathy: the Charcot foot, in Frykberg RG, editor: *The high risk foot in diabetes mellitus*, New York, 1991, Churchill Livingstone.

72. Scales JT: Pathogenesis of pressure sores, in Bader DL, editor: Pressure sores—clinical practice and scientific approach, New York, 1990, MacMillan.

73. Schaff PS, Cavanagh PR: Shoes for the insensitive foot: the effect of a "rocker bottom" shoe modification on plantar pressure distribution, *Foot Ankle* 11:129–140, 1990.

74. Shiang TY, Cavanagh PR: Finite element analysis of the foot-shoe interface in diabetic patients [abstract], Biomedical Engineering in the 21st Century, 1992 International Symposium, Sept 23–26, 1992, Taipei.

75. Simoneau GG, Cavanagh PR, Becker MB: Design and preliminary testing of a device to quantify proprioceptive function during weightbearing [abstract], in Woollacott, M, Horak F, editors: *Posture and gait: control mechanisms*, Portland, 1992, University of Oregon Books, vol I.

76. Simoneau GG, Ulbrecht JS, Becker MB, et al: Instability during quiet standing among patients with diabetic neuropathy [abstract], *Diabetes* 41:141A, 1992.

77. Sims DS, Birke JA: Effect of rocker sole placement on plantar pressures [abstract], Proceedings of the 20th Annual Meeting of the USPHS Professional Association, Atlanta, 1985.

78. Sinacore DR, Mueller MJ, Diamond JE, et al: Diabetic plantar ulcers treated by total contact casting: a clinical report, *Phys Ther* 67:1543–1549, 1987.

79. Sosenko JM, Kato M, Soto R, et al: Comparison of quantitative sensory-threshold measures for their association with foot ulceration in diabetic patients, *Diabetes Care* 13:1057–1061, 1990.

80. Stehr M, Dietz HG, Morlock MM: Clinical application of pressure distribution measurements during full gait, Proceedings of the Second EMED Users Meeting, Nov 1–3, 1991, Vienna.

81. Stokes IAF, Faris IB, Hutton WC: The neuropathic ulcer and loads on the foot in diabetic patients, *Acta Orthop Scand* 46:839–847, 1975.

82. Tappin JW, Pollard JP, Beckett EA: Method of measuring "shearing" forces on the sole of the foot, *Clin Phys Physiol Meas* 1:83–85, 1980.

83. Thompson DE: The effects of mechanical stress on soft tissue, in Levin ME, O'Neal LW, editors: *The diabetic foot*, ed 4, St Louis, 1988, Mosby-Year Book.

84. Tooke JE: Microvascular haemodynamics in hypertension and diabetes, *J Cardiovasc Pharmacol* 18:S51–S53, 1991.

85. Veves A, Masson EA, Fernando DJS, et al: Sustained pressure relief under the diabetic foot with experimental hosiery, and comparison of different padding densities [abstract], *Diabetic Med* 6:3A, 1989.

86. Veves A, Masson EA, Fernando DJS, et al: Use of experimental padded hosiery to reduce abnormal foot pressures in diabetic neuropathy, *Diabetes Care* 12:653–655, 1989.

87. Wainwright SA, Biggs WD, Currey JD, et al: Principles of the strength of materials: phenomenological description, in Wainwright SA, Biggs WD, Currey JD, editors: *Mechanical design in organisms*, London, 1976, Edward Arnold.

88. *Webster's ninth new collegiate dictionary*, Springfield, Mass, 1986, Merriam-Webster.

89. Young MJ, Cavanagh PR, Thomas G, et al: The effect of callus removal on dynamic plantar foot pressures in diabetic patients, *Diabetic Med* 9:55–57, 1992.

## APPENDIX 9–A

### Glossary

A number of terms are defined below as they are used in the chapter. This is not intended to be a comprehensive list but more a guide to some of the less frequently used biomechanical terms.

**compressive stress** Stress that tends to cause the material to reduce the dimension along the direction in which the stress is applied. (See also tensile stress.)

**deformation** Change in configuration of a material under the action of a force.

**dynamic range** Range defined by the minimum and maximum values of a quantity that can be accurately measured by a particular instrument.

**force platform** Device that measures the total force acting under the foot during contact with the ground. (Compare with pressure platform.)

**frequency response** Ability of an instrument to measure quantities that change rapidly (e.g., impulsive force).

**hysteresis** Property of viscoelastic materials during material testing (and in real use) in which the value of stress at a given strain is different depending on whether the material is being loaded or unloaded. (See also viscoelastic.)

**linearity** A device is said to be linear within a certain range if there is a straight line relation between input and output (e.g., a given change in force results in the same change in voltage in different regions of the force range).

**N** Symbol for Newton, the International System (SI) unit of force; 1 lb = 4.46 N, 1 kg = 9.81 N.

**normal** At right angles to the surface. In the context of force or pressure this is often used to mean "vertical," because the surface is assumed to be horizontal.

**Pa (kPa, MPa)** Symbol for Pascal, the International System (SI) unit of pressure. Prefixes k for kiloPascal (Pascals/1,000) and M for megapascal (Pascals/1,000,000) invariably are used in biomechanics because the Pascal is a very small unit); 1 lb/sq inch = 6.9 kPa, 1 kg/cm$^2$ = 98.1 kPa.

**pressure** Force applied divided by area of application. (See also stress.)

**pressure platform** Device that can measure pressure at many sites under the foot (typically there are at least two sensors per square centimeter). (See also spatial resolution and force platform.)

**sampling rate** Number of times per second that an instrument makes a measurement. Force and pressure platforms typically have sampling rates between 50 and 500 samples per second.

**Scotch cast boot** Technique to immobilize the foot yet allow the subject to remove the device for sleeping. (See also total contact cast.)

**shear** Force or stress applied at right angles to the normal load (see normal), usually in the plane of the floor. This can be resolved into components, usually in the anteroposterior and mediolateral directions.

**spatial resolution** Size of the sensors in a pressure platform or in-shoe system that defines the minimum distance between adjacent measurement sites; typical values are 0.5 cm.

**strain** Deformation that a material undergoes as a result of applied stress, calculated as change in length divided by original length. It therefore has no units. Must not be used interchangably with stress.

**stress** Force applied divided by area of application. International System (SI) unit is the Pascal. Must not be used interchangably with strain.

**support phase** Time during which the foot is in contact with the ground during gait (as contrasted with swing or nonsupport phase).

**tensile stress** Stress that tends to cause the material to increase the dimension in the direction of the applied stress. (See also compressive stress.)

**total contact cast** Cast used to immobilize the foot yet allow ambulation during ulcer healing or Charcot fracture. (See also Scotch cast boot.)

**viscoelastic** Material properties that exhibit damping and time dependence (such as creep or hysteresis). Perfectly elastic materials are not viscoelastic but many materials used in footwear and insole manufacture are.

# CHAPTER 10

# Etiopathogenesis and Management of Abnormal Foot Pressures

**Andrew J.M. Boulton, M.D.**

**Aristidis Veves, M.D.**

**Matthew J. Young, M.D.**

Foot ulceration remains a serious problem in diabetic patients, and during the last 20 years considerable work has focused on the identification of the contributory risk factors and on developing intervention techniques that help to prevent, as well as treat, this condition.[4] Abnormally high foot pressure during walking is one factor that has been extensively studied, and there is now sufficient evidence to suggest that it plays an important role in the development of foot ulceration. The underlying mechanisms for the development of high plantar pressures in the diabetic neuropathic patient and their management forms are discussed in this chapter.

## ETIOPATHOGENESIS OF HIGH PLANTAR PRESSURES IN DIABETES

Diabetic neuropathy has been identified as one of the main etiopathogenic factors for the development of high foot pressures. A mixture of sensorimotor and autonomic nerve dysfunction in the foot and lower limb is probably responsible for disrupting the normal gait cycle and disturbing the foot-ground sequence (Fig 10–1).[12] Motor neuropathy leads to small muscle atrophy, and the consequent imbalance between flexors and extensors results in the "intrinsic minus" foot, which is characterized by clawing of the toes and prominent metatarsal heads (Fig 10–2).[22] This, together with the altered loading under the foot, is associated with subluxation of the fat pads which normally protect the metatarsal heads and metatarsophalangeal joints. As a result, high pressure usually develops under these prominent metatarsal heads during both walking and standing. Repetitive stresses, such as those during walking, in these areas of moderately elevated pressures lead to inflammatory autolysis of the skin and foot ulceration.[9]

Autonomic dysfunction results in dry, brittle skin and callus formation. Callus plaques are commonly found in areas of high plantar pressure, and the frequency of preulcerative and ulcerated lesions below them suggests that they may act as a foreign bodies. It has now been demonstrated that removing plantar callosities can significantly reduce the plantar pressure, and this would also tend to support this view.[35] Finally, sensory neuropathy permits the develop-

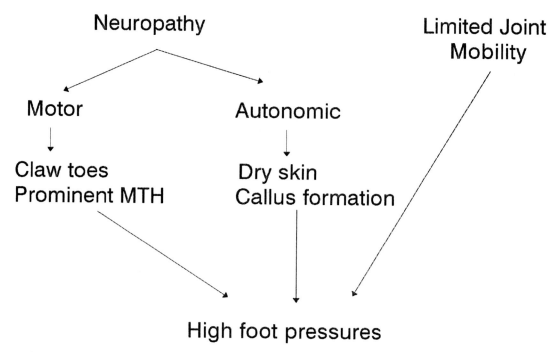

FIG 10–1.
Etiopathogenetic factors for high foot pressures.

ment of painless ulceration, often hidden under a callus, without the patient being aware of its existence.[3]

Limited joint mobility is the other major etiopathogenic factor of high foot pressures. It is usually attributed to thickening of the skin, which results in the loss of full extension of the fingers and other joints. Patients with this condition are usually unable to oppose their palmar surfaces and are said to exhibit the "prayer sign." Although its etiopathogenesis is not fully understood, the principle mechanism is believed to be nonenzymatic glycosylation of skin and joint capsule collagen.[21] An association between limited joint mobility and foot ulceration was

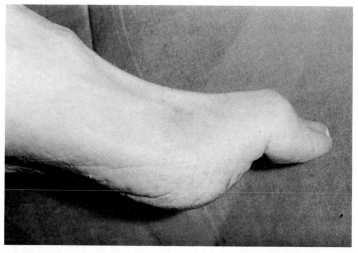

FIG 10–2.
Intrinsic minus foot with claw toes and prominent metatarsal heads.

originally shown and attributed to subtalar joint involvement by Delbridge et al.[17] Foot pressures were not measured in this study, but the authors suggested that limited mobility of the subtalar joint resulted in high pressures under the foot and subsequent foot ulceration. In a subsequent study, the direct relationship between limited joint mobility and abnormal foot pressures was examined in diabetic patients with and without neuropathy.[19] Strong correlations between plantar foot pressures and subtalar joint mobility were found, and a history of previous foot ulceration was present in 65% of patients with neuropathy and limited joint mobility, suggesting that limited joint mobility is a major factor in causing abnormally high foot pressures and contributes to the etiopathogenesis of foot ulceration in the susceptible neuropathic foot.

## Foot Structure

It has now been shown that foot structure, as defined by weight-bearing standing radiographs, plays a large part in determining the plantar pressure exerted by the foot during walking.[14] Metatarsal inclination and a reduction in the thickness of the metatarsal head soft tissue cushioning, measured directly from foot radiographs, are directly related to the plantar pressure as measured using a dynamic optical pedobarograph. These findings offer some explanation for

the mechanisms underlying high plantar pressures in the intrinsic minus foot outlined earlier.

## Other Factors

Weight does not seem to play an important role in foot pressure levels despite initial reports that suggested the opposite.[16, 27] Studies on both healthy subjects and diabetic patients have failed to show any significant contribution of weight to the measured pressures, suggesting that the foot can redistribute and therefore adapt to increased weight without significant change in the foot pressure.[13, 29] Age also does not have any significant importance in foot pressure measurements.

Previous amputation in diabetic patients is a risk factor for foot problems in the remaining limb, and such patients are at great risk for having a contralateral amputation.[2] Diabetic amputee patients, fully mobilized with the use of an artificial limb, were recently shown to have higher foot pressures when they were compared with a matched group of nondiabetic amputees and healthy controls.[34] In contrast, when they were compared with a group of diabetic patients without amputation but with similar degree of neuropathic involvement, no difference was found in the mean peak pressure or the number of feet with abnormally high pressures. Similarly, no difference existed be-

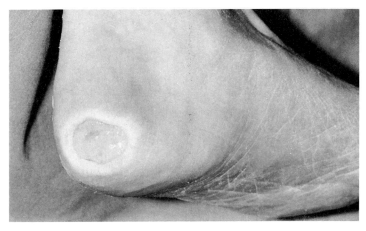

**FIG 10–3.**
Heel ulcer caused by prolonged bed rest.

tween nondiabetic amputees and healthy subjects. This study suggests that amputation and prosthetic usage themselves are not risk factors for the development of high pressures under the remaining foot, but in diabetic patients it is the coexisting neuropathy that accounts for this.

### Extrinsic Pressure

Although primarily concerned with plantar foot pressure, a significant number of pressure ulcers form because of extrinsic pressure. The purely neuropathic foot is generally well perfused, but nutritive skin flow may be reduced. In addition to this, vascular disease frequently coexists. Thus relatively low sustained pressure can cause skin necrosis and autolysis leading to ulceration. This is commonly manifested in the dorsal ulcers on clawed toes and the lateral fifth toe ulceration because of tight shoes. This mechanism is at its most devastating when unprotected heels are left pressing down on a surface, causing craterous ulcers that improve only slowly, if at all (Fig 10–3). This is sadly still a problem for patients confined to bed or during operations if adequate heel protection is not employed.

## PREVALENCE OF HIGH FOOT PRESSURES IN DIABETES

The prevalence of high foot pressure in diabetic patients and healthy subjects was studied for the first time using an optical pedobarograph by Boulton et al.[8] They reported that 31% of the feet of neuropathic patients without ulceration had abnormally high peak pressures compared with 17% of nonneuropathic feet and 7% of healthy subjects. In a subsequent study by the same group, foot pressure studies were performed in diabetic patients without clinical neuropathy, and they were found to be abnormal in 36%.[5] Veves et al.[29] screened a large number of diabetic patients with and without clinical neuropathy who attended a hospital based diabetic clinic and compared them with age-matched healthy subjects using the

same technique as the previous studies. They reported that high foot pressures were found under 30% of all diabetic feet or 39% of neuropathic feet and 15% of nonneuropathic feet, whereas in healthy subjects the prevalence of high pressures (14%) was similar to that of nonneuropathic patients.

It seems therefore reasonable to conclude from these studies that abnormally high foot pressures are common in diabetic patients, especially those with diabetic neuropathy, in whom more than one third of feet may be abnormal. This last fact also indicates that neuropathy is the major etiopathogenic factor in the development of high foot pressures.

An association between diabetic nephropathy and an increase in foot pressure was reported by Fernando et al.[20] Foot pressures and peripheral nerve function measurements were performed in diabetic patients with microalbuminuria, with albuminuria (creatinine clearance > 40 mL/minute), chronic renal failure (clearance < 40 mL/minute), in diabetic patients without nephropathy, and in healthy subjects. The mean peak pressure in all three nephropathic groups was higher compared with controls, whereas those with albuminuria and chronic renal failure had higher pressure than patients with microalbuminuria. The peripheral nerve function was also reduced in the three nephropathic groups, whereas a history of previous plantar ulceration increased from 5% in the diabetic control group to 10% in the microalbuminuria and albuminuria groups and to 40% in the renal failure group.

## DISTRIBUTION OF PEAK PRESSURES UNDER THE FOOT

A lateral shift of maximum loads under the foot was reported in one of the first studies to measure foot pressures quantitatively in diabetic patients and healthy subjects.[27] In contrast, in a subsequent study, a medial shift of maximum loads was found by a different group of investigators.[16] The most recent study of the peak pressure distribution under the feet of neuropathic diabetic pa-

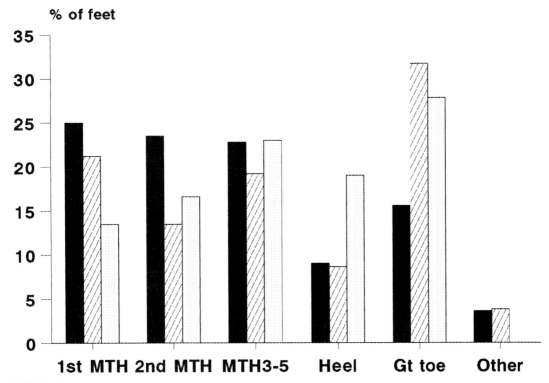

**FIG 10–4.**
Distribution of peak pressure under various areas of the foot in diabetic neuropathic patients *(black area),* diabetic nonneuropathic patients *(hatched area),* and healthy subjects *(stippled area).* No significant difference under the third, fourth, and fifth metatarsal head (MTH) were found, but in neuropathic subjects peak pressure was more often seen under the first MTH and less often under the great toe, suggesting a transfer of pressure from toe to the metatarsal heads. In nonneuropathic patients, peak pressures under the heel were less frequently observed when compared with healthy subjects, indicating that pressure transfer to the forefoot may occur at the early stages of subclinical neuropathy. *(Data from Veves A, Fernando DJS, Walewski P, et al:* Foot *1:89–92, 1991.)*

tients, nonneuropathic diabetic patients, and healthy subjects showed that there was no difference in the distribution of peak pressures under the lateral foot (third, fourth, and fifth metatarsal heads) in any of the groups, but neuropathic patients had a higher frequency under the first metatarsal head and a lower frequency under the great toe (Fig 10–4).[29] Peak pressures under the heel were found more frequently in healthy subjects compared with both nonneuropathic and neuropathic patients. These results suggest that early changes under the diabetic foot, even before the development of clinical neuropathy, include a rise of pressure under the forefoot and a subsequent transfer of peak pressures from the heel to the metatarsal heads. With the development of neuropathy there is a further transfer of

load from the toes, obviously related to clawing, to the metatarsal heads, but no transfer from one side of the foot to the other seems to take place.

## NATURAL HISTORY OF FOOT PRESSURES

The natural history of foot pressures in diabetic patients remains obscure, and very few longitudinal studies have been conducted to investigate their development and progress. A cross-sectional study of diabetic patients without clinical evidence of neuropathy has shown that patients with high pressures had significantly abnormal nerve function assessed by vibration perception threshold and sural sensory nerve conduction velocity when compared with an age-matched group of patients with normal foot pressures.[5] This strongly suggests that abnormalities of foot pressure occur in early sensory neuropathy and may even precede clinical abnormalities, but other coexisting factors that could have been responsible for the high pressures, such as limited joint mobility, were not examined.

In the first longitudinal study of foot pressures in neuropathic diabetic patients, foot pressures were repeated after a mean period of 3 years.[6] The results showed that there was no difference in the number of feet with abnormally high foot pressures at baseline and follow-up measurements, but important changes occurred in the distribution of pressure under the metatarsal heads and the level of the abnormal pressure under the same site.

These findings have been confirmed in a prospective study that examined the changes in the foot pressure in diabetic patients with clinical neuropathy, nonneuropathic patients, and healthy subjects.[33] All patients had their pressures measured at the beginning and the end of the study after a mean follow-up period of 30 months. Mean peak pressure was higher at the follow-up visit when compared with baseline measurements in both neuropathic and nonneuropathic groups but was stable in the control subjects. Despite this, similar numbers of patients had high foot pressures at follow-up and baseline in both neuropathic and nonneuropathic groups. The area under which the peak pressure was found was different in 59% of the feet, suggesting that it changes over a short period.

## RELATIONSHIP BETWEEN HIGH FOOT PRESSURES AND FOOT ULCERATION

The relationship between high foot pressures and foot ulceration has been studied more extensively than the natural history in recent years. The first study was published by Barrett and Mooney[1] in 1973 and used the Harris mat and the Brand slipper sock. They reported that in neuropathic diabetic patients, foot ulcers often occurred at sites

of high loading, and they speculated that points of high pressure should be considered as at risk of ulceration. When the slipper sock was used, high pressures were found under the metatarsal heads, and in some cases, they were higher than walking barefoot. In a subsequent study by Stokes et al.[27] quantitative methods were used to measure the load distribution under the foot of diabetic patients and healthy subjects. They found that ulcers occurred at sites of maximum load and that the toe loading in patients with ulcers was reduced. Similar results were found in a subsequent study,[16] namely that foot ulcers occurred at the sites of maximum load and that patients with ulceration were heavier compared with those without ulceration and normal subjects. It must be noted that the last two studies did not match groups for either age or weight and that the spatial resolution of the systems used to measure foot pressures was relatively low, which could affect their reliability in measuring foot pressures under specific areas of the foot, such as the areas with previous ulceration. Using the optical pedobarograph with a satisfactory reliability and high resolution, Boulton et al.[8] studied matched groups of patients with and without neuropathy and nondiabetic controls. They showed that a significantly higher number of patients with diabetic neuropathy had abnormally high foot pressures and that patients with previous ulceration had high pressures at the ulcer sites.

All of these studies were cross-sectional, and although they are suggestive, they do not have the power of a prospective study to support any final conclusions about the role of high foot pressures in the etiopathogenesis of foot ulceration. The first prospective study of diabetic patients with high foot pressures has recently been reported. In this study, diabetic patients with and without clinical neuropathy were followed prospectively for a mean period of 30 months.[33] Foot pressures were measured at the beginning and the end of the study, and all of the ulcers that occurred during the study were recorded. Plantar ulcers developed in 17% of all diabetic patients, and abnormally high foot pressures were present at baseline in all

(100%) of these patients, whereas neuropathy was present in 93% of patients at baseline and in all (100%) of patients who had developed a plantar ulcer at the end of the study. Looking from a different angle, 35% of all patients with high pressures and 45% of neuropathic patients with high pressures at baseline developed an ulcer during the study. Therefore, foot pressure measurement was found in this study to have a sensitivity of 100%, a specificity of 61%, and a predictive value for foot ulceration over 30 months of 35% for all diabetic patients and 45% for neuropathic diabetic patients. The exact area of foot ulceration could not be predicted, however, because only one half of the ulcers developed under areas with high pressures at baseline (Fig 10–5). These findings confirm the etiopathogenic role of high foot pressures in foot ulceration and suggest

that foot pressure measurement is a reliable screening test to identify patients at risk of ulceration.

However, isolated high foot pressures, in the absence of established clinical neuropathy, although important contributary etiopathogenic factors for foot ulceration, do not lead directly to foot ulcer formation, because intact pain perception will protect the otherwise high-risk foot. This is best seen in patients with rheumatoid arthritis who, because of tissue disruption and foot deformity, may also have high foot pressures. Despite the frequent existence of a mild neuropathy of vasculitic origin, pain perception in such patients is usually not seriously affected, and foot ulceration is rare.[24] In a direct comparison of a group of patients with rheumatoid arthritis and a group of diabetic patients with similar foot abnormali-

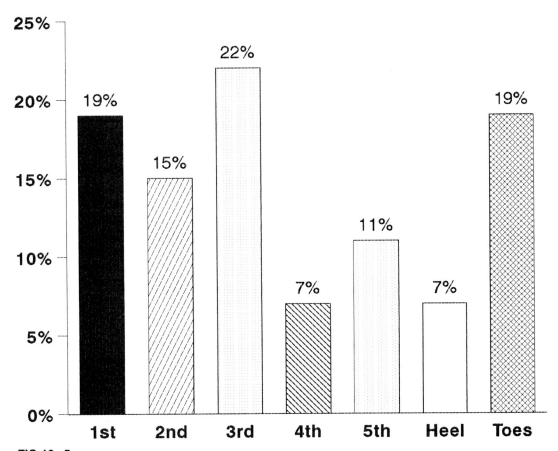

**FIG 10–5.**
Distribution of foot ulcers under various areas of the foot of diabetic patients who were prospectively followed up for a mean of 30 months. The most frequent area was under the third metatarsal head, followed closely by the first metatarsal head. *(Data from Veves A, Murray HJ, Young MJ, et al:* Diabetologia *34(suppl 2:A40); 1991.)*

ties on clinical examination, Masson et al.[23] reported that almost one third of diabetic patients but none of the rheumatoid patients had a history foot ulceration. The mean peak pressure and the frequency of abnormal high pressure were similar in both groups, and peripheral nerve function measurements were significantly reduced in the diabetic patients, whereas none of the rheumatoid patients had clinically severe neuropathy. These studies therefore suggest that both neuropathy and high foot pressures must be present for the development of foot ulceration and that if one of these factors is absent or can be normalized, the risk of foot ulceration may be reduced.

## MANAGEMENT OF HIGH FOOT PRESSURES IN DIABETES

It is clear that in addition to patient education, any treatment or device capable of producing a reduction in high plantar pressures should be tried in an effort to reduce plantar ulceration, because at present there is no effective treatment that can influence established diabetic neuropathy. Avoidance of applying any kind of pressure on the foot would virtually guarantee that no foot ulcer would occur, but of course such drastic treatment is not feasible and hardly can be recommended to any patient. Bed rest is thought to be of paramount importance when patients with neuropathic ulceration are treated, but its impracticalities have led to the development of nonweight-bearing total contact casts[15] or pressure-reducing fiberglass cast boots[11] to produce freedom from plantar pressure while maintaining mobility. Diabetic patients with high foot pressures, especially in the presence of neuropathy, should be considered at risk of ulceration and should be especially targeted for education and proper footwear in an effort to prevent rather than treat foot ulcers. This is best accomplished in the setting of a diabetic foot clinic that includes a foot educator nurse, pedorthist or orthotist, podiatrists, diabetologists, and vascular and orthopedic surgeons.[18, 28] The rationale and the methods of identifying at-risk patients using pedobarographic systems are described elsewhere in this book. The purchase and routine use of such devices are, however, still difficult to recommend in routine clinical practice. Pedobarographic systems are expensive and time consuming to use, and apart from research uses, the information they provide is also largely superfluous. For most purposes at-risk high-pressure areas can be identified by routine clinical examination of the foot shape, callosities, shoe wear pattern, and previous ulcer sites. This can then be supplemented with a Harris mat either on the ground or by cutting to shape even in-shoe to obtain a semiquantitative assessment of high-pressure areas to facilitate the use of appropriate pressure-reduction systems. These include socks, insoles, and shoes, and each of them has an important role to play in reducing and redistributing the abnormally high pressures.

### Stockings

The majority of people wear some kind of stockings in their daily life, and therefore stockings with pressure-relieving properties have the potential of being easily accepted as an intervention technique. In a recent study a specially designed sock (Thor-Lo, Statesville, N.C.) with extra-thick padding under the heel and the forefoot was compared with ordinary socks and barefoot walking in a group of diabetic patients with abnormal dynamic pressures.[31] A significant reduction of 26% of the mean peak pressure was achieved by the specially designed socks where no difference existed between the patients own socks and barefoot walking (Fig 10–6).

These special socks could also be protective for the dorsum of the clawed toes because they covered them with extra-thick padding. In a subsequent longitudinal study,[32] a group of neuropathic diabetic patients was followed for 6 months of regular use of these socks. At the end of the study, the socks continued to provide significant pressure relief, although not as high as at baseline; nevertheless, it can be claimed that each pair can be used continuously for at least 2 months without losing their beneficial

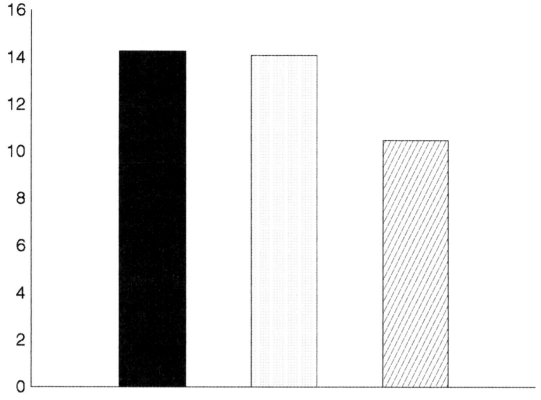

**FIG 10-6.**
Foot pressure measurements in diabetic neuropathic patients walking barefoot *(black area),* wearing their own socks *(hatched area),* and wearing a specially designed sock with extra-thick padding (Thor-Lo, Statesville, N.C.). Significant pressure relief is provided by the experimental sock, but no difference is seen between patients walking barefoot or wearing their own socks.

effects. A problem with these socks is that they are more bulky than ordinary socks, and therefore larger shoes are usually needed to avoid the risk of dorsal or lateral foot ulceration. This problem is ideally solved if patients have their feet measured when they are wearing the socks before they buy shoes.

Patient satisfaction with these socks was very high, and all patients who took part in the longitudinal study elected to continue to wear them after the study had finished. The degree of comfort provided by these socks is very difficult to test in diabetic neuropathic patients in whom pain perception is reduced or absent. In contrast, patients with rheumatoid arthritis also have high foot pressures but with normal pain perception and are therefore an ideal model for assessing whether increased comfort is provided by these socks. In a group of such "surrogate" patients, it was found that along with the

foot pressure reduction, the hosiery also provided significant pain relief of 51%, suggesting that it may be useful in reducing foot discomfort in all syndromes of painful feet either in diabetic patients in whom the pain perception is not severely affected or in nondiabetic patients.[30]

## Insole Materials

The insole has provided the mainstay of in-shoe pressure relief for diabetic patients over the past century.[10] The new synthetic materials, such as closed-cell polyethylene foam (Plastazote) and open-cell urethane polymer (PPT, Poron), have different mechanical properties and allow the production of custom sculpted insoles to relieve pressure in individual patients or as sheets of material to provide a generic insole for most patients. The pressure-relieving properties of these materials have been demonstrated in a number of studies either with the insole between the foot and the pedobarograph[7] or in-shoe below the pressure-measuring device.[26]

Insole materials come in various thicknesses. They should always be used in in-depth shoes so that the thickest possible insole that can be accommodated within the shoe can be provided, because with plantar pressures greater than 10 kg/cm$^2$, thin insoles will tend to bottom out and lose their pressure-relieving capability. For this reason, when a custom insole is designed for a diabetic patient, often to a cast of the patient's foot, it may be better to build up the insole in the arch area rather than cut away the insole in areas of prominence on the plantar surface to provide the maximum cushioning for the whole of the foot. This does not preclude the common practice of providing wells of softer materials below prominent areas in an insole of more resilient material, but we would suggest that these wells be sufficiently deep to fulfill their intended role.

### Shoes

The design of shoes for diabetic patients has changed radically over the years from simple moccasin-like shoes to complex arrays of shoes with rigid soles, rocker bottoms, and flared heels (see Chapters 24 and 25). In general, a shoe for a neuropathic diabetic patient should be measured individually for each foot, made of soft leather to accommodate any minor prominences without exerting undue pressure, and designed to allow any further pressure-relieving systems to be employed. If possible, they should be cosmetically acceptable to the patient, because expensive shoes, no matter how well designed and comfortable, will remain unworn if patients feel that they cannot wear them because they are "ugly."

The neuropathic diabetic patient with a normal foot outline, although usually with the changes of the intrinsic minus foot as described earlier, should be provided with two pairs of in-depth shoes. These shoes provide adequate toe space to accommodate marked clawing and other abnormalities, such as minor hallux valgus. This then lessens the risk of extrinsic pressure on the foot from shoes, which is the commonest cause of dorsal and lateral toe ulceration that we see. They also allow room for the provision of insoles and the wearing of padded socks to further reduce the plantar pressure. These shoes are less expensive than custom-made footwear while providing excellent protection for most patients. The provision of two pairs allows for a longer shoe life and means that the patient is never without proper footwear should any repairs be needed. It also allows for the patient to change the shoes regularly to avoid constant pressure within a given shoe. Although few patients are able to follow Brand's advice and change their shoes in the middle of the day, alternating the shoes is certainly to be advised.[10]

The design and manufacture of custom footwear is a specialized task and requires close cooperation between the diabetologist,

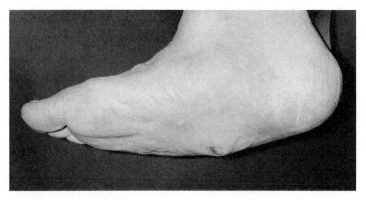

**FIG 10–7.**
Rocker bottom foot caused by Charcot neuroarthropathy.

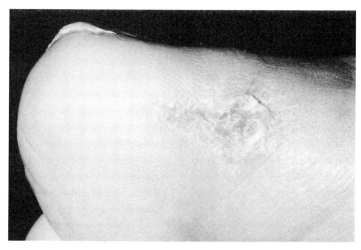

**FIG 10–8.**
Ridge of callus caused by hallux rigidus. This toe has recently ulcerated at the site of this callus after a missed appointment for debridement.

podiatrist, the pedorthist or orthotist, and the cobbler. These shoes are particularly expensive and tend to be reserved for patients with abnormal foot shapes, such as patients with Charcot neuroarthropathy or amputations of the toes or metatarsals. The same basic principles apply to these shoes but are often complicated by the need to accommodate these deformities. For example, a patient with Charcot neuroarthropathy with a "rocker bottom" foot (Fig 10–7) requires a shoe with considerable depth, with room for a thick insole to cradle the foot to relieve the exceptionally high pressures that can occur under the midfoot and a shoe rise on the sole on the other side so that the sole is level for walking.

Hallux rigidus is a common problem in the diabetic foot; a ridge of hard callus forms on the inferomedial border of the toe, and ulceration is a frequent complication (Fig 10–8). Rocker and roller bottom shoes are designed to take the excess load from the toes during the toe-off phase of walking. The sole of a rocker or roller bottom shoe is rigid, often with a steel plate inserted in it, and the angulation or curve, respectively, that is incorporated into the sole allows for heel lift to occur, simulating the normal gait pattern. They are believed to reduce shear stress, and pedobarographic studies of rocker bottom shoes have shown that when individually and correctly made, they can effectively reduce plantar pressures at the hallux. However, if the rocker is in the wrong place, either too far anterior or posterior on the sole of the shoe, it can actually increase hallux or midfoot loading. Careful initial follow-up of patients supplied with these shoes is recommended to ensure that the rocker is performing correctly.

## Callus Removal

The underlying causes of callus development on the diabetic foot are poorly understood, but we now know that callosities act as foreign bodies on the plantar surface of the diabetic foot. Debridement of these lesions has been shown to be an effective way of reducing plantar pressures.[35] A small study that has followed patients after callus debridement has also shown that the pressures increase steadily as the callus returns, and therefore debridement should be performed at regular intervals to maintain them at a lower level.

## Casts

Although used primarily for healing plantar ulcers, there is a role for casts, particularly the lightweight, removable, fiberglass-type boot, in helping to maintain the integrity of a patient's foot long after the ulcer has healed. Some patients' feet, despite the best efforts of pedorthist or orthotist, podiatrist, and diabetologist, will continue to breakdown and reulcerate when they are wearing shoes all of the time. These patients will often have very high pressures in certain areas of the foot, perhaps related to an amputation or foot deformity. In these patients, wearing a fiberglass-type boot in the home and shoes for work or social occasions can keep their feet free from ulcers and thus allow them to remain active in their lives and the community.

Fiberglass-type boots can be used for heel protection in bed-resting patients, but conventional heel troughs and padded booties are probably more cost effective and practical in the majority of cases.

## Surgical Reduction of High Pressures

Surgery is never to be contemplated lightly in diabetic patients, particularly because those with neuropathy and high foot pressures may have other associated diabetic complications, such as nephropathy. However, in the absence of significant vascular disease, considerable pressure relief can be obtained from selective orthopedic surgery. Selective surgery is the key, however; for example, the straightening of a hallux valgus can produce considerable benefits by

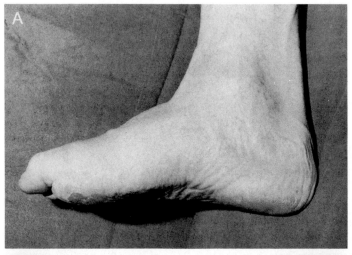

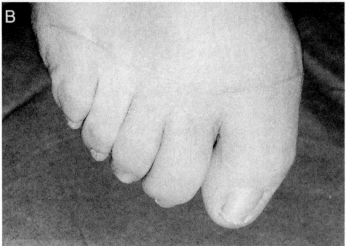

**FIG 10–9.**
**A,** intrinsic minus foot corrected by Fowler operation. **B,** dorsal scar from Fowler operation.

reducing ulceration over the bunion, but if it is inappropriately performed, by producing a rigid great toe, may lead to high pressures below the hallux, callus formation and recurrent ulceration at this site instead.

Numerous operations are described for the diabetic foot.[25] The two main operations used to reduce plantar pressures with repeated success are Fowler's operation (excision of the metatarsal heads and part of the metatarsal shafts, producing a new flatter metatarsal contact area for the forefoot; (Fig 10–9) and lumpectomy for patients with Charcot neuroarthropathy with a rocker bottom foot (see Fig 10–7). Both of these operations are effective at reducing foot pressure and should be considered in suitable patients.

## CASE HISTORIES

Mr W is 48 years old with type II diabetes diagnosed 11 years ago. He has had peripheral neuropathy for 5 years and frequently suffered plantar ulceration. His foot peak metatarsal pressure is 14.4 kg/cm$^2$. With padded socks this is reduced to 11.8 kg/cm$^2$, and a 9-mm sheet of Plastazote laid on the pedobarograph produces a further reduction to 10.2 kg/cm$^2$ in measured pressure. Since referral to our clinic and wearing padded socks in extra-depth shoes with flat-sheet insoles, he has been ulcer free for 3 years (see Fig 10–6).

Mr H is 63 years old. He had bilateral intrinsic minus feet and recurrent ulcers at the site of the first metatarsal on the left. A Fowler operation was carried out on the left foot, which remained ulcer free. When the right foot ulcerated, it too was referred for surgery. Before surgery the peak metatarsal pressure was 15.3 kg/cm$^2$. After surgery the pressure is 10.5 kg/cm$^2$, and the foot is ulcer free after nearly 1 year. (See Fig 10–9.)

## CONCLUSION

The development of foot ulceration in diabetic patients is intimately associated with the development of high plantar pressures. By careful assessment and the appropriate application of the available pressure-reduc-

ing systems and treatments, it may be possible to reduce the incidence of foot ulcers and hopefully achieve a significant reduction in amputations resulting from diabetes.

## REFERENCES

1. Barrett JP, Mooney V: Neuropathy and diabetic pressure lesions, *Orthop Clin North Am* 4:43–47, 1973.

2. Bild D, Selby J, Sinnock P, et al: Lower-extremity amputation in people with diabetes: epidemiology and prevention, *Diabetes Care* 12:24–31, 1989.

3. Boulton AJM: The diabetic foot, *Med Clin North Am* 72:1513–1530, 1988.

4. Boulton AJM: The diabetic foot: neuropathic in aetiology? *Diabetic Med* 7:852–858, 1990.

5. Boulton AJM, Betts RP, Franks CI, et al: Abnormalities of foot pressure in early diabetic neuropathy, *Diabetic Med* 4:225–228, 1987.

6. Boulton AJM, Betts RP, Franks CI, et al: The natural history of foot pressure abnormalities in neuropathic diabetic subjects, *Diabetes Res* 5:73–77, 1987.

7. Boulton AJM, Franks CI, Betts RP, et al: Reduction of abnormal foot pressures in diabetic neuropathy using a new polymer insole material, *Diabetes Care* 1:113–124, 1984.

8. Boulton AJM, Hardisty CA, Betts RP, et al: Dynamic foot pressure and other studies as diagnostic and management aids in diabetic neuropathy, *Diabetes Care* 6:26–33, 1983.

9. Brand PW: *Insensitive feet: a practical handbook on foot problems in leprosy*, London, Leprosy Mission, 1977.

10. Brand PW: The diabetic foot, in Ellenberg M, Rifkin H, editors: *Diabetes mellitus, theory and practice*, ed 3, New York, Medical Exam Publishing Co, 1983, pp 829–849.

11. Burden AC, Jones GR, Jones R, et al: Use of the 'Scotch-cast' boot in treating diabetic foot ulcers, *Br Med J* 286:1555–1557, 1983.

12. Cavanagh PR, Derr JA, Ulbrecht JS et al: Problems with gait and posture in insulin dependent diabetes, *Diabetic Med* 7(suppl 2):29A, 1990.

13. Cavanagh PR, Sims DS Jr, Sanders LJ: Body mass is a poor predictor of peak plantar pressure in diabetic men, *Diabetes Care* 14:750–755, 1991.

14. Cavanagh PR, Young MJ, Adams JE, et al: Correlates of structure and function in neuropathic diabetic feet, *Diabetologia* 34(suppl 2);A39, 1991.

15. Coleman WC, Brand PW, Birke JA: The total contact cast: a therapy for plantar ulceration on insensitive feet, *J Am Podiatr Med Assoc* 11:548–550, 1987.

16. Ctercteko GC, Dhanendram M, Hutton WC, et al: Vertical forces acting on the feet of diabetic patients with neuropathic ulceration, *Br J Surg* 68:608–614, 1981.

17. Delbridge L, Perry P, Marr S, et al: Limited joint mobility in the diabetic foot: relationship to neuropathic ulceration, *Diabetic Med* 5:333–337, 1988.

18. Edmonds ME, Blundell MP, Morris ME, et al: Improved survival of the diabetic foot: the role of a specialised foot clinic, *Q J Med* 60:763–771, 1986.

19. Fernando DJS, Hutchison A, Veves A, et al: Relationship of limited joint mobility to abnormal foot pressures and diabetic foot ulceration, *Diabetes Care* 14:8–11, 1991.

20. Fernando DJS, Masson EA, Veves A, et al: Risk factors for non-ischaemic foot ulceration in diabetic nephropathy, *Diabetic Med* 8:223–225, 1991

21. Goodfield MJD, Millard LG: The skin in diabetes mellitus, *Diabetologia* 31:567–575, 1988.

22. Lippmann HI, McLellan GE, Klenerman L: The neuropathic foot of the diabetic, *Bull NY Acad Med* 52:1159–1178, 1976.

23. Masson EA, Hay EM, Stockley I, et al: Abnormal foot pressures alone may not cause ulceration, *Diabetic Med* 6:426–428, 1989.

24. Nakano KK: Neurologic complications of rheumatoid arthritis, *Orthop Clin North Am* 6:861–880, 1975.

25. Nicklas BJ: Prophylactic surgery in the diabetic foot, in Fryckberg RG, editor: *The high risk foot in diabetes*, New York, 1991, Churchill Livingstone.

26. Smith L, Plehwe W, McGill M, et al: Foot bearing pressures in patients with unilateral diabetic foot ulcers, *Diabetic Med* 6:573–575, 1989.

27. Stokes IAF, Furis IB, Hutton WC: The neuropathic ulcer and loads on the foot in diabetic patients, *Acta Orthop Scand* 46:839–847, 1975.

28. Thomson FJ, Veves A, Ashe H, et al: A team approach to diabetic foot care—the Manchester experience, *Foot* 1:75–82, 1991.

29. Veves A, Fernando DJS, Walewski P, et al: A study of plantar pressures in a diabetic clinic population, *Foot* 1:89–92, 1991.

30. Veves A, Hay EM, Boulton AJM: The use of specially padded hosiery in the painful rheumatoid foot, *Foot* 1:175–177, 1992.

31. Veves A, Masson EA, Fernando DJS, et al: The use of experimental padded hosiery to reduce abnormal foot pressures in diabetic neuropathy, *Diabetes Care* 12:653–655, 1989.

32. Veves A, Masson EA, Fernando DJS, et al: Studies of experimental hosiery in diabetic patients with high foot pressures, *Diabetic Med* 7:324–326, 1990.

33. Veves A, Murray HJ, Young MJ, et al: The risk of foot ulceration in diabetic patients with high foot pressure: a prospective study, *Diabetologia* 35:660–663, 1992.

34. Veves A, Van Ross ERE, Boulton AJM: Foot pressure measurements in diabetic and non-diabetic amputees, *Diabetes Care* 15:905–907, 1992.

35. Young MJ, Cavanagh PR, Thomas G, et al: The effect of callus removal on dynamic plantar foot pressures in diabetic patients, *Diabetic Med* 9:55–57, 1992.

# CHAPTER 11

# Growth Factors and Repair of Diabetic Wounds

**David R. Knighton, M.D.**
**Vance D. Fiegel, B.S.**

Normal wound repair results from a complex interplay between the various cell types found in the wound space and their capacity to both produce and respond to an array of growth factors. These growth factors modulate cellular migration, proliferation, extracellular matrix production, enzyme activity, and the production of additional growth factors. Thus, the repair process is believed to be regulated largely by locally acting growth factors.

This chapter reviews the process of wound repair, with emphasis on the roles of the locally acting growth factors. In addition, the use of growth factors in diabetic wound repair is discussed and the current clinical data are reviewed.

## MORPHOLOGY OF NORMAL WOUND REPAIR

Cutaneous wounds can be divided into three major categories: (1) partial thickness, (2) full thickness, and (3) complex wounds (Fig 11–1).[1] A partial thickness wound describes a defect that removes the most superficial part of the skin, the epidermis, leaving the lower layers largely intact. A simple abrasion is a partial-thickness wound, as is the donor site from a split-thickness skin graft. To repair this injury,

part of the dermis, epidermis, and keratin layers need to be replaced. This is accomplished by migration of keratinocytes from the edge of the wound and from the hair follicles and sweat glands.[2] Keratinocytes first migrate across the wound, divide to form the epidermis, and finally stratify and produce keratin to form new skin.

In full-thickness wounds, both epidermis and dermis are lost, uncovering the subcutaneous tissue, fascia, or muscle. To repair this type of wound, vascularized connective tissue grows from the wound edge in a characteristic sequence (Fig 11–2).[3, 4] Fibroblasts begin to migrate into the wound space from connective tissue at the wound edge within 24 hours. As they move, fibroblasts produce matrix molecules (collagen and glycosaminoglycans) that form an extracellular matrix. Capillary buds are seen in the perfused microcirculation at the wound edge by 48 hours after wounding. These buds grow into the wound space and provide a new capillary network for the wound connective tissue. Fibroblast proliferation and migration and capillary growth continue as a unit until the wound space is completely filled with new tissue. The newly formed granulation tissue is then covered with epithelium. Keratinocytes from the cut edge of the skin migrate and divide to form a new epithelial covering. The leading edge of the epithelium

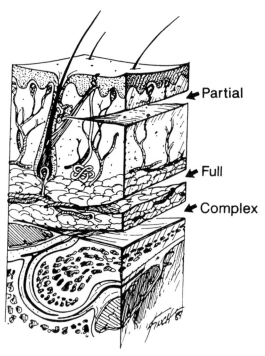

**FIG 11–1.**
Cross-sectional diagram of the dermis and underlying connective tissue indicating the depth at which partial, full, and complex wounds occur. *(From Knighton DR, Fiegel VD, Doucette MM: Chronic wound care: a clinical source book for healthcare professionals, 1990, Health Management Publications, pp 431–445. Used by permission.)*

is one cell layer thick. As the process progresses, the single layer of epithelium thickens through proliferation, and eventually, keratinocytes mature and produce keratin, forming a protective layer over the epithelium.[2] This neoepithelium consists of epidermis only. Dermal appendages such as sweat glands and hair follicles do not regenerate after full-thickness wounds. Full-thickness wounds also close by contraction, which occurs through cellular forces pulling the edges of the wound toward its center. Contraction accounts for large portions of wound closure in areas of loose skin (abdomen, nape of neck, loose skinned animals).

A "complex" wound penetrates to tendons, ligaments, bones, and internal organs. These wounds also heal by granulation tissue formation and epithelization, but when tendons and ligaments are injured and then reapproximated surgically, they tend to fuse into the mass of granulation tissue that closes the remainder of the wound.[3] Early, active movement of the tendons by the patient aids them in becoming independent of the mass of granulation tissue, allowing functional movement to resume.

## GROWTH FACTORS AND REPAIR

The cellular activities associated with wound repair appear to be regulated by locally acting growth factors. These biomolecules, usually small polypeptides, stimulate cell proliferation, movement, and biosynthetic activity. They can act as paracrine (produced by one cell type to act on another in the local area) or autocrine (produced by a cell acting on itself) factors. This is a rapidly changing field, and new growth factors with potential roles in wound repair are continually being isolated and characterized.

Locally acting growth factors can be grouped into three large categories: (1) mitogens, which signal cells to proliferate, (2) chemoattractants, which stimulate cellular migration; and (3) transforming growth factors, which alter the phenotypic state of the cell.

Mitogens can be divided into "competence" and "progression" factors. To divide, cells must be stimulated to progress from the resting state ($G_0$) to a state of readiness to replicate DNA and divide ($G_1$). So-called competence factors appear to stimulate cells to make this transformation. Once cells enter $G_1$, progression through the division cycle seems to require the presence of progression factors (Fig 11–3).[5] Platelet-derived growth factor (PDGF) and epidermal growth factor (EGF) are examples of competence factors. Known progression factors include insulin-like growth factor (IGF-1) and the other somatomedins. These progression factors circulate in plasma and are readily available to cells stimulated to enter $G_1$ by the competence factors. There is also evidence that they are secreted by cells in wounds and in this way act as autocrine factors.

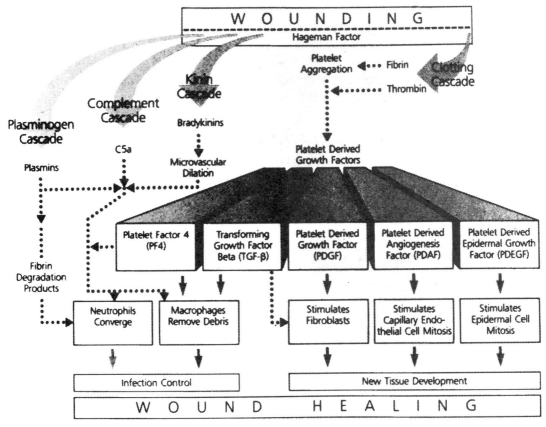

**FIG 11–2.**
Wounding unleashes a series of events culminating in accumulation of inflammatory cells and growth factors in the wound. This in turn results in stimulation of cell division, leading to new tissue formation and eventual healing of the wound. *(From Knighton DR, Fiegel VD, Doucette, MM:* Chronic wound care: a clinical source book for healthcare professionals, *1990, Health Management Publications, pp 431–445. Used by permission.)*

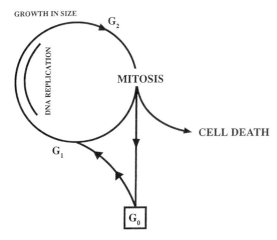

**FIG 11–3.**
Schematic depicts the cell cycle. In response to PDGF and EGF, cells at resting state *(G₀)* are stimulated to a state of readiness to replicate DNA and divide *(G₁).*

Chemoattractants can be divided into chemotactic factors and chemokinetic factors. Chemotactic factors work through cell surface receptors, which, on reaching one side of a cell in higher concentrations than the other, cause the target cell to move in a given direction. Examples of chemotactic factors are C5a, which is a chemoattractant for neutrophils, and PDGF, which is a chemoattractant for fibroblasts.[6, 7] Chemokinetic factors increase the rate of cell migration but not in a directional manner.[8] An example of chemokinesis is the effect of albumin on neutrophil migration.[9] Many growth factors act as both mitogens and chemoattractants, depending on concentration and target cell.

Transforming growth factor β (TGF-β) has been the most studied, and is reported to have a variety of activities, dependent on the cell type affected and the microenvironment in which it is acting.[10] In certain concentrations, it inhibits fibroblast division and stimulates increased production of matrix molecules (collagen and glycosaminoglycans). It also induces the production of PDGF in certain cells. Transforming growth factor α (TGF-α) shares considerable homology with EGF, binds to the same receptor, and evokes many of the same responses as EGF.[11, 12]

A summary of the biochemical and biologic activities of the certain growth factors presently thought to play a role in the regulation of wound repair follows.

## Platelet-Derived Growth Factor

Platelet-derived growth factor is a 30,000 to 32,000-dalton glycoprotein made up of two disulfide-linked subunits.[13] Originally discovered in platelets, this competence factor has been found in monocytes, smooth muscle cells, endothelial cells, and various transformed cells.[14-17] It binds to high-affinity receptor sites, is active in the picomolar range, and is a potent mitogen for most mesenchymally derived connective tissue cells.[18] As mentioned earlier, it is both a chemotactic molecule and a competence factor.

## Epidermal Growth Factor

Epidermal growth factor is a 6,000-dalton protein made up of a single chain of 53 amino acids.[19] It binds to high-affinity receptors and is found in platelets, salivary glands, duodenal glands, and urine.[20-23] It is a competence factor for many epithelial and mesenchymal cells and stimulates epidermal regeneration after partial thickness injuries.[24]

## Angiogenesis Factors

Angiogenesis is the process of new capillary formation. It is poorly understood in terms of the actual growth factor regulation because the potential list of "angiogenesis factors" is long and continues to grow. Angiogenesis involves at least five cellular events: (1) endothelial cell protease production, (2) endothelial cell migration, (3) endothelial cell proliferation, (4) endothelial cell tube formation, and (5) extracellular matrix synthesis. Ultrastructural studies on capillary proliferation demonstrate that capillary endothelial cell migration with enzyme production is the first activity seen, followed by endothelial cell proliferation.[25]

## Fibroblast Growth Factors

Fibroblast growth factors (FGFs) appear to be the best candidate for the mitogen that produces endothelial cell proliferation after migration has occurred. It is present in acidic (aFGF) and basic (bFGF) forms and binds to high-affinity receptors. The acidic form has a molecular weight of 16,000 daltons, and the basic form is 18,000 daltons. Both forms are heat and acid labile and are single polypeptide chains.[26] It is a potent mitogen for mesodermal and endothelial cells.[27] It stabilizes the phenotypic expression of cells in culture and is purported to cause neovascularization in vivo.[28, 29] It is produced by endothelial cells and is bound to the basement membrane.[30] FGF does not have a signal peptide that allows it to be secreted by a cell, so the mechanism by which FGF exits the cell is still unknown.

With progress in angiogenesis research, it is becoming clear that capillary formation involves two and possibly three different growth factors. The chemoattractant factor from platelets or macrophages triggers the process of capillary growth by stimulating endothelial cell migration. The capillary endothelial cell must break through the basement membrane to migrate, so proteolytic enzymes must be produced.[31, 32] A very low molecular weight factor has been isolated from platelets that induces plasminogen activator synthesis in capillary endothelial cells and may be responsible for the increase in proteolytic enzyme production seen in stimulated capillary endothelium. FGF also stimulates production of proteolytic enzymes by capillary endothelial cells.[33]

## Transforming Growth Factor β

Transforming growth factor β is a 25,000-dalton protein made up of two chains. It is secreted from the cell as a high molecular weight precursor that is cleaved at low pH.[34, 35] It is acid and heat stable and binds to high-affinity receptors on the target cell. It is found in many cells, including platelets, macrophages, and lymphocytes.[10] It inhibits cellular proliferation, is a monocyte chemoattractant, stimulates macrophages to produce many monokines, and stimulates collagen and fibronectin production from fibroblasts and keratinocytes.[36–40] In vitro it has been shown to stimulate endothelial cells to form tubelike structures.[41]

## Factors Regulating Collagen Synthesis

Collagen production by fibroblasts provides the molecular structure that gives tensile strength to the healing wound. The time course of collagen deposition, biochemical details of collagen production, and interplay between synthesis and lysis in wound repair are all well known. The regulatory mechanisms controlling the rate of collagen production, type of collagen produced, and proportion of collagen in the extracellular matrix are largely unknown. The role of growth factors in the regulation of wound healing collagen synthesis is intimately linked to fibroblast biology. Growth factors such as PDGF that regulate fibroblast proliferation and migration affect collagen synthesis by increasing the number of fibroblasts in the wound.[42] Growth factors also affect the rate of collagen synthesis per fibroblast. TGFβ significantly increases the collagen production/cell, as well as stimulates an increase in RNA levels for type I, III, and V collagen.[39, 43]

## CHRONIC NONHEALING DIABETIC WOUNDS

As described in the previous section, the process of wound repair is orderly and timely. When this process is stalled or interrupted, resulting in delay or complete cessation of the healing process, a chronic wound results. With this definition, a chronic wound could occur in any tissue of the body. We will focus on chronic wounds involving the skin.

## Pathobiology of Chronic Cutaneous Wounds

There are many reasons why the healing process is interrupted, resulting in a nonhealing cutaneous ulcer. A complete discussion is beyond the scope of this chapter. Essentially there are four main reasons why wounds do not heal: (1) infection, (2) ischemia, (3) repeated trauma, and (4) medications. Many patients have all four problems, resulting in a complex interaction that must be completely understood and treated before wound repair can occur. Others have only one problem, which when corrected, results in prompt repair.

Patients with diabetes commonly have all four problems, but even when they are all addressed clinically, the diabetic still has difficulty healing compared with nondiabetics. Documentation of this deficit in wound repair is best seen in animal experiments of wound repair. When genetically diabetic mice and rats made diabetic with streptozotocin are used, models of full-thickness wounds and incisional wounds have delayed repair compared with nondiabetic controls.[42, 44, 45] The exact mechanism by which diabetes delays repair is not yet known. There are multiple hypotheses such as glycosilation of important structural proteins and growth factors, decrease in oxygen delivery because of microvascular basement membrane thickening, and possibly a deficit in specific growth factor production or release into the wound.

## Infection

All cutaneous wounds are exposed to bacteria. During the process of successful wound repair, the original bacterial inoculum is destroyed by the nonspecific, neutrophil-monocyte based, host defense system.

When the patient is unable to effectively control and eliminate the bacterial innoculum, the normal process of wound repair is either delayed or stopped. If the bacterial proliferation goes unchecked, the resulting infectious necrosis of the periwound tissue can significantly increase the total wound burden.

The presence of increasing numbers of bacteria in the wound space and periwound tissue, along with the effects of the host response to clear the infection, can affect both oxygen delivery and blood flow. The increased oxygen demand resulting from infection and the neutrophil response to that infection increase the total oxygen and nutrient demand. In a patient with impaired blood flow, impaired oxygenation, or both, the increased demand may not be met by increased delivery, resulting in a negative feedback loop. The end result is often massive tissue necrosis or sepsis. Controlling the infection to decrease the oxygen and nutrient demand is often as important as increasing blood flow or tissue oxygenation. Often the infection cannot be effectively controlled until adequate blood flow and oxygenation is established.

In addition, recent experimentation with human chronic wounds shows that the chronic wound can be its own worst enemy. Wound fluid from nonhealing wounds degrades the fibronectin in the wound to fragments that are unable to function as matrix for cell mobility and proliferation.[46] Wound fluid from healing wounds has intact fibronection with no evidence of breakdown. Other experiments show that cellular division is inhibited by wound fluid from nonhealing wounds and stimulated by wound fluid from healing wounds.[47] These clinical studies support the role of wound excision to remove the chronically compromised tissue, creating an environment that has the capability to heal.

## Ischemia and Hypoperfusion

The process of wound repair requires energy. Any pathologic process that interrupts delivery of oxygen and nutrients to the cells involved in normal repair can result in de-

layed healing. Decreased oxygen and blood flow can result from a deficiency in any portion of the oxygen-blood flow biology, which extends from the alveolus to the arterial, to the capillary and venous circulation, and, finally, across the extracellular space to the cell and its energy machinery. Common areas of impairment include inadequate oxygenation because of chronic lung disease and congestive heart failure, deficient delivery because of arterial stenosis or obstruction, impaired cellular delivery because of increased tissue edema from venous disorders, or decreased capillary perfusion because of increased tissue pressure, and deficient cellular nutrient-oxygen utilization because of enzyme deficiency or pharmacologic manipulation. Restoring adequate flood flow and oxygen-nutrient delivery is critical if healing is to occur.

## Repeated Trauma

The process of wound repair requires an orderly sequence of cellular events. If during the healing process repeated injury continually destroys the new tissue, a nonhealing wound can result. The repeated injury could be caused by repeated excessive tissue pressure that interrupts blood flow, resulting in tissue ischemia and necrosis. Repeated injury resulting in continual breakdown of the protective epithelial barrier can lead to persistent invasive infection. Uncontrolled inflammation caused by a connective tissue disorder or foreign body can create a cellular microenvironment that prevents connective tissue formation and wound repair.

## Medications

Administration of topical or systemic medication often affects or impairs a critical event in wound repair. Many of the topical antimicrobials are toxic to connective tissue cells. Their use may decrease the superficial bacterial content of the wound but significantly delay the repair process. Medications that modulate the inflammatory process, such as corticosteroids and nonsteroidal anti-inflammatory agents significantly delay repair by impairing the necessary early signals that start wound healing. Chemotherapeutic agents used to treat cancer and some connective tissue disorders affect wound repair by killing the rapidly dividing cells necessary for prompt wound repair.

Chronic nonhealing wound repair is a complex and dynamic process involving four main pathologic conditions that change over time, depending on the therapeutic intervention and patient compliance with the intervention. To determine the effect of a particular intervention, such as growth factor administration, on wound repair requires careful monitoring of the state of ischemia, infection, trauma, and patient compliance, along with the wound repair endpoints, including infection control, granulation tissue formation, and epithelialization. At present, the most completely studied and used growth factors in diabetic wounds are the naturally occuring mix of growth factors from the α-granule of the platelet. This mixture of growth factors, protease inhibitors, and matrix molecules is called platelet-derived wound healing formula (PDWHF).

PDWHF is an autologous solution made from the patient's own blood. Blood is withdrawn from the patient and sent to a special processing laboratory. The platelets are extracted from the blood, and the growth factors are extracted from the platelets. The growth factors are resuspended in a solution that allows them to stay active. The PDWHF is then dispensed to the patient in single tube doses. One blood draw on the average produces enough growth factor for the entire treatment course of approximately 10 weeks.

To apply the growth factors to the wound, the patient saturates gauze with the single-dose PDWHF. The gauze is then packed into the wound, making sure that the solution is in contact with all the open wound area. This is covered with petrolatum-impregnated gauze to avoid evaporation and held in place with an appropriate dressing. The PDWHF is applied for 12 hours, usually before the person goes to bed at night. For the alternate 12 hours, a dressing of normal saline solution or a triple antibiotic solution, depending on the pathologic

condition of the wound, is kept in place. To keep the growth factors viable, the tubes of PDWHF need to be frozen. The tube to be used for the dressing is thawed in the refrigerator overnight before using.

PDWHF contains at least five locally acting growth factors from α-granulates: PDGF,[48] platelet-derived angiogenesis factor (PDAF),[49] platelet-derived epidermal growth factor (PDEGF),[50] TGF-β,[51] and platelet factor 4 (PF-4).[48]

### Clinical Trials

Three separate clinical trials have documented the effectiveness of this comprehensive approach to the diabetic foot ulcer:

1. Retrospective study of 88 diabetic patients with 124 plantar and metatarsal head ulcers.[52]
2. Prospectively randomized double-blind placebo controlled trial of PDWHF in which roughly half of the patients had diabetes.[53]
3. Two limb salvage studies: one in patients recommended for amputation, and a second study in which a panel of experts on amputation analyzed case reviews to determine the severity of the wound and predict whether amputation was necessary.[54]

The retrospective study examined 88 diabetic patients with 124 plantar and metatarsal head ulcers.[52] Their wounds were in existence for an average of 30 weeks. Forms of treatment during this time included dressings (72%), soaks (69%), oral antibiotics (52%), debridement (46%), intravenous antibiotics (31%), topical creams (30%), peroxide (28%), and whirlpool (20%). None of the wounds healed with these treatment modalities. The patients were then admitted to the Outpatient Wound Healing and Limb Salvage Clinic.

On admission to the clinic, the average wound volume was 11,996 mm$^3$. The average glycosylated hemoglobin was 8.9% (normal 3.4%–6.1% of total Hgb). Besides neuropathy, 24% of the limbs were ischemic, as evidenced by transcutaneous oxygen pressure (TcPo$_2$). Limbs with TcPo$_2$ less than 30 mm

Hg were considered ischemic. The average wound grade according to the Wound Care Center (WCC) wound grading system was 3; a full-thickness ulcer that involves tendon, bone, ligament, and/or joint. Twenty-six percent of the ulcers also had abscess, osteomyelitis, or both.

The patients then participated in the new comprehensive wound management program. Twenty-four percent of the limbs were revascularized, 75% of the wounds were surgically debrided, and all of the patients (100%) treated the wounds topically with PDWHF for an average of 65 days. The outcome of this treatment protocol was that 115 (93%) of the 124 wounds achieved 100% epithelialization in an average of 7.8 weeks. The wounds were followed for 12 months, and there was no breakdown during that time.

### Double-blind, Randomized, Crossover, Placebo-controlled Trial

To test the independent efficacy of PD-WHF, a double-blind, crossover, placebo-controlled trial was performed.[53] A total of 32 patients were randomized into treatment and control groups. All patients received standard wound care as described earlier. The placebo was the platelet buffer combined with microcrystalline collagen without platelet $\alpha$-granule release products. Patients randomized to the control group had their blood drawn and the PDWHF stored for use after the crossover period. Both groups were treated for 8 weeks, and then the placebo patients were crossed over to the positive arm of the study, treatment with PDWHF.

When the patient populations in each group were analyzed and wounds graded using the wound grading system, the two groups were matched except for the area measurement. Patients randomized to the control group had a higher area measure than control because of two patients with very large wounds.

A total of 13 patients finished the positive arm. Eleven patients finished the control arm. In the positive arm, 17 out of 21 total wounds achieved 100% epithelialization in an average of 8.6 weeks. In the placebo group of 11 patients, 2 out of 13 wounds (15%) healed during the initial 8 weeks of placebo treatment, and 11 of 13 wounds (85%) failed to heal in 8 weeks and were crossed over to the positive group. After crossover, all 11 nonhealed wounds achieved 100% epithelization in an average of 7.1 weeks. When analyzed statistically, there is a high degree (p < 0.0002) of significance between the two groups.

### Limb Salvage Study

Many of the patients referred to the clinic have threatened limbs because of ischemic nonhealing wounds. We retrospectively studied 24 of these patients to determine if treatment in the clinic under defined protocols with the use of PDWHF resulted in limb salvage.[54]

Patients were studied if they had ischemic nonhealing extremity ulcers that required amputation according to their referring physician. Recommended amputations at the transmetatarsal (TMA) level or higher were included. Minor amputations of the toes were not included. Success was defined as 100% epithelialization of the wound, progressive epithelial maturation, and the ability to tolerate limited weight bearing.

The patients ranged in age from 28 to 80 years, with 9 patients (38%) 65 years or older. The primary diagnosis was diabetic mellitus in 21 patients (88%), atherosclerotic peripheral vascular disease in 2 patients (8%), and rheumatoid arthritis in 1 patient (4%). All patients older than age 65 had diabetes mellitus.

Eleven patients had 15 prior amputations, 7 patients had 10 previous vascular procedures, and 6 of these 7 patients had vascular reconstructions in the limb that was now threatened.

The referring physician recommended transtibial amputation (TTA) below the knee in 18 patients, transmetatarsal amputation (TMA) in 5 patients, and a ray amputation in 1 patient (this patient was included because he needed a TTA on our evaluation).

The patients had 26 ulcers. The mean duration of conventional unsuccessful therapy was 26 weeks, with a range of 3 to 43 weeks.

As far as other factors are concerned, 46% (11 of 24) of the patients smoked, and

21% (5 of 25) were taking corticosteroids (4 for renal transplantation and 1 for severe rheumatoid arthritis).

Arteriograms were performed in 13 of 24 patients (54%), 11 of 24 patients (45%) underwent vascular reconstruction, and 20 of 24 patients (83%) had operative wound debridement before beginning PDWHF therapy.

The patients were followed for an average of 15 months, with a range of 7 to 29 months. Follow-up data were obtained from their last clinic visit or telephone conversation.

Of the 24 patients, 4 required amputation. Two patients' wounds did not heal. One required a transfemoral (above the knee) amputation, the other a TTA amputation. The other two patients' wounds were healing. One had a clotted vascular bypass resulting in amputation, and the other developed necrotizing soft tissue infection from walking on a plantar surface ulcer; both required TTA amputations.

In all, 19 of 24 patients (79%) healed 21 of 26 wounds. Two patients' wounds recurred after healing; one of these patients' wounds healed a second time by the end of the study. Two patients were still healing at the end of the study, leaving a total of 18 of 24 patients (75%) healed with 20 of 26 wounds (77%) healed. Most important, 17 of 18 patients who healed are ambulatory, with one healed patient unable to ambulate because of a previous stroke. The two patients who were still healing are on restricted ambulation. Of the four amputees, two ambulate on prostheses and two are nonambulatory.

A second study on amputation prevention involved an independent review panel composed of an orthopedic surgeon, a vascular surgeon, and an endocrinologist. They conducted a blinded retrospective review of 71 diabetic patients with 124 wounds on 81 limbs. Based on their expertise, the review panel classified the wound severity and identified the limb's risk for amputation. Their judgment was compared with the actual outcome.

The review panel predicted 65 (80%) of the limbs would be salvaged and 16 (20%) would be amputated. The actual outcome was that 75 (93%) of the limbs were salvaged and 6 (7%) were amputated (p < 0.005). This study demonstrated that the combination of aggressive revascularization and debridement, infection control, and unweighting of plantar ulcers, along with the use of PDWHF, was effective in amputation prevention.

Two other clinical trials using recombinant growth factors in patients with pressure sores and split-thickness skin grafts have been recently published.[55, 56] To date, there have been no other published studies on recombinant growth factors and diabetic ulcer healing.

## CONCLUSION

Growth factors play a pivotal role in normal wound repair. Currently available data suggest that their role in the care of diabetic ulcers will be to complement aggressive wound care, which includes wound excision, revascularization, infection control, and protection.

## REFERENCES

1. Maibach HI, Rovee DT: Epidermal wound healing, St Louis, 1972, Mosby-Year Book.

2. Pang SC, Daniels WH, Buck RC: Epidermal migration during the healing of suction blisters in rat skin: a scanning and transmission electron microscopic study, *Am J Anat* 153:177–191, 1978.

3. Hunt TK: *Wound healing and wound infection: theory and surgical practice*, New York, 1980, Appleton-Century-Crofts.

4. Clark RAF: Cutaneous tissue repair: basic biologic considerations, *J Am Acad Dermatol* 13:701–725, 1985.

5. Deuel TF: Polypeptide growth factors: roles in normal and abnormal cell growth, *Ann Rev Cell Biol* 3:443–492, 1987.

6. Snyderman R, Phillips J, Mergenhagen SE: Polymorphonuclear leukocyte chemotactic activity in rabbit serum and guinea pig serum treated with immune complexes: evidence for C5a as the major chemotactic factor, *Infect Immunol* 1:521–525, 1970.

7. Seppa H, Grotendorst G, Seppa S, et al: Platelet-derived growth factor is chemotactic for fibroblasts, *J Cell Biol* 92:584–588, 1982.

8. Wilkinson PC: Chemotaxis and chemokinesis: confusion about definitions, *J Immunol Methods* 110:143–144, 1988.

9. Wilkinson PC, Allan RB: Assay systems for measuring leukocyte locomotion: An overview, in Gallin JI, Quie PG, editors: *Leukocyte chemotaxis: methods, physiology and clinical implications*, New York, 1978, Raven Press, pp 1–24.

10. Sporn MB, Roberts AB, Wakefield LM, et al: Some recent advances in the chemistry and biology of transforming growth factor-beta, *J Cell Biol* 105:1039–1045, 1987.

11. Massague J: Epidermal growth factor-like transforming growth factor: isolation, chemical characterization, and potentiation by other transforming factors from feline sarcoma virus transformed rat cells, *J Biol Chem* 258:13606–13620, 1983.

12. Derynck R, Roberts AB, Winkler ME, et al: Human transforming growth factor alpha: precursor structure and expression in *E. coli*, *Cell* 38:287–297, 1984.

13. Raines EW, Ross R: Platelet-derived growth factor I: high yield purification and evidence for multiple forms, *J Biol Chem* 257:5154–5160, 1982.

14. Martinet Y, Bitterman PB, Mornex JF, et al: Activated human monocytes express the c-sis protocogene and release a mediator showing PDGF-like activity, *Nature* 319:158–160, 1986.

15. Walker LN, Bowen-Pope DF, Ross R, et al: Production of PDGF-like molecules by cultured arterial smooth muscle cells accompanies proliferation after arterial injury, *Proc Natl Acad Sci USA* 83:7311–7315, 1986.

16. DiCorleto PE, Bowen-Pope DF: Cultured endothelial cells produce a platelet-derived growth factor-like protein, *Proc Natl Acad Sci USA* 80:1919–1923, 1983.

17. Deuel TF, Huang JS: Platelet-derived growth factor: structure, function and roles in normal and transformed cells, *J Clin Invest* 74:669–676, 1984.

18. Ross R, Raines EW, Bowen-Pope DF: The biology of platelet-derived growth factor, *Cell* 45:155–169, 1986.

19. Taylor JM, Mitchell WM, Cohen S: Epidermal growth factor: physical and chemical properties, *J Biol Chem* 247:5928, 1972.

20. Oka Y, Orth DN: Human plasma epidermal growth factor/β-urogastrone is associated with blood platelets, *J Clin Invest* 72:249, 1983.

21. Kasselberg AG, Orth DN, Gray ME, et al: Immunocytochemical localization of human epidermal growth factor/urogastrone in several human tissues, *J Histochem Cytochem* 33:315–322, 1985.

22. Olsen PS, Poulsen SS, Kirkegaard P: Adrenergic effects on secretion of epidermal growth factor from Brunner's glands, *Gut* 26:920–927, 1985.

23. Gregory H: Isolation and structure of urogastrone and its relationship to epidermal growth factor, *Nature* 257:325–327, 1975.

24. Brown GL, Nanney LB, Griffen J, et al: Enhancement of wound healing by topical treatment with epidermal growth factor, *N Engl J Med* 321:76–80, 1989.

25. Folkman J: Angiogenesis, in Jaffe EA, editor: *Biology of endothelial cells*, Boston, 1984, Martinus Nijhoff Publishers, pp 412–428.

26. Fox GM: Fibroblast growth factor, in Clark RAF, Henson PM, editors: *The molecular and cellular biology of wound repair*, New York, 1988, Plenum Press, pp 265–271.

27. Gospodarowicz D, Greenberg G, Bialecki H, et al: Factors involved in the modulation of cell proliferation in vivo and in vitro: the role of fibroblast and epidermal growth factors in the proliferative response of mammalian cells, *In Vitro* 14:85–118, 1978.

28. Vlodavsky I, Johnson LK, Greenburg G, et al: Vascular endothelial cells maintained in the absence of fibroblast growth factor undergo structural and functional alterations that are incompatible with their in vivo differentiated properties, *J Cell Biol* 83:468–486, 1976.

29. Gospodarowicz D, Bialecki H, Thakral TK: The angiogenic activity of the fibroblast and epidermal growth factor, *Exp Eye Res* 28:501–514, 1979.

30. Baird A, Ling N: Fibroblast growth factors are present in the extracellular matrix produced by endothelial cells in vitro: implications for a role of heparinase-like enzymes in the neovascular response, *Biochem Biophys Res Commun* 142:428–439, 1987.

31. Gross JL, Moscatelli D, Rifkin DB: Increased capillary endothelial cell protease activity in response to angiogenic stimuli in vitro, *Proc Natl Acad Sci USA* 80:2623–2627, 1983.

32. Kalebic T, Garbisa S, Glaser B, et al: Basement membrane collagen: degradation by migrating endothelial cells, *Science* 221:281–283, 1983.

33. Moscatelli DA, Presta M, Rifkin DB: Purification of a factor from human placenta which stimulates capillary endothelial cell protease production, DNA synthesis and migration, *Proc Natl Acad Sci USA* 83:2091–2095, 1986.

34. Pircher R, Jullien P, Lawrence DA: Beta-transforming growth factor is stored in human blood platelets as a latent high molecular weight complex, *Biochem Biophys Res Commun* 136:30–37, 1986.

35. Lawrence DA, Pircher R, Jullien P: Conversion of a high molecular weight latent beta-TGFβ from chicken embryo fibroblasts into a low molecular weight active beta-TGFβ under acidic conditions, *Biochem Biophys Res Commun* 133:1026–1034, 1985.

36. Moses HL, Tucker RF, Leof EB, et al: Type beta

transforming growth factor is a growth stimulator and a growth inhibitor, *Cancer Cells* 3:65–71, 1985.

37. Wahl SM, Hunt DA, Wakefield LM, et al: Transforming growth factor type beta induces monocyte chemotaxis and growth factor production, *Proc Natl Acad Sci USA* 84:5788–5792, 1987.

38. Wiseman DM, Polverini PJ, Kamp DW, et al: Transforming growth factor-beta (TGFβ) is chemotactic for human monocytes and induces their expression of angiogenic activity, *Biochem Biophys Res Commun* 157:793–800, 1988.

39. Ignotz R, Massague J: Transforming growth factor-β stimulates the expression of fibronectin and collagen and their incorporation into the extracellular matrix, *J Biol Chem* 261:4337–4345, 1986.

40. Wikner NE, Persichitte KA, Baskin JB, et al: Transforming growth factor-β stimulates the expression of fibronectin by human keratinocytes, *J Invest Dermatol* 91:207–212, 1988.

41. Madri JA, Pratt BM, Tucher AM: Phenotypic modulation of endothelial cells by transforming growth factor b depends upon the composition and organization of the extracellular matrix, *J Cell Biol* 106:1375–1384, 1989.

42. Grotendorst GR, Martin GR, Pencev D, et al: Stimulation of granulation tissue formation by platelet-derived growth factor in normal and diabetic rats, *J Clin Invest* 76:2323–2329, 1985.

43. Ignotz R, Endo T, Massague J: Regulation of fibronectin and type I collagen mRNA levels by transforming growth factor β, *J Biol Chem* 262:6443–6446, 1987.

44. Goodson WH III, Hunt TK: Deficient collagen formation by obese mice in a standard wound model, *Am J Surg* 138:692–694, 1979.

45. Knighton DR, Fiegel VD: Unpublished data.

46. Wysocki AB, Grinnel F: Fibronectin profiles in normal and chronic wound fluid, *Lab Invest* 63:825–831, 1990.

47. Schultz G, Rotatori S, Clark W: EGF and TGF-α in wound healing and repair, *J Cell Biochem* 45:346–352, 1991.

48. Kaplan KL, Broekman MJ, Chernoff A, et al: Platelet alpha-granule proteins: studies on release and subcellular localization, *Blood* 53:604–618, 1979.

49. Michaeli D, Hunt TK, Knighton DR: The role of platelets in wound healing: demonstration of angiogenic activity, in Hunt TK, Heppenstall RB, Pines E, et al, editors: Soft and hard tissue repair: biological and clinical aspects, New York, 1984, Praeger, pp 380–394.

50. Oka Y, Orth DN: Human plasma epidermal growth factor/beta-urogastrone is associated with blood platelets, *J Clin Invest* 72:249–259, 1983.

51. Assoian RK, Sporn MB: Type-beta transforming growth factor in human platelets: release during platelet degranulation and action on vascular smooth muscle cells, *J Cell Biol* 102:1217–1223, 1986.

52. Fylling CP, Knighton DR, Gordinier RH: The use of a comprehensive wound care protocol including topical growth factor therapy in treatment of diabetic neuropathic ulcers, in Ward J, Goto Y, editors: *Diabetic neuropathy*, New York, 1990, John Wiley & Sons.

53. Knighton DR, Ciresi K, Fiegel VD, et al: Stimulation of repair in chronic nonhealing cutaneous ulcers: a prospectively randomized blinded trial using platelet-derived wound healing formula, *Surg Gynecol Obstet* 170:56–60, 1990.

54. Knighton DR, Fylling CP, Fiegel VD, et al: Amputation prevention in an independently reviewed at-risk diabetic population using a comprehensive protocol and platelet-derived wound healing formula, *Am J Surg* 160:466–471, 1990.

55. Brown GL, Nanney LB, Griffin J, et al: Enhancement of wound healing by topical treatment with epidermal growth factor, *N Engl J Med* 321:76–79, 1989.

56. Robson MC, Phillips LG, Thomason A, et al: Platelet derived growth factor-BB for the treatment of chronic pressure ulcers, *Lancet* 339:23–25, 1992.

# CHAPTER 12

# Local Aspects of Diabetic Foot Ulcer Care: Assessment, Dressings, and Topical Agents

**Oscar M. Alvarez, Ph.D., M.D.**

**Greta Gilson, R.N., M.S.**

**Michael J. Auletta, M.D.**

## ENVIRONMENT FOR HEALING

Throughout history, wounds have been dressed in an attempt to prevent gross contamination and potential infection. Nonetheless, recently as the 1960s many of the products used would have been familiar to the physician or surgeon of the 19th century.[37] In the past decade, however, dressing design and usage have changed considerably. The principal function of modern wound dressing is to provide an optimum healing environment. Because major changes take place in the wound environment at different stages of healing, several types of dressings have been designed to optimize each stage of the repair process.

In the first phase of wound healing, acute inflammatory events limit damage, setting the stage for subsequent repair. Wounds must be protected from further damage, infection controlled, and debris cleared. During this phase, wounds are most vulnerable to infection, especially in the diabetic host.[69] In the second, or proliferative, phase, formation of fibrovascular granulation tissue is followed by epithelialization. At this point, an optimal wound environment should facilitate connective tissue formation (repair) and epidermal migration (regeneration). Also, the worst is now over, because a well-granulated wound is much more difficult to infect. The healing process is then completed by remodeling and maturation of scar tissue. During this third phase, the clinician should start planning for the prevention of reinjury.

## ULCER ASSESSMENT AND DEBRIDEMENT

An adequate and uniform assessment of the patient and the foot ulcer is essential in the design of an effective standardized program for local management. Assessment of the foot ulcer should guide management principles by helping to determine whether the wound is clinically infected, whether minor or major sharp debridement is indicated, approximately how long it will take for the ulcer to heal by secondary intention, and what type of dressing should be used as healing progresses.

A physical examination, detailed history and diagnostic procedures designed to rule out osteomyelitis and determine the etiology of ulcer development (neuropathy, ischemia, venous hypertension, necrobiosis, etc.) are essential. Each ulcer should be classified by wound morphology, severity, and location. In Table 12–1 a format for ulcer assessment

**TABLE 12–1.**
Diabetic Foot Ulcer Assessment*

---

I. General wound parameters
  A. Periwound erythema: Congestive or exudative redness surrounding wound caused by engorgement of the capillaries in the lower layers of the skin.
    1. None: Blanches on digital pressure.
    2. Mild: Redness that does not blanch with digital pressure; may or may not be warm to the touch.
    3. Marked: Prominent redness or bluish coloration; usually warm to the touch.
  B. Periwound edema: An excessive accumulation of tissue fluid in the tissue surrounding the wound.
    1. Graded none, mild, or marked.
  C. Wound purulence: A viscous, yellowish white or green fluid formed in the infected tissue.
    1. Graded none, mild, or marked.
  D. Wound fibrin: A yellowish white meshwork not removable with a sterile swab or gauze. It adheres to the wound but can be removed with a scalpel blade by gentle scraping.
    1. Graded none, mild, or marked.
  E. Limb pitting edema: Localized excessive accumulation of interstitial fluid.
    1. None: Absent
    2. Mild: Digital pressure leaves a small but rebounding (within a few seconds) depression at the site.
    3. Marked: Digital pressure for 30 seconds leaves a persistant depression site.
  F. Limb brawny edema: A solid woodlike appearance to the lower limbs.
    1. None: Absent.
    2. Mild: Appears in a limited area.
    3. Marked: Whole leg involvement.
  G. Wound granulation: Formation of small, granular masses in the base of the wound that have a beefy-red appearance.
    1. None: Absent.
    2. Mild: Beginning to fill in and may not be epithelialized.
    3. Marked: Epithelialized and filling in.
II. Anatomic considerations
  A. Dorsalis pedis pulse: Artery is usually palpable in the groove between the first tendons on the medial side of the dorsum of the foot.
    1. 0–1+: Not palpable or barely present.
    2. 2+: Present, but diminished.
    3. 3–4+: Normal.
III. Wound measurements
    1. Size (cm$^2$): A standard metric circle template (Berol RapiDesign) is used to approximate the area of the ulcer.
    2. Depth (mm): Measure the wound at its deepest part at a 90-degree angle to the skin. Use a sterile swab as an aid. Graded < 5, 5–10, 10–20 mm.
    3. Undermining (mm): Measure the deepest part of any tunneling or shearing. Use a sterile swab as an aid. Graded 0, < 2, 2–5, >5 mm.
    4. Duration: Calculate the approximate duration from the wound's onset (break in the skin) to the date of assessment.

*Data from Pecoraro RE, Reiber GE: Wounds 2:65–73, 1990; Knighton DR, Fiegel VD, Doucette MM, et al: Pract Diabetol 8:5–10, 1989; Wagner FW Jr: A classification and treatment program for diabetic neuropathic and dysvascular foot problems, in American Academy of Orthopaedic Surgeons: Instructional Course Lectures, vol 28. St Louis, 1979, Mosby-Year Book.*

is presented.[81] It incorporates steps that correspond directly with all levels of the widely used but less comprehensive Wagner[106] and Knighton et al.[58] wound classifications. A systematic description of wound and limb appearance, including edema, erythema, exudation, granulation, and the presence of fibrin or eschar, is documented. In addition, ulcer area, depth of granulation, degree of undermining, and duration of nonhealing status should be recorded.

Thorough debridement should be performed with a scalpel at the initial visit. This includes removal of necrotic tissue, elimination of undermining, and cutting back to bleeding and seepage at the wound margin. At each follow-up visit, minor debridement should be performed to remove callosity surrounding the ulcer, entirely exposing the wound margins. Very little reliable information exists on the use of hydrotherapy or other pressurized mechanical methods of wound debridement. Often the antiseptics and preservatives used in the whirlpool, temperature, or the force of the jets may cause unnecessary harm to the delicate healing tissues.[66]

## FUNCTION OF WOUND DRESSINGS

First and foremost, a wound must be isolated from the external environment before healing can begin. The simple act of covering a wound mimics the barrier functions of the epithelium and enhances hemostasis and the dissipation of microorganisms and toxins.[37] For example, a simple compression dressing promotes hemostasis, limits edema, reduces pain, and improves gas and solute exchange between blood and tissue.[24] The nonspecific nature of inflammation results in tissue damage. Associated vascular leakage, release and activation of lytic enzymes, free radical generation, oxygen consumption, and the sensitization of nerve endings all are disruptive to tissue.[99] Any measure that limits inflammation, therefore, should promote wound healing, provided that it compromises neither the ability to resist infection nor essential macrophage function.

Infected wounds do not heal as quickly or as simply as noninfected wounds.[28, 86] Significant numbers ($10^3$–$10^4$) of commensal microflora are found in a normal healing wound,[76] apparently without adverse effect. Chronic dermal wounds such as pressure ulcers and venous stasis ulcers have been noted to heal in the presence of gross contamination (pathogenic bacterial populations exceeding $10^5$/g of wound tissue). In occluded wounds, these numbers increase ($10^6$–$10^8$) with a shift to gram-negative flora, and yet those that do not show the clinical signals of infection continue to heal at an apparently normal rate.[9, 35, 40] The distinction between "contamination" and "infection" will determine whether or not healing takes a complicated course. Infection is defined as contamination by pathogens that cannot be controlled by body defenses. Precisely what converts a grossly contaminated wound into an infected wound is not yet known. Practically, it has been shown in acute wounds and grafts that wound sepsis occurs when more than $10^5$ pathogens/g of wound tissue are present,[86] impairing healing.[61] In general, infection impedes wound healing by damaging tissue and promoting inappropriate and excessive inflammation. The ability to resist infection is compromised by bacterial toxins. Bacterial cell wall products and enzymes fix complement, destroy tissue, and activate or recruit neutrophils and macrophages.[99] Wound debris may be removed by mechanical debridement, irrigation, and absorption of exudate by a dressing. This reduces the requirement for phagocytic and autolytic debridement and removes a potential substrate for microbial growth. Thus, although a dressing cannot sterilize a wound, it may create the conditions for reducing the pathogenic load by preventing overgrowth and colonization or by delivering antimicrobial agents to the wound.

Subsequent to major surgical debridement of a foot ulcer in a diabetic patient, one should consider a dressing regimen that does not promote bacterial growth, absorbs exudate (especially during the first couple of days), prevents desiccation, and reduces pain. During this phase, a combination of a topical antibiotic ointment or cream (Table 12–2) applied once or twice daily and cov-

**TABLE 12–2.**

Commonly Used Topical Antibacterial Agents

| Agent | Vehicle | Comments/Administration |
|-------|---------|-------------------------|
| Silver sulfadiazine 1% | Water miscible cream | Effective against staphylococci, streptococci, *Pseudomonas* sp., and yeast; contraindicated for patients with history of hypersensitivity to silver sulfadiazine potential of cross-sensitivity with other sulfonamides; once daily × 2 wk |
| Polymyxin B sulfate–bacitracin zinc | White petrolatum ointment | Active against staphylococci and streptococci; limited effectiveness against *Pseudomonas* sp.; ointment base helps to prevent wound dessication; once daily × 2 wk |
| Polymixin B sulfate–bacitracin zinc, neomycin | White petrolatum ointment | Increased activity against *Pseudomonas* sp.; neomycin can cause skin sensitization; once daily × 2 wk |
| Gentamicin sulfate | Cream or petrolatum ointment | Activity directed to *Pseudomonas* sp.; prolonged use may create resistant strains; once daily × 1 wk |
| Mupuricin 2% | Polyethylene glycol ointment | Active against Staphylococci and streptococci; not effective against *Pseudomonas* sp. |

ered with an inexpensive absorbent, nonadhesive, nonocclusive (sleeve) dressing would be a good choice (Table 12–3). The proper topical antibiotic agent will assist in maintaining a moist environment, help reduce bacterial count, and serve as a chemical barrier for exogenous pathogens. The absorbent dressing should impede maceration, absorb excess exudate, and be easy to change without wound injury during removal. This dressing regimen should continue for approximately 2 to 3 weeks or until the wound space is filled with healthy, well-vascularized granulation tissue.

## CONTROL OF WOUND ENVIRONMENT DURING GRANULATION

### Occlusion (Wound Fluid Healing)

Dressing design for the second and third phases of wound healing is based principally on the manipulation of hydration and oxygen tension within the wound. Occlusion is a concept central to the evolution of wound dressings. It refers to the relative ability of a wound dressing to transmit gases and water vapor from a wound surface to the atmosphere. Numerous comparisons have been

**TABLE 12–3.**

Available Dressings*†

| Dressing | Type Name and Manufacturer | Description‡ |
|---|---|---|
| Adherent, absorbent, nonocclusive | | Many absorbent woven and nonwoven products are available; gauzes are based on cotton and/or rayon (regenerated cellulose) |
| Nonadherent, nonabsorbent, nonocclusive | Adaptic (Johnson & Johnson Medical, Inc.) | Knitted cellulose acetate impregnated with petrolatum emulsion |
| | Aquaphor (Beiersdorf) | Impregnated gauze |
| | Jelonet (Smith & Nephew) | Paraffin tule gras gauze |
| | N-Terface (Winfield) | Polyethylene-based mesh |
| | Transite (Smith & Nephew) | Fenestrated film |
| Nonadherent, absorbent occlusive, hydrocolloid dressings | Comfeel Ulcus (Coloplast) | Absorbent carboxymethylcellulose adhesive layer backed by a polyurethane film; also available as powder and paste containing guar, xanthan, and carboxymethylcellulose |
| | DuoDERM (Convatec) | Hydrocolloid layer composed of gelatin, pectin, sodium carboxymethylcellulose, and adhesive polyisobutylene; truly occlusive to gases and bacteria; backed hydrophobic foam |
| | Other hydrocolloid dressings include Intact (Bard), Intrasite (Smith & Nephew), Restore (Hollister), and Ultec (Sherwood) | |
| Composite dressings | Tegaderm Pouch Dressing (3M) | Inner fenestrated film; exudate accumulates in pouch formed by outer film layer, which transmits water vapor only at high levels; not strictly an "absorbent" dressing, although it has the same effect (i.e., displaces wound exudate away from wound) |
| | Viasorb (Sherwood) | Cotton polyester pad contained within a polyurethane sieeve; wound surface is slit fenestrated urethane |
| | Other composite dressings include Lyofoam (Acme, United), and Transigen (Smith & Nephew) | |
| Hydrogel dressings (occlusive) | Geliperm (Geistlich-Pharma/ Fougera) | Hydrogel of polyacrylamide and agar (96% water); moist sheet, dry material, and gel; tape required for fixation |
| | Vigilon (Bard) | Cross-linked polyethylene oxide hydrogel (95% water) between two polyethylene films; nonadherent, gas permeable; both film layers can be removed to enhance evaporation but may not exclude bacteria; tape required for fixation |

*(Continued.)*

**TABLE 12–3 (cont.).**

Available Dressings*†

| Dressing | Type Name and Manufacturer | Description‡ |
|---|---|---|
| | Other hydrogel dressings include Cutinova Gelfilm (Beiersdorf), and Elastogel (Southwest Technologies), and Nu-Gel (Johnson & Johnson Medical, Inc.) | |
| Hydrogel (nonocclusive); a number of hydrogels are available that are applied to (poured on) the wound, inhibit wound desiccation, dressing reinjury, and are somewhat occlusive; they may be irrigated on dressing change and require a secondary dressing | Carrington Dermal Wound Gel (Carrington) | Acemannan containing hydrogel |
| | Geliperm Granulat (Geistlich-Pharma/Fougera) | Milled hydrogel, polyacrylamide and agar |
| | Intrasite Gel (Smith & Nephew) | Starch copolymer |
| Semiocclusive/occlusive, nonabsorbent | Bioclusive (Johnson & Johnson Medical, Inc.) | Transparent polyurethane film with acrylic adhesive |
| | Blisterfilm (Sherwood) | Polyurethane film with perimeter adhesive for atraumatic removal and increased moisture vapor transmission rate |
| | Opsite (Smith & Nephew) | Polyurethane film with polyether adhesive |
| | Tegaderm (3M) | Polyurethane film, acrylic adhesive |
| | Other products in this category include Acuderm (Acme United), Co Film (Sherwood), Uniflex (Howmedica/Pfizer), and Visulin (Beghin Say) | |
| Biologic dressings | Biobrane (Woodroof Laboratories) | Silicone-nylon/collagen bilayer composite; depending on chosen porosity can be used on heavily or lightly exudative wounds |
| | E.Z. Derm (Genetic Labs) | Porcine xenograft, cross-linked collagen, stable at room temperature; contains silver as antimicrobial; recommended for use as a short-term dressing (i.e., daily changes) until adherence, when it may be allowed to slough off spontaneously |
| Medicated dressings | Odor Absorbent Dressing (Hollister) | Tea bag–like containing activated charcoal deodorant |
| | Scarlet Red Dressing (Sherwood) | Lanolin/olive oil/petrolatum impregnated gauze, containing scarlet red |
| | Tegaderm Plus (3M) | Contains iodophor |
| | Xeroform (Sherwood) | Absorbent gauze impregnated with bismuth tribromophenate in petrolatum base |

Available Dressings*†

| Dressing | Type Name and Manufacturer | Description‡ |
|---|---|---|
| Hemostats, absorbable | Collagen Hemostats include Avitene (Alcon), Helistat (Helitrex), Hemopad (Astr), Instat (Johnson & Johnson Medical, Inc.), Oxycell (Parke-Davis) (oxidized cellulose), Surgicell, and Nu-Knit (Johnson & Johnson Medical Inc.) (oxidized regenerated cellulose) | |
| Powders and pastes | A number of available absorbent powders and pastes are poured into the wound, absorb exudate, are somewhat occlusive, and may later be irrigated from the wound; these include Bard Absorption Dressing (Bard), Comfeel Granules (Coloplast), Debrisan Wound Cleaning Beads and Debrisan Wound Cleaning Paste (Johnson & Johnson Medical Inc.), DuoDERM Granules (Squibb) | |

*Adapted from Weisman D, Rovee D, Alvarez O: Wound dressings: design and use in wound healing, in Cohen K, Diegleman R, Linblad W, editors: Biochemical and clinical aspects, Philadelphia, 1922, WB Saunders, pp 562–580.
†This list is not complete and does not include every dressing sold in the United States.
‡The authors have attempted to give accurate descriptions of composition and use of commercially available wound dressings. We do, however, advise that the manufacturer should be consulted as to the precise composition and licensed usage of their products. The products described may be trademarks or registered trademarks of their respective companies.

made between occluded and exposed wounds.[11, 20, 47, 87] Occlusion affects both epidermis and dermis. Exposed wounds are more inflamed and necrotic than occluded wounds in early stages of repair. Later, the dermis of exposed wounds is more fibroplastic, fibrotic, and scarred. Dermal collagen synthesis is enhanced in occluded wounds.[11] Epithelial cell migration is enhanced by occlusion, although the magnitude and duration of the epithelial mitotic response are decreased.[88] Perhaps the most important function of an occlusive dressing is the limitation of tissue desiccation and secondary damage (Fig 12–1).[108] By maintaining a moist environment epidermal barrier, function is rapidly restored in superficial wounds.[110] An eschar (scab) forms when serous exudate dries, incorporating inflammatory cells, wound debris, and a layer of desiccated dermal tissue. The eschar bonds wound and dressing surfaces, making dressing removal painful and traumatic.[110, 113]

Epithelialization is delayed in open wounds because epithelial cells are forced to migrate below the eschar, through the difficult terrain of dehydrated dermis, instead of taking the easy route of a moist occluded wound bed.[109] This moist environment is also conducive to the migration of defensive and reparative cells such as polymorphonuclear leukocytes and macrophages.[25] Research evidence has been accumulated demonstrating that an occlusive wound environment, where the granulating wound is bathed by its exudate, promotes reepithelialization,[11, 109] granulation,[11, 62] autolytic debridement,[9, 35, 40] angiogenesis,[28, 60] and fibrinolysis.[72]

Occlusion, however, must be carefully controlled. In diabetic patients, it should be limited to the management of superficial wounds or full-thickness wounds that exhibit healthy granulation tissue (Fig 12–2). Diabetic patients whose foot ulcers are managed with occlusive dressings need to be followed

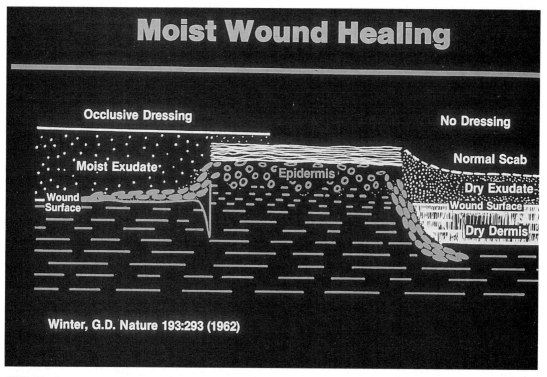

**FIG 12–1.**
Diagrammatic representation of epidermal migration in a moist vs. dry environment. *(Adapted from Winter GD, Scales JT: Nature 197:91–92, 1963.)*

closely (once weekly) and with more frequent dressing changes (once daily). The same environment that enhances healing may enhance pathogenic growth. Thus, occlusion is contraindicated in infected and draining wounds. The benefits and potential dangers of occlusive wound therapy are outlined in Table 12–4. Maceration is probably the most frequent complication of foot ulcers,[15] especially those occurring on the plantar surface in the neuropathic patient (Fig 12–3). Hutchinson and Lawrence[52] conducted a retrospective survey of the literature comparing the reported rates of clinical infection with occlusive and classical dressing regimens. The survey concluded that in most wound types (partial-thickness donor sites, pressure ulcers, and leg ulcers) significantly more infections were recorded when classical dressing regimens (wet to dry gauze, gauze alone, sleeve dressings) were used than when occlusive dressings (semipermeable plastic films, hydrocolloid, and hydrogels) were used. Hydrocolloids had the fewest reported infections. This survey,

however, did not include enough information on diabetic foot ulcers. Occlusive wound therapy is much less risky in a patient population that is less prone than diabetics to develop a serious infection.[33, 69]

Large numbers of microorganisms may be found in occluded wounds.[9, 35, 40, 76] Even on normal skin, bacterial growth occurs beneath occlusion.[13] In deliberately inoculated, experimentally induced human skin wounds, occlusion supported bacterial growth, although without apparent detri-

**TABLE 12–4.**

Advantages and Disadvantages Associated With Occlusive Dressings on Foot Ulcers

| Advantages | Disadvantages |
| --- | --- |
| Reduced pain | Maceration |
| Rapid healing | Accumulation of pus |
| Autolytic debridement | Adherence to healthy/new tissue |
| Increased granulation | Increased number of bacteria |
| Reduced friction | May promote anaerobe growth; difficult to apply |

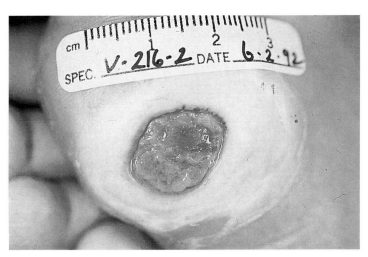

**FIG 12–2.**
Maceration of healthy epidermis surrounding a neuropathic ulcer in a diabetic patient. Maceration was caused by an occlusive nonabsorbent polyurethane dressing (changed once daily for 7 days).

ment to healing.[55] In an uncomplicated wound such as a donor site, occlusion may decrease the incidence of infection slightly.[74] Control of wound pH under occlusion may be a key to controlling pathogens: a low pH (5.8–6.6) may be desirable[105] and may have a positive influence on epithelialization.[36]

It is commonly stated that diabetic patients are more susceptible to infection than normal individuals. Reduced leukocyte mobilization has been reported in patients with diabetes mellitus,[22] and a neutrophil bactericidal defect has been reported in nonketotic adult diabetics.[98] Impaired granulocyte bactericidal activity has also been demonstrated in alloxan-induced diabetic animals.[84] Epidemiologic studies, on the other hand, have produced conflicting results.[33] There is no convincing evidence that immunologic competence is impaired in patients with diabetes mellitus,[91] nor is there any significant difference in antibody responses of alloxan-treated and normal mice.[69] Despite the absence of data showing a greater susceptibility to or severity of infection, it has been proposed that effective antibiotic therapy for infection is second only to the availability of insulin in significantly increasing the life span of diabetic patients.[102] Although investigators cannot agree on a specific biochemical defect in diabetics that makes them more susceptible to infection, there is general accord that once an infec-tion of the foot becomes established, it is more severe and refractory in the diabetic patient.[69, 102]

## OXYGEN

Perfusion and oxygenation of wounded tissue are vital to repair. Oxygen inhibits anaerobic growth and is required by phagocytes for the generation of bactericidal free radicals,[51] although it also inhibits macrophage angiogenic function.[59] Thus, the requirement for oxygen seems to conflict with that for hypoxia. Because it is practical to raise tissue $P_{O_2}$ only at the wound edges, the enhanced delivery of oxygen has the following effects: (1) microbial clearance from the wound is facilitated, and (2) fibroblast metabolism is promoted. Neither central wound hypoxia nor central wound macrophage angiogenic activity is altered. Enhancement of tissue $P_{O_2}$ by adequate perfusion, hydration, and the inspiration of hyperbaric oxygen has been advocated for wound treatment and has been suggested to be as effective as antibiotics in reducing infection.[19, 51] Although the beneficial effects of local oxygen administration have been discussed,[39, 56, 96] this treatment is controversial and raises further questions about the requirement for oxygen permeability in a dressing. Oxygen diffusion into normal adult human dermis

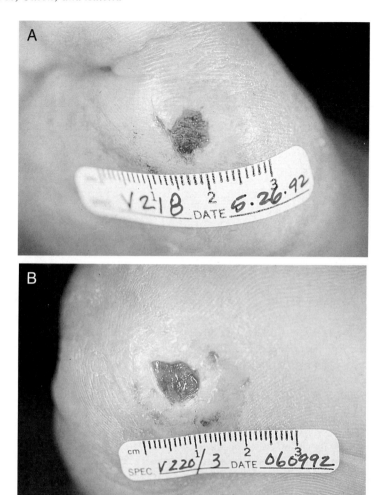

**FIG 12–3.**
Examples of diabetic foot ulcers (neuropathic) where occlusive therapy is indicated. **A,** superficial ulcer. **B,** ulcer with well-vascularized marked granulation tissue.

from the atmosphere is insufficient to raise $P_{O_2}$, although it may be sufficient in small mammals. Furthermore, wound exudate and active leukocytes present a formidable barrier to oxygen diffusion.[96] Leslie et al.[63] assessed the benefit of topical, so-called hyperbaric oxygen for the treatment of diabetic foot ulcers. Topical oxygen was no more successful in wound healing than dressing changes alone. A prospective randomized study to evaluate the effects of topical oxygen on the healing of experimentally induced uniform partial thickness donor site type wounds in healthy volunteers was recently conducted.[5] No significant differences were found in the healing rates between topical oxygen treated (at 1 hour daily and 2 hours

daily) and sham-treated control wounds. In vitro studies have shown that optimal epidermal cell growth occurs at atmospheric oxygen concentrations of 10% to 50%,[49] suggesting that increased epithelial oxygenation might enhance epithelialization. In full-thickness wounds, the $P_{O_2}$ values under oxygen-permeable polyurethane films were only slightly raised compared with those under totally occlusive hydrocolloid dressings (4.5 vs. 0 mm Hg).[105] What difference does topical oxygen make to the rate of epithelialization? Rates of epithelialization under dressings correlate inversely with their moisture vapor transmission rates but not with their known oxygen permeabilities.[111] Thus, it appears that oxygen permeability is not an essential attribute of a dressing. The ability of an oxygen-permeable dressing to prevent anaerobic infection is controversial, because the oxygen permeability of plastic films (especially those coated with adhesive) is dramatically reduced in vivo compared with in vitro. It must be emphasized that occlusive dressings should be used only on clean granulating wounds in patients whose underlying pathologic condition has been addressed and who are receiving concomitant supportive care (including non–weight bearing techniques and proper shoe gear).

## EFFECT OF WOUND TEMPERATURE

Heat losses are limited by the insulating effect of a dressing, which may be beneficial because low temperature may have a deleterious effect on healing per se, as a result of a decrease in metabolic activity and to vasoconstriction. Healing in human partial-thickness wounds occurs optimally at 37° C to 39° C, whereas below 26° C there is little epithelialization, and above 42° C there is cell death.[42] A raised ambient temperature also has the effect of increasing skin surface $Po_2$.[96] Thus, a warm environment is desired throughout the regenerative phase.

## PATIENT COMFORT

Studies are not available to verify whether dressing-induced analgesia is clinically important in the neuropathic patient. However, the documented reduction of pain by dressings[38, 74, 111] is a benefit that should not be undervalued. The mechanism of analgesia by dressings is unclear, although reduction of inflammation and the protection of nerve endings may be important factors.

Toxicity, allergenicity, and overall safety are also important considerations in dressing design. Lint granulomata have been associated with the use of surgical swabs.[23, 103] However, refinements in woven and nonwoven technology, as well as the trend away from the use of cotton materials as primary dressings, has reduced this problem.

## TYPES OF WOUND DRESSINGS

The terminology used to describe the many wound dressings available can be confusing. These terms are based on composition, physical properties, or usage and are not necessarily mutually exclusive. Figure 12–4 illustrates the design of several types of dressings. Table 12–3 classifies commercially available dressings using the terms described in the discussion that follows. Table 12–5 incorporates this classification to summarize the appropriate uses of each dressing (also see the section on matching the dressing to the wound).

### Primary and Secondary Dressings

All dressings can be classified as either primary or secondary. A primary dressing is placed in direct contact with the wound and may provide absorptive capacity while preventing desiccation, reducing the possibility of infection, and enhancing reepithelialization. A secondary dressing is placed over a primary dressing to provide further protection, absorptive capacity, compression, occlusion, or simply adhesion. The selection of materials for primary or secondary dressings is governed by the particular application. Cotton or rayon is most commonly used. They are inexpensive and can be manufactured in many configurations such as bandages, sponges, gauzes, tubular bandages, and stockings.

### Absorbent Dressings

The accumulation of wound fluid to the point of flooding has severe consequences, including maceration and bacterial overgrowth.[93] Thus, an absorbent dressing should imbibe exudate without losing its integrity. If the edge-seal between the skin and dressing is broken, a channel is formed for microorganisms to enter the wound from the outside. Cotton, wool, hydrophilic polyurethane foam, sponge, and moss all have been used as absorbent dressings. Even sawdust has been used to absorb pus and to pack abscesses because of the presence of antimicro-

## NONADHERENT, NONABSORBENT DRESSING

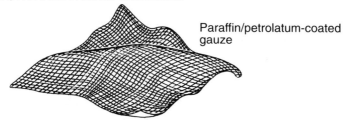

Paraffin/petrolatum-coated gauze

## NONADHERENT, ABSORBENT DRESSING

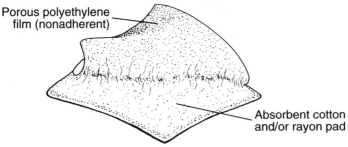

Porous polyethylene film (nonadherent)

Absorbent cotton and/or rayon pad

## NONADHERENT, ABSORBENT, OCCLUSIVE DRESSING (HYDROCOLLOID)

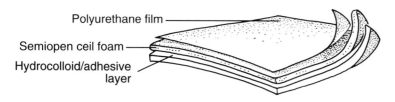

Polyurethane film

Semiopen ceil foam

Hydrocolloid/adhesive layer

## NONADHERENT, ABSORBENT, OCCLUSIVE DRESSING (HYDROGEL)

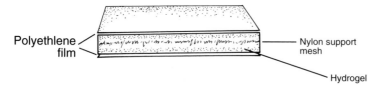

Polyethlene film

Nylon support mesh

Hydrogel

## NONADHERENT, ABSORBENT, SEMIOCCLUSIVE DRESSING (COMPOSITE)

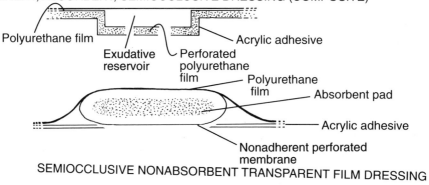

Polyurethane film

Acrylic adhesive

Exudative reservoir

Perforated polyurethane film

Polyurethane film

Absorbent pad

Acrylic adhesive

Nonadherent perforated membrane

## SEMIOCCLUSIVE NONABSORBENT TRANSPARENT FILM DRESSING

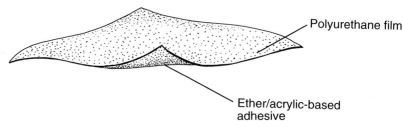

Polyurethane film

Ether/acrylic-based adhesive

bial resins within the particles. Other absorbent materials that have been used include chitin and chitosan (from the exoskeletons of crustaceans),[17] alginates, pectin, gelatin, gels of the pluronics series (triblock polymers of poly[oxypropylene] and poly[ethylene oxide]), carboxymethylcellulose, karaya gum, and starch acrylonitriles.[32, 79, 94] An absorbent dressing should be designed to match the exudation characteristics of the wound it is meant to cover. Acute wounds or freshly debrided chronic ulcers exude maximally at about 24 hours after injury. Chronic wounds (e.g., leg ulcers, pressure ulcers) exude slowly at first and then at a maximal plateau starting at 48 to 72 hours until the wound has granulated. Thus, hydrocolloid dressings, which do not absorb rapidly at first, are of little use in an acute exudative wound or after sharp debridement.

## Nonadherent Dressings

Nonadherent dressings are designed to not stick to the wound. Gauze is often impregnated with paraffin, petroleum jelly, or surgical lubricating jelly for use as a nonadherent dressing. However, the impregnate may wear off, necessitating a dressing change.[44] A secondary dressing should be used with a nonadherent dressing to seal the wound edge to prevent desiccation and the entrance of pathogens. In addition to the impregnated gauze type, nonadherent dressings often consist of an absorbent pad faced by a perforated nonadherent film layer. Such dressings may occasionally adhere to the wound, perhaps because of epithelial ingrowth through the holes in the film layer or via the polymerization of fibrin, forming a bridge between the wound and the dressing. Such adherence may be reduced by keeping the dressing moist at all times, even at the expense of some absorbency. Alternatively, the use of an ointment or a cream underneath the dressing may prevent adherence

by inhibiting desiccation. A distinction should be made between adherence to dry and to wet surfaces. Some "adhesive"-backed film dressings do not stick to the wet wound surface, whereas adherence to dry regenerated epithelium may cause disruption on removal. Thus, film dressings should be allowed to separate spontaneously from the healed wound.[53, 113] Plain gauze dressings will adhere to exudative wounds, and this property has been used traditionally as a means of debridement by removing the debris-encrusted dressing (wet or dry). This practice may be counterproductive, because granulation tissue and regenerated epithelium are also removed in the process. Often, wet to dry dressings are removed before they are completely dry and therefore do not remove the unwanted fibrin slough. Wet to dry compresses should be applied after gently rubbing the ulcer until it oozes. An unfolded damp (not wet) gauze sponge is then applied and secured with another dry sponge held in place by taping the edges only (taping over the wound will inhibit desiccation). When thoroughly dry, the gauze should be pulled away from the wound. This form of debridement should be performed until approximately one half of the wound has healthy granulation tissue three or four times.

## Occlusive and Semiocclusive Dressings

The terms occlusive, semiocclusive, and semipermeable are often used interchangeably when, in fact, they are not synonymous. Nevertheless, some water vapor permeability is desirable to prevent exudate puddling, although this may be aspirated from beneath the dressing. Occlusive-semiocclusive dressings provide an excellent environment for a clean, minimally exudative wound, and can be used to protect uninvolved tissue from an exudative wound. Experimentally, polyvinylidene (Saran) and polyethylene (Glad) films increase epidermal

**FIG 12–4.**
Dressing construction and design. *(Modified from Wiseman DM, Rovee DT, Alvarez OM: Wound dressing design and use, in Cohen K, Diegelmann R, Linblad W, editors:* Wound healing: biochemical and clinical aspects, *Philadelphia, 1992, WB Saunders, p 568.)*

**TABLE 12–5.**
Matching Dressing to Wound*

| Foot Ulcer | Full-thickness; Granulation None or Mild | Superficial or Marked Granulation; No Undermining | Ischemic Ulcer; Toes or Dorsum | Localized Infection Erythema, Edema; Culture and Treat Systemically | Miscellaneous Ulcer Palpable Pulses; Granulation None–Mild | Acute Surgical Procedure; Primary or Secondary Closure |
|---|---|---|---|---|---|---|
| Absorbent powders and pastes | *Cover with nonadherent absorbent (once daily)* | | | | *Cover with nonadherent absorbent (once a day)* | *Paste only* |
| Nonadherent, nonadhesive | | | | | | |
| Nonadherent, nonabsorbent | | | | | | |
| Nonadherent, absorbent | *Use with topical antibiotic (once daily)* | | *Use with topical antibiotic* | *Use with topical antibiotic* | *Use with topical antibiotic* | *Use with topical antibiotic* |
| Hydrocolloids | | *Daily dressing change; frequent follow-up; attention to signals of infection* | | | | |
| Occlusive absorbent composites | | *Daily dressing change; frequent follow-up; attention to signals of infection* | | | | *Use with topical antibiotic* |
| Occlusive nonabsorbent | | *Daily dressing change; frequent follow-up; attention to signals of infection* | | | | *Use with topical antibiotic* |
| Hydrogels: occlusive | | *Daily dressing change; frequent follow-up; attention to signals of infection* | | | | |
| Hydrogels: nonocclusive | *Cover with nonadherent absorbent* | *Cover with nonadherent absorbent* | *Cover with nonadherent absorbent* | Cover with nonadherent absorbent | *Cover with nonadherent absorbent* | Cover with nonadherent absorbent |

*italics signify recommendation.

healing by 31 % and 24% respectively, in superficial wounds compared with untreated controls.[111] Adhesive polyurethane film dressings are probably the most common type in this category.[101] They increase epidermal healing by 18% to 30% compared with untreated or wet to dry dressing in both animal studies and trials in humans.[5, 11] Film dressings are waterproof and impervious to microorganisms but permeable to water vapor and oxygen. They are prone to wrinkling, with the formation of channels that allow microorganisms to enter the wound from its margins.[77] Thus, it is important to obtain an "edge seal" around the wound by degreasing and drying the skin surrounding the wound and framing the wound with at least 2 in. of dressing.[1, 107] This is sometimes difficult to accomplish in ulcers of the foot. These polyurethane films are very thin and hard to handle. Patients should be allowed to practice dressing their ulcer while under supervision so that proper technique is followed. Hand washing immediately before dressing application is imperative because the wound contact surface of the dressing may be contaminated by touching. The tissue beneath a film dressing may have a yellow gelatinous appearance. Unless the wound is infected (showing the signs of infection, i.e., erythema, edema, induration), this appearance reflects healthy autolytic debridement of the moist wound bed and not pus. Adhesive films have also been used to protect areas vulnerable to friction injury (skin tears). Hydrocolloid dressings are usually totally occlusive, as are a number of tapes used to fix gauze in place.

## Hydrophilic and Hydrophobic Dressings

Hydrophilic and hydrophobic are terms often used to describe components of composite dressings. A primary hydrophilic layer is designed to absorb exudate either directly or by capillary transposition to an absorbent layer. A hydrophobic backing renders the dressing waterproof and averts penetration. In trilayered dressings, with a hydrophilic layer sandwiched between two hydrophobic layers, the wound contact layer is moisture (or moisture vapor) permeable and nonadherent.

## Hydrocolloid and Hydrogel Dressings

Hydrocolloid and hydrogel dressings attempt to combine the benefits of occlusion and absorbency. One approach has been the use of absorbent, hydrophilic hydrocolloids or hydrogels ("gels") formulated as sheets or pastes. Hydrocolloids and hydrogels form complex structures with the dispersion of discrete particles around which water molecules and solvated ions form a shell-like structure. Fluid absorption occurs principally by particle swelling and enlargement of this structure. The hydrocolloid mass of these dressings consists of gumlike materials such as guar or karaya, sodium carboxymethylcellulose, and pectin bound by an adhesive such as polyisobutylene. Hydrocolloid dressings display wet tack (adhesion to a wet surface) because of particle swelling. This property facilitates atraumatic removal. The dry tack (adhesion to a dry surface) of hydrocolloid dressings is caused by an adhesive such as polyisobutylene that is inactivated by moisture. The dry tack retained by the dressing around the wound preserves the edge seal. Exudate absorption by most hydrocolloid dressings results in a yellow-brown gelatinous mass that remains on the wound after dressing removal. This should not be confused with pus and may be irrigated from the wound. Hydrogels are complex lattices in which the dispersion medium is trapped rather like water in a "molecular" sponge.[85] The hydrogel is typically a cross-linked polymer such as polyvinylpyrrolidone or polyethylene oxide. Hydrogel dressings are nonadherent and have a high water content. Backed by a semipermeable film, hydrogels allow a high rate of evaporation without compromising wound hydration, which makes them useful in burn treatment, superficial dermabrasions, and shallow wounds where the epidermis has been denuded.

Hydrogels and hydrocolloids have been reported to increase epidermal healing by 30% to 36% compared with untreated and dry gauze–treated partial-thickness wounds[4, 11] and in full-thickness wounds.[62] Hydrocolloids and hydrogels can be supported by a foam or film layer and can be truly occlusive.[101] In liquefying, hydrogels and hydrocolloids conform to the wound, and their removal is atraumatic. There have, however, been anecdotal reports of epithelial damage on removal of hydrocolloid dressings, and it is probably inadvisable to use adhesive hydrocolloid dressings (but not hydrogels) on wounds located on hairy surfaces or on partial-thickness wounds shortly after reepithelialization. One report by Lithner[68] describes adverse effects of a highly adhesive hydrocolloid dressing on diabetic foot ulcers in two patients. In one case, a hydrocolloid dressing was left for 7 days on a superficial granulating wound in an ischemic diabetic patient. On dressing removal, the wound had become deeper and was infected with β-streptococci. In another instance, the same hydrocolloid was left on a foot fissure in a diabetic patient for 6 weeks, resulting in a deep wound infection. These experiences emphasize that the use of occlusive hydrocolloid dressings should be limited to healthy granulating wounds with frequent follow-up and dressing changes.

## Bioabsorbable Materials

Bioabsorbable materials are degraded in vivo. Particularly useful in bleeding open wounds as hemostatic agents, these materials include collagen, gelatin, oxidized cellulose, and oxidized regenerated cellulose.[16, 24] Collagen sponges and ground collagen (powder) have been used as wound dressings,[62, 114] and gelatin is a component of some hydrocolloid dressings. Increased bacterial growth has been reported on collagen matrix material when used in wounds.[62] Collagen may also be rapidly degraded by enzymes present in the wound. Calcium alginate dressings derived from seaweed and transformed into matrixlike sheets or ropes are a recent addition to the dressing family. Although they have been used in the United Kingdom for several years, they were not introduced in the United States until late 1989. Controlled, clinical investigations documenting

their effectiveness compared with other moist wound healing therapies in the healing of chronic dermal ulcers are not available. It is believed that the sodium from the wound exudate interacts with the calcium from the alginate to form a gel-like mass that stimulates repair. These are recommended for use in highly exudative wounds and when there is some bleeding because these alginates possess hemostatic properties. When used in wounds that do not exude a great deal of fluid, the alginate fibers may attach and remain embedded in the wound bed. Although this side effect has been reported previously, it does not seem to induce granuloma formation.[54]

## Medicated Dressings

The use of gauze dressings impregnated with bismuth tribromophenate (Xeroform) and scarlet red in lanolin, olive oil, and petrolatum has been reported in the wound healing and burn literature. Their use is predominantly limited to partial-thickness skin donor site care. There is no evidence available on the ability of either of these impregnated gauze dressings to help prevent infection or decrease the bacterial burden. There is one animal study in which scarlet red delayed wound healing.[4] A metronidazole-containing gel has recently been introduced. This product has been used for the treatment of rosacea and has been shown to reduce the odor of pressure ulcers. It has not been demonstrated to inhibit or reduce the growth of anaerobes in chronic wounds.

## Matching Dressing to Wound

The use of classical materials in wound management may be described as "passive" because an environment is being created for a wound to heal itself. Correct selection from the wide choice of dressings is essential for optimal healing. Dressing selection is based on overall wound care strategy and consideration of the likelihood of drainage and infection. The classification by Cruse and Foord[31] is particularly helpful in the case of infection. Dressing changes should be made as frequently as demanded by the accumulation of fluid and debris, overload of absorbent materials, degree of infection, and exhaustion or inactivation of medicaments. A list and classification of commercially available dressings is presented in Table 12–3. We have compiled a chart suggesting the selection of a particular dressing type to match the wound (see Table 12–5). This is not necessarily based on the product license defined by the U.S. Food and Drug Administration. In all cases, the manufacturer should be consulted as to the precise composition and usage of their particular products.

### Skin Grafts, Biologic Dressings, and Skin Equivalents

The skin graft shares many of the problems of the other types of organ graft: the use of an autograft is traumatic to an already compromised patient, donor or cadaver homografts are frequently rejected, and pigskin grafts usually are removed after several days. Several types of artificial skin are under investigation: composites of connective tissue elements and synthetic materials,[112] grafts of epidermal cells,[83] dermal cells,[30] or biosynthetic tissue substitutes (for a complete discussion of artificial skin, see Boykin and Molnar[21]).

Sponges of type I collagen have been used experimentally[62] and clinically[114] as wound dressings and artificial skin in full-thickness but not partial-thickness wounds. These sponges reduced wound contraction and scarring and increased the rate of epithelialization. The mechanism of healing enhancement seems to be related to the physical rather than the chemical form of the sponge because milled collagen powder is ineffective.[4, 62] Human amnionic membrane has been used as a treatment for burns and chronic leg ulcers.[92] Amnionic membrane possesses many ideal features of a dressing: it is somewhat occlusive, is highly conforming, and releases a number of growth and angiogenic factors.[27] However, because it must be purified of viral and bacterial contaminants, its use is impractical.

## ANTISEPTIC CLEANSERS AND TOPICAL AGENTS

Most commonly used antiseptics have been shown to be harmful to several cell types vital to the healing process.[66] Some have even been proved to delay normal wound healing in well-established animal models.[4, 82] However, very little clinical data exists to support the in vitro and animal experiments. Iodophor-containing agents (povidone-iodine) have little value in reducing the number of bacteria when a large population already exists in a wound.[75, 82] In addition, in draining wounds or in the presence of serum, iodophors are neutralized and lose their antiseptic properties.[50] Commonly used concentrations of acetic acid (0.25%), sodium hypochlorate solution (Dakin's solution 0.13%), and hydrogen peroxide (3%) are toxic to normal wounds despite their desirable antimicrobial or cleansing actions. Table 12–6 lists commonly used antiseptic cleansers and their effect on the rate of repair in normal healing wounds.

Many available topical agents have been evaluated in controlled studies using well-established wound healing experimental models.[34] Nearly all of the topical agents demonstrated to affect healing in such controlled studies have been confirmed by observations or clinical trials.[34] Physiologic saline solution or clean tap water are effective cleansers and should be used to irrigate the wound at every dressing change. Pressurized irrigation or hydrotherapy is not necessary, provided that the wound is effectively surgically debrided and free of necrotic tissue. Even the so-called inert topical agents or inactive bases (vehicles) may affect healing. Skin wounds are missing the natural cellular barrier (stratum corneum) that protects us from the external environment. Therefore, agents that are inactive on unwounded skin may have significant biochemical effects on cutaneous wounds. Many lotions, creams, and ointments have agents within them that have been shown to be irritants and sensitizers to the skin.[12] Patients with chronic wounds may develop allergies to the compounds used on the ulcers. The agents most often associated with irritation and allergic response are

## TABLE 12–6.

Agents That Delay Wound Healing

| Agent | Relative Rate of Healing (0%)* |
|---|---|
| Synthetic or fluorinated corticosteroids | 34 |
| Nitrofurazone | 30 |
| Liquid detergent | 28 |
| Neomycin sulfate | 5 |
| Chlorhexidine 2% | 7 |
| Povidone-iodine solution (10%) | 10 |
| Dakins solution (0.25%) | 15 |
| Acetic acid solution (0.25%) | 12 |
| Hydrogen peroxide (3%) | 8 |

*Compared with untreated, air-exposed control wounds. Data obtained from swine studies conducted on partial-thickness wounds.[4, 34] Relative rate of healing was calculated as*

$$\frac{HT_{50}\ untreated \times HT_{50}\ experimental}{HT_{50}} \times 100$$

*where $HT_{50}$ is healing time in which 50% of wounds are completely healed.*

preservatives, fragrances, and dyes. Several antibiotics such as neomycin and bacitracin zinc have also been demonstrated to be sensitizers as well.[12, 48]

The use of topical corticosteroids should be limited to lower-strength hydrocortisone-containing ointments. Synthetic corticosteroids such as triamcinolone acetonide and probably other moderate-, as well as high-strength, fluorinated anti-inflammatory corticosteroids will retard epidermal resurfacing and dermal collagen synthesis.[7] Bacitracin zinc, silver sulfadiazine, and some topical triple antibiotics (containing bacitracin zinc, polymyxin B, and neomycin) speed repair in wounds healing normally.[41] Several viscous ointments and creams can enhance healing simply by providing an occlusive (moist) environment.

There are several effective topical antibacterial agents[48]; however, because controlled clinical trials on chronic wounds are not available, their use in diabetic foot ulcers and other contaminated wounds remains unclear. Table 12–2 lists several commonly used antibacterial agents, their vehicle base, and recommended use. There is no general agreement on length of use, sequence of administration, prophylaxis, or the creation of resistant organisms. If infection is a consideration, they should not replace systemic antibiotics. The effectiveness of a topical antibiotic agent in treating a chronic wound infection is unknown. They may be quite effective, however, in preventing infection by providing a chemical barrier to exogenous pathogens or reducing the bacterial burden.[12, 48] If topical antibiotics are considered for the treatment of a localized wound infection, the use should be based on initial culture results.

Silver sulfadiazine is bactericidal for many gram-negative and gram-positive bacteria, as well as yeast. Polymyxin B and bacitracin zinc compounds are effective against most gram-positive and gram-negative bacilli, such as hemolytic streptococci and *Pseudomonas aeruginosa*. Neomycin-containing triple antibiotics may be more effective against certain resistant bacterial infections, but they occasionally cause skin sensitization. Topical gentamicin ointment is very effective against gram-positive and gram-negative bacteria, including certain penicillin-resistant strains. There is a risk, however, of creating bacteria resistant to this important aminoglycoside if this topical antibiotic is used for a prolonged period. Mupuricin (2% pseudomonic acid) is an antibiotic produced by fermentation by the organism *Pseudomonas fluorescens*. It is effective against infections caused by *Streptococcus pyogenes* and *Staphylococcus aureus* (including methicillin-resistant and beta-lactamase-producing strains). It is the only topical antibiotic agent that has documented clinical efficacy against penicillin-resistant *S. aureus* wound infections.[12, 48]

Although significantly less common than bacterial infections, opportunistic or deep fungal infections should be considered in immunosuppressed patients especially if the wound does not respond to antibacterial therapy. The suspicion of fungal infection should be validated by direct microscopic examination of clinical material and confirmed by culture. Antifungal treatment should be directed toward the suspected organism.

## CONCLUSION

Local care for diabetic foot ulcers should commence with a complete history and phys-

**TABLE 12–7.**

Ulcer Care Strategy

1. Address underlying pathologic condition.
2. Do sharp debridement to healthy bleeding tissue, eliminate undermining, and assure hemostasis.
3. Assess ulcer (general wound parameters), anatomic considerations and measure wound (see Table 12–1).
4. Apply topical antibiotic ointment (silver sulfadiazine, polymyxin B–bacitracin zinc, mupuricin 2%) once daily for 2 weeks.
5. Select nonadherant, nonocclusive absorbent dressing (dressing change once daily).
6. As soon as wound is granulated and well vascularized, occlude with synthetic dressing that keeps wound moist. Make sure dressing changes are at least once daily and patient follow-up is once weekly. Advise patient to notify office if they notice the clinical signs of infection.
7. Once wound has healed plan strategy for protection.

ical examination. Diagnostic procedures should be aimed at exclusion of osteomyelitis, dysvascular problems, extent of neuropathy, electrolyte imbalance, high or low blood glucose levels, nutritional defects. Oral antibiotics should be prescribed empirically after a wound culture is taken. Antibiotic use should be based on initial Gram's staining and clinical signs of active soft tissue infection. Antibiotics should be continued for 2 weeks as long as there is clinical improvement, but specific coverage should be reconsidered based on culture results if the infection does not respond.[80] Medical therapy for heart failure or other known cause of edema should be optimized because of reversible adverse effects of edema on cutaneous oxygenation.[80] An ulcer care strategy for local management is presented in Table 12–7. Other recommendations are to eliminate or minimize ambulation and, when necessary, to wear protective temporary footgear.

## Acknowledgments

I thank Timothy Oswold and Brenda Silverman for editorial assistance.

## REFERENCES

1. Alling P, North AF: Polyurethane film for coverage of skin graft donor sites, *J Oral Surg* 39:970–971, 1981.

2. Alper JC, Welch EA, Ginsberg M, et al: Moist wound healing under a vapor permeable membrane, *J Am Acad Dermatol* 1987; 8:437.

3. Altemeier WA, Burke JF, Pruitt BA, et al: *Manual on control of infection in surgical patients*, Philadelphia, JB Lippincott, 1976.

4. Alvarez OM: Pharmacological and environmental modulation of wound healing, in Vitto J, Parejda AJ, editors: *Connective tissue disease, molecular pathology of the extracellular matrix*, New York, 1987, Marcell Dekker, p 367.

5. Alvarez OM, Auletta M, O'Hara L, et al: A model for the clinical evaluation of partial thickness wound healing in healthy human subjects: the effects of an acemannan hydrogel, occlusive dressings and topical hyperbaric oxygen [abstract], fifth annual symposium on advanced wound care and medical research forum on wound repair, April 23–25, 1992.

6. Alvarez OM, Goslen JB, Eaglstein WH, et al: Wound healing, in Fitzpatrick IM, Eisen AZ, Wolff K, et al, editors: *Dermatology in general medicine*, ed 3, New York, 1987, McGraw-Hill, pp 321–336.

7. Alvarez OM, Levendorf KD, Smerbeck RV, et al: Effect of topically applied steroid and nonsteroidal anti-inflammatory agents on skin repair and regeneration, *Fed Proc* 1984; 43:2793.

8. Alvarez OM, Massac E, Brown B, et al: Evaluation and staging of pressure ulcers, *Fam Pract* 12:60–75, 1990.

9. Alvarez OM, Massac E, Brown B, et al: Management issues in the critical care of pressure ulcers, *Fam Pract* 12:78–104, 1990.

10. Alvarez OM, Massac E, Brown B, et al: Prevention, initial assessment, and supportive care of pressure ulcers, *Fam Pract* 12:15–35, 1990.

11. Alvarez OM, Mertz PM, Eaglstein WH: The effect of occlusive dressings on collagen synthesis

and epithelialization in superficial wounds, *J Surg Res* 35:142–148, 1983.

12. Aly R, Maibach HI: Commonly used drugs: anti-bacterial agents, in *Bacterial and fungal infections of the skin*, Aly R, Maibach HI, editors: Somerville, NJ, Hoechst Roussel Press, 1987, pp 26–34.

13. Aly R, Shirley C, Cunico B, et al: Effect of prolonged occlusion on the microbial flora, pH, carbon dioxide and transepidermal water loss on human skin, *J Invest Dermatol* 71:378–381, 1978.

14. Apelquist J, Castenfors J, Larsson J, et al: Wound classification is more important than site of ulceration in the outcome of diabetic foot ulcers, *Diabetic Magazine* 6:526–530, 1989.

15. Apelqvist J, Larsson J, Stenstrom A: Topical treatment of necrotic foot ulcers in diabetic patients: a comparative trial of DuoDERM and MeZinc, *Br J Dermatol* 123:787–792, 1990.

16. Arand AG, Swaya R: Intraoperative chemical hemostasis in neurosurgery, *Neurosurgery* 18:223–233, 1986.

17. Balassa LL, Prudden JF: Application of chitin and chitosan in wound healing acceleration, in Muzzarelli RAA, Parne ER, editors: *Proceedings of the 1st International Conference on Chitin and Chitosan*, Cambridge, Mass, 1978, MIT Press.

18. Barnett A, Berkowitz RL, Vistnes LM: Comparison of synthetic adhesive moisture vapor permeable and fine mesh gauze dressings for split thickness skin graft donor sites, *Am J Surg* 145:379–381, 1983.

19. Bass BH: The treatment of varicose leg ulcers by hyperbaric oxygen, *Postgrad Med J* 46:407–408, 1970.

20. Bothwell JW, Rovee DT: The effect of dressings on the repair of cutaneous wounds in humans, in Harkiss KJ, editor: *Surgical dressings and wound healing*, London, 1971, Crosby Lockwood, pp 78–79.

21. Boykin JV, Molnar JA: Burn scar and skin equivalents, in Cohen K, Diegelmann R, Linblad W, editors: *Wound healing: biochemical and clinical aspects*, Philadelphia, 1992, WB Saunders, pp 523–540.

22. Brayton RG, Stokes PE, Schwartz MS, et al: Effect of alcohol and various diseases on leukocyte mobilization, phagocytosis, and intracellular bacterial killing, *N Engl J Med* 282:123, 1970.

23. Brittan RF, Studley JGN, Parkin JV, et al: Cellulose granulomatous peritonitis, *Br J Surg* 71:452–453, 1984.

24. Browder, IW, Litwin MS: Use of absorbable collagen for hemostasis in general surgical patients, *Am Surg* 52:492–494, 1986.

25. Buchan IA, Andrew JK, Lang SM: Clinical and laboratory investigation of the composition and properties of human skin wound exudate under semipermeable dressings, *Burns* 7:326–332, 1981.

26. Bucknall TE, Cox PJ, Ellis H: Burst abdomen and incisional hernia-prospective study of 1129 major laparotomies, *Br Med J* 284:931–933, 1982.

27. Burgos H: Angiogenic factor from human term placenta: purification and partial characterization, *Eur J Clin Invest* 16:486–493, 1986.

28. Cherry GW, Ryan TJ: Enhanced wound angiogenesis with a new hydrocolloid dressing, in Role of Occlusion, Royal Society of Medicine International Congress and Symposium, Series No. 88, London. *R Soc Med* 1985; 61–68.

29. Conway H, Griffith BH: Plastic surgery for closure of decubitus ulcers in patients with paraplegia: based on experience with 1000 cases, *Am J Surg* 91:946, 1956.

30. Cooper M: Studies in Dermagraft for full thickness wounds, Fourth Annual International Symposium on Wound Healing and Wound Management, Chicago, October 1989.

31. Cruse PJ, Foord R: The epidemiology of wound infection: a ten year prospective study of 62979 wounds, *Surg Clin North Am* 60:27–40, 1980.

32. De Riel S: Assessment of burn wound therapy systems, in Wise DL, editor: *Burn wound coverings*, Boca Raton, Fla, 1984, CRC Press, vol I, pp 1–38.

33. Diabetes mellitus and polynephritis [editorial]. *N Engl J Med* 261:1247, 1959.

34. Eaglstein WH, Mertz PM, Alvarez OM: Effect of topically applied agents on healing wounds, *Clin Dermatol* 2:112–115, 1985.

35. Eaglstein WH, Mertz PM, Falanga V: Occlusive dressings, *Am Fam Phys* 35:211–216, 1987.

36. Eisinger M, Soo Lee J, Hefton JM, et al: Human epidermal cell culture: growth and differentiation in absence of dermal components or medium supplements, *Proc Natl Acad Sci USA* 76:5340–5344, 1979.

37. Elliott IMZ: *A short history of surgical dressings*, London, 1964, Pharmaceutical Press.

38. Falanga V: Occlusive wound dressings, *Arch Dermatol* 124:872–877, 1988.

39. Fischer BH: Topical hyperbaric oxygen treatment of pressure sores and skin ulcers, *Lancet* 2:407–408, 1969.

40. Friedman SJ, Su WPD: Management of leg ulcers with hydrocolloid occlusive dressings, *Arch Dermatol* 120:1329–1336, 1984.

41. Geronimus RG, Mertz PM, Eaglstein WH: Wound healing: the effects of topical antimicrobial agents, *Arch Dermatol* 1979; 15:1311.

42. Gimbal NS, Farris W: Skin grafting, *Arch Surg* 92:554–557, 1966.

43. Goslen JB, Kobayaski GS: Mycologic infections, in Fitzpatric TB, Eisen AZ, Wolfe K, editors: *Dermatology in general medicine*, New York, 1987, McGraw-Hill, p 2193.

44. Harkiss KJ: Cost analysis of dressing materials used in venous leg ulcers, *Pharm J* 235:268–269, 1985.

45. Haury B, Rodeheaver G, Vensko J, et al: Debridement: an essential component of traumatic wound care, *Am J Surg* 1978; 135:238.

46. Hien NT, Prawer SE, Katz HI: Facilitated wound healing using transparent film dressing following Mohs micrographic surgery, *Arch Dermatol* 124:903–906, 1988.

47. Hinman CD, Maibach HI: Effect of air exposure and occlusion on experimental human skin wounds, *Nature* 200:377–378, 1963.

48. Hirschman JV: Topical antibiotics in dermatology, *Arch Dermatol* 1988; 124:1691.

49. Horikoski T, Balin AK, Carter DM: Effect of oxygen on the growth of human epidermal keratinocytes, *J Invest Dermatol* 86:424–427, 1986.

50. Hugo WH, Newton JM: The antibacterial activity of complex of iodine and a nonionic surface active agent, *J Pharm Pharmacol* 1964; 16:189.

51. Hunt TK, Halliday B, Knighton DR, et al: Impairment of microbicidal function in wounds: correction with oxygenation, in Heppenstall RB, Hunt TK, Pines E, et al: *Soft and hard tissue repair: biological and clinical aspects*, New York, Praeger, 1984, pp 455–468.

52. Hutchinson JJ, Lawrence JC: Wound infection under occlusive dressings, *J Hosp Infect* 17:83–94, 1991.

53. James JH, Watson AC: The use of Opsite, a vapor permeable dressing, on skin graft donor sites, *Br J Plast Surg* 28:107–110, 1975.

54. Jeter KF, Tintle TE: Wound dressings in the nineties: indications and contraindications, in Albert SF, Mulder GD, editors: *Clinics in podiatric medicine and surgery*, Wound healing edition, Philadelphia, 1991, WB Saunders, pp 799–816.

55. Katz S, McGinley K, Leyden JJ: Semipermeable occlusive dressings: effects on growth of pathogenic bacteria and reepithelization of superficial wounds, *Arch Dermatol* 122:58–62, 1986.

56. Kaufman T, Alexander W, Nathan P, et al: Microclimate wound chamber: topical treatment of deep burns with humidified oxygen, *Surg Forum* 33:607–609, 1982.

57. Kerstein MD: *Management of surgical infection*, Mount Kisco, NY, 1980, Futura.

58. Knighton DR, Fiegel VD, Doucette MM, et al: Platelet extracts in the treatment of nonhealing diabetic ulcers, *Pract Diabetol* 8:5–10, 1989.

59. Knighton DR, Oredsson S, Banda M, et al: Regulation of repair: hypoxic control of macrophage meditated angiogenesis, in Hunt TK, Heppenstall RB, Pines E, et al: *Soft and hard tissue repair: biological and clinical aspects*, New York, 1984, Praeger, pp 50–66.

60. Knighton DR, Silver IA, Hunt TK: Regulation of wound healing angiogenesis: effect of oxygen gradients and inspired oxygen concentration, *Surgery* 90:262–270, 1981.

61. Krizek TJ, Robson MC, Kho E: Bacterial growth and skin graft survival, *Surg Forum* 18:518–519, 1967.

62. Leipziger LS, Glushko V, DiBernardo B, et al: Dermal wound repair: role of collagen matrix implants and synthetic polymer dressings, *J Am Acad Dermatol* 12:409–419, 1985.

63. Leslie CA, Sapico FL, Ginunas VJ, et al: Randomized controlled trial of topical hyperbaric oxygen for treatment of diabetic foot ulcers, *Diabetes Care* 11:111–115, 1988.

64. Levenson SM, Kan-Gruber D, Gruber C, et al: Wound healing accelerated by *Staphylococcus aureus*, *Arch Surg* 118:310–320, 1983.

65. Leyden JJ, Stewart R, Kligman AM: Updated in vivo methods for evaluating topical anti-microbial agents on human skin, *J Invest Dermatol* 72:165–170, 1979.

66. Lineaweaver W, Howard R, Soucy D, et al: Topical antimicrobial toxicity, *Arch Surg* 120:267, 1985.

67. Linsky CB, Rovee DT, Dow T: Effect of dressings on wound inflammation and scar tissue, in Dineen P, Hildick-Smith G, editors: *The surgical wound*, Philadelphia, 1981, Lea & Febiger, pp 191–205.

68. Lithner F: Adverse effects on diabetic foot ulcers of highly adhesive hydrocolloid dressing [letter], *Diabetes Care* 13:814–815, 1990.

69. Little JR, Vobayashi GS: Infection of the diabetic foot, in Levin ME, O'Neil LW, editors: *The diabetic foot*, ed 4, St Louis, 1988, Mosby–Year Book, pp 104–118.

70. Ljungh A, Wadstrom T: Occlusive dressings and wound infection [letter]. *J Infect Dis* 155:831, 1987.

71. Lobe TE, Anderson GF, King DR: An improved method of wound management for pediatric patients, *J Pediatr Surg* 15:886–889, 1980.

72. Lydon MJ, Cherry GW, Cederholm-Williams SA, et al: Fibrinolytic activity of hydrocolloid dressings, in Ryan TJ, editor: *Beyond occlusion: wound care proceedings*, Royal Society of Medicine Services International Congress and Symposium, series no 136, London, 1988, Royal Society of Medicine, pp 9–17.

73. Majno G: *The healing hand*, Cambridge, Mass, 1975, Harvard University Press.

74. May SR: Physiology, immunology and clinical efficacy of an adherent polyurethane wound

dressing OP-site, in Wise DL, editor: *Burn wound coverings*, Boca Raton, Fla, 1984, CRC Press, vol II, pp 53–78.

75. Mertz PM, Alvarez OM, Smerbeck V, et al: A new in vivo model for the evaluation of antiseptics on superficial wounds: the effect of 70% alcohol and povidone iodine solution, *Arch Dermatol* 120:58, 1984.

76. Mertz PM, Eaglstein WH: The effect of a semiocclusive dressing on the microbial population in superficial wounds, *Arch Surg* 119:287–289, 1984.

77. Mertz PM, Marshall DA, Eaglstein WH: Occlusive wound dressings to prevent bacterial invasion and wound infection, *J Am Acad Dermatol* 12:662–668, 1985.

78. Mueller MJ, Diamond JE, Sinacore DR, et al: Total contact casting in treatment of diabetic plantar ulcers: controlled clinical trial, *Diabetes Care* 12:384–388, 1989.

79. Nalbandian RM, Henry RL, Balko KW, et al: Pluronic F-127 gel preparation as an artificial skin in the treatment of third degree burns, *J Biomed Mater Res* 21:1135–1148, 1987.

80. Pecoraro RE, Ahroni JH, Bayco EJ, et al: Chronology and determinants of tissue repair in diabetic lower extremity ulcers, *Diabetes* 40:1305–1313, 1991.

81. Pecoraro RE, Reiber GE: Classification of wounds in diabetic amputees, *Wounds* 2:65–73, 1990.

82. Peterson AF, Rosenberg A, Alatory SD: Comparative evaluation of surgical scrub preparations, *Surg Gynecol Obstet Pharmacol* 16:198, 1964.

83. Phillips TJ: Treatment of skin ulcers with cultured autografts, *J Am Acad Dermatol* 21:191–195, 1989.

84. Qvist R, Larkins RG: Diminished production of thromboxane $B_2$ and prostaglandin E by stimulated polymorphonuclear leukocytes from insulin treated diabetes subjects, *Diabetes* 32:622, 1983.

85. Rawlins EA: *Bentley's textbook of pharmaceutics*, ed 8, London, 1977, Balliere-Tindall.

86. Robson MC, Heggars JP: Quantitative bacteriology and inflammatory mediators in soft tissue, in Hunt TK, Heppenstall RB, Pines E, et al, editors: *Soft and hard tissue repair: biological and clinical aspects*, New York, 1984, Praeger, pp 483–507.

87. Rovee DT, Kurowsky CA, Labun J: Local wound environment and epidermal healing, *Arch Dermatol* 106:330–334, 1972.

88. Rovee DT, Miller CA: Epidermal role in the breaking strength of wounds, *Arch Surg* 96:43–52, 1968.

89. Rowbotham JL, Gibbons GW, Gray M, et al: Local treatment of the diabetic foot, in Kozak GP, Hoare CS, Rowbotham JL, et al, editors: *Management of Diabetic Foot Problems*, Philadelphia, 1984, WB Saunders, pp 113–121.

90. Rudolph R: Wound treatments, nostrums and hokums, in Rudolph R, Noe JM, editors: *Chronic problem wounds*, Boston, 1983, Little Brown, pp 47–51.

91. Sabin JA: Bacterial infections in diabetes mellitus, *Br J Dermatol* 91:481, 1974.

92. Sawhney P: Amnionic membrane as a biological dressing in the management of burns, *Burns* 15:339–342, 1989.

93. Scales JT, Towers AG, Goodman N: Development and evaluation of a porous surgical dressing, *Br Med J* 2:962–968, 1956.

94. Schmolka I: Artificial skin: I, preparation and properties of Pluronic F-127 gels for treatment of burns, *J Biomed Mater Res* 6:571582, 1972.

95. Shah SV, Wallin JD, Eilen SD: Chemoluminescence and superoxide anion production by leukocytes from diabetic patients, *J Clin Endocrinol Metab* 57:402, 1983.

96. Silver IA: Oxygen tension and re-epithelialization, in Maibach HI, Rovee DT, editors: *Epidermal wound healing*, Chicago, 1972, Mosby-Year Book, pp 291–305.

97. Sirvio LM, Grussing DM: The effect of gas permeability of film dressings on wound healing, *J Invest Dermatol* 93:528–531, 1989.

98. Tan JS, Anderson TC, Watanakunakoi C, et al: Neutrophil dysfunction in diabetes mellitus, *J Lab Clin Med* 85:26, 1975.

99. Taussig M: *Processes in pathology and microbiology*, ed 2, Boston, 1984, Blackwell.

100. Thomas S, Loveless P: Moisture vapour permeability of hydrocolloid dressings, *Pharm J* 241:806, 1988.

101. Thomas S, Loveless P, Hay NP: Comparative review of the properties of six semipermeable film dressings, *Pharm J* 240:785–787, 1988.

102. Thornton GF: Infections and diabetes, *Med Clin North Am* 55:931, 1971.

103. Tinker, MA, Teicher I, Burdman D: Cellulose granulomas and their relationships to intestinal obstruction, *Am J Surg* 133:134–139, 1977.

104. Unger DH, Lucca M: The role of hyperbaric oxygen therapy in the treatment of diabetic foot ulcers and refractory osteomyelitis, *Clin Podiat Med Surg* 7:403–492, 1990.

105. Varghese MC, Balin AK, Carter M, et al: Local environment of chronic wounds under synthetic dressings, *Arch Dermatol* 122:52–57, 1986.

106. Wagner FW Jr: A classification and treatment program for diabetic neuropathic and dysvascular foot problems, in *American Academy of Orthopaedic Surgeons: Instructional Course Lectures, vol 28*. St Louis, 1979, Mosby-Year Book.

107. Weymuller EA: Dressings for split thickness skin graft donor sites, *Plast Laryngol* 91:652–653, 1981.

108. Winter GD: Formation of the scab and the rate of epithelisation of superficial wounds in the skin of the young domestic pig, *Nature* 193:293–294, 1962.

109. Winter GD: Healing of skin wounds and the influence of dressings on the repair process, in Harkiss KJ, editor: *Surgical dressings and wound healing*, London, 1971, Crosby Lockwood, pp 46–60.

110. Winter GD, Scales JT: Effect of air drying and dressings on the surface of a wound, *Nature* 197:91–92, 1963.

111. Wiseman DM, Rovee DT, Alvarez OM: Wound dressings: design and use, in Cohen R, Diegelmann R, Lindblad WJ, editors: *Surgical aspects of wound healing*, Philadelphia, 1992, WB Saunders, pp 562–580.

112. Yannas IV, Burke LF, Warpehoski M, et al: Prompt long term functional replacement of skin, in Wise DL, editor: *Burn wound coverings*, Boca Raton, 1984, CRC Press, vol II, pp 1–26.

113. Zitelli JA: Delayed wound healing with adhesive wound dressings, *J Dermatol Surg Oncol* 10:709–710, 1984.

114. Zitelli JA: Wound healing for the clinician, *Adv Dermatol* 2:243–268, 1987.

# CHAPTER 13

# Total-Contact Casting in the Treatment of Neuropathic Ulcers

**David R. Sinacore, Ph.D., P.T.**

**Michael J. Mueller, M.H.S., P.T.**

Multiple clinical reports* and one controlled clinical trial[22] suggest that no treatment is as effective as total-contact casting in healing grade 1 or 2 neuropathic ulcers. Few reports, however, have adequately described the method of total-contact cast application. The purpose of this chapter is to summarize the effectiveness, indications, and contraindications of total-contact casting and to detail a method of application in the treatment of select diabetic neuropathic ulcerations. In addition, some variations of the procedure are discussed to emphasize the clinical usefulness of this type of casting.

## HISTORY AND THEORY

The early use of casting for trophic ulcerations dates back to Dr. Joseph Kahn in India in the 1930s.[19] He described an ambulatory technique for the treatment of plantar ulcers occurring in patients with Hansen's disease (leprosy) as an alternative to prolonged, expensive periods of bed rest in the hospital. The technique was adapted in this country by Dr. Paul Brand in the early 1960s and popularized by him and his associates at the Gillis W. Long Hansen's Disease Center in Carville, Louisiana. The use of contact casting as a treatment for plantar surface ulcerations has since been expanded

to a variety of conditions involving insensitivity of the feet, including patients with diabetes mellitus, syringomyelocele, Charcot-Marie-Tooth disease,[7, 26] tabes dorsalis, chronic alcoholism, and herniated nucleus pulposus resulting in compression of $S_1$ and $S_2$ nerve roots, leading to motor and sensory neuropathy.

It is now well recognized that the primary factor in the cause of diabetic plantar surface ulcerations is the presence of peripheral neuropathy leading to diminished or absent sensation. This insensitivity allows excessive and prolonged stresses and pressures to occur in the diabetic foot, which ultimately results in tissue breakdown.[1, 5, 6, 12] If the tissue breakdown (ulcer) goes unnoticed or untreated, infection is imminent, and major amputation is likely.[23]

The main purpose of treating neuropathic plantar ulcerations by total-contact casting is to reduce the excessive mechanical stress and pressures (both vertical and horizontal shear) on the plantar surfaces of the feet as advocated by Brand[5, 6] and Ctercteko et al.[10] while maintaining ambulation (see also Chapters 9 and 10). The reduction of mechanical stress and relief of excessive pressures in the areas of ulceration allows healing to occur. The cast is fabricated to reduce excessive pressure at the ulcer site by spreading forces over an increased surface area of the foot and leg, thus allowing the ulcer to heal rapidly and completely. One

References 4, 13, 14, 16, 17, 21, 24, 26, 30, 31.

group[3] reported a 75% to 84% reduction in peak pressure at the first and third metatarsal heads, respectively, when a person walked in the total-contact cast compared to normal shoes. The metatarsal head region and great toe are the most frequent and susceptible areas to develop ulcerations in the diabetic patient.[7]

## EFFECTIVENESS

Total-contact casting not only has been demonstrated to be effective in reducing excessive plantar pressures but has also been shown to be an effective, ambulatory method for healing diabetic neuropathic ulcers.[4, 14, 26] Several studies[9, 14, 24–26] report the average time of healing to be 36 to 42 days. Many patients report having had a plantar surface ulcer for a number of years that would not heal until a TCC was applied. Two studies[25, 26] report patients who had chronic plantar ulcers for an average of 11 months (ranging from 1 week–13 years) despite other forms of treatment, such as daily dressing changes, antibiotic therapy, frequent callus shaving and debridement, and multiple skin grafts (Figs 13–1 and 13–2).

We[22] have conducted a controlled clinical trial that compared total-contact casting with a control group receiving traditional treatments including daily wound care, dressing changes, and footwear modifications. Nineteen of 21 (91%) ulcerations treated with total-contact casting healed in a mean time of 42 days compared with a healing rate of 32% in a mean time of 65 days in the control group. In addition, none of the casted ulcers developed an infection, whereas 26% (5 of 19 patients) of the traditional therapy group developed serious infection that required hospitalization. Of the five hospitalized patients, two required a subsequent forefoot amputation. The results of this prospective study confirm earlier descriptive studies and support our contention that total-contact casting is superior to traditional treatment methods in the rates of healing and the prevention of serious infection.

## INDICATIONS AND CONTRAINDICATIONS

The indication for total-contact casting is a grade 1 or 2[31] plantar ulcer in the presence of insensitivity (i.e., diminished or absent protective sensation on the plantar surface of the feet). Plantar ulcers that are classified as grade 1 are superficial, whereas grade 2 lesions are full thickness and may penetrate the subcutaneous fat to muscle, tendon, ligament, or bone but have not produced deep infection.[31] Some ulcerations, although not technically on the plantar surface, may actually be weight-bearing ulcers and respond well to this pressure-relieving therapy. For example, the patient with an ulcer on the lateral border of the foot secondary to a severe varus deformity may respond well to this form of therapy.

There are some distinct contraindications to total-contact casting. The presence of a deep infection (wound grades 3–5 involving deep abscess, osteomyelitis, purulent tendonitis or synovitis, or gangrene[31]) should not be casted. Antibiotic therapy and bed rest until the acute infection has subsided has been recommended.[6] If the ulcer depth is greater than the ulcer width, the ulcer should be opened to allow the deeper layers to heal and prevent premature superficial closing.

The patient with excessively fragile skin (e.g., seen with chronic corticosteroid use or stasis ulcers) either on the dorsum of the foot or leg are more likely to develop skin breakdown or abrasions with total-contact casting than patients with normal skin. Excessive edema must be treated before total-contact cast application. Fluctuating edema presents a difficult problem because total uniform contact between the cast and the limb is the essential element to success. If the foot and leg become loose in the cast, shear pressure caused by movement of the skin in the cast may delay healing and cause additional skin breakdown.

Any patient who is unsafe, unable to keep regularly scheduled follow-up visits, opposed to having a cast on the limbs, or unable to adhere to the cast precautions and instructions should not be casted. Although

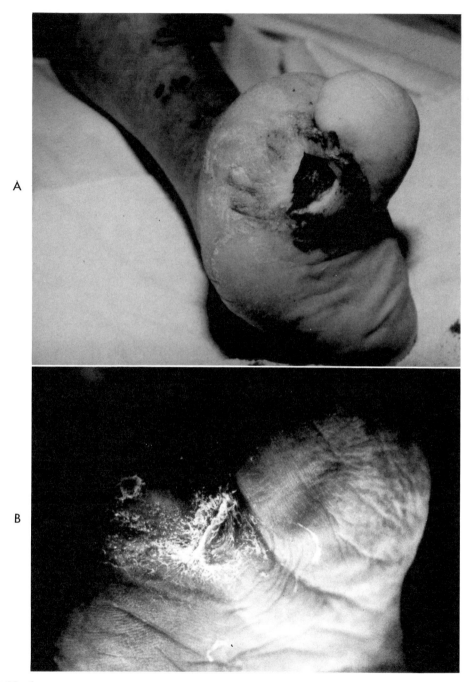

**FIG 13–1.**
**A,** 65-year-old diabetic with chronic ulcer on distal weight-bearing surface after transmetatarsal amputation. Ulcer had been present 18 months. Multiple skin grafts to area did not close the ulcer. Note thickened callus (remnants of skin grafts) surrounding perimeter of ulcer, which was debrided and pared. **B,** same ulcer after total-contact casting for 36 days. Ulcer is adequately closed but callus remains.

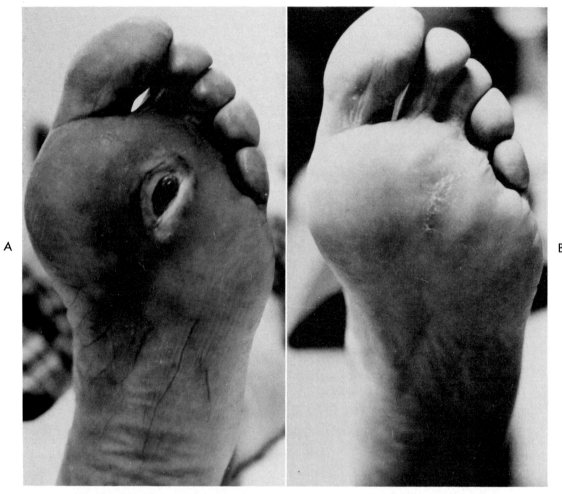

A

B

**FIG 13–2.**
**A,** ulcerated region over third metatarsal head of a 68-year-old man. This patient has been diabetic for 25 years. Ulcer had been present for 36 months despite daily dressing changes. **B,** ulcer closed after 49 days in total-contact cast. After fitting with Plastazote inserts and rocker-bottom shoes, foot shows no signs of recurrent ulceration.

total-contact casting is not strictly contraindicated in patients who are blind, ataxic, or obese, some additional caution is required. In these patients, alternative methods of therapy should be explored.

## ADVANTAGES

The major advantages to total-contact casting include the following:

1. Maintains ambulation.
2. Reduces excessive plantar pressures.
3. Protects foot from further trauma.
4. Immobilization helps localize and prevent spread of infection.

5. Controls edema.
6. Requires minimum patient compliance.

Above all, total-contact casting allows the patient to be ambulatory and eliminates the lengthy and expensive hospital costs associated with complete bed rest and nursing care. In most cases, below-knee total-contact casting allows the patient to remain working in more sedentary jobs, thereby minimizing income loss for the individual. Patients whose jobs require prolonged weight bearing (e.g., standing or walking) must limit their activity by taking leave or temporary reassignment to more sedentary duties.

The cast is fabricated to reduce excessive pressures on the plantar surface of the foot and spread the peak forces uniformly throughout the leg and entire foot. The even distribution of pressure helps eliminate or reduce edema in the limb as well. Immobilization in a cast may help to localize any minor infection and prevent the spread to adjacent tissues.[14, 22] In addition, casting will protect the insensitive foot from trauma while healing occurs.

Finally, total-contact casting requires little daily compliance by the patient or family members. There is no need for daily wound care and dressing changes. The cost of the cast is often less than the cost of dressing supplies and topical antiseptic agents.

## DISADVANTAGES

The major disadvantages of total-contact casting include the following:

1. Joint stiffness and muscle atrophy if immobilization is prolonged.
2. Possible skin abrasions or new ulcerations if cast is poorly applied or not monitored.
3. Foul odor if drainage is excessive.

If immobilization with casting is prolonged, side effects such as joint stiffness and muscular atrophy may ensue. These side effects can be minimized with proper flexibility and strengthening exercises at cast changes and after the cast is removed. Other side effects, such as bone atrophy and neuropathic (Charcot) joints have been reported, although it is not clear if these changes are consequent to the immobilization or are osseous sequelae to diabetes mellitus.[28]

If care is not taken when the cast is applied and removed, skin breakdown and new ulcerations may result. Patients who do not limit ambulation and remain full weight bearing are prone to skin abrasions. These obviously can be minimized through skill acquisition and precise cast-wearing instructions, as well as regularly scheduled follow-up visits. Even with optimal application of the cast and compliance by the patient, skin abrasions[4, 22] and fungal infections[22] can develop. In our experience, skin abrasions as a result of total-contact casting typically are

on non-weight-bearing areas and heal quickly with cessation of casting. Superficial fungal infections (most commonly *Trichophyton rubrum*) have been reported to occur on the foot or leg in approximately 15% of casted patients[22] and should be treated immediately with a topical antifungal cream such as Lotrimin cream (Schering Corp., Kenilworth, N.J.). These minor complications do not appear to delay healing of the primary ulcer. Casting should be discontinued with severe fungal infections. Casted ulcers with moderate amounts of drainage can have foul odors that are socially unacceptable. Delaying casting until drainage is minimal, or more frequent cast changes with cleaning the ulcer will minimize this problem.

## CAST APPLICATION
### Patient Preparation

The ulcer must be thoroughly evaluated for any evidence of sinuses. If the ulcer is deeper than it is wide, the ulcer should be opened to at least a width equal to its depth to ensure adequate drainage and healing of the wound's inner layers and prevent premature superficial healing. The ulcer should be cleaned with removal of all necrotic tissue. The surrounding callus should be removed or pared to reduce pressure and rigidity at the margins of the ulcer (see Chapter 2).

The ulcer size and depth are measured by a millimeter rule and depth gauge. The perimeter of the ulcer also may be traced onto clean exposed radiographic film using an indelible ink marker and placed in the patient's record for subsequent comparison measurements (Fig 13–3). We have found this a reliable and useful method of quantifying the size of the ulcer because it gives the patient visual feedback regarding the effectiveness of total-contact casting, helping to overcome any reluctance to continue the casting procedure.

After the ulcer has been evaluated, a saline solution–soaked fine mesh gauze is placed over the ulcer, covered with a dry thin dressing, and secured with paper tape (Fig 13–4). The dressing should be kept as

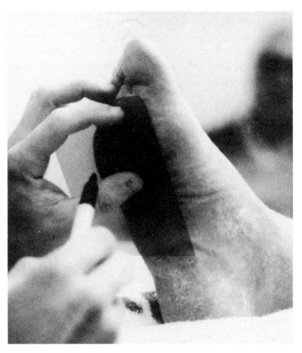

**FIG 13-3.**
Tracing size of ulcer on clean exposed radiographic film for permanent record of size of ulcer.

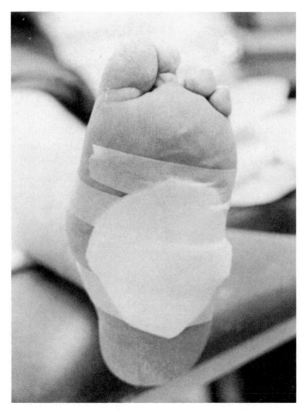

**FIG 13-4.**
Thin dressing is used to cover the ulcer in the cast.

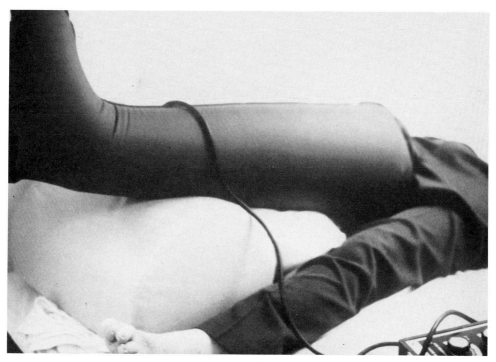

**FIG 13-5.**
Reducing edema in leg and foot using Jobst compression pump immediately before casting.

thin and small as possible to avoid excessive pressures from the dressing on the ulcer in the cast. If the ulcer is deep, a loosely packed gauze may be used to fill the ulcer to the surface, and then the thin dressing is applied. In the past, we[22] and others[31] have applied a dressing along with a topical antiseptic (povidone-iodine solution), but this is unnecessary and no longer advised.

It is common in diabetic patients with chronic plantar ulcers to have excessive foot and lower limb edema. It may be necessary to elevate the edematous foot and leg before casting to reduce the swelling. Using the Jobst compression pump (Jobst Inst., 653 Toledo, Ohio) for 30 to 60 minutes is effective in transiently reducing moderate to extensive edema (Fig 13-5).

To apply a total-contact cast, place the patient in the prone position with the affected knee and ankle flexed to 90 degrees, with the plantar surface of the ulcerated foot parallel to the floor. This position prevents further edema, takes the stretch off the gastrocnemius muscle, and allows the limb to be held up easily while the inner layers of the cast are forming, thus preventing

dents or other high-pressure areas in the cast. Patients often are unable to comfortably assume the prone position because of hip flexor tightness, low back pain, or obesity. In these patients, it is necessary to modify the position by placing a number of pillows under the abdomen or pelvis. We have found that adjustable tables, which allow one half of the table to be lowered, thus accommodating slight hip flexion, afford a comfortable position during the casting procedure (Fig 13-6).

A small amount of cotton padding or lamb's wool is placed loosely between adjacent toes to absorb any moisture and prevent maceration. A 3-in wide, closely fitting cotton stockinette is rolled over the foot and leg up to the knee. The toe end of the stockinette should be sewn closed or can be folded into the toe sulcus and taped closed. The stockinette is pulled tight so it is wrinkle free. Wrinkles occurring at the dorsum of the ankle are cut, and the edges are overlapped and taped with paper tape to prevent a seam (an area of high pressure) when the plaster is applied (Fig 13-7).

Next, a layer of foam (½-in. adhesive-

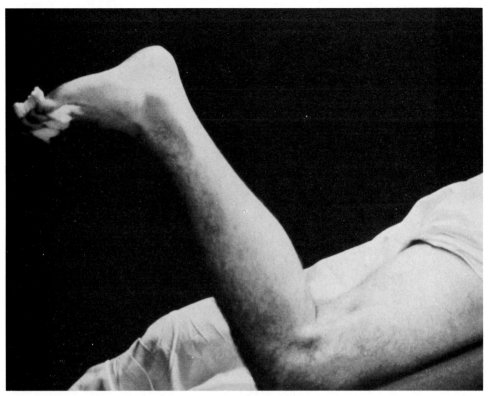

**FIG 13−6.**
Cast is applied with patient in prone position with affected limb flexed at knee and dorsiflexed at ankle. Adjustable tables modify prone position for patients unable to maintain complete hip extension. Note cotton padding placed between adjacent toes.

backed Sifoam [Omni Medical Specialties, San Diego, Calif]) or felt is applied to cover and protect all the toes. This foam layer should be placed over the closed stockinette and extended dorsally from the metatarsophalangeal area around the toes to the toe sulcus on the plantar surface (Fig 13−8). The edges of the foam should be trimmed medially and laterally and beveled to minimize pressure. The toes in the total-contact cast are enclosed in plaster to protect the insensitive foot and prevent damage to the toes from striking objects or from objects becoming lodged in the cast.

The leg should now be supported by an assistant and the foot and ankle held stable in the neutral position (90 degrees at the ankle), with the toes passively dorsiflexed only slightly. Many diabetic patients are unable to achieve the neutral, or 90-degree, position of the ankle joint secondary to joint or muscle limitations. Attempts to achieve this position passively may result in abnormal

pronation and a prominent talus or navicular bone medially. Bony prominences in the abnormally pronated foot may cause areas of high pressure in the cast, so excessive pressure to achieve the neutral position is not recommended. A small amount of equinus can be accommodated in the cast by building up the posterior portion of the sole of the cast with plaster to level the weight-bearing surface.

Two circular pieces (approximately 2 in. in diameter) of 1/8- to 1/4-in. adhesive-backed felt are then placed over the malleoli on the stockinette. The felt pieces should be beveled along the edges to reduce the pressure along the felt-plaster interface. Another felt pad 18 to 20 in. long and 2 in. wide is beveled along the edges and placed along the anterior aspect of the leg and dorsum of the foot from just below the tibial tuberosity distal to the metatarsal heads (Fig 13−8). This felt pad protects the prominent tibial crest and facilitates cast removal. The felt pads

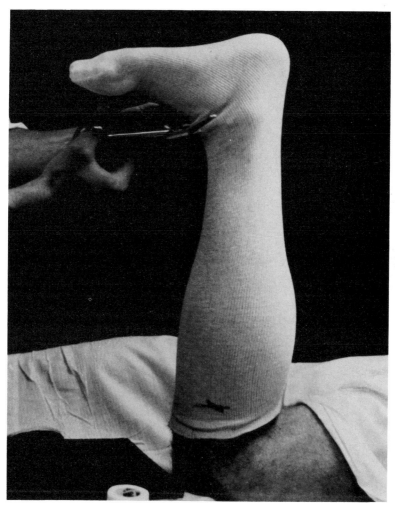

**FIG 13–7.**
Wrinkles in stockinette over dorsum of ankle are cut and edges overlapped and taped.

prevent the cast from rubbing on bony prominences. Occasionally additional bony prominences such as the styloid process of the fifth metatarsal or talonavicular area may be padded, depending on the foot type. No other padding is used.

One or two layers of extra fast–setting, creamy plaster bandage (Gypsona II [National Patent Development Corp, Dayville, Conn., Chaston Med., Melville, N.Y.]) are wrapped quickly and without tension around the lower leg and foot from the proximal to the distal aspect. The plaster bandage should commence below the previously marked fibular head (approximately 1 to 1½ inches distal) and continue distally to beyond the metatarsal heads. Care must be taken to avoid any wrinkles in the plaster.

The bandage is then rubbed continuously to conform to the shape of the foot and leg until it has set. The plaster is molded into every crevice and around bony prominences and pads (Fig 13–9). Particular attention should be given to molding the plaster to the contours of the sole of the foot. This thin layer of plaster is the most critical part of the contact cast. The patient should be instructed not to move the foot or leg once this "eggshell" layer has been applied. The assistant supporting the leg and foot should not move the foot or apply pressure to the plaster, which could distort it and cause potential areas of high pressure. The inner layer should be allowed to fully set before any more plaster is applied.

Once the inner eggshell layer of plaster

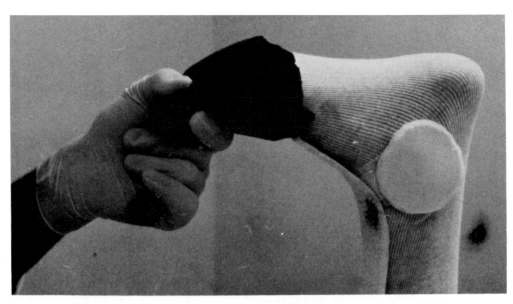

**FIG 13–8.**
Foam layer covers toes, which are enclosed in cast for protection. Felt padding is applied over malleoli and tibial crest to protect bony prominences. Felt strip along tibial crest facilitates cast removal.

has set (approximately 5 minutes), additional layers should be added for reinforcement. Plaster splints (five layers thick) approximately 30 in. long are applied anteriorly to posteriorly (Fig 13–10,A) from the dorsal surface of the toes around to the plantar aspect of the foot and up to posterior aspect of the leg. A second set of splints are wrapped in a medial to lateral direction around the calcaneus and up the proximal sides of the leg (Fig 13–10,B). These splints reinforce the plantar and posterior portions of the cast.

The cast is completed by incorporating a rubber walking heel in the plantar surface of the cast. A ¼-in. plywood board is used between the walking heel and the cast to minimize the danger of cracks in the sole of the cast from pressure on the heel. The ¼-in. plywood board should be cut smaller than the length of the foot (Fig 13–11). It should extend from the heel to the toe sulcus and be slightly narrower than the foot's width. The area between the contoured sole of the foot and the board should be filled with a plaster roll to level the plantar surface.

The placement of the walking heel is critical. The walking heel is placed on the board just behind the transverse midline of the foot (Fig 13–12). Placing the heel too far forward on the foot will cause the patient to have difficulty with balance and may cause excessive movement of the foot and leg in the cast. Placing the heel too far posteriorly will cause the patient to roll forward onto the toe of the cast. This may allow contact with the ground, breaking the toe of the cast. The walking heel is attached to the cast, and the toes are fully enclosed by an additional one or two rolls of plaster. Every attempt should be made to keep the anterior portion of the cast thin to facilitate removal. We use fiber glass tape (3M Orthopedic Products, Irving, Calif.) to attach the heel and complete the outer layers (Fig 13–13). This material is light weight, durable, quick setting, and water resistant. However, fiber glass tape is more expensive and is not molded as easily to the limb, making it unsuitable for the inner layers. We recommend the use of this material, particularly with patients who may need to bear weight soon after application.

The completed cast should be allowed to dry thoroughly. As an added precaution, the patient is instructed not to bear weight for at least 24 hours after application to allow the inner layers to harden. Before the patient is dismissed, the cast should be checked for proper fit and instructed in proper cast care and precautions.

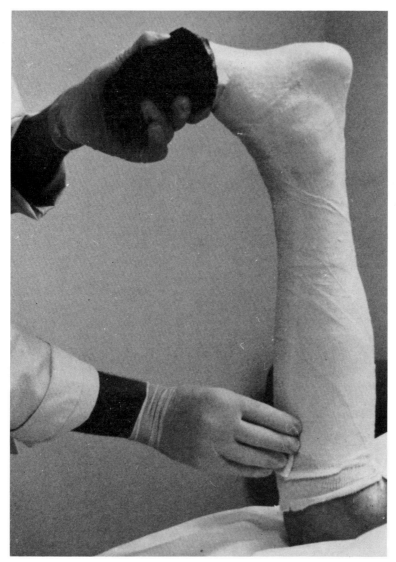

**FIG 13–9.**
First layer of plaster is continuously molded around bony prominences to conform to foot and leg until it has set.

## Instructions to Patients

The patient with a total-contact walking cast should be given meticulous instruction in the care and monitoring of the cast. Because the foot lacks protective sensation, the patient must be instructed to watch for signs of intolerance and problems. We routinely obtain written informed consent before casting to ensure the patient understands the purpose of total-contact casting and to explain the risks involved and all precautions to be taken. We have found that providing detailed, written instructions to be useful, including an explanation of the purpose of the cast and how it differs from an ordinary below-knee cast. An emergency telephone number for contact, should problems occur, must be provided to all patients. An example of these written instructions and some helpful reminders regarding the care of the cast are provided in Figure 13–14. If the patient experiences any one or a combination of the following signs, the cast should be removed and the ulcer inspected immediately:

1. Excessive swelling of the leg or foot, causing the cast to become too tight.

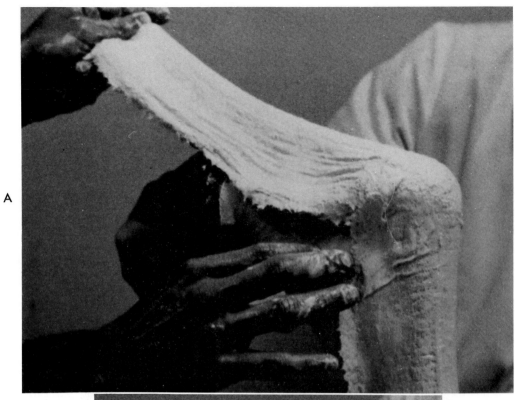

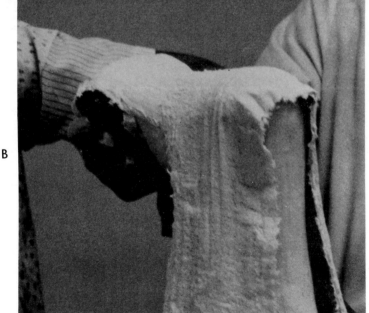

**FIG 13–10.**

**A** and **B,** layers of plaster splints are applied to medial, lateral, posterior, and plantar walls of cast for strength.

2. Excessive mobility of the foot in the cast.
3. Drainage through the cast.
4. Deep cracks or soft spots in the cast.
5. Sudden tenderness in the inguinal lymph nodes.
6. Sudden increase in body temperature.
7. Complaints of discomfort or pain.

In addition to instruction in the warning signs, the patient should be taught proper ambulation, with emphasis on limitation of

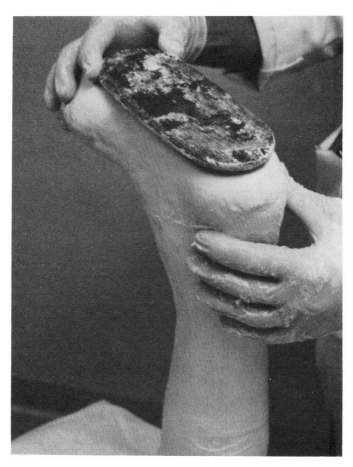

**FIG 13–11.**
A ¼-in. plywood board is placed between walking heel and cast. Space between board and contoured cast is filled with plaster for support and to level plantar surface for walking.

walking distance and frequency. The less the patient walks, the less stress on the foot. In the absence of excessive stress, the ulcer will heal quickly. The patient is encouraged to avoid fast walking, shorten stride length, avoid excessive push-off in late stance, and to limit ambulation to one third of the normal daily routine. We routinely issue crutches or a walker to decrease weight bearing and improve balance. If patients develop low back pain or leg pain, a temporary lift may be added to the opposite shoe to level the pelvis.

## FOLLOW-UP VISITS

The initial cast is left on no more than 5 to 7 days. The cast should be changed even earlier if it becomes loose. Moderate or excessive edema at the time of the initial cast application will decrease, leaving the cast too loose to provide the needed total-contact fit. The cast is removed using a standard cast saw and spreaders. Cuts are made along the anterior surface from proximal to distal along the felt strip, then medial to lateral at the level of the ankle (Fig 13–15). It should be remembered that the anterior wall of the cast is thin compared with the other walls, so caution must be taken.

At the first cast change, the ulcer is re-evaluated. The perimeter of the ulcer is re-traced on the exposed radiographic film to document any change in ulcer size. The first cast change also provides the opportunity to evaluate the patient's response to the cast.[9] Skin temperature checks will detect any local inflammation caused by the cast rubbing on the skin,[9] so future modifications can be made.

This first cast change also provides the opportunity to begin preparation for definitive footwear for the diabetic patient. Cus-

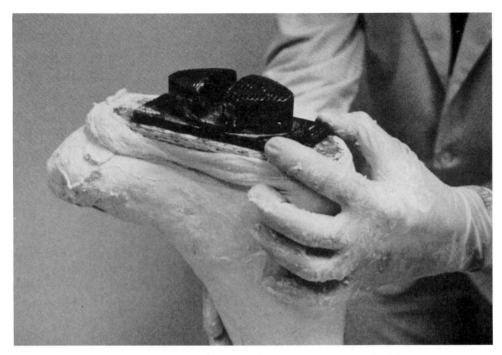

**FIG 13–12.**
Placement of walking heel on board just behind tranverse midline of foot.

tom shoes and insole fabrication require a negative mold of the foot. Because edema should be resolved, the foot can be casted at this time to allow time for fabrication. Although this practice is time consuming, it will ultimately save time and expense and provide protection when the ulcer is healed.

The cast may now be reapplied as previously described. The next cast may be left in place for up to 2 weeks. Casts should be changed more frequently in the presence of significant edema or drainage. At each cast change, the ulcer should be evaluated and the cast reapplied if healing is incomplete. For individuals whose compliance is questionable, more frequent monitoring and cast changes are recommended.

If the ulcer has healed, the patient should be placed immediately in appropriate therapeutic footwear (see Chapter 25). Custom-molded insoles with rigid rocker bottom shoes are recommended for forefoot ulcers.[5] In addition to the appropriate footwear, the patient must be carefully instructed in monitoring the newly healed ulcer. Brand[5] points out that the newly healed ulcer is particularly susceptible to reulceration within the first month after healing. This is because of the poor capacity of scar tissue to accommodate shear stress.[5] The diabetic patient with a newly healed ulcer should be instructed to increase weight-bearing activities slowly, continue using ambulatory aids, and frequently check skin temperature to identify local warm spots on the feet that may indicate inflammation. Frequent follow-up visits *after* the cast is removed are mandatory to educate the patient and reinforce the roles of excessive pressure and insensitivity.

## PRECAUTIONS

The methods of cast application just described should be detailed enough to replicate; however, caution is necessary. Thorough training and practice in the cast application are requisite to ensure success and to minimize the potential side effects and sequelae of immobilizing an insensitive foot.[4] The application of total-contact casts on an insensitive foot requires considerable skill. We recommend visiting a facility or medical center that regularly performs total-contact casting to observe, learn, and practice the application of these casts before one

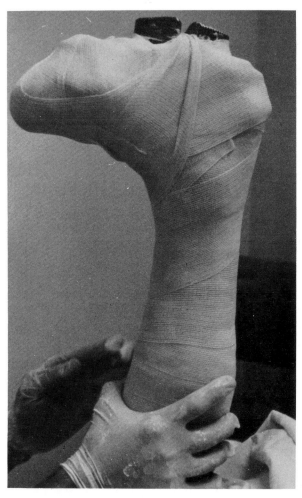

**FIG 13–13.**
Completed cast. Weight bearing should be delayed 24 hours to allow inner layers to thoroughly set.

attempts them alone. An excellent videotape depicting this method is available on a 2 weeks' loan basis from the U.S. Public Health Service.* The treatment of diabetic neuropathic ulcers by this method requires a strong commitment and willingness on the part of the diabetic foot care team members (or individuals applying the cast) to respond quickly to patients' complaints or problems at any time.

The keys to minimizing potential side effects and successful management by this method are close and frequent monitoring of the ulcer and the patient's tolerance to the casting procedure. Strict patient compliance with subsequent follow-up visits are paramount. If patients are unable or unwilling to

*The videotape is available from Gillis W. Long Hansen's Disease Center, Dept. of Education and Training, 5445 Point Clair Rd, Carville, LA 70721-9607.

be followed up regularly as outpatients, development of complications from the casts are inevitable, and this method should not be employed.

## MODIFICATION OF BELOW-KNEE WALKING CAST

Several modifications to the original total-contact below-knee walking cast have been suggested.[2, 8, 11, 18] The molded double-rocker plaster shoe is one such modification (Fig 13–16).[11, 18] The plaster shoe is molded over the entire foot but ends at the ankle (below the malleoli). The wooden double-rocker platform is attached to the molded foot, and the medial and lateral arches are filled with plaster to complete the weight-bearing surface. As with the below-knee cast, placement of the double-rocker plat-

## Total-Contact Cast Instructions

You have had a total-contact cast applied to your foot for the purpose of healing the ulcer (sore) on your foot. These ulcers do not heal because of the extremely high pressures on the sole of the foot during walking. The cast was made to decrease the pressure on the ulcer, thereby allowing the ulcer to heal. In addition to the pressure relief, the cast is designed to be very snug fitting with the toes enclosed for protection.

For the total contact cast to be effective, you must know how to take care of your cast. The following is a list of what to do and *not* to do.

- Do not bear weight or walk on your cast until you are told to do so by the person putting the cast on your foot. Usually no weight bearing is allowed for 24 to 48 hours after the cast is applied. This allows the inner layers of plaster to dry thoroughly.
- After 24 to 48 hours, you may resume walking. We recommend you limit your walking and standing to one third of the normal daily routine or walking distance.
- Never use the cast to strike or hit objects. Dents, cracks, or softened areas of the cast may cause excessive pressure on your foot in the cast and should be reported immediately.
- Keep the cast dry at all times. Water will destroy your cast. Sponge bathing is recommended instead of showering while in your cast. Use a rubberized short leg disposable sleeve to protect the cast when bathing. *Do not submerge your cast in water.* If the cast does become wet, dry it immediately with a towel or hair dryer set to "cool." If it rains, cover the cast with a plastic bag.
- Your cast may be inconvenient, and you may have difficulty sleeping. This is not uncommon. You may try wrapping the cast in a towel or placing it on a pillow while in bed.
- After you have been wearing the cast several days, perspiration and dirt may cause itching of the skin inside the cast. This is common. You must ignore it. Do not stick pencils or coat hangers or other objects in the cast to scratch the skin.
- Inspect the entire cast daily. Look and feel for deep cracks or soft spots on the cast. Use a small hand mirror to inspect the sole of the cast or have a family member check the sole of the cast.
- Never attempt to remove your cast by yourself.

REMOVING YOUR CAST

We have a specially designed saw to remove the cast with little discomfort. It should be removed only by a health care professional. After removal, your skin may be flaky and dry, and your joint may feel stiff. Apply a thick cream or oil for several days to moisten and soften the skin. Your therapist will show you exercises to decrease the stiffness in your foot.

You will need to have your specially made shoes ready to wear immediately after the cast is removed to prevent your foot from getting another ulcer.

You should continue to use crutches or a walker for several weeks after the ulcer is healed to help protect your foot. Be sure and talk to your doctor or therapist about protecting the foot after the cast is removed.

WARNING SIGNS:

*If any of the following signs or symptoms occur call (phone number).*

1. Excessive swelling of the leg or foot if the cast becomes too tight.
2. The cast becomes too loose and your leg can move up or down in the cast greater than 1/4 inch.
3. The cast has any deep cracks or soft spots.
4. Any drainage of pus or blood on the outside of the cast. This will appear brownish or dark yellow.
5. Any foul-smelling odor of the cast.
6. You experience any excessive tenderness in your groin or the casted foot.
7. Any excessive leg pain or annoying pressure in the ankle or foot which will not go away.
8. You notice any sudden onset of fever or an unusual elevation in your blood sugar. We highly recommend daily self-monitoring of your blood glucose during casting if you are not already doing so.

*If any of the above conditions exist, do the following:*

1. Notify appropriate professional personnel at once (provide phone number).
2. Do not walk on your cast. Keep your leg elevated.
3. Use crutches or a walker and keep the casted foot off the ground until seen by professional personnel.

**FIG 13–14.**
Initial contact cast instructions.

form on the sole is critical. It should be placed so that the center of the posterior rocker bar is aligned with the center of the medial malleolus and the front edge of the anterior rocker bar is immediately behind the first metatarsal head.

We believe the primary use for the rocker-bottom plaster shoe is for patients with superficial plantar ulcers who have fragile skin or concomitant stasis ulcers on the lower leg (i.e., who may not tolerate a below-knee cast) (see Fig 13–17). Several de-

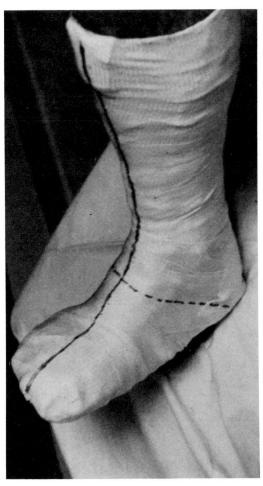

**FIG 13–15.**
Lines on cast indicate where cuts should be made when removing cast. Single cut is made along felt strip. Additional cuts (if necessary) may be carefully made on either side of ankle.

scriptive studies report favorable healing rates and quick healing times with this method.[8, 11, 18, 25] These reports also are quick to point out that the molded double-rocker plaster shoes were more socially acceptable, less costly to fabricate, and may have less risk associated with them than the below-knee cast.

Another alternative to total-contact casting is a walking splint or a padded ankle-foot orthosis.[2] A walking splint is fabricated using a method similar to the total-contact cast except that the anterior portion of the cast is removed. The splint is secured to the foot and leg with elastic bandages. Birke et al.[2] indicate that use of the walking splint is advisable in patients with hypotrophic skin,

active infection, poor circulation, or fear of being casted. The obvious advantage of the walking splint is that it can be removed to frequently and easily observe the skin and ulcer. A potential disadvantage is that the patient may not comply with reapplication of the splint. An alternative to a plaster walking splint is a prefabricated padded ankle-foot orthosis (Fig 13–18). The plantar healing orthosis, an orthosis similar to the one in Figure 13–18, is available commercially (Alimed, Inc., Dedham, Mass.). We agree that alternative methods to below-knee total-contact casting are indicated when complicating factors are present. However, if total-contact casting is not contraindicated, our experience indicates these alternative methods may not have as rapid healing rates as treatment with below-knee total-contact casting. Further research is needed to determine if healing rates with removable splints and other alternative methods are comparable with healing rates using below-knee total-contact casting.

## Case Study

A 55-year-old man with type II diabetes mellitus (reported 22 years' duration) had bilateral plantar ulcerations beneath the right first metatarsal head and left third metatarsal head (Fig 13–19,A). Each grade 1 ulcer measured approximately 5 $cm^2$ and was 1 to 2 mm deep. Both ulcers had been reported present for 18 months. This patient demonstrated severe sensory neuropathy in both feet, as evidenced by an inability to sense the 6.10 Semmes-Weinstein monofilament. Peripheral pulses were present and palpable on both feet. Bilateral Doppler ankle-arm indices were 1.0. We typically cast the foot with the larger ulcer first, because patients do not tolerate bilateral casts because of difficulty with ambulation. A total-contact cast was initially applied to the right foot, and dressing changes were continued on the left foot. He was instructed in the use of a walker. The initial cast was changed in 1 week. Subsequent casts were changed every 2 weeks, with complete healing in 65 days (Fig 13–19,B). He was immediately fit with a rigid rocker-bottom shoe containing an accommodative, total-contact insert for the newly healed ulcer.

The ulcer on the left foot did not significantly change in size during casting of the right foot.

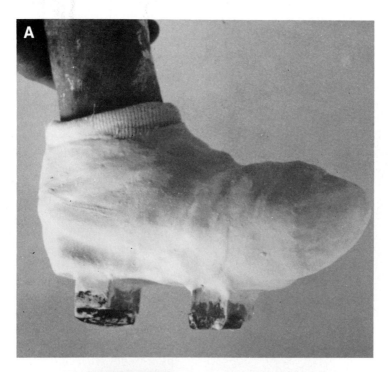

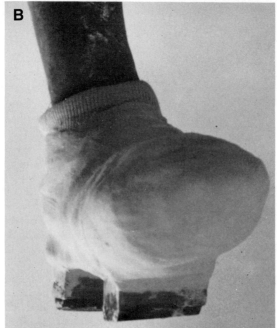

**FIG 13–16.**
Molded double rocker shoe. **A,** lateral view. **B,** oblique view.

---

**FIG 13–17.**
**A,** chronic neuropathic ulcer in cuneiform metatarsal region of 66-year-old diabetic woman. Ulcer had been present for 10 months before casting. **B,** after 39 days in molded double-rocker plaster shoe. Ulcer is well healed.

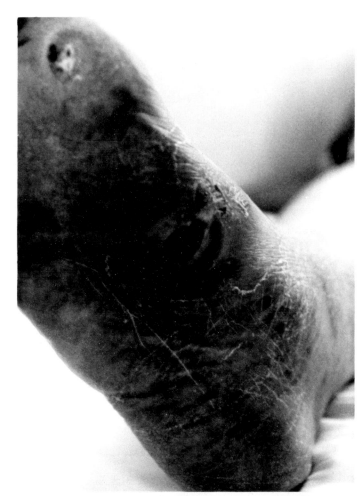

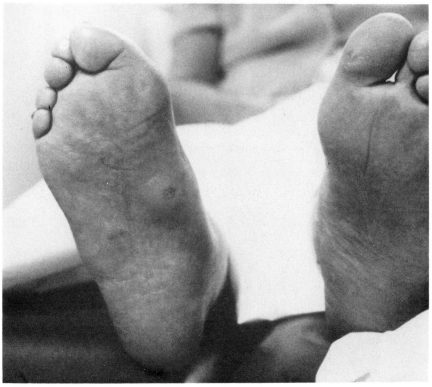

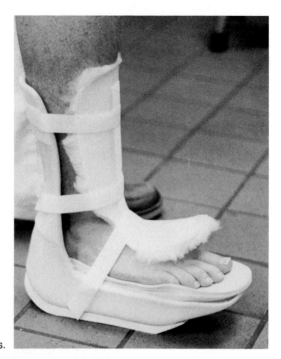

**FIG 13–18.**
Prefabricated total-contact posterior ankle-foot orthosis.

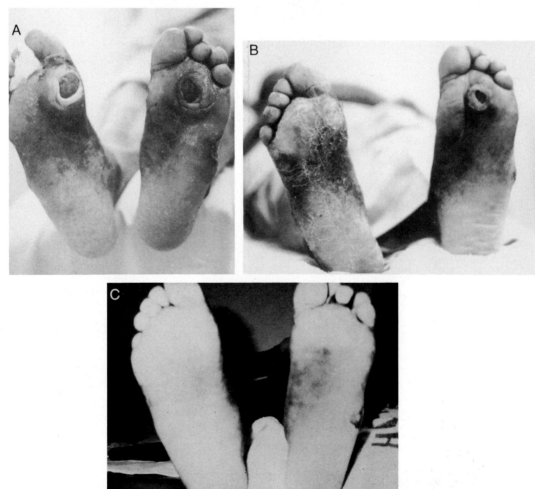

Casting then was begun on the left foot after a similar procedure. Healing of the ulcer on the left foot was complete in 42 days. After the left plantar ulcer healed (Fig 13–19,C), the patient was fit with another rocker-bottom shoe and total-contact accommodative insert. After both plantar ulcers were healed, we encouraged him to continue to use the walker and to remain partial weight bearing on the left foot for an additional 2 weeks to allow further maturation of the recently healed ulcer. After 2 weeks, this patient ambulated independently without ulcers or an assistive device.

## SUMMARY

Total-contact casting is an effective, rapid, and ambulatory therapy for healing the diabetic neuropathic plantar ulcer. The skill and technique of application appear to be worth mastering, because the reported benefits greatly outweigh potential complications. In addition, with growing pressures for shortened hospital stays, the total-contact casting method provides an effective and cost-prudent alternative to prolonged, expensive periods of bed rest in the hospital.

## Acknowledgment

We thank The late Steven J. Rose, P.T., Ph.D., for early guidance and support; Ronna S. Delitto, M.H.S., P.T., for assistance with the photographs used in this chapter; and Jay E. Diamond, M.H.S., P.T., for his contributions to and critical review of the manuscript.

## REFERENCES

1. Bauman JH, Girling JP, Brand PW: Plantar pressures and trophic ulceration: an evaluation of footwear, *J Bone Joint Surg* 45:652, 1963.

2. Birke JA, Novick A, Graham SL, et al: Methods of treating plantar ulcers, *Phys Ther* 71:116–122, 1991.

3. Birke JA, Sims DA, Buford WL: Walking casts: effect of plantar foot pressures, *J Rehabil Res Dev* 22:18, 1985.

4. Boulton AJM, Bowker JH, Gadia M, et al: Use of plaster casts in the management of diabetic neuropathic foot ulcers, *Diabetes Care* 9:149–152, 1986.

5. Brand PW: The insensitive foot, in Jahss MM, editor: *Disorders of the foot*, Philadelphia, 1982, WB Saunders, vol 2.

6. Brand PW: The diabetic foot, in Ellenberg M, Rifkin H, editors: *Diabetes mellitus*, Garden City, NY, 1983, Medical Examination Publishing Co.

7. Brenner MA: An ambulatory approach to the neuropathic ulceration, *J Am Podiatr Assoc* 64:862, 1974.

8. Burden AC, Jones GR, Jones R, et al: Use of the "Scotchcast boot" in treating diabetic foot ulcers, *Br Med J* 286:1555, 1983.

9. Coleman WC, Brand PW, Birke JA: The total contact cast: a therapy for plantar ulceration on insensitive feet, *J Am Podiatr Assoc* 74:548, 1984.

10. Ctercteko GC, Dhanendran M, Hutton WC, et al: Vertical forces acting on the feet of diabetic patients with neuropathic ulceration, *Br J Surg* 68:608, 1981.

11. Diamond JE, Sinacore DR, Mueller MJ: Molded double-rocker plaster shoe for healing a diabetic plantar ulcer, *Phys Ther* 67:1550–1552, 1987.

12. Ellenberg M: Diabetic neuropathic ulcer, *J Mt Sinai Hosp* 35:585, 1968.

13. Gleckman RA, Roth RM: Diabetic foot infections—preventions and treatment, *West J Med* 142:263, 1985.

14. Helm PA, Walker SC, Pullium G: Total contact casting in diabetic patients with neuropathic foot ulcerations, *Arch Phys Med Rehabil* 65:691, 1984.

15. Holstein P, Larsen K, Sager P: Decompression with the aid of insoles in the treatment of diabetic neuropathic ulcers, *Acta Orthop Scand* 47:463, 1976.

16. Jacobs RL: Neuropathic foot in the diabetic patient, in Bateman JE, editor: *Foot science*, Philadelphia, 1976, WB Saunders.

17. Jacobs RL, Karmody AM: Office care of the insensitive foot, *Foot Ankle* 2:230, 1982.

18. Joseph B, Joshua S, Fritschi EP: The molded double-rocker plaster shoe in the field treatment of plantar ulcer, *Lepr Rev* 54:39, 1983.

19. Kahn JS: Treatment of leprous trophic ulcers, *Lepr India* 11:19, 1939.

20. Larsen K, Christiansen JS, Ebskov B: Prevention and treatment of ulcerations of the foot in unilaterally amputated diabetic patients, *Acta Orthop Scand* 53:481, 1982.

**FIG 13–19.**
Bilateral plantar surface ulcers in a 55-year-old patient with type II diabetes mellitus. **A,** before total-contact casting. **B,** after 65 days of total-contact casting to right foot only. **C,** after 42 days of total-contact casting to left foot. See text for full case history.

21. Lee EH, Bose K: Orthopedic management of diabetic foot lesions, *Ann Acad Med* 14:331, 1985.

22. Mueller MJ, Diamond JE, Sinacore DR, et al: Total contact casting in treatment of diabetic plantar ulcers: controlled clinical trial, *Diabetes Care* 12:384–388, 1989.

23. Pecoraro RE, Reiber GE, Burgess EM: Pathways to diabetic limb amputation: basis for prevention, *Diabetes Care* 13:513–521, 1990.

24. Pollard JP, LeQuesne LP: Method of healing diabetic forefoot ulcers, *Br Med J* 286:436, 1983.

25. Pring DJ, Casiebanca N: Simple plantar ulcers treated by below-knee plaster and molded double-rocker plaster shoe—a comparative study, *Lepr Rev* 53:261, 1982.

26. Sinacore DR, Mueller MJ, Diamond JE, et al: Diabetic neuropathic ulcers treated by total contact casting, *Phys Ther* 67:1543–1549, 1987.

27. Soderberg G: Follow-up of application of plaster-of-paris casts for non-infected plantar ulcers in field conditions, *Lepr Rev* 41:184–190, 1970.

28. Staple TW: Radiography of the diabetic foot, in Levin ME, O'Neal LW, editors: *The diabetic foot*, ed 3, St Louis, 1983, Mosby-Year Book.

29. Tappin JW, Pollard J, Beckett EA: Method of measuring "shearing" forces on the sole of the foot, *Clin Phys Physiol Meas* 1:83, 1980.

30. Walker SC, Helm PA, Pullium G: Total contact casting and chronic diabetic neuropathic foot ulcerations: healing rates by wound location, *Arch Phys Med Rehabil* 68:217–221, 1987.

31. Wagner FW: Treatment of the diabetic foot, *Compr Ther* 10:29, 1984.

# CHAPTER 14

# Adjunctive Hyperbaric Oxygen Therapy in Treatment of Diabetic Foot Wounds

**Paul Cianci, M.D.**

**Thomas K Hunt, M.D.**

Diabetes mellitus affects 5% to 6% of the population (half of cases are undiagnosed).[10] The annual cost of care exceeds $20.4 billion. At any given time perhaps 1 million diabetic patients have lower limb ulcers. Twenty percent of hospital admissions of diabetics are because of lower limb problems.[6] The incidence of amputation is 6 per 1,000. Diabetics accounted for 50% to 70% of the 118,000 amputations performed in the United States in 1983. Nine percent required amputation of a foot, 31% of the lower leg, and 30% lost at or above the knee.[47] The cost of a primary amputation was recently reported to be in excess of $40,000.[54] Medicare reimbursement for primary amputation is approximately $12,500. The morbidity and mortality associated with amputation are significant. Ipsilateral, often higher amputation will occur in 22% of cases. Contralateral amputation occurs at a rate of approximately 10% per year. Sixty-eight percent of elderly amputees will be alive at 4 years,[25] and only 40% to 50% will be rehabilitated.[19] The length of hospital stay for primary amputation varies widely but has been reported to average 40.3 days.[6] Six to 9 months may be necessary to maximize walking ability.[45] The cost of amputation is in excess of $1.5 billion yearly. Readmission within 2 years for stump modi-

fication or reamputation represents an additional $1 billion expenditure.[14]

Clearly, primary amputation is far from an expeditious solution to the problem of foot wounds in diabetics. An aggressive, multidisciplinary team approach to diabetic foot management can result in improved salvage and significant cost savings.[14] We have used this approach at our community hospital since 1983. Patients are quickly evaluated, are seen by appropriate specialists, revascularized aggressively, and, when indicated, receive hyperbaric oxygen therapy as an adjunct to their medical and surgical care. This chapter is a comment on this experience.

## DIABETIC FOOT

The diabetic foot is characterized by sensory, motor, and autonomic neuropathy and macrovascular disease. These may lead to ulceration, infection, gangrene, and amputation. Motor neuropathy may lead to alteration of pressure distribution. Foot deformities and altered sensation can lead to ulceration. The classical plantar ulcer is caused by the loss of sensation and painless trauma. This can occur in the absence of ischemia and frequently heals with conservative measures such as unweighting and aggressive wound management (see Chapter 2). Primary management is directed to patient education and foot care. Autonomic neuropathy may cause alterations in blood flow and diversion of nutritive flow, resulting in cutaneous ischemia.[26] Ulcers associated with cutaneous ischemia may be associated with pathophysiologic alterations involving small cutaneous vessels in addition to the contribution of arterial insufficiency. Many diabetics have areas of low flow and hypoxia in their feet and ankles even in the presence of palpable pulses. Contributing factors may be increased blood viscosity, platelet aggregation, and accelerated capillary endothelial growth.[1, 2, 58] Recently it has been suggested that capillary hyperfusion and vasodilatation lead to injury via subendothelial deposition of macromolecules.[92] Progressive capillary wall hyalinization leads to capillary obstruction.[28, 84] Surgical revascularization can often provide the necessary substrate for wound healing. Some wounds, however, fail to heal, even in the presence of restored circulation and when tissue perfusion appears adequate.[89] Defective wound healing appears to be a major factor contributing to limb loss.[70] Thrombosis also predisposes to ulceration and gangrene. "In the diabetic, response to local tissue stresses is thrombosis and necrosis as opposed to inflammatory response in nondiabetics."[43] Some investigators believe that tight control of blood glucose concentration may slow or even reverse this process.[66, 69, 74] Regardless of mechanism, however, the net result of this pathologic condition is a focal hypoxia that involves regions of the foot or ankle, often toes, or the lateral side of the foot. Hyperbaric oxygen therapy, therefore, may favorably influence outcome.

Hyperbaric oxygen (HBO) therapy is not new, having been used since 1943.[20] Modern therapy dates to the early 1960s, when Dutch investigators demonstrated the efficacy of HBO therapy in gas gangrene and anemic states.[7, 8] Hyperbaric oxygen therapy is presently used as primary treatment for decompression sickness (the bends), air embolism, and severe carbon monoxide poisoning.[29, 46, 90] Adjunctive indications include clostridial myonecrosis,[8, 34, 38] crush injury and traumatic ischemias,[78, 80, 82] enhancement of healing in selected problem wounds,[22] necrotizing soft tissue infections,[4, 31, 75] refractory osteomyelitis,[21, 22, 61, 78] radiation damage to soft or hard tissue,[56, 63] compromised skin grafts or flaps,[44, 82, 93] and burns.[13, 15, 16, 33] All of these conditions have focal hypoperfusion, hypoxia, or both in common.

## RATIONALE FOR THERAPY: ROLE OF OXYGEN IN HEALING

Injuries damage microvasculature and initiate several chemattractant and growth factor pathways, including coagulation, platelet degranulation, and complement generation. Consequently, inflammatory cells (which consume oxygen) collect at the site. In this manner, most injuries and infections create "energy-poor" environments characterized by low oxygen tensions, low pH, and high lactate concentrations. Macrophages, which release lactate aerobically and anaerobically, sense this environment and because of it release potent growth factors resulting in a brisk angiogenesis and multiplication of fibroblasts at the wound margins.[49] The primary stimulator of growth factor secretion by inflammatory cells appears to be the high lactate concentration. As macrophages move into the injured area, fibroblasts begin to multiply and migrate after them. Endothelial buds then appear from venules and follow the fibroblasts into the hypoxic, highly lactated area. Under the influence of the lactate, fibroblasts transcribe collagen genes and synthesize collagen.

Most, and perhaps all, of these events can proceed in very low oxygen tensions.[51] However, fibroblasts must modify the collagen they synthesize so that it can be polymerized and secreted into the extracellular space. This vital step can be accomplished only when oxygen is present at rather high partial pressures (Fig 14–1).[72]

Thus, collagen is deposited most rapidly when both lactate and oxygen concentra-

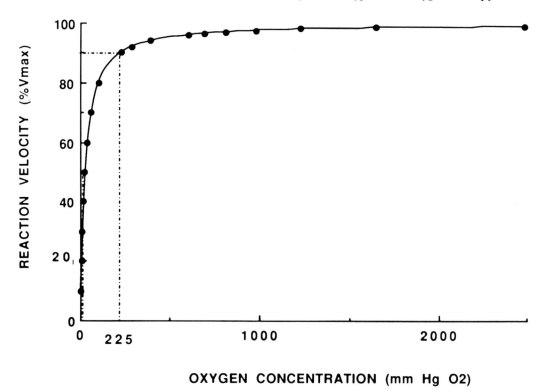

**FIG 14–1.**
Kinetics of prolyl hydroxylase (Km = 25 mm Hg). Reaction velocity of prolyl hydroxylase depends on the concentration of oxygen in the endoplasmic reticulum, with half maximal velocity (*Km*) at about 20 mm Hg. Normally the $P_{O_2}$ there varies between a few to perhaps 50 mm Hg. Normal mean probably is in the region of 30 to 40 mm Hg. In foot lesions in diabetics the number of focal areas at which $P_{O_2}$ is zero increases markedly, and the mean may fall close to zero. Clearly there is better collagen deposition at somewhat higher levels.

tions are high. The idea that process can be initiated by "energy deficit" and accelerated by hyperoxia is not paradoxical because macrophages release lactate even in well-oxygenated environments and continue to produce it in well-oxygenated wounds. The stimulus to collagen production, lactate, remains, therefore, even during hyperoxia. The need for oxygen persists well into the healing process because "new collagen" must be deposited as "old collagen" is lysed. Production must accommodate to degradation if wounds are to heal and maintain strength.

The mechanism of the oxygen effect rests at least partly on one important step in collagen biosynthesis, the hydroxylation of proline and lysine residues in procollagen. In the synthetic pathway of collagen, proline and lysine are incorporated into the growing peptide chain and are hydroxylated later when the peptides enter the endoplasmic reticulum. These hydroxylations are necessary for polymerization and cross-linkage of procollagen strands and transport of collagen molecules to the extracellular space. This process proceeds at one half maximal rate at $P_{O_2}$ 20 mm Hg and 90% maximal rate at about 200 mm Hg (see Fig 14–1). Thus, collagen *deposition*, the process that fills tissue defects and supports new blood vessels, proceeds in proportion to transcutaneous oxygen pressure ($tcP_{O_2}$) throughout and even beyond the whole physiologic range.[68]

Cell replication also requires oxygen. Fibroblast and vascular endothelial cells replicate most rapidly at about 40 mm Hg, whereas epidermal cells replicate best at about 700 mm Hg![59]

Any interference with oxygen delivery to wounds also increases susceptibility to infection. Raising $P_{O_2}$ levels, conversely, enhances resistance. In a sense, this has been obvious to surgeons for centuries. Wounds of the extremities are often infected, whereas those in tissues that have higher blood flow and tissue oxygen tensions, such as the tongue or face, rarely are. The difference is blood flow and consequently the $P_{O_2}$ in the wounds. Leukocytes kill most effectively when supplied with abundant oxygen (Fig 14–2).[55] Phagocytosis stimulates a huge, often 20-fold increase in oxygen consumption, the so-called respiratory burst, which produces superoxide, peroxide, and other active oxygen species (oxygen radicals) that, when released into phagosomes, are lethal to many bacteria. This oxidative mech-

anism is at its best in high oxygen tensions, even up to several hundred millimeters of mercury.[73] The key enzyme that converts oxygen to superoxide has kinetics similar to those of prolyl hydroxylase. It fails rapidly as tissue oxygen tensions fall to less than 30 to 40 mm Hg. Oxidative killing and antibiotic killing of bacteria are independent mechanisms and are additive in wounds (Fig 14–3).[40, 48]

Well-perfused and oxygenated myocutaneous flaps are resistant to infection and infectious gangrene. Random flaps, which have low distal oxygen tensions (analogous

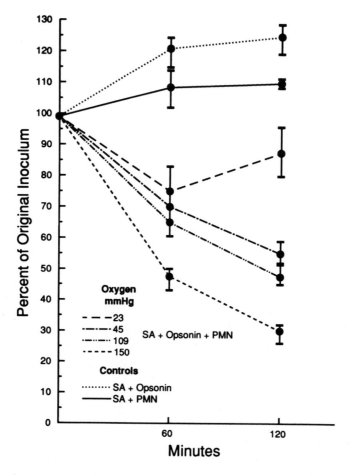

**FIG 14–2.**
This study reinforces the validity of the kinetic approach noted in Figure 14–1. Mean (± SE [*brackets*]) phagocytic killing of *staphylococcus aureus (SA)* under different oxygen tensions. *SA*, rabbit peritoneal leukocytes *(PMN)*, and opsonin (10% normal human serum) were tumbled for 30 minutes at 4° C in a total volume of 1 mL. Each tube was decanted into a culture dish so that the suspension was 1 mm thick; an aliquot was removed for determination of the number of colony-forming units (CFUs) of SA. Dishes were placed under different oxygen tensions at 37° C, and removed after 60 or 120 minutes, when the number of CFUs of the initial inoculum was counted. At least six separate experiments at each oxygen tension were performed, each in duplicate. As oxygen tension increases staphylococcal survival decreases, reflecting increased killing by PMNs. *(Courtesy of Jon Mader.)*

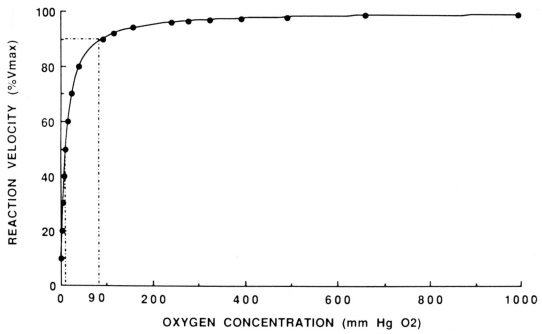

**FIG 14–3.**
Kinetics of NADPH-linked oxidase of leukocytes. Curve describing NADPH-linked oxidase conversion of molecular oxygen to superoxide ($O_2^-$) (compare with Fig 14–1). Km is variously estimated at 8 and 25 mm Hg. Thus the $V_{max}$ will vary from approximately 80 to 250 mm Hg. The oxidative antibacterial system is particularly directed at the usual wound pathogens, such as *staphylococcus, streptococcus, and Escherichia coli.*

to the low oxygen tensions measured near diabetic foot ulcers),[76] are susceptible to infection and suffer a high degree of necrosis secondary to infection.[11, 30, 42, 71] Oxygen administration to elevate $Po_2$ values to more than 100 mm Hg minimizes infectious necrosis.

## ANGIOGENESIS

Stimulation and regulation of angiogenesis are similar in principle to those of collagen synthesis. Increased lactate concentration stimulates macrophages to produce angiogenic substance or substances that are mainly chemattractants to endothelial cell migration. Removing the lactate removes the stimulus. The effect occurs in the presence of oxygen, and there is no doubt that angiogenesis occurs most rapidly when it proceeds from a high oxygen tension to a low one and from a low lactate environment to a high one.[49, 56] What is known of the mechanism is compatible with clinical observations of increased angiogenesis during HBO therapy.

## HYPERBARIC OXYGEN THERAPY

The Undersea and Hyperbaric Medical Society, an international scientific organization and the leading authority for diving and hyperbaric medicine in the United States, defines HBO therapy as the intermittent administration of 100% oxygen *inhaled* at pressure greater than sea level. The technique may be implemented in a walk-in (multiplace) chamber (Fig 14–4) compressed to depth with air while the patient breathes 100% oxygen via head tent, face mask, or endotracheal tube (Fig 14–5). Alternatively the patient may be treated in a one-person (monoplace) chamber (Fig 14–6) pressurized to depth with oxygen. In either case, the arterial partial pressure of oxygen will approach 1,500 mm Hg at the pressure equivalent of 33 ft of seawater (2 atmospheres absolute [ATA], 10 m).

### Topical Oxygen Therapy

Topical oxygen therapy rendered in small limb–encasing devices is not considered

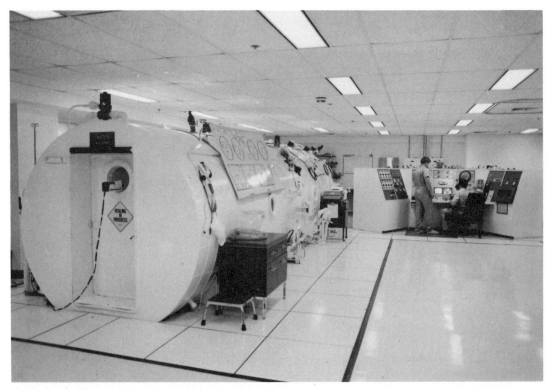

**FIG 14–4.**
Multiplace chamber with capacity for concurrent treatment of multiple patients. Hands-on capability and provision of critical care are advantages in this type of unit. *(Courtesy of Dean Heimbach, M.D., Ph.D., San Antonio, Tex.)*

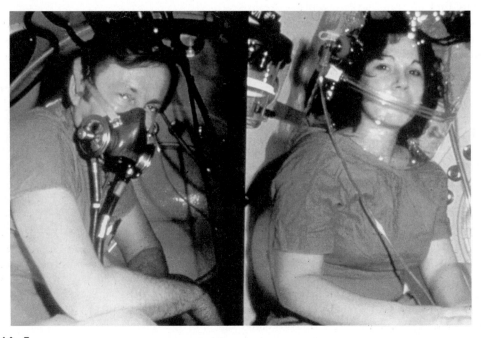

**FIG 14–5.**
In multiplace chambers patients breathe 100% oxygen through a mask, head tent, or endotracheal tube. Chamber is pressurized to treatment depth with compressed air.

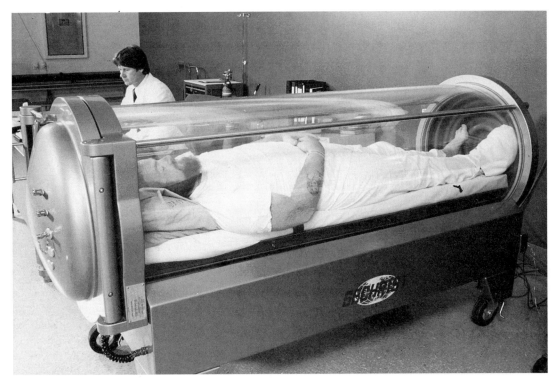

**FIG 14–6.**
Patient being treated in a monoplace chamber pressurized with 100% oxygen. No mask or head tent is necessary.

HBO therapy and has been demonstrated to be ineffective. It may, in fact, decrease oxygen delivery to the affected limbs.[18, 50]

## Mechanisms of Action

Oxygen inhaled at pressure dissolves in plasma. At the pressure equivalent of 3 atm, an arterial $Po_2$ of nearly 2,200 mm Hg may be achieved. Up to 6.9 vol% of oxygen may be forced into solution, a quantity sufficient to maintain life in the absence of hemoglobin.[7]

With HBO therapy, tissue oxygen tensions can often be raised to the relatively moderate levels necessary for fibroblast replication, development of a collagen matrix, and the ingress of capillaries into avascular areas. This can occur because wounds actually consume relatively little oxygen. Therefore, the added dissolved oxygen can increase $Po_2$ values in them. Diffusion of oxygen away from functional capillaries is independent of hemoglobin and is increased twofold to fourfold at the pressure equivalent of 3 atm. This may be of vital impor-

tance in preserving marginally viable tissue and enhancing collagen deposition, angiogenesis, and bacterial killing in wounds. A marked increase of tissue oxygen tension may be achieved only with HBO therapy (Table 14–1).[9, 41, 55, 83, 86]

## Neovascularization

Restoration of abnormally low tissue oxygen tensions to physiologic values assists in capillary proliferation and advancement into the wound space. Increased angiogenesis after HBO therapy has been noted by many therapists, but the mechanism is unknown. The data of Knighton and Marx[48, 57] suggest that angiogenesis is proportional to the gradient of $Po_2$ from capillary to wound space. This, in turn, is consistent with clinical experience.

## Vasoconstriction

Exposure to oxygen at pressure results in a 20% reduction in blood flow in normal tissue. This effect is offset by the tenfold to 15-

**TABLE 14–1.**

Tissue Oxygen Tension With Increasing Inspired Oxygen Pressure*

| ATA $O_2$ (mm Hg) | | Subject | | | | | |
|---|---|---|---|---|---|---|---|
| | Rat Brain[65] | Rabbit Tibia[55] | | Human (Clostridial Myonecrosis) | Human (Subcutaneous)[67] | |
| | | Normal | Osteo | Phlegmon[66] | Muscle | Tissue |
| 0.2 | 34 | 45 | 21 | 50 | 29 + 3 | 37 + 6 |
| 1.0 | 90 | — | — | 110 | 59 + 13 | 53 + 10 |
| 2.0 | 244 | 321 | 104 | 250 | 221 + 72 | 221 + 72 |
| 3.0 | 452 | — | — | 330 | — | — |

*ATA = 1 atmosphere absolute; $O_2$ = oxygen.

fold increase in oxygen content of plasma. This vasoconstriction may favorably effect the neurogenic edema seen in the feet of diabetics.[5] Hyperoxia probably does not cause vasoconstriction in ischemic or hypoxic tissues.[76]

## Rheologic Effects

Recently pharmacologic agents have been used to increase red blood cell (RBC) flexibility with the goal of improving oxygen delivery through compromised microvasculature.[60] Hyperbaric oxygen therapy has been shown to improve RBC deformability and may even act synergistically with pharmacologic agents.[57, 64]

## Toxicity and Side Effects

Risks involved in the use of HBO therapy are related to pressure changes and the toxic effects of oxygen. They include barotrauma to the ears or sinuses, pulmonary overpressure accidents with pneumothorax, and pulmonary toxicity. Trauma to the ears or sinuses can be averted by slow compression, the use of decongestants, and patient education. Occasionally myringotomy is necessary. Pulmonary overpressure accidents are very rare, perhaps 1 in 50,000 treatments,[4] and can be avoided by careful pretreatment screening for pulmonary blebs, air trapping caused by bronchospasm or secretions, and the presence of preexisting pneumothorax secondary to chest compression, central lines, ventilatory support, or other forms of

trauma.[62] An undetected pneumothorax at sea level can be converted to a tension pneumothorax on ascent as ambient pressure decreases. Treatment is immediate insertion of a chest tube. Additional minor side effects are a transient change in visual acuity that reverts to baseline within a few weeks to months after treatment. There is no evidence that the protocols presently used in the United States predispose to cataract formation.

## Oxygen Toxicity

Oxygen itself has definite toxic effects as a result of overdosage, usually affecting the brain or lungs. Exposure to oxygen at depth may cause grand mal seizures, possibly related to interference with γ-aminobutyric acid (GABA) metabolism.[87, 88, 91] Susceptibility varies widely. As the $Po_2$ value rises, so does the risk of seizures. For this reason, oxygen treatments are limited to a maximum depth of 3 ATA (66 ft of seawater, 20 m). (Fig 14–7) Fever and certain medications can predispose this complication, and careful attention to potential drug enhancement is mandatory. Oxygen seizures are, in fact, rare, occurring in perhaps 1 in 10,000 to 12,000 treatments.[20] They are self-limited and treated by cessation of oxygen therapy. Hyperbaric oxygen treatment may be reestablished after seizure activity has ceased.

Damage to lung tissue, manifested by a decrement in vital capacity and irritation to the large airways, is a predictable complication of oxygen exposure at depth. The mechanism is believed to be loss of surfactant and

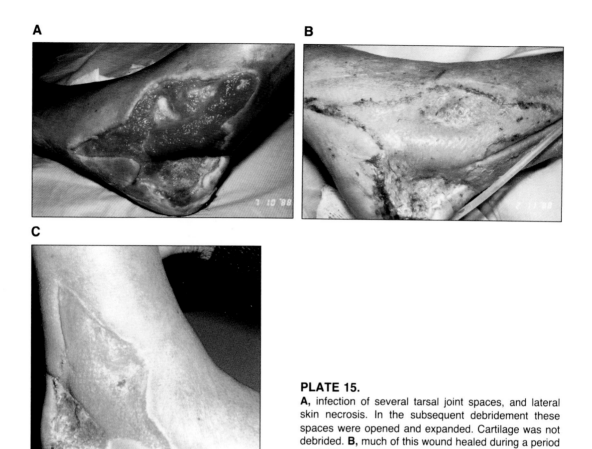

**PLATE 15.**

**A,** infection of several tarsal joint spaces, and lateral skin necrosis. In the subsequent debridement these spaces were opened and expanded. Cartilage was not debrided. **B,** much of this wound healed during a period in which the patient breathed oxygen at sea level. After several weeks of HBO therapy skin grafts were placed. **C,** wound remains healed and the patient ambulant 1½ years later.

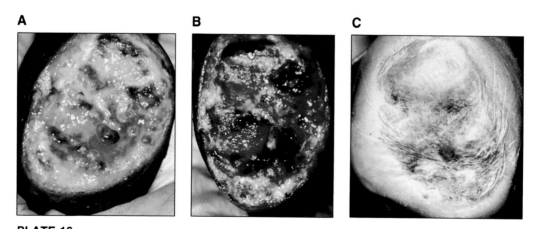

**PLATE 16.**

**A,** unhealed transmetatarsal wound in a 55-year-old man 5 weeks after extensive debridement and successful revascularization of viable tissue. Standard wound care was provided, but failed. **B,** angiogenesis after 10 days of wound care and HBO treatment. **C,** wound remains healed after split-thickness mesh grafting at 27 months follow-up. The contralateral limb was paralyzed.

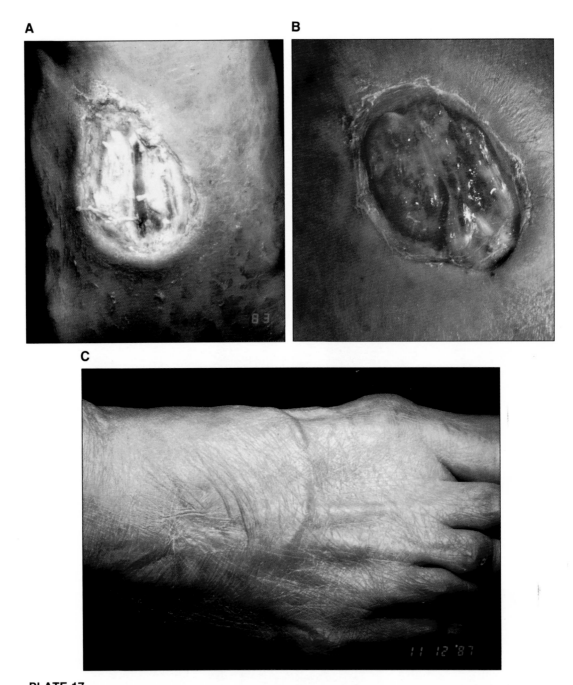

**PLATE 17.**
**A,** unhealed, painful dorsal foot lesion in a 70-year-old woman 6 weeks after successful revascularization. Wound showed no evidence of healing with standard care. **B,** 3 weeks later after 38 hyperbaric treatments. Note extensive granulation tissue. **C,** lesion closed without further surgical intervention, and remained healed at 4-year follow-up.

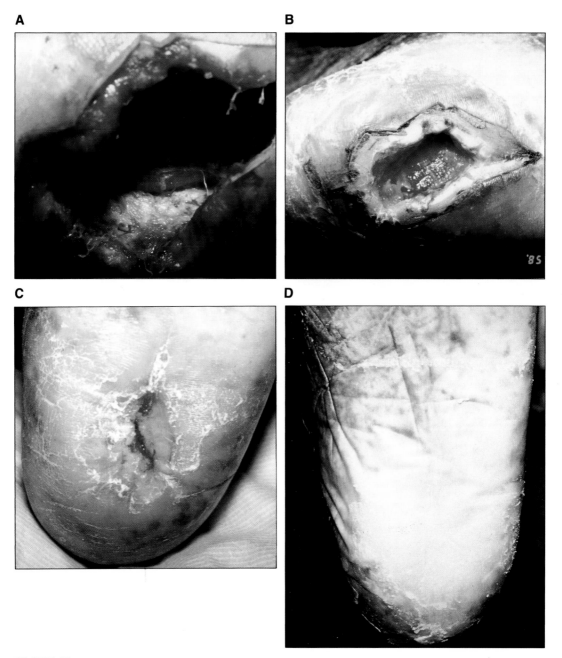

**PLATE 18.**

**A,** deep calcaneal lesion 2 days after successful revascularization and debridement of necrotizing heel lesion. Because of infection, compromised host, and a limb-threatening lesion, adjunctive HBO therapy was initiated early. **B,** 50% reduction of wound diameter and volume after 278 days of wound care and adjunctive HBO treatment. **C,** healed lesion after 28 HBO treatments. **D,** at 4-year follow-up, lesion remains healed. Patient lost opposite limb during interim.

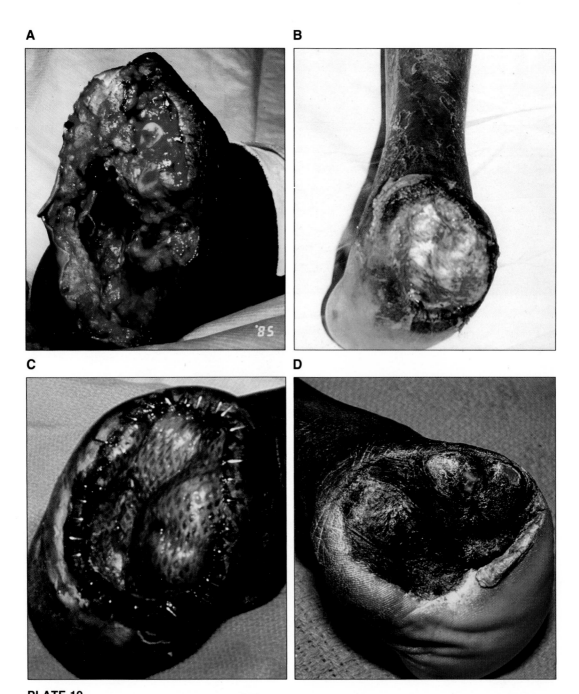

**PLATE 19.**
**A,** forefoot amputation status after revascularization in a 70-year-old man with diabetes mellitus, renal failure, and necrotizing infection. Because of limb-threatening lesion and prior contralateral limb amputation, adjunctive HBO therapy was initiated in the postoperative period. **B,** lesion 3 weeks later, after 21 HBO treatments and aggressive wound care. Note extensive healing. **C,** lesion 50 days after radical debridement and split-thickness mesh graft was placed. **D,** foot remains healed at 1-year follow-up.

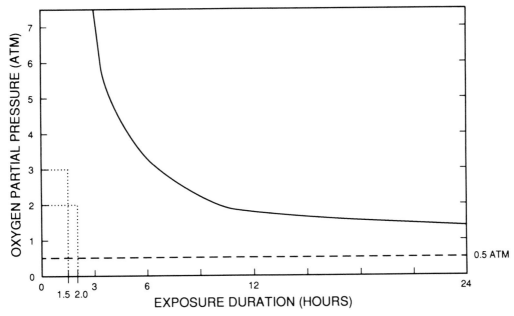

**FIG 14–7.**
Central nervous system and pulmonary toxicity as a function of depth and time of exposure. Treatment protocols are designed to stay within acceptable limits of tolerance. Oxygen is not administered at depths greater than 66 ft. Most clinical exposures are 2 to 2.4 atm for 90 minutes once or twice daily.

changes in the pulmonary macrophages.[3, 39] Because toxicity is related to the depth and duration of exposure, treatment protocols are designed to use the shallowest depth consistent with the desired results (see Fig 14–7). In practice, pulmonary toxicity from currently used wound healing protocols is virtually unheard of.[20, 35]

## Confinement Anxiety

Although not a complication of treatment, claustrophobia may be a problem for patients being treated in hyperbaric chambers. Sedation and reassurance usually remedy the problem. A small percentage of patients cannot tolerate treatment.

## Use of Hyperbaric Oxygen Therapy in Treatment of Diabetic Foot

Restoration of $tcPo_2$ to normal or slightly raised levels enhances epithelialization, fibroplasia, collagen deposition, angiogenesis, and bacterial killing. Controversy remains as to whether specific cellular immunity is diminished in diabetics in the absence of hyperglycemia, but no one argues that hypoxia

increases morbidity of infection, resulting in sepsis, loss of life or limb, or both.

Hyperbaric oxygen greatly increases tissue oxygen levels, and even though treatment is brief (2–3 hours daily), oxygen tension values may remain elevated in the subcutaneous tissue for several hours after exposure (Fig 14–8).[65, 88]

In the long run, the effect on angiogenesis may be the fundamental one. Sheffield[76] has elegantly demonstrated the improvement in capillarity, measuring transcutaneous oxygen levels over healing tissue in diabetic feet. His experience clearly documents the slow improvement in blood flow over the first 3 weeks of therapy, as evidenced by rising oxygen tensions in the tissue, especially during HBO therapy sessions. Marx et al.[56] have demonstrated the same changes in ischemic irradiated tissues.

## Clinical Results

Several groups have reported increased limb salvage with HBO.[12, 67, 81] Baroni et al.[5] reported a statistically significant reduction in morbidity (amputation) in HBO-treated patients. Sixteen of 18 patients in

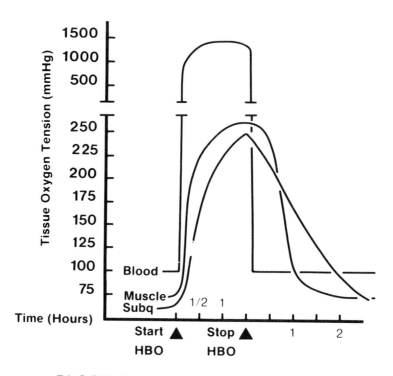

## BLOOD, SUBCUTANEOUS, & MUSCLE OXYGEN TENSIONS WITH HBO

**FIG 14–8.**
Rapidity of rise of oxygen tension after the onset of HBO is proportional to the capillary density of the organ at which the oxygen is transferred, either in the blood or to the peripheral tissue. The decline also is proportional to the height of the peak and to the rate of oxygen consumption. Subcutaneous tissue consumes little oxygen. Height of the peak is lower and the decline rather more rapid in inflamed tissue. *Solid circles*=patients who healed; *open circles*=patients who did not heal. *(Courtesy of George Hart, M.D.)*

their treated group healed, whereas only 1 in 10 in the controls did. The amputation rate was 40% in the controls vs. 12.5% in the treated group (p < 0.001). Hyperbaric oxygen–treated patients were improved sufficiently to be discharged in 62 days, and 16 went on to complete healing. Nine of ten of the controls had not healed 82 days later. In a continuation of this study,[67] 62 patients in the treated group were compared with 18 controls. A 95% salvage rate was achieved in the HBO-treated group in which there were three amputations (4.8%). The control group suffered six amputations (33%, p < 0.001). The incidence of amputation in the untreated group was essentially unchanged from a group of patients treated nearly 10 years earlier without adjunctive HBO therapy. There were no statistical differences in any of the groups relating to age, glycemic control, or diabetic complications. In 1988

our group[14] (P.C.) reported a series of 19 diabetics as a subset of 39 patients with lower limb lesions. We noted a salvage rate of 89%. Forty-two percent of these patients had undergone successful revascularization and were referred to us because of infection or nonhealing wounds. Salvage was defined as bipedal ambulation (if two limbs were originally present) and wound coverage for at least 1 year. Hyperbaric oxygen costs were $12,668 and were reflected in total hospital charges of $34,370, with an average stay of 35 days.

Our group[17] has recently analyzed another series of 41 diabetic patients averaging 63 years in age. Thirty-nine patients (97%) were believed to have limb-threatening lesions. Eighteen patients (55%) had undergone revascularization. The average Wagner score was 4 (gangrene of the toes or forefoot). Thirty-one patients' extremities were salvaged (78%). Hyperbaric charges were $15,900, total hospital charges $32,000, and the average length of stay 27 days.[17] These costs compare favorably with the cost of primary amputation, which has been previously reported as more than $40,000.[54] Avoidance of perhaps another $40,000 to 50,000 in rehabilitation costs[14] and the additional savings involved in prevention of reamputation or stump revision have been an additional benefit. Despite early doubts, the effects appear to be durable. Twenty-five salvaged patients have been followed for 1 to 6 years, averaging 30 months. Twenty-three patients (92%) remain ambulatory without further lesions or problems. Two patients have suffered below-knee amputations (8%) (Table 14–2).

These studies are encouraging, but as with all other therapeutic interventions in the diabetic foot, adequacy of control data remains a problem.[32, 71] One cannot escape, however, the reality that there is no such thing as a "control chronic wound" in humans. Fortunately, the large number of controlled studies in animals is convincing.

## Patient Selection

Shallow ulcers, particularly of neuropathic origin, unless grossly infected, will usually respond to more conservative treat-

**TABLE 14–2.**

Analysis and Follow-up of 40 Diabetic Lower Limb Lesions*

| | | |
|---|---|---|
| No. of Patients | 40 | |
| Mean age (yr) | 63 | |
| Wagner score (mean) | 4 | |
| Mean HBO treatments | 40 | |
| Mean HBO cost ($K) | 16.0 | |
| Average hospital charges ($K) | 32.3 | |
| Average length of stay (day) | 29 | |
| Average no. of days before HBO treatment/delay | 5 | |
| Average no. of days in HBO treatment | 33 | |
| Vascular surgery | 20 | (50%) |
| Limb-threatening lesion | 37 | (93%) |
| Salvage/success | 31 | (78%) |
| Follow-up | 25 | (81%) |
| Limb intact | 23 | (92%) |
| Average follow-up (mo) | 30 | (12–84) |

*HBO = hyperbaric oxygen.*

ment. Patients with class 3, 4, or 5 Wagner lesions are considered for treatment based on assessment of blood flow. Patients without adequate arterial flow are referred for angiograms and revascularization as indicated. Transcutaneous $Po_2$ is a useful, noninvasive method for evaluation of perfusion and selection of patients for vascular referral.[37] This measurement is widely available and can be helpful in patient selection for HBO therapy. Patients with transcutaneous periwound $tcPo_2$ values greater than 30 to 40 mm Hg on room air may heal without intervention. Patients with readings less than 20 mm Hg while breathing air have a poor prognosis.[70] An increase to 40 mm Hg or greater while breathing 100% oxygen by tight-fitting mask or while in the hyperbaric chamber at 1 atm indicates perfusion is adequate for oxygen therapy to benefit.[76] If periwound transcutaneous $O_2$ levels are low and unresponsive, angiography may be helpful in selecting those patients who might benefit from revascularization. In cases where $tcPo_2$ level is low and revascularization is not possible, the prognosis is very guarded. In these instances, a trial of therapy may be indicated on a case by case basis if limb loss is the only alternative. More recently Wattel et al.[85] have reported that patients who show transcutaneous oxygen values of 100 mm Hg in the vicinity of the wound while breathing pure oxygen at 2.5 ATA heal 75% of the time, whereas patients with lower values will go on to amputation (Fig 12–9). Hart et al.[36] have reported data that support this hypothesis. As more data become available, patient selection criteria will become more precise.

## Treatment Protocols

Treatment protocols vary depending on the severity of the problem and the type of chamber used. In larger, multiplace chambers, treatments are rendered at 2 to 2.4 atm for 90 to 120 minutes once or twice daily. In monoplace configurations, most centers use treatment at 2 atm.

Patients with serious infections are hospitalized for intravenous antibiotics and tight diabetes control. Hyperbaric oxygen treat-

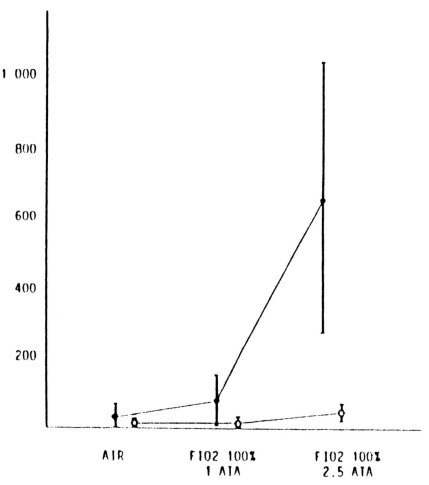

**FIG 14–9.**
Measurement of periwound transcutaneous oxygen level while one breathes 100% oxygen in a hyperbaric chamber appears to be a good predictor of healing. *(Courtesy of Wattel, M.D.)*

ment in such cases is usually rendered twice daily for 90 minutes. As soon as feasible, patients are transferred to an in-house skilled nursing facility or to home health care where daily wound care, debridement, and HBO treatments can be continued in the outpatient setting. In such instances, HBO is administered once daily for 2 hours, usually right after whirlpool or debridement. After a suitable capillary bed has been established, split-thickness mesh grafts or other plastic techniques are used to effect rapid wound closure. In our experience early application of grafts, when appropriate, can significantly shorten morbidity, hospital stay, and cost of care. With proper coordination, this program has proved cost effective, even in this era of severe fiscal constraint.[14, 17] Recent preliminary data suggest

in selected cases, wound growth factors and HBO therapy may be synergistic and lead to even further shortening of healing times.[24] It is ironic that the federal reimbursement for amputation, which involves a much greater long-term cost, is 30% greater than that provided for attempts at limb salvage.[53]

## SUMMARY

Hyperbaric oxygen therapy given in specially designed chambers is an adjunct to current medical and surgical treatment of frequently discouraging and difficult problems of healing failure in diabetics. Recent investigations have demonstrated that adequate tissue oxygen tension is an essential factor in wound healing. Frequently, adequate levels can be reached only through adjunctive HBO treatment. This results in more normal fibroblast proliferation, angiogenesis, collagen deposition, epithelization, and enhancement of bacterial killing. Although HBO therapy is costly, the ability to preserve a functional extremity can reduce the high cost of disability resulting from amputation. The shortened healing time for chronic wounds will reduce the cost of frequent, repeated surgical procedures. As part of a multidisciplinary program of wound care, it can be cost effective.

## CASE ILLUSTRATIONS (PLATES 16 TO 20)

Revascularization often can provide the substrate necessary for healing. However, historically limbs have been lost to necrotizing infections, even in the presence of adequate circulation and excellent wound care. We use adjunctive HBO therapy early when there is extensive soft tissue infection, which often necessitates extensive radical debridement. Adjunctive HBO therapy can speed the healing process in the severely compromised limb.

### Acknowledgment

We thank Sharon Drager, M.D., for suggestions in preparation of this chapter.

## REFERENCES

1. Aagenaes O, et al: Light- and electron-microscope study of skin capillaries of the diabetic, *Diabetes* 10:253–259, 1961.

2. Arenson OJ, et al: Neuropathic angiopathy and sepsis in the diabetic foot: part 2, angiopathy, *J Am Podiatr Med Assoc* 71:661–665, 1981.

3. Armbruster S: Surfactant in pulmonary oxygen toxicity, *Adv Exp Med Biol* 215:345–349, 1987.

4. Bakker DJ: Pure and mixed aerobic and anaerobic soft tissue infections, *Hyperbar Oxygen Rev* 6:65–96, 1985.

5. Baroni G, et al: Hyperbaric oxygen in diabetic gangrene treatment, *Diabetes Care* 10:81–86, 1987.

6. Block P: The diabetic foot ulcer: a complex problem with a simple treatment approach, *Milit Med* 146:644, 1981.

7. Boerema I, et al: Life without blood: a study of the influence of high atmospheric pressure and hypothermia on dilution of blood, *J Cardiovasc Surg* 1:133–146, 1960.

8. Brummelkamp WH, et al: Considerations on hyperbaric oxygen therapy at three atmospheres absolute for clostridial infections type welchii, *Ann NY Acad Sci* 117:688–699, 1965.

9. Brummelkamp WH, et al: Treatment of anaerobic infections (clostridial myositis) by drenching the tissues with oxygen under high atmospheric pressure, *Surgery* 49:299–302, 1961.

10. Centers for Disease Control: *Diabetes in the United States: a strategy for prevention*, Atlanta, May 1991, Centers for Disease Control.

11. Chang N, et al: Comparison of the effect of bacterial inoculation in musculocutaneous and random-pattern flaps, *Plast Reconstr Surg* 70:1–10, 1982.

12. Cianci P: Adjunctive hyperbaric oxygen in the treatment of problem wounds, an economic analysis, in Kindwall E, editor: *Proceedings of the eighth international congress on hyperbaric medicine*, San Pedro, Calif, 1984, Best Publishing, pp 213–216.

13. Cianci P, et al: Adjunctive hyperbaric oxygen reduces the need for surgery in 40–80% burns, *J Hyperbar Med* 3:97–101, 1988.

14. Cianci P, et al: Salvage of the problem wound and potential amputation with wound care and adjunctive hyperbaric oxygen therapy: an economic analysis, *J Hyperbar Med* 3:127–141, 1988.

15. Cianci P, et al: Adjunctive hyperbaric oxygen reduces length of hospitalization in thermal burns, *J Burn Care Rehab* 10:432–435, 1989.

16. Cianci P, et al: Adjunctive hyperbaric oxygen in the treatment of thermal burns an economic analysis, *J Burn Care Rehab* 11:140–143, 1990.

17. Cianci P, et al: Adjunctive hyperbaric oxygen in the salvage of the diabetic foot, *Undersea Baromedical Res* 18(suppl):108, 1991 (paper presented at the UHMS Annual Scientific Meeting, San Diego).

18. Cotto-Cumba C, et al: Transcutaneous oxygen measurements in normal subjects using topical HBO control module, *Undersea Baromedical Res* 18(suppl):109, 1991 (presented at the UHMS Annual Scientific Meeting, San Diego).

19. Couch NP, et al: Natural history of the leg amputee, *Am J Surg* 133;469–473, 1977.

20. Davis JC: Refractory osteomyelitis, in Davis JC, Hunt TK, editors: *Problem wounds: the role of oxygen*, New York, Elsevier, 1988, pp 125–142.

21. Davis JC: Hyperbaric oxygen therapy, *Intensive Care Med* 4:55–57, 1989.

22. Davis JC, et al: Chronic nonhematogenous osteomyelitis treated with adjuvant hyperbaric oxygen, *J Bone Joint Surg* 68A:1210–1217, 1986.

23. Davis JC, et al: *Problem wounds: the role of oxygen*. New York, Elsevier, 1988.

24. Dunn J, et al: Personal communication, 1992.

25. Ebskov G, et al: Incidence of reamputation and death after gangrene of the lower extremity, *Prosthet Orthotics Int* 4:77–80, 1980.

26. Edmonds ME, et al: Improved survival of the diabetic foot: the role of the specialized foot clinic, *Q J Med* 60:763–771, 1986.

27. Foster DW: Diabetes mellitus, in Wilson JD, Braunwald E, Isselbacher KJ, et al, editors: *Harrison's principles of internal medicine*, ed 12, New York, 1991, McGraw-Hill.

28. Friederici HHR, et al: Observations on small blood vessels of skin in the normal and in diabetic patients, *Diabetes* 15:233–250, 1960.

29. Goodman MW, et al: Oxygen-breathing approach of treatment of decompression sickness in divers and aviators, Washington, DC, Bureau of Medicine and Surgery, BuShips Project SF0110606, Task 11513-2, Research Rep 5-65, 1965.

30. Gottrup F, et al: Properties of tissue oxygen in healing flaps, *Surgery* 95:527–536, 1984.

31. Gozal D, et al: Necrotizing fasciitis, *Arch Surg* 121:233–235, 1986.

32. Grunfeld C: Diabetic foot ulcers: etiology, treatment, and prevention, in Stollerman GH, et al, editors: *Advances in internal medicine*, St Louis, 1991, Mosby-Year Book, vol 37, pp 103–132.

33. Hart GB, et al: Treatment of burns with hyperbaric oxygen, *Surg Gynecol Obstet* 139:693–696, 1974.

34. Hart GB, et al: Gas gangrene, *J Trauma* 23:991–1000, 1983.

35. Hart GB, et al: Vital capacity of quadraplegic patients treated with hyperbaric oxygen, *J Am Paraplegia Soc* 7:91–92, 1984.

36. Hart GB, et al: Transcutaneous partial pressure of oxygen measured in a monoplace hyperbaric chamber at 1, 1.5, and 2 atm abs oxygen, *J Hyperbar Med* 5:223–229, 1990.

37. Hauser CJ, et al: Assessment of perfusion in the diabetic foot by regional transcutaneous oximetry, *Diabetes* 33:527–531, 1984.

38. Heimbach RD: Gas gangrene: review and update, *Hyperbar Oxygen Rev* 1:41–61, 1980.

39. Holm BA, et al: Pulmonary physiological and surfactant changes during injury and recovery from hyperpoxia, *J Appl Physiol* 59:1402–1409, 1985.

40. Hunt TK: The physiology of wound healing, *Ann Emerg Med* 17:1265–1273, 1988.

41. Jamieson D, et al: Measurement of oxygen tensions in cerebral tissues of rats exposed to high pressures of oxygen, *J Appl Physiol* 18:869–876, 1963.

42. Jonsson K, et al: Effect of environmental oxygen on bacterial-induced tissue necrosis in flaps, *Surg Forum* 35:589–591, 1984.

43. Joseph WS, et al: The pathogenesis of diabetic foot infection immunopathy, angiopathy, and neuropathy, *J Foot Surg* 26:S7–S11, 1987.

44. Kaelin CM, et al: The effects of hyperbaric oxygen on free flaps in rats, *Arch Surg* 125:607–609, 1990.

45. Kihn RB, et al: The geriatric amputee, *Ann Surg* 176:305–314, 1972.

46. Kindwall EP: Carbon monoxide and cyanide poisoning, *Hyperbar Oxygen Rev* 1:115–122, 1980.

47. Knighton DR, et al: Oxygen tension regulates the expression of angiogenesis factor by macrophages, *Science* 221:1283–1285, 1983.

48. Knighton DR, et al: Oxygen as an antibiotic: the effect of inspired oxygen on infection, *Arch Surg* 119:199–204, 1984.

49. Knighton DR, et al: Amputation prevention in an independently reviewed at-risk diabetic population using a comprehensive wound care protocol, *Am J Surg* 160:466–472, 1990.

50. Leslie CA, et al: Randomized controlled trial of topical hyperbaric oxygen for treatment of diabetic foot ulcers, *Diabetes Care* 11:52, 1988.

51. Levene CI, et al: The activation of protocollagen proline hydroxylation by ascorbic acid in cultured 3T6 fibroblasts, *Biochem Biophys Acta* 338:29, 1974.

52. LoGerfo FW, et al: Vascular and microvascular disease of the foot in diabetes, *N Engl J Med* 311:1615–1619, 1984.

53. Lorenz EW: *The physician's DRG working guidebook 1988*, 1988, St Anthony Hospital Publications.

54. Mackey WC, et al: The cost of surgery for limb-threatening ischemia, *Surgery* 99:26–35, 1986.

55. Mader JT, et al: A mechanism for the amelioration by hyperbaric oxygen of experimental staphylococcal osteomyelitis in rabbits, *J Infect Dis* 142:915–922, 1980.

56. Marx RE, et al: Relationship of oxygen dose to angiogenesis induction in irradiated tissue, *Am J Surg* 160:519–524, 1990.

57. Mathieu D, et al: Erythrocyte filterability and hyperbaric oxygen therapy, *Med Sub Hyperbar* 3:100–104, 1984.

58. McMillan DE, et al: Forearm skin capillaries of diabetic, potential diabetic and non-diabetic subjects: changes seen by light microscopy, *Diabetes* 15:251–257, 1966.

59. Medawar PB: The cultivation of adult mammalian skin epithelium, *Q J Microbial Sci* 89:187, 1948.

60. Monteiro DT, et al: The influence of pentoxifylline on skin flap survival, *Plast Reconstr Surg* 77:271–281, 1986.

61. Morrey BF: Hyperbaric oxygen and chronic osteomyelitis, *Clin Orthop* 144:121–127, 1979.

62. Murphy DG, et al: Tension pneumothorax associated with hyperbaric oxygen therapy, *Am J Emerg Med* 9:176–179, 1991.

63. Myers RAM, et al: Use of hyperbaric oxygen in postradiation head and neck surgery, *NCI Monogr* 9:151–157, 1990.

64. Nemiroff PM: Synergistic effects of pentoxifylline and hyperbaric oxygen on skin flaps, *Arch Otolaryngol Head Neck Surg* 114:977–981, 1988.

65. Niinikoski J, et al: Combination of hyperbaric oxygen, surgery, and antibiotics in the treatment of clostridial gas gangrene, *Infect Surg* 2:23–27, 1983.

66. O'Hare JA, et al: Poor metabolic control, hypertension and microangiopathy independently increase the transcapillary escape rate of albumin in diabetes, *Diabetologia* 25:260–263, 1983.

67. Oriani G, et al: Hyperbaric oxygen therapy in diabetic gangrene, *J Hyperbar Med* 5:171–175, 1990.

68. Pai MP, et al: Effect of varying oxygen tensions on healing of open wounds, *Surg Gynecol Obstet* 135:756–758, 1972.

69. Parving HH, et al: The effect of metabolic regulation on microvascular permeability to small and large molecules in short-term juvenile diabetes, *Diabetologia* 12:161–166, 1976.

70. Pecoraro RE: The nonhealing diabetic ulcer—a major cause for limb loss, *Prog Clin Biol Res* 365:27–43, 1991.

71. Pecoraro RE, et al: Chronology and determinants of tissue repair in diabetic lower extremity ulcers, *Diabetes* 40:1305–1313, 1991.

72. Prokop DJ, et al: Biosynthesis of collagen and its disorders, *N Engl J Med* 301:13–23, 1979.

73. Rabkin J, et al: Infection and oxygen, in Davis JC, Hunt TK, editors: *Problem wounds: the role of oxygen*, New York, 1987, Elsevier.

74. Rashkin P, et al: The effect of diabetic control on the width of skeletal-muscle capillary basement membrane in patients with type I diabetes mellitus, *N Engl J Med* 309:1546–1550, 1983.

75. Riseman JA, et al: Hyperbaric oxygen therapy for necrotizing fasciitis reduces mortality and the need for debridements, *Surgery* 108:847–850, 1990.

76. Sheffield PJ: Tissue oxygenation measurements, in Davis JC, Hunt TK, editors: *Problem wounds: the role of oxygen*, New York, 1988, Elsevier.

77. Skyhar MJ, et al: Hyperbaric oxygen reduces edema and necrosis of skeletal muscle in compartment syndromes associated with hemorrhagic hypotension, *J Bone Joint Surg* 68A:1218–1224, 1986.

78. Slack WK, et al: Hyperbaric oxygenation in chronic osteomyelitis, *Lancet* 1:1093–1094, 1965.

79. Strauss MB, et al: Reduction of skeletal muscle necrosis using intermittent hyperbaric oxygen in a model compartment syndrome, *J Bone Joint Surg* 68A:656–662, 1983.

80. Strauss MB, et al: Crush injury and the role of hyperbaric oxygen, *Top Emerg Med* 6:9–24, 1984.

81. Strauss MB, et al: Salvaging the difficult wound through a combined management program, in Kindwall E, editor: *Proceedings of the eighth international congress on hyperbaric medicine*, San Pedro, Calif, 1984, Best Publishing.

82. Tan CM, et al: Effects of hyperbaric oxygen and hyperbaric air on the survival of island skin flaps, *Plast Reconstr Surg* 73:27–28, 1984.

83. Thom SR: Hyperbaric oxygen therapy. *J Intens Care Med* 4:58–74, 1989.

84. Vracko R, et al: Basal lamina of abdominal skeletal muscle capillaries in diabetics and nondiabetics, *Circulation* 35:690–700, 1967.

85. Wattel F, et al: Hyperbaric oxygen therapy in chronic vascular wound management, *Angiology* 41:59–65, 1990.

86. Wells CH, et al: Tissue gas measurements during hyperbaric oxygen exposure, in Smith G, editor: *Proceedings of the sixth international conference on hyperbaric medicine*, 1977, Aberdeen, University Press, pp 118–124.

87 Wood JD: GABA and oxygen toxicity: a review, *Brain Res Bull* 5:777–780, 1980.

88. Wood JD, et al: Sensitivity of GABA synthesis in human brain to oxygen poisoning, *Aviat Space Environ Med* 46:1155–1156, 1975.

89. Wyss CR, et al: Relationship between transcutaneous oxygen tension, ankle blood pressure, and clinical outcome of vascular surgery in diabetic and nondiabetic patients, *Surgery* 101:56–62, 1987.

90. Yarbrough OB, et al: The treatment of compressed air illness utilizing oxygen, *J Indus Hyg Toxicol* 21:6, 1939.

91. Yoneda Y, et al: Modulation of synaptic GABA receptor binding by membrane phospholipids: possible role of active oxygen radicals, *Brain Res* 333:111–122, 1985.

92. Zamboni WA, et al: The effect of acute hyperbaric oxygen therapy on axial pattern skin flap survival when administered during and after total ischemia, *J Reconstr Microsurg* 5:343–347, 1989.

93. Zatz A, et al: Pathogenesis of diabetic microangiopathy: the hemodynamic view, *Am J Med* 80:443–453, 1986.

# CHAPTER 15

# Noninvasive Testing: Practical Knowledge for Evaluating Diabetic Patients

Joseph J. Hurley, M.D.

John J. Woods, Jr., M.D.

Falls B. Hershey, M.D.

The noninvasive vascular laboratory along with careful history taking, physical examination, and, in many instances, angiography continues to assume an integral role in the evaluation of peripheral arterial ischemic disease in patients with diabetes mellitus. Its appropriate application requires an understanding of the variations in the history, physical examination, and physiology between patients with and without diabetes mellitus. The information obtained in the noninvasive testing is not intended to stand alone but to supplement the information revealed by history taking and physical examination.

Peripheral arterial insufficiency in persons with diabetes mellitus, whether insulin dependent or not, is an especially onerous condition, having serious implications regarding morbidity and mortality. Reunanen et al.[23] noted intermittent claudication in 4.3% of diabetic individuals aged 30 to 59 years vs. only 2.0% in nondiabetics of the same age range. Although diabetic persons account for only approximately 5% to 6% of the general population, they constitute 16% of patients with diagnosis of intermittent claudication,[10] 30% to 50% of patients operated on for peripheral vascular disease, and 60% to 70% of patients undergoing vascular reconstruction below the popliteal artery.[6, 24] In another collected series[5] of 2,323 patients undergoing lower limb amputation for vascular insufficiency, 54% were individuals with diabetes mellitus, more than ten times the expected rate. In this same series, 20% of the individuals had had a prior contralateral amputation, with only 37% of the entire series (diabetic and nondiabetic alike) surviving for 5 years. McDaniel and Cronenwett[16] noted even with only the diagnosis of intermittent claudication, mortality was significant after 5 years, revealing a 23% mortality in nondiabetic individuals vs. a 49% mortality in those patients with diabetes mellitus.

## CLINICAL DIAGNOSIS

The possibility of lower limb arterial insufficiency is usually first encountered in the clinical situation. Various aspects of the history, supplemented by a careful physical examination, lead to a desire for further delineation of the presence and extent of peripheral arterial occlusive disease. The symptoms noted with inadequate lower limb circulation are progressive, from intermittent claudication, through rest pain, ending with frank tissue necrosis.

Unfortunately, because many persons with diabetes mellitus also have significant neuropathy, the stage of rest pain is frequently absent, with patients giving the history of claudication leading directly to the unheralded appearance of tissue loss.

The presence of a critical stenosis in the peripheral arteries is related to the degree of narrowing (fixed) and the volume of flow (variable). The degree of stenosis and the associated decrease in flow in a steady volume per unit of time varies logarithmically (Table 15–1). At 50% stenosis a 15% decrease in flow might occur, whereas at 90% stenosis an 80% decrease in flow has occurred. Couple with this the fact that active exercise can increase the flow demands 10- to 15-fold, and the basis for intermittent claudication becomes apparent. The work of moving one's body climbing a hill or stairs as opposed to ambulation on level ground adds additional flow demands on the lower limb circulation. The symptoms of claudication, although often described as painful, can also be recognized as weakness, heaviness, or even of a crampy nature. The level of these symptoms usually reveals the level of the narrowing or blockage. Thigh and buttock claudication suggests an aortoiliac location with proximal femoral involvement affecting the thigh and lower femoral, popliteal, and tibial vessel disease yielding calf claudication. Normally the presence of impotence would be highly suggestive of aortoiliac arterial occlusive disease, but in diabetic patients the possibility of a neurogenic cause for impotence has to be strongly considered. When the flow of blood is affected to a degree that is significant at rest, the necessary oxygen and nutrition requirements are not being met, and rest pain supervenes. Usually two-level severely stenotic or totally occluded arterial segments are required to produce rest pain. The discomfort of rest pain is much more likely to be described as pain that occurs within 1 or 2 hours of assuming a recumbent position. The area involved is the distal forefoot, and this discomfort is commonly relieved by dangling the foot over the side of the bed, short-distance ambulation, or actually sleeping in the sitting position. With rest pain, there is inadequate blood pressure, hence flow to perfuse the distal 3 to 4 in. of the forefoot in the recumbent position.

Physical findings are detected by observation and palpation. The ischemic foot will display changes in color with elevation and dependency because of a decrease in autonomic control of blood flow. A ruborous foot on dependency blanches rapidly when elevated 12 to 18 in. above the heart level. The rubor is a result of dilated subcutaneous capillaries trying to increase oxygen extraction. Hypoxemia is the greatest stimulus to vasodilation known.

Assessment of the pulses in the femoral, popliteal, and pedal locations should be graded as normal, diminished, or absent. Absence of a dorsalis pedis pulse can be a congenital variant and does not necessarily imply a pathologic condition. If there is doubt as to whether one is feeling one's own pulse or the patient's, a check against the patient's radial pulse quickly settles the ques-

**TABLE 15–1.**

Correlation Between Diameter, Area, and Flow Reduction for Arterial Stenosis*

| 2/5 × 100 = 40% or 60%<br>Stenosis by Diameter (%) | (2/5)² × 100 = 16% or 84%<br>Stenosis by Area (%) | 30% Reduction of Flow (%) |
|---|---|---|
| 0 | 0 | 0 |
| 30 | 51 | >0 |
| 40 | 64 | ≤20 |
| 60 | 84 | ~30 |
| 70 | 91 | ~40 |
| 85 | 98 | ~70 |

*A lateral, two-dimensional 60% stenosis actually represents an 84% cross-sectional area obliteration. This nevertheless results in only a 30% reduction of resting flow.

tion. Finally, auscultation of the aortoiliac and femoral regions for a bruit should be performed. A narrowing of 50% or more (but < 90%) usually produces a bruit, providing a valuable clue as to location and severity of arterial occlusive disease.

The natural progression of arterial insufficiency in persons with diabetes mellitus was reported in a prospective, 24-month minimal follow-up study of Bendick et al.[3] Using the noninvasive laboratory to detect the presence of peripheral arterial insufficiency (ankle-arm index [AAI] < 0.9), monophasic waveforms, or evidence of progression (drop in AAI of ≥ 0.15) in following the course of arterial insufficiency, they discovered that less than 10% of patients initially displaying a normal study developed any criteria of arterial insufficiency during the study, whereas greater than 75% of those identified as having arterial insufficiency at the start of the trial demonstrated progression of arterial insufficiency. They believe that the strongest indication of atherosclerotic arterial progression is preexisting arterial disease, with the potential for significant progression to occur in a relatively short time span.

Marinelli et al.[14] performed a prospective clinical noninvasive screening of 458 patients with diabetes mellitus using segmental blood pressure measurements, treadmill exercise, and Doppler velocimetry (waveform analysis). Their screen revealed that nearly one third of the patients who gave no history of intermittent claudication were found to have measureable arterial disease, whereas one fifth of the patients considered to be normal by physical examination also had abnormal results by noninvasive testing.

There seems to be ample evidence that inclusion of noninvasive testing in the initial work-up in patients with diabetes mellitus is justified to allow accurate identification of those individuals at higher risk for progression of arterial insufficiency, possibly to limb loss, and even death.

## PATHOPHYSIOLOGY

In the resting state only high-grade stenosis or total occlusion of a vessel results in abnormal changes recorded at the ankle level. Arterial narrowing or obstruction forces the blood to follow collateral arteries, which are usually high-resistance pathways. The greater the number of sequential critical stenoses or occlusions, the greater the degree of total impairment that will be detected at the most distal assessment point.

Besides a generalized yes or no answer regarding the presence of arterial obstructive disease, segmental pressure measurements allow some attempt at accurate identification of the anatomic location of the obstruction (Fig 15–1). Strandness et al.,[27] however, caution that inaccuracies are most likely to occur when there is multilevel involvement. They further note the following specific problems: (1) high thigh pressures may be abnormally low in the presence of an occluded proximal superficial femoral artery, and gradients between high thigh and low thigh may be "normal" in patients with superficial femoral obstructions when there is significant aortoiliac disease; and (2) disease below the knee will not be recognized consistently unless the obstruction is quite severe and involves all three vessels. The authors mention these problems not to condemn this approach but to point out that pressure measurements may be more reliable than arteriograms as a guide to the surgeon in selecting therapy, because they more accurately reflect the *physiologic* magnitude of the disease.

Even more information can be obtained when the response to a demand for maximum flow in the limb is obtained. The data of Strandness and Bell[26] and others demonstrate that exercise in the presence of occlusive arterial disease proximal to the blood supply of the calf muscles results in a transient decrease in blood pressure at the ankle. Furthermore, it has been shown that this fall in the ankle pressure may be used as an objective test for assessing and following the course of the disease in patients with obliterative arterial disease of the lower extremities. Increases in heart rate, systolic blood pressure, cardiac output, oxygen consumption, and limb blood flow are the normal responses to exercise. The magnitude of these changes is a direct function of the work performed. In addition, the duration

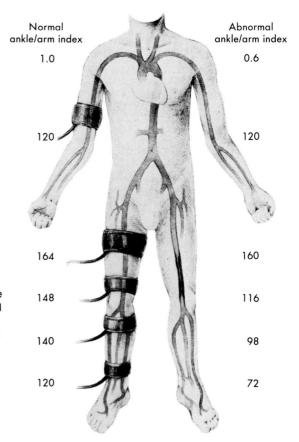

Normal
ankle/arm index

1.0

120

164

148

140

120

Abnormal
ankle/arm index

0.6

120

160

116

98

72

**FIG 15–1.**
Normal condition on right side of body with ankle systolic pressure equal to brachial systolic pressure. Ankle pressure divided by arm pressure determines AAI, in this case 1.0. On left side, AAI is 0.6, indicating only 60% of expected normal flow at rest. In addition, any gradient greater than 30 mm Hg between two successive cuffs indicates high-grade stenosis or occlusion. Here 44 mm Hg high thigh gradient localizes diseased segment to superficial femoral artery. *(From Arizona Heart Institute: Cerebrovascular and peripheral vascular disease: advanced noninvasive diagnostic techniques.)*

of increased blood flow after exercise (reactive hyperemia) is a valuable mark of the amount of work performed and a mark of the vascular system's ability to respond adequately to such demands (Fig 15–2). Normal individuals display postexercise reactive hyperemia of very short duration, lasting only a few minutes in response to normal exercise loads. In contrast, those patients with critical arterial stenosis or occlusions display markedly prolonged periods of decreased blood flow in response to even minimum exercise demands. The magnitude of the decrease in ankle pressure and its time course are rough guides to the extent of the impairment to blood flow after exercise or induced hyperemia.[25] Reactive hyperemia can be assessed in those individuals unable to exercise by inflating a thigh cuff 50 mm Hg greater than systolic pressure for 3 minutes and then recording the drop in pressure on release of the cuff. This is referred to as "induced reactive hyperemia." It is impor-

tant to emphasize that the response of each patient's ankle pressure to exercise is specific and permits the patient's other ankle to serve as a control. This has important implications for follow-up purposes, particularly if the physician is aware of the factors that tend to change it.

Progression of arteriosclerotic lesions or recurrent distal embolism will increase stenosis or cause occlusion of the vascular tree. Hypertension, diabetes mellitus, hyperlipidemia, and tobacco use clearly encourage arteriosclerosis. Control of the first three conditions and total cessation of smoking, on the other hand, when coupled with a walking program and the passage of time, can lead to collateral channel development. Although collateral pathways are high-resistance pathways, their development can improve distal blood flow. This is usually detected first by exercise testing after prolonged walking time; positive signs are a smaller drop in pressure after exercise and a more rapid rise of the pressure to preexercise baselines.

Moore and Malone,[19] in a series of canine experiments, using multiple in-line arteriovenous fistulas, which provided a wide range of iliac artery blood flow, demonstrated that (1) the percentage of decrease in blood pressure was the same as the percentage of decrease in blood flow (i.e., blood pressure and blood flow vary directly), and (2) the greater the flow the less stenosis necessary to create the same incremental decrease in pressure (Table 15–2). One additional difficulty in interpreting angiography is the relationship between the actual three-plane cross-sectional area changes and the lumen size as determined by two-plane angiograms.

## NONINVASIVE EVALUATION

In the past 15 years there has been a series of new instrumentation introduced in an effort to develop the ideal noninvasive test that would allow an ability to predict healing of wounds or determine appropriate levels of amputation in diabetic individuals.[1] Early efforts began with measurement of pressures at the ankle and toe level. This has progressed from transcutaneous oxygen determinations, laser Doppler velocimetry, and

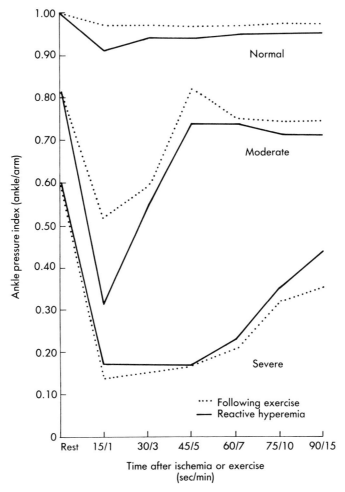

**FIG 15–2.**
Effect of increasing blood flow demands on normal patients and those with moderate and severe peripheral arterial disease. Note correlation between exercise measured in minutes and reactive hyperemia measured in seconds.

**TABLE 15–2.**
Determination of Critical Stenosis*

| Condition of measurement | Avg Blood Flow (mL/min) | Critical Stenosis Determined by 10% Drop in Flow (%) | Critical Stenosis Determined by 10% Drop in Pressure (%) |
|---|---|---|---|
| Iliac artery | 144 | 85 | 86 |
| Iliac artery + 1 AV fistula | 456 | 75 | 74 |
| Aorta + 1 AV fistula | 314 | 86 | 86 |
| Aorta + 2 AV fistulas | 593 | 79 | 79 |
| Aorta + 3 AV fistulas | 886 | 73 | 73 |

*This table demonstrates the pathophysiology of arterial stenotic disease. Increasing the flow by opening a progressively larger number of arteriovenous (AV) fistulas causes a progressively lesser amount of stenosis necessary to initiate a 10% drop in flow. The validity of using noninvasive pressure measurements to determine flow changes is seen by comparing the last two columns. (Courtesy of Dr. Wesley Moore, Tucson, Ariz.)*

duplex arterial imaging to, most recently, magnetic resonance–derived flow measurements. We review the methods, costs, and benefits of these studies in relationship to one another.

In 1979, Gibbons et al,[7] employing ankle systolic blood pressure measurements, evaluated 150 diabetic patients seeking a decisive number to predict success in selecting an amputation level. Their conclusion—"In the diabetic patient, clinical judgement continues to provide the most accurate and reliable information by which the type of amputation and the likelihood of its success can be judged"—was well supported by their clinical material. Mehta et al.[17] confirmed the fallibility of ankle pressures in predicting healing of transmetatarsal amputations in diabetics, whereas Barnes et al.[2] did likewise for the healing of the below-knee amputations. Bone and Pomajzl[4] suggested the value of indexing the potential of healing forefoot amputations using toe pressures derived photoplethysmographically. In their study, 8 limbs with digital pressure less than 45 mm Hg failed to heal, 2 of 8 (25%) failed to heal in the range of 45 to 55 mm Hg, and all 14 patients subjected to forefoot amputation with a pressure greater than 55 mm Hg healed. They also demonstrated the unreliability of ankle systolic blood pressure (ASBP) in predicting amputation success.

## INSTRUMENTATION

We use several pieces of equipment to determine the hemodynamic status of our pa-

tients in an entirely noninvasive fashion: the photoplethysmograph, Doppler velocity flowmeters and probes, and a set of 12-cm blood pressure cuffs. An automatic cuff insufflator and a strip chart recorder increase the ease of performance and provide a permanent hard copy of the waveform for the patient's file. More recently we have added Duplex scanners, which help clarify proximal superficial femoral artery occlusions, as well as provide information on the number and status of nonstenotic or occluded tibial vessels.

## Photoplethysmography

Photoplethysmography employs a transducer that transmits infrared light from an emitting diode into the tissue. Part of the transmitted light is reflected back from the blood within the cutaneous microcirculation and is received by an adjacent phototransistor. The amount of reflected light varies with the blood content of the microcirculation. The output of the phototransistor is A/C, coupled to an amplifier for recording as a pulsatile analog waveform. This phototransducer is taped to the end of the toe with double-faced cellophane tape while a small digital blood pressure cuff is placed at the base of the digit. Figure 15–3 demonstrates the instrumentation. The pressure at which the waveform obliterates corresponds to the digital systolic pressure. The pressure may also be measured using a digital strain gauge or a peripherally placed Doppler probe. The photoplethysmograph, however, is the easiest to use, making it our

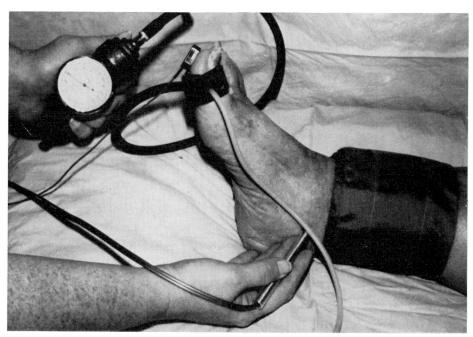

**FIG 15–3.**
Measurement of both posterior tibial ankle pressure and great toe pressure is demonstrated using Doppler ultrasound device and photoplethysmography.

preferred procedure for obtaining digital recordings.

## Doppler Ultrasound

The Doppler ultrasound device consists of two piezoelectric crystals mounted in a probe. By stimulating one of the crystals with an electrical charge, sound waves of various frequencies (all beyond the range of human hearing) are emitted. The second crystal receives the sound waves reflected from moving particles, producing a voltage change. This change can be amplified and converted to analog waveforms or sound. The higher the frequency emitted by the crystal, the less the depth of penetration and the narrower the width investigated. A frequency of 5 MHz gives deep penetration and comparatively broad beam especially suited for monitoring deep blood vessel flow in the vena cava or iliac veins or for examining peripheral veins. An operating frequency of 10 MHz is less penetrating but permits a sharper focus and is ideal for blood velocity detection in arteries and veins of limbs and digits. The Doppler probe is coupled to the skin with acoustical gel and held at an appropriate angle to the vessel being examined. This angle varies in accordance with the specifications of the individual manufacturers, ranging from 38 to 52 degrees.[1] A good seal between the probe and the skin is critical because the sound waves travel poorly through the air. Because there is no ideal probe angle for optimum recording, using a large amount of acoustical coupling gel allows one to vary the angle of insonation to find that point where the audible sound is clearest. A beam of ultrasound travels to the underlying vessel where it is reflected from red blood cells and shifted in frequency by an amount proportional to the flow velocity of erythrocytes in that vessel. The pitch of the audiofrequency signal produced by the receiving crystal is therefore proportional to the average velocity of the blood flowing within the vessel under study. The Doppler does not record the flow velocity itself but a phase shift. The recorded Doppler signal is used in two ways: (1) to measure segmental systolic pressure and (2) to produce flow velocity waveform patterns for analysis.

## Segmental Pressures

Pressure cuffs, 12 cm wide, are placed at the high thigh level, above the knee, below the knee, and at the ankle level. By listening with the Doppler probe over one of the pedal vessels (dorsalis pedis, posterior tibial, or lateral tarsal arteries), one can obtain the pressure at the level of the inflated cuff. An index is obtained by dividing the segmental systolic pressure by the brachial systolic pressure. The usual index recorded is that of the ankle (ankle pressure/brachial pressure), which should be 1 or just slightly higher. Pressure changes correlate directly with flow as previous discussed; thus an index of 0.5 represents only 50% of the expected blood flow. A gradient of 40 mm Hg or greater between the levels being compared suggests an occlusion or highly stenotic segment. In normal situations, the high thigh pressure is 1.3 times the brachial systolic pressure.

## Toe Pressures

The role of toe pressures in predicting the potential for ulceration healing or for successful treatment of gangrenous skin conditions of the feet using primary amputation is extremely pertinent when one is dealing with the diabetic foot.[10, 11] Holstein et al.[9] have demonstrated that absolute toe pressures provide a highly accurate method for determining the likelihood of success in the healing of an ulcer or in minor amputation. This prevents the need for a more proximal, major, potentially disabling amputation in an effort to heal an ulcer or relieve rest pain.[23] Barnes et al.[2] agree that toe pressures in diabetes are predictive of minor amputation healing. A toe pressure of 30 to 40 mm Hg seems to represent the watershed below which healing is doubtful.

## Waveform Evaluation

The peripheral arterial tree is largely a muscular bed and therefore has high resistance. Waveforms from normal subjects obtained at the common femoral, popliteal, dorsalis pedis, posterior tibial, and some-times lateral tarsal artery levels reflect this fact. Many approaches to quantitative analysis of waveforms have been suggested, but all have seemingly added little, if any, value over a rapid, subjective, qualitative evaluation.[14] The waveform in the normal state shows a rapid systolic upstroke and usually a peaked appearance. The actual magnitude of the waveform can be affected by the depth of the artery (e.g., decreased in obese persons), by probe pressure that actually compresses a thin patient's artery, by the probe angle in relation to the artery, or even by the consistency of the vessel being evaluated (e.g., a prosthetic graft will give a distorted picture even when fully patent). Thus, no comparison of the height of the peak should be attempted. In addition, a normal peripheral waveform will usually show a reversed component as the initial diastolic portion, followed by a small second forward component, as in Figure 15–8. The reverse segment is the result of distal resistance, followed by the elastic recoil of the vessel wall. This can sometimes be absent in the normal subject at the ankle level. Deterioration of the waveform can be seen just proximal to an obstructing lesion; distal to the lesion the waveform is always abnormal with a loss of the normal rapid systolic upstroke so that the slope is the same as that of the downstroke. In addition, even before these changes, early milder stenosis will cause loss of the diastolic components at the popliteal or femoral levels. As the flow deteriorates, waveforms become flattened and then undulating before they totally disappear. Flow and viability may exist despite absent waveforms, because the Doppler probes rarely detect flow at less than 6 mL/min. Comparing pressures and waveforms helps to avoid errors in interpretations, especially at the high thigh level.

Exercise can lead to a 10- to 20-fold increase in blood flow requirements in the muscular beds. As is apparent in Table 15–2, increased flows can lower the degree of stenosis necessary to create a given drop in flow or pressure. In addition, limiting factors other than claudication are sometimes demonstrated. A standard treadmill test is done on an incline of 12 degrees at 2 mph.[29]

The treadmill test is limited to a maximum of 5 minutes or the onset of chest discomfort, shortness of breath, dizziness, or severe leg pain. The cuffs placed before stress to determine the resting ankle pressure remain in place during the study. Immediately when the stress is stopped, at 2½ minutes and again at 5 minutes, ankle pressures are determined. The level of exercise necessary to validate claudication is much less than would be routinely encountered in cardiac stress testing. Nevertheless, caution is urged in patients who have coronary artery disease, and it is our policy to have a well-trained nurse or technician in attendance at all times.

In patients with recent contralateral amputations, painful infections, ulcers, digital necrosis, or recent surgery, reactive hyperemia can be induced. The high thigh pressure cuff is inflated to 50 mm Hg over the previously determined resting high thigh pressure. The patient is supine for this study, and the cuff remains inflated for 3 minutes. Ankle pressures are again measured immediately after release of the high thigh pressure cuff and at 15-second intervals for 3 to 5 minutes. Figure 15–2 shows the configuration of curves obtained in this way for cases with moderate and severe arterial obstruction compared with normal individuals. Although the curves are similar in shape, note that the response is rapid with induced reactive hyperemia and slow—a matter of minutes—after exercise testing.

Ouriel et al.[21] performed a critical evaluation of stress testing in the diagnosis of peripheral vascular disease. They studied 218 patients (372 limbs) and 25 normal subjects (50 limbs) with resting ankle index (RAI), treadmill exercise (TE), and postocclusive reactive hyperemia (PORH) to determine reliability and descrimination. They concluded that RAI was a simple, accurate, and reproducible test and that routine stress testing was not cost effective, adding little diagnostic information whether one is dealing with claudicants or patients harboring rest pain, ulceration, or gangrene. They suggested that stress testing should be reserved for the small subset of symptomatic patients with normal RAI. They also noted that walking distance was not a reproducible measure and that only a weak correlation existed between walking distance and the severity of disease as assessed by RAI.

A gradual decrease in the use of stress testing has been experienced. It nevertheless can prove useful in those situations where symptoms seemingly contradict physical findings and resting ankle/arm indices. At times, other etiologies for decreased ambulatory ability are clearly elucidated when the patient reproduces symptoms while undergoing testing.

We reviewed the predictive value of AAIs and absolute digital systolic pressures in diabetic and nondiabetic patients. In 120 limb salvage patients the average AAI preoperatively in diabetics was 0.53, increasing to 0.97 postoperatively, with a very wide scatter. This index appeared more reliable in nondiabetic persons: 0.34 preoperatively (Fig 15–4,A) and rising to 1.03 postoperatively, with a narrower scatter (Fig 15–4,B). Photoplethysmographically derived digital pressures (PDDPs) were much more predictable and precise in both diabetic and nondiabetic patients. In the diabetic population, only four patients demonstrated a pressure greater than 40 mm Hg preoperatively (Fig 15–5,A), whereas only five remained below this range (only one < 30 mm Hg) after successful revascularization (Fig 15–5,B). More recently, McCollum et al.[15] confirmed the value of PDDP in the assessment of severe ischemia but cautioned that appropriate warming of the foot permitting adequate foot vasodilation was essential to allow accurate conclusions to be drawn and to allow meaningful interpretation of results. Appropriate testing conditions are critical to every method of noninvasive testing to be reported on. Vincent et al.[28] reported on the use of PDDP toe/brachial index, noting in patients with chronic ulcerations toe pressures were higher in diabetics than nondiabetics. They believed during pressure measurements, attention must be directed to the patient's state of relaxation, digital skin temperature, and toe position relative to the level of the heart. They emphasized that systolic pressure fluctuated with respiration and activity (e.g., talking). Nielson[20] demonstrated that

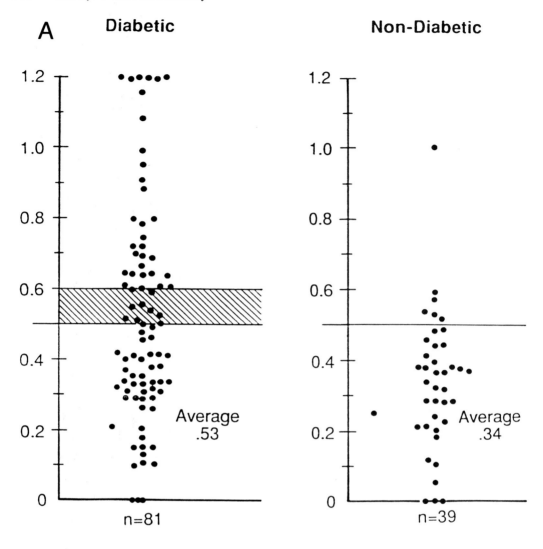

incompressible or >1.2 AAI will be recorded as 1.2

**FIG 15–4.**
**A,** preoperative ankle-arm pressure indices (AAIs) display a wide range in diabetic as compared with nondiabetic patients, because of medial calcinosis of the vessels causing incompressibility. (Incompressible or incompressability >1.2 AAI recorded as 1.2.) **B,** postoperative indices in nondiabetic patients display a significant change from preoperative levels. The same change to a lesser degree is seen with diabetic individuals.

skin temperature variation from 33°C to 24°C caused an average change of 10 mm Hg in toe systolic pressures secondary to changes in vasomotor tone. Finally, the same authors revealed diminished toe pressure as a result of hydrostatic forces when measurements were obtained with the patient supine.

### Regional Tissue Perfusion Measurements

Efforts to improve noninvasive evaluation after ankle and toe pressure testing have

centered on regional microcirculation using transcutaneous oximetry.

Tissue oxygen tension, a reflection of the adequacy of the circulatory system, is an absolute number on which a possible etiology of symptoms and the likelihood of healing can be based. The transcutaneous oxygen pressure (tcPo$_2$) monitors containing a chemical electrode are placed in peripheral (10 cm above the knee, 5 cm below the knee, and on the dorsum of the foot) and central or reference positions (5 cm below the middle left clavicle) to obtain readings. After

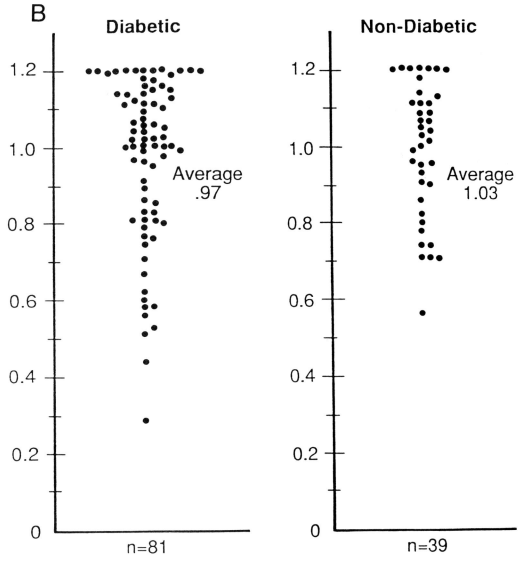

**FIG 15–4** (cont.).

patients have remained supine 10 to 15 minutes to allow equilibration, readings are then obtained at 3- to 5-minute intervals with the patient standing. Accuracy in testing depends on multiple systemic (fractional concentration of oxygen in inspired gas [$FIO_2$], lung function, blood hemoglobin level, and cardiac output) and local (skin thickness, capillary formation and density, and the presence of inflammation or edema) factors.

The ability to discriminate severity of disease, likelihood of ulcer healing, or the appropriate amputation level was claimed for transcutaneous oximetry by Hauser et al.[8] in 1984. They employed positional changes of the foot. They derived a regional perfu-sion index (RPI) for each limb as the ratio of foot $tcPO_2$/chest $tcPO_2 \times 100$. These were determined in the supine, standing, and leg-elevated positions. They found claudicants could be discerned from normal patients best with leg elevation, but with rest pain and gangrene, RPI values were quite similar in the supine and elevated positions, diverging in the dependent position. They compared transcutaneous oxymetry to ankle systolic blood pressure measurements and found superiority at a statistically significant ($p < 0.001$) level. They believed regional transcutaneous oximetry to be the only non-invasive test of limb perfusion consistently accurate in diabetics.

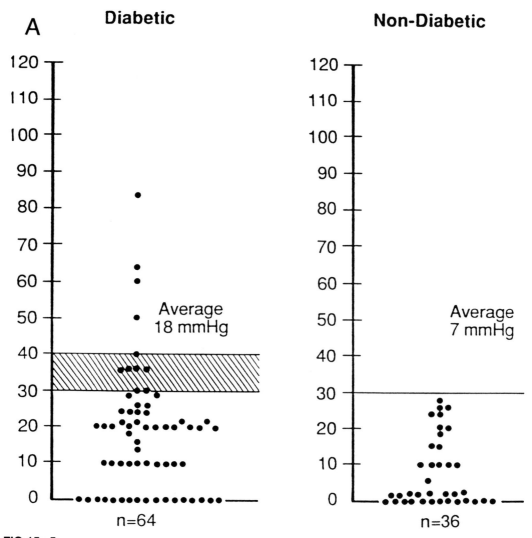

**FIG 15–5.**
**A,** absolute toe pressure measurements obtained photoplethysmographically in preoperative diabetic and nondiabetic limb salvage patients reveal only four patients with a value > 40 mm Hg in the diabetic group and none with > 30 mm Hg in nondiabetic patients. **B,** absolute photoplethysmographically obtained pressure measurements in postoperative assessment reveal three patients with values < 30 mm Hg and only five patients with < 40 mm Hg in the diabetic group. This degree of improvement is not observed in the nondiabetic patient.

Subsequent to attempts to use transcutaneous oximetry, the employment of laser Doppler velocimetry (LDV) alone or in conjunction with tcPo$_2$ was reported. The LDV device emits a monochromatic helium-neon laser beam at a frequency of 632.8 nm that is conducted to the skin through a plastic fiberoptic probe. The basis of LDV is that a collumated beam becomes diffusely scattered, absorbed, and broadened when applied to the skin, resulting in Doppler shifts that may be detected by a sensitive photodetector. The Doppler shift is linearly related to the mean velocity of RBCs within skin capillaries and varies with the angle of the probe to the tissue being monitored. Measurements reflect an average over a semisphere of skin approximately 1 mm in radius. The photo-detected reflected signal is fed into an analog signal processor, and values are expressed in millivolts. The normal LDV tracing is fairly characteristic, whereas ischemic tissues generate pulse waves of lesser magnitude and amplitude. Kram et al.[12] performed LDV measurements in 29 patients (16 diabetic individuals) before they

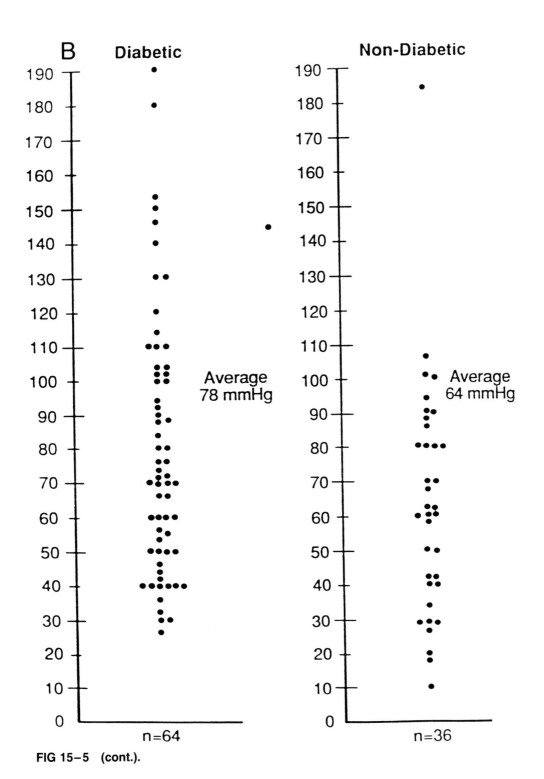

**FIG 15–5** (cont.).

underwent below-knee amputations. Anterior and posterior calf LDV values greater than or equal to 20 mV were associated with successful below-knee amputation wound healing in 25 of 26 patients; all three patients with either anterior or posterior calf LDV values less than 20 mV had below-knee amputations that failed to heal.

Karanfilian et al.[11] combined $tcPo_2$ and LDV measurements in predicting healing of ischemic forefoot ulcerations and amputations in diabetic and nondiabetic patients. Fifty-nine limbs, 63% of which were nondiabetic patients, were studied. Either transmetatarsal amputations or debridement with or without skin grafting were performed. Criteria for successful healing included a $tcPo_2$ value of more than 10 mm Hg, laser Doppler pulse wave amplitude of more than 4 mV, and an ankle systolic pressure of more than 30 mm Hg. With these criteria, the outcome was predicted correctly in 53 of 56 limbs (95%) by $tcPo_2$, in 46 of 53 limbs (87%) with LDV, and in 31 of 59 limbs (52%) with Doppler ankle pressures. They concluded that the estimation of skin blood flow by the $tcPo_2$ and LDV is significantly better than Doppler ankle pressure measurements in predicting the healing of forefoot ulcerations and amputations in diabetic and nondiabetic patients. The absolute number derived with $tcPo_2$ level measurement alone is unclear. The Pecoraro et al.[22] series indicated that at 22 mm Hg there was extremely low probability of healing. An absolute number to predict healing does not currently exist.

## Duplex Scanning of Peripheral Arterial Tree

Duplex scanning combines B-mode capabilities of revealing the anatomic and the Doppler-derived velocity recordings, indicating the degree of vessel lumen stenosis. Gating the Doppler signal on the B-mode imagery allows the arterial blood flow to be analyzed at selective levels within the lumen, as well as at progressive sites along the vessel course. Introduction of color imaging has greatly aided the interogation of vessels, allowing easier, more rapid identification of

high-flow (hence, stenotic) areas. Duplex imaging requires the use of probes capable of deep penetration, such as 2.25 and 3.5 MHz, as well as 5- and 8-MHz heads. Low-megahertz, high-penetrative probes are necessary for interogration of vessels deep in obese patients. These studies are significantly impeded by increased depth of penetration needed, bone, intestinal gas, and cutaneous problems, preventing the direct application of the probes. Duplex imaging, much like arteriograms, can give the anatomic assessment of the arterial tree, as well as the severity of multiple areas of stenosis, but fail to give a bottom line evaluation of the severity of distal ischemia. Hence, this study is an adjunct but realistically cannot stand alone in determining the severity of ischemia in the lower limbs.

Moneta et al.[18] discussed the accuracy of lower limb arterial duplex mapping (LLADM) from the aortic bifurcation to the ankle in 150 consecutive patients. They compared the noninvasive results to angiography in a standard fashion. The LLADM visualized 99% of arterial segments proximal to the tibial vessels, with overall sensitivities for detecting a 50% or greater lesion ranging from 89% in the iliac vessels to 67% at the popliteal artery. Stenosis was successfully distinguished from occlusion in 98% of cases. In the tibial vessels, LLADM was better at visualizing anterior tibial and posterior tibial arterial segments (94% and 96%) than peroneal artery segments (83%) ($p < 0.001$).

Duplex imaging of the iliac vessels has proved to be helpful in assessing those patients who might be percutaneous angioplasty candidates. Regional pressure measurement of the aortoiliac segments noninvasively is not possible, because no successful method exists to compress these vessels. Using the modified Bernoulli equation ($P = 4 V_{max}$) a pressure gradient can be calculated.[13] This calculated pressure gradient correlates closely with arterial "pull-through" pressures obtained during arteriography.

Computer software calculates velocity (using the Doppler equation) obtained by sound spectrum analyzed Doppler signals derived at B-mode localized retroperitoneal segments. A correction is made in the computer for the angle of insonation. A significant gradient of at least 30 mm Hg alerts the angiographer of a lesion potentially suitable for angioplasty. The area in question can then be subjected to closer scrutiny through multiple angiographic views to resolve the question of significant stenosis.

## Magnet Resonance Flowmetry

Magnetic resonance flow measurements application to peripheral arterial insufficiency is a relatively new modality having been released for commercial use only in 1989. Its early development began in 1979 with a successful operating unit not available until 1984.

The basic unit includes a 0.1 tesla field producing magnet weighing 5,300 lb in a table-line work station. In addition, either electric or magnetic shielding in a dedicated room is required. Likewise, temperature control between 17.8°C and 29°C Farenheit is critical. Any patient having a cardiac pacemaker is categorically excluded. Magnetic resonance flow measurements are still in the early stages of evaluation but may be of value in diabetic patients, because it measures flow and not pressure and theoretically should not be affected by noncompressible vessels. The ability to accurately and precisely directly measure blood flow in the lower limbs may allow better discrimination between claudication and those patients with rest pain, ulceration, and gangrene. Stress testing has not appeared to be essential with magnetic resonance flow measurements to obtain adequate results. Unfortunately, the time and cost factors of this modality will require dramatically superior results to other noninvasive modalities to justify its application in other than research areas. Much more information regarding magnetic resonance force measurements should be forthcoming during the next few years.

## Peripheral Noninvasive Investigation

Two questions need to be addressed in regard to noninvasive investigation and dia-

betic patients. First, on which patients should these studies be performed? Second, which studies should be employed in these investigations? The former question is resolved by history and physical examination, whereas the latter requires understanding of the effectiveness, cost, and effort required of each study.

Clinical examination can usually detect those patients who have no deficit in their pulses at rest. If a pulse can still be easily palpated after ambulation down a hallway, walking in place, or repeated toe stands, it is doubtful that symptoms come from peripheral arterial disease. Such patients rarely require further evaluation except as baseline screening or as a prelude to invasive procedures such as angiography, cardiac catheterization, or aneurysm repair.

Those patients with physical findings, femoral bruits, or diminished or absent pulses benefit from physiologic quantification of their status. Data from asymptomatic or mildly symptomatic patients will serve as a baseline and anatomic localizer for future progression of peripheral arterial occlusive disease. Those patients with superficial femoral artery occlusions who show minimal or no change in the pressure level after 5 minutes of treadmill exercise or an equivalent period of reactive hyperemia testing have adequate collateral circulation. A plan of watchful waiting is then the appropriate course to recommend. A follow-up of patients participating in an exercise program or receiving hemorrheologic agents is best pursued with exercise stress testing results because these tests provide objective evidence of improvement, a result that is encouraging to patient and physician alike.

What is the best noninvasive study to employ in investigating lower limb peripheral arterial insufficiency in diabetic individuals? The study employed depends on the data required. The question of a hemodynamically significant iliac stenosis or the likelihood of a digital amputation succeeding are two vastly different situations requiring different noninvasive procedures. Ankle systolic blood pressures, because of the high incidence of arterial medial calcinosis in diabetes mellitus, have clearly been shown to be unreliable. Magnetic resonance flowometry, because of extremely high costs ($375,000 for equipment and additional expenses for the physical facility) and current meager data of effectiveness, cannot substantiate the use of this method. Only duplex imaging can evaluate the severity and treatability of iliac arterial stenosis. Although admittedly this comprises only 5% to 10% of those diabetic patients with peripheral arterial insufficiency, the noninvasive knowledge obtained can prevent unnecessary angiograms. At the same time it may allow a beneficial correction of stenosis-related claudication in patients who might not have otherwise had angiography performed. The resolution of the vicissitudes of severe peripheral ischemia then rely on three studies: (1) photoplethysmograpically derived digital pressures, (2) transcutaneous oximetry, and (3) laser Doppler velocimetry. Interestingly enough, all three are capable of generating the information needed to make these determinations. Likewise, it is significant that transcutaneous oximetry and LDV were compared with Doppler-derived ankle systolic blood pressures rather than PDDP in spite of extensive evidence invalidating ankle systolic blood pressure as a reliable study at the time these comparisons were being undertaken. Clearly, comparison with PDDP would have been much more revealing. All three studies are repeatable. The range of cost in equipment is $1,000 to 3,000 for PDDP equipment, $8,000 to 10,000 for LDV equipment, and $10,000 to 12,000 for tcP$o_2$ equipment. Photoplethysmographically derived digital pressures can be obtained most quickly—approximately 10 minutes, whereas tcP$o_2$ studies require 30 to 40 minutes of time and LDV examinations fall somewhere in between.

Careful attention to testing conditions, including ambient temperature, patient's state of relaxation, positioning of the limb, coupled with skillful application of the noninvasive techniques, allow any of these modalities to be repeatable, reliable, and valuable in decision making in the face of severe ischemia.

Understanding of the limitations of the various noninvasive modalities likewise is necessary when the interpretation of these studies is applied. Unrecognized ischemia can occur for two main reasons: patient error or physician error. Patient error centers around physical findings often in hard to examine areas (plantar surface, heel, interdigital areas) where significant tissue damage is obscured by severe peripheral neuropathy, as reported by Boulten (see Chapter 10).

Physician error also can stem from inadequate interpretation of noninvasive studies because of a lack of sophistication in their application. Most often, near-normal or extremely high ankle systolic blood pressure is equated with no risk of distal ischemia. As we have pointed out, AAI greater than 1.0 can be associated with limb salvage conditions. The Foot Council of the American Diabetic Association reminds all physicians to have the shoes and socks off of all diabetic patients and inspect the feet whenever they are seen in consultation. To this wise admonition should be added: also understand the applications and limitations of noninvasive testing.

Physicians can also, at times, easily overlook physical changes even when inspecting the feet unless a careful, systematic routine is followed.

### Examples

The practicality of noninvasive studies is best explained with examples of the role they have played in the management of patients who have undergone surgery for correction of peripheral arterial insufficiency. Figure 15–6 shows normal waveforms in a diabetic man who has calcified arteries causing elevated segmental pressures. The toe pressure is normal. Figure 15–7 depicts the findings in a 58-year-old diabetic man with a nonhealing traumatic ulcer of the left shin. Pressures and waveform analysis correlate well with the arteriographic findings of occluded iliac and superficial femoral arteries. After aortofemoral and femoropopliteal grafting (Fig 15–8), his AAI index is more than 1, the waveforms are normal (except for the absence of diastolic reversal), and

Right arm = 144

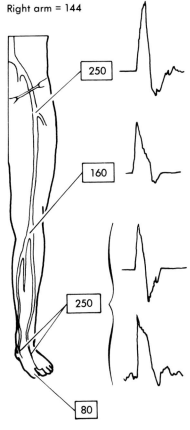

**FIG 15–6.**
Diabetics with patent vessels frequently have abnormally high ankle pressure because of medial calcification, which requires extremely high pressures to occlude. In addition, waveforms display early diastolic reversed flow, reliable indicator of patency when present. Note that highest brachial systolic pressure is 144 mm Hg.

Left arm = 166

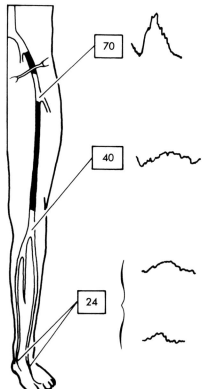

**FIG 15–7.**
Note abnormally low thigh pressure indicative of proximal occlusion or stenosis, coupled with postobstructed waveform. Additional 30 mm Hg gradient between high thigh and knee levels with further deterioration of waveforms at this level indicates severe stenosis or occlusion of superficial femoral arterial segment. Brachial systolic pressure is 166 mm Hg, yielding ankle-arm index of 0.15, or 15%, of expected resting ankle blood flow.

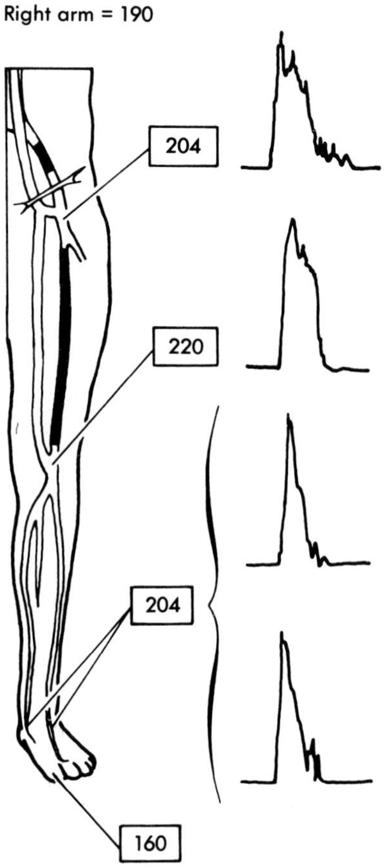

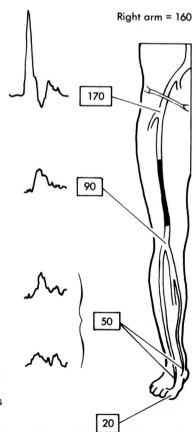

Right arm = 190

204

220

204

160

**FIG 15-8.**
Verification of operative success in patient in Figure 15-7 is seen following aortofemoral and femoropopliteal bypass. Ankle pressure (204) mm Hg) is now greater than brachial pressure (190 mm Hg). Characteristically, normal early diastolic reversed flow is absent following use of proximal synthetic Dacron conduit.

Right arm = 160

170

90

50

20

**FIG 15-9.**
Example of occlusion of superficial femoral artery. Gradient of 80 mm Hg confirms location. High thigh pressure (170 mm Hg) greater than brachial pressure (160 mm Hg), coupled with normal waveform at this level, confirms clinical impression of lack of any significant inflow abnormality.

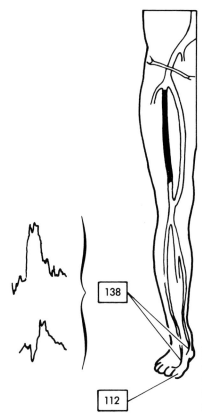

Right arm = 150

138

112

**FIG 15–10.**
After femoropopliteal vein graft bypass on patient in Figure 15–9, marked improvement in ankle pressure is noted. That ankle-arm index remains less than 1 confirms presence of significant stenotic disease of distal tibial vessels.

his great toe pressure of 160 mm Hg is normal. The ulcer healed after skin grafting. Finally, Figure 15–9 shows the results of an isolated superficial femoral artery occlusion in a 48-year-old woman with diabetes and severe claudication. The proximal thigh pressure and waveform are normal, whereas distal pressures are low and the waveforms are distinctly abnormal. After a saphenous vein femoropopliteal bypass graft, her ankle pressure is much improved, the waveform is more normal, and her great toe pressure is normal (Fig 15–10). The claudication resolved.

## REFERENCES

1. Baker WH, Barnes RW: Minor forefoot amputation in patients with low-angle pressure, *Am J Surg* 133:331, 1977.

2. Barnes RW, Thornhill B, Nix L, et al: Prediction of amputation wound healing, *Arch Surg* 116:80, 1981.

3. Bendick PJ, Glover JL, Kuebler TW, et al: Progression of atherosclerosis in diabetics, *Surgery* 9316:834, 1983.

4. Bone GE, Pomajzl MJ: Toe blood pressure by photoplethysmography: An index of healing in forefoot amputation, *Surgery* 89:569, 1981.

5. DeFrang RD, Taylor LM, Porter JM: Basic data related to amputations: basic data underlying clinical decision-making in vascular surgery, *Ann Vasc Surg* 2:62, 1988.

6. Duj JJ, Jimes RA: The role of diabetes in the development of degenerative vascular disease: with special reference to the incidence of retinitis and peripheral vasculitis, *Ann Intern Med* 14:1902, 1941.

7. Gibbons GW, Wheeloch FC, Siembreda C, et al: Noninvasive predictions of amputation level in diabetic patients, *Arch Surg* 114:1253, 1979.

8. Hauser CJ, Klein SR, Hehringer CM, et al: Superiority of transcutaneous oximetry in non-invasive vascular diagnosis in patients with diabetes, *Arch Surg* 119:690, 1984.

9. Holstein P, Noer I, Tonneses KH, et al: Distal blood pressure in severe arterial insufficiency, in Bergan J, James Y: *Gangrene and severe ischemia of the lower extremities*, New York, 1978, Grune & Stratton.

10. Jonason T, Ruggvist I: Diabetes mellitus and intermittent claudication: relation between peripheral vascular complications and location of the occlusive atherosclerosis, *Acta Med Scand* 218:217, 1985.

11. Karanfilian RG, Lynch TG, Zirul VT, et al: The value of laser Doppler velocimetry and transcutaneous oxygen tension determination in predicting healing of ischemic forefoot ulcerations and amputations in diabetic, *J Vasc Surg* 4:511, 1986.

12. Kram HB, Appel PL, Shoemaker WC: Prediction of below-knee amputation wound healing using noninvasive laser Doppler velocimetry, *Am J Surg* 158:29, 1989.

13. Langsfeld M, Nepute J, Binnington HB, et al: The use of deep duplex scanning to predict hemodynamically significant aorto-iliac stenoses, *J Vasc Surg* 7:395, 1988.

14. Marinelli MR, Beach KW, Glass MJ, et al: Noninvasive testing vs clinical evaluation of arterial disease: a prospective study, *JAMA* 241:2031, 1979.

15. McCollum PT, Stanley ST, Kent P, et al: Assessment of arterial disease using digital systolic pressure measurements, *Ann Vasc Surg* 5:349, 1991.

16. McDaniel MD, Cronenwett JL, Basic data underlying history of intermittent claudication: basic data underlying clinical decision making in vascular surgery, *Ann Vasc Surg* 2:1, 1988.

17. Mehta K, Hobson RW, Jamil Z, et al: Fallibility of Doppler ankle pressures in predicting healing of transmetatarsal amputations, *J Surg Res* 28:466, 1980.

18. Moneta GL, Yeager RA, Antonovic R, et al: Accuracy of lower extremity arterial duplex mapping, *J Vasc Surg* 5:275, 1991.

19. Moore WS, Malone JM: Effect of flow rate and vessel caliber on clinical arterial stenosis, *J Surg Res* 26:1, 1979.

20. Nielson PE: Digital blood pressure in normal subjects and patients with peripheral arterial disease, *Scand J Clin Lab Invest* 36:731, 1976.

21. Ouriel K, McDonnell AE, Metz CE, et al: A critical evaluation of stress testing in the diagnosis of peripheral vascular disease, *Surgery* 91:686, 1982.

22. Pecoraro RE, Ahroni JH, Boyko EJ, et al: Chronology and determinants of tissue repair in diabetic lower extremity ulcers, *Diabetes* 40:10, 1991.

23. Reunanen A, Takkunen H, Aromaa A: Prevalence of intermittent claudication and its effect on mortality, *Acta Med Scand* 211:249, 1982.

24. Rosenblood MS, Flanigan DP, Schuler JJ, et al: Risk factors affecting the natural history of intermittent claudication, *Arch Surg* 123:867, 1988.

25. Strandness DE: Abnormal exercise responses after successful reconstructive arterial surgery, *Surgery* 59:325, 1966.

26. Strandness DE, Bell IW: An evaluation of the hemodyncamic response of the claudicating extremity to exercise, *Surg Gynecol Obstet* 59:325, 1966.

27. Strandness DE, Priest RE, Gibbons GE: Combined clinical and pathologic study of diabetic and non diabetic peripheral arterial disease, *Diabetes* 13:366, 1964.

28. Vincent DG, Salles-Cunha SX, Bernhard VM, et al: Noninvasive assessment of toe systolic pressures with special reference to diabetes mellitus, *J Cardiovasc Surg* 24:22, 1983.

29. Ad Hoc Committee on Reporting Standards, Society for Vascular Surgery, North American Chapter, International Society for Cardiovascular Surgery: Suggested standards for reports dealing with lower extremity ischemia. *J Vasc Surg* 4:80, 1986.

# CHAPTER 16

# Imaging of the Diabetic Foot

Kevin W. McEnery, M.D.

Louis A. Gilula, M.D.

David C. Hardy, M.D.

Tom W. Staple, M.D.

A variety of imaging studies may contribute greatly to the diagnosis and treatment of diseases of the diabetic foot. The neurologic and vascular problems of the diabetic foot have been amply reviewed in other chapters. Imaging examinations are valuable adjuncts to physical examination of the foot, helping to demonstrate the extent and severity of the disease process. Gangrene of a toe or soft tissue ulceration is a common indication for evaluation of the diabetic foot. Such changes in the skin may be caused by vascular insufficiency, diabetic neuropathy, infection, or a combination of these factors. Skeletal changes in diabetic feet may be manifested by several findings, including (1) generalized demineralization, (2) focal osteolysis, (3) Charcot joint, or (4) infection. Although conventional radiography is the most cost effective and readily available way of imaging the diabetic foot, other methods may be very useful in resolving specific clinical problems in selected cases.

## SKELETAL CHANGES NOT DIRECTLY ASSOCIATED WITH DIABETES MELLITUS

Causes of foot pain not related to diabetes are discovered occasionally when patients with suspected diabetic skeletal changes are evaluated. Although usually clinically apparent, hallux valgus deformity (Fig 16–1) may produce secondary changes in the metatarsophalangeal joint and the surrounding bursae, producing both pain and redness. Diffuse idiopathic skeletal hyperostosis (DISH) is relatively common in diabetic and obese patients.[16, 23, 27] Although the process is most commonly associated with spinal abnormalities, bony excrescences of the foot and heel are present in most patients or may be present in diabetic patients without DISH.[52] For example, subungual exostoses (Fig 16–2) and spurs of the os calcis (Fig 16–3) are particularly important causes of foot pain not directly related to diabetes. Subungual exostoses may produce ulceration of the nail bed or the surrounding tissue and may simulate tumor.[45] Chronic infection has been reported in 34% to 60% of patients with subungual exostoses. Even without ulceration or redness, the pain of a subungual exostosis may simulate vascular insufficiency.[32] The pain produced by spurs of the os calcis is well known.

Another somewhat uncommon lesion is demonstrated in a 60-year-old woman who for 3 weeks before seeing her physician experienced pain and swelling in her left foot without a previous traumatic incident. There was

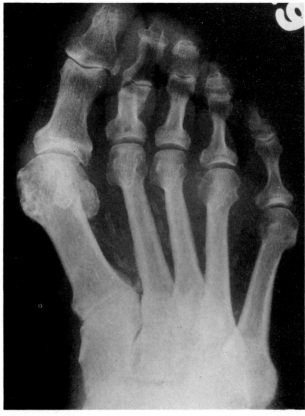

**FIG 16–1.**
Hallux valgus deformity and vascular calcification in a diabetic foot with medial bowing at first metatarsophalangeal joint. Joint has mild degenerative changes. Parallel streaks of densities between metatarsal shafts are typical arterial calcifications.

tenderness but no redness over the second metatarsal. A foot radiograph (Fig 16–4,A) demonstrated considerable periosteal new bone about the second metatarsal shaft. The attending physician was rightfully concerned about the possibility of a malignant tumor. However, the radiologist believed that the radiographic findings, along with the 3-week clinical history, were characteristic of a stress fracture and suggested conservative management rather than a biopsy. A reexamination 3 weeks later (Fig 16–4,B) showed maturation of the callus and progressive healing consistent with a fracture. Four weeks later the foot pain had completely abated.

## GENERALIZED DEMINERALIZATION AND FOCAL OSTEOLYSIS

While interpreting the results of plain film radiographic examination, one should keep in mind that avascular bone cannot be resorbed. When bone underlying impending or actual gangrene has been destroyed, sufficient bony vascular supply remains to produce the observed resorption, as was pointed out by Phemister[47] many years ago. Therefore the destructive bone changes associated with diabetes are found in the patient with an adequate vascular supply to the foot.

Resorption of bone can take a number of forms. All of the foot bones may be diffusely demineralized, and this change can be entirely independent of disuse (Fig 16–5). On the other hand, osteolysis may begin as focal forefoot defects. The defects typically are sharply outlined local defects 1 to 5 mm in diameter, most often in the phalanges and the metatarsal heads (Fig 16–6,A). They may remain unchanged for many years or may progress to massive osteolysis in a relatively short time (see Fig 16–6,B–D). The osteolysis generally begins in the metaphysis as an ill-defined loss of cortex and spreads

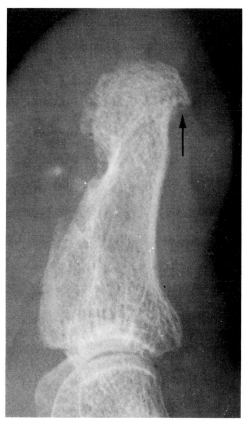

**FIG 16–2.**
Subungual exostosis in great toe (*arrow*) was source of pain in this diabetic patient. *(Courtesy of O.L. Lippard, M.D., St. Louis.)*

through the remaining metaphysis and then into the epiphysis, sparing the diaphysis. The end of the diaphysis may at first be ragged, but as the lesion progresses, it becomes pointed, producing a candlestick or pencil-like configuration (see Fig 16–6, B–D). Later the surface becomes smooth and the remaining bone sclerotic (Fig 16–6,C and D).

Considerable doubt has been raised regarding the etiology of erosive or resorptive changes about the phalangeal tufts and the metatarsal heads. Some authors[66] believe that such changes are present only in the diabetic patient with peripheral neuropathy, foot ulcerations, and soft tissue and bone infections. There is, however, no question that these changes may be of noninfectious origin. Localized forefoot osteolysis is therefore poorly understood but is probably related to ischemia, infection, or neurologic deficiency, either alone or in combination. In some patients the condition will be found in the absence of proof of any of these conditions.[51]

The process of osteolysis may be self-limiting, destroying only one bone, thus producing a shortened digit with a pencil-like base of a proximal phalanx and a slightly irregular metatarsal head (see Fig 16–6,C and D). Usually the articular surface is the last resorbed.

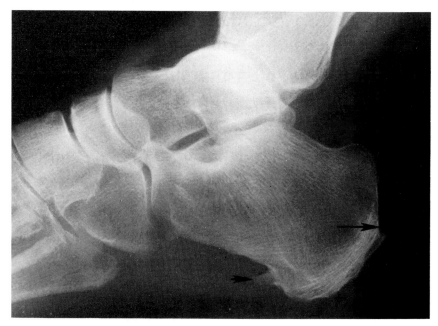

**FIG 16–3.**
Spurs extend from os calcis in Achilles tendon (*arrow*) and plantar fascia (*arrowhead*).

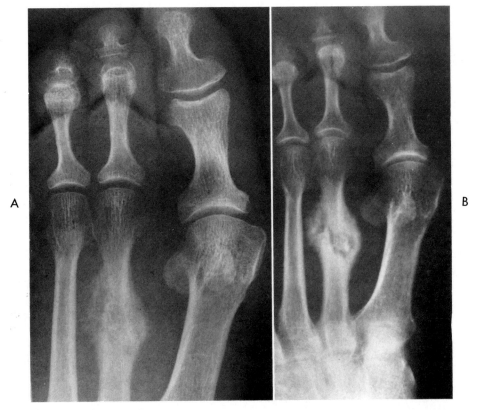

**FIG 16–4.**
Stress fracture. **A,** shaft of second metatarsal contains irregular periosteal proliferation. **B,** 3 weeks later some bone has been resorbed, making fracture line evident, and the callus has assumed mature organized appearance.

**FIG 16–5.**
Diffuse demineralization in diabetic foot.

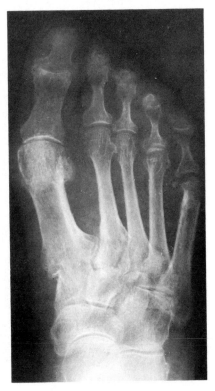

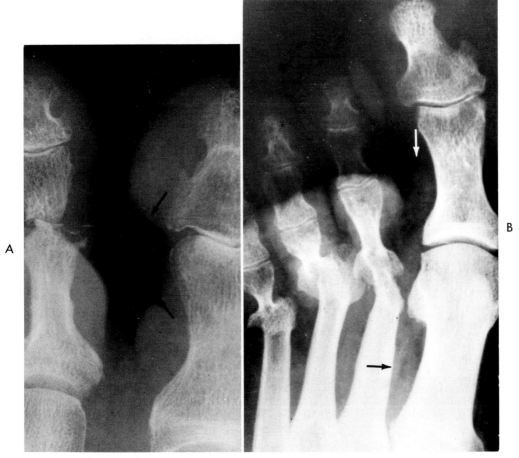

**FIG 16–6.**
Diabetic osteopathy. **A,** involvement of proximal interphalangeal joint of second toe. Base of middle phalanx shows early penciling. Both sides of head of proximal phalanx are eroded. Skin over second toe is intact. Soft tissue of medial aspect of first toe is ulcerated (*arrows*). **B,** heads of second and fourth metatarsals are eroded, and proximal phalanges of second and fourth metatarsals are dislocated ventrally at metatarsophalangeal joints. Shaft of second metatarsal has early pencil-point deformity. Lucency in webs between toes is subcutaneous air secondary to infection (*arrows*). (Continued.)

Similarly, the tips of the phalanges may be resorbed (see Fig 16–6,E). When associated with soft tissue infection in the tip of a digit, the change may be difficult to differentiate from osteomyelitis. Again, radiographic demonstration of bone destruction should not be the sole basis of a decision concerning amputation of a digit or an extremity.

Meltzer et al.[36] reviewed the foot radiographs of 32 diabetic patients with soft tissue necrosis. Without any further history they placed 17 patients with no radiographic evidence of osseous resorption into an ischemic limb category. Of these 17, only three had palpable dorsalis pedis and posterior tibial artery pulses. Intermittent claudication was present in 70%, and two had clinical diabetic neuropathy. All of these patients with soft tissue necrosis but no bone resorption required major amputation within 1 week to 3 months because the soft tissue lesions progressed or failed to heal.

The other 15 patients had bone resorption and were classified as nonischemic. The pulses about the ankle were palpable in 13 patients, and claudication was found in only two patients. Eleven patients had gangrene of one or more toes, and four patients had trophic ulcers, abscesses, and cellulitis in various combinations. None of these patients required a major amputation despite radiographic evidence of bone resorption. Conservative management such as debridement, oscillating bed, antibiotic therapy, and dia-

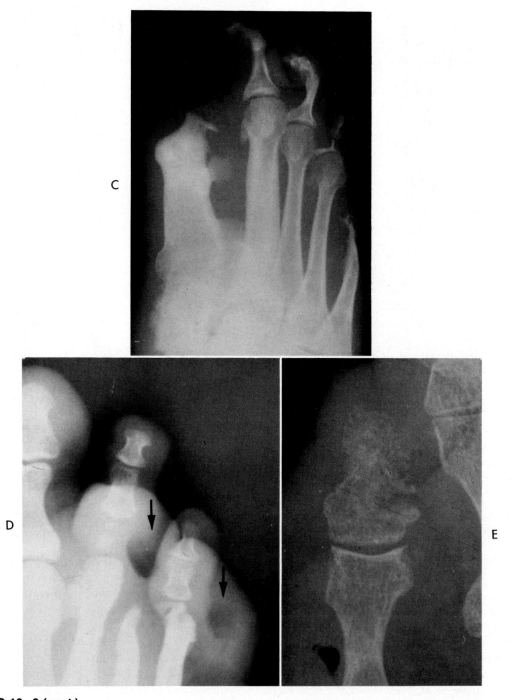

**FIG 16–6 (cont.).**
**C,** penciling of proximal phalanx of fourth toe and first and fifth metatarsals. First and fifth toes were amputated because of infection. **D,** penciling and sclerosis of third metatarsal. Large portions of proximal phalanges of second and fourth toes have been resorbed. Soft tissue lucencies adjacent to metatarsal heads are trophic ulcers on plantar aspect of foot (*arrows*). **E,** parts of distal and middle phalanges of little toe have been resorbed. *(Courtesy of Dr. O.L. Lippard, St. Louis.)*

betic control produced healing in seven patients. Minor surgery, usually amputation of the phalanx, affected adequate healing in the remainder, as indicated in clinical follow-up of 2 months to 10 years.

## DIABETIC NEUROPATHY

The radiographic appearance of the diabetic neuropathic joint cannot be differentiated from the neuropathic joint of syringomyelia, syphilis, or congenital insensitivity to pain. However, there are clinical and radiographic findings that indicate the diabetic joint destruction is neuropathic in origin. The classic radiographic appearance of neuropathic joint is one of extensive bone destruction with little or no demineralization. In fact, the bones may be sclerotic. There may be massive destruction with the joint greatly swollen, and small fragments of bone may be scattered throughout the swollen soft tissue (see Fig 16–7,C and D). Histologic examination shows these fragments of bone embedded within the synovium of the distended joint. The ligaments and capsule contain areas of fibroblastic and small round cell infiltration and edema. The articular cartilage shows varying degrees of degeneration replaced by fibrous tissue. The subchondral bone is necrotic, fragmented, and avascular. Separate fragments of dead bone are also usually present.[48] Localized, mature-appearing periosteal proliferation along the proximal second through fourth metatarsals is very common in patients with diabetes.[8] The precise cause of this finding is uncertain but is believed to be related to neuropathic changes.[20, 30]

Severe joint pain is not a hallmark of the neuropathic joint. In fact, the patient with such a joint often has been walking on the extremity. Therefore, the bone is well mineralized despite severe destruction because no bone atrophy of disuse has occurred. The

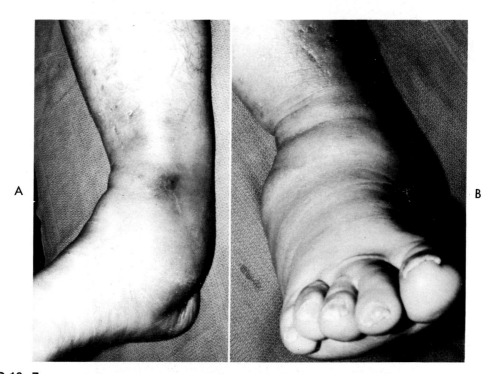

**FIG 16–7.**
Neuropathic ankle joint. **A** and **B,** swelling and deformity about the ankle, with subluxation of foot. **C** and **D,** multiple fragments of distal tibia, with some fragments embedded in synovium. Bone shows increased density, contrary to what usually occurs in such severe injuries in nondiabetic patients. **E,** at this time soft tissue about os calcis was normal. **F,** 4 weeks later, a trophic ulcer had developed on heel. Disruption and loss of normal thickness of soft tissues are evident. *(Courtesy of Edward Lansche, M.D., St. Louis.)* (Continued.)

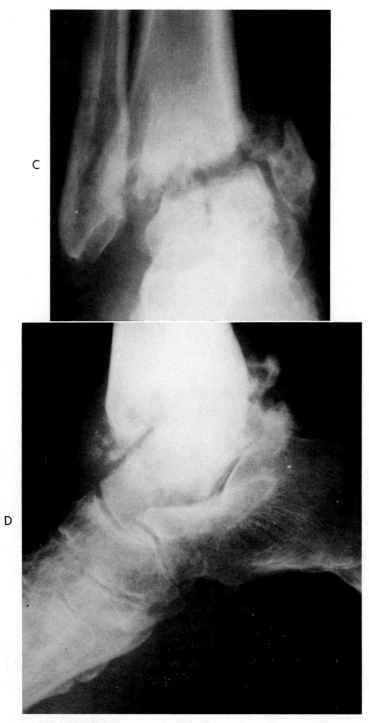

**FIG 16–7 (cont.).**

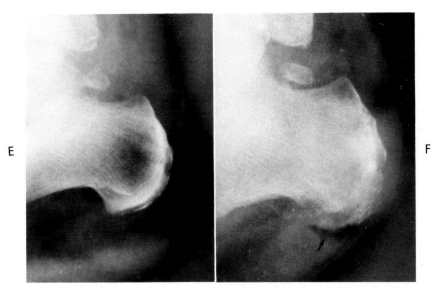

E     F

**FIG 16–7 (cont.).**

neuropathic joint and destruction by pigmented villonodular synovitis are the primary conditions in which severe destruction will fail to result in demineralization of the associated structures.

A 64-year-old man whose foot is shown in Figure 16–7 had diabetes with posterior column disease and neuropathy for 15 years. Three weeks before the examination he twisted his ankle while mowing his lawn. It became swollen and deformed. His pain was not sufficient to compel him to seek care at that time, but a persistent slight discomfort and deformity caused him to visit his physician. By then considerable swelling and deformity had developed about the ankle (see Fig 16–7,A and B). Radiographs showed a fracture dislocation at the ankle joint and sclerosis of the affected bones (see Fig 16–7,C and D). Some loose fragments were embedded in the capsule of the distended joint. The findings were typical of a Charcot joint. A cast was applied. Approximately 4 weeks later a gradually enlarging ulceration appeared over the heel (see Fig 16–7,E and F). Six months later only a small ulceration persisted, and the ankle joint had become stable.

The subtalar joint may be similarly affected. The findings may be more subtle but identical to those in other joints. The opposing joint surfaces become fragmented, and

the fragments of bone may be extruded to the side of the os calcis and the talus (Fig 16–8).

The neuropathic foot is somewhat more subject to fractures and dislocations. Small periarticular fractures are a common early manifestation of diabetic neuroarthropathy. When the changes of neuroarthropathy become severe with resultant changes in the normal biomechanical function of a joint, fracture, subluxation, or dislocation may occur.[42] In some diabetic patients spontaneous fracture, subluxation, or dislocation will occur with no definite abnormality in the underlying bony structure.[12, 31] These neuropathic changes may be a factor in the etiology of avascular necrosis of the fourth metatarsal head, also known as Freiberg's disease in diabetic patients.[44] Fractures of the os calcis, for example, have been reported in diabetics who have not sustained any severe injury.[10] In addition, large avulsion-type fractures of the superior tuberosity of the calcaneous are characteristic of diabetes.[28] Fracture may be the first sign of a neuropathic joint and may, in fact, play an important role in initiating neuroarthropathic joint changes.[9, 26] Insensitivity to pain probably is a contributing factor in this phenomenon.[4] Repetitive exercise is probably the most common cause of this fracture. Fractures that develop in diabetic patients

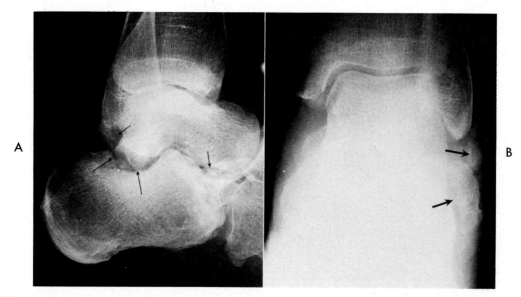

**FIG 16–8.**
Neuropathic subtalar joint. **A,** lateral view. Posterior articular facet of os calcis is eroded (*long arrows*). Bone fragments have extruded anteriorly and posteriorly (*short arrows*). **B,** anteroposterior view. Bone fragments have been extruded laterally (*arrows*).

without a history of significant trauma have a poor prognosis.

It is not uncommon for a patient with neuropathic joint to visit a physician because of dissatisfaction with the deformed extremity rather than because of pain. The radiographs of some of these patients have been misinterpreted as showing a malignant tumor because of the extensive destruction. However, malignant primary bone tumors, even when large, seldom destroy both sides of the joint. Furthermore, a malignant lesion of such extent is accompanied by considerable pain. Even though pain is present in approximately 50% of patients with a Charcot joint, it is seldom of any great severity. Disuse of the extremity with a malignant tumor produces diffuse demineralization directly adjacent to the lesion in contrast to the bones of the neuropathic joint, which show little, if any, demineralization and usually osteosclerosis.

In some patients radiographic examination will be performed after diabetic neuropathic osteoarthropathy has healed. Features that suggest healed diabetic arthropathy in the foot include well-corticated deformity of the metatarsal heads, shortening of the first proximal phalanx (usually as a result of either prior articular destruction or fracture deformity), and ankylosis of joints (especially the interphalangeal joints).[50]

## INFECTION

Osteomyelitis in the distal foot may be exceedingly difficult to differentiate radiographically from diabetic osteopathy. The destruction of diabetic osteopathy may appear radiographically identical to osteomyelitis in a bone underlying ulcerated skin, but if the skin is intact, the destruction is more likely to be diabetic osteopathy than osteomyelitis. A recent study demonstrated that in asymptomatic patients with foot ulcer, underlying osteomyelitis was present in 68%.[43]

An example of diabetic osteopathy appearing radiographically identical to osteomyelitis is shown in Figure 16–6,A. The patient was in his early sixties and had been diabetic for about 10 years. The skin of the second, third, and fourth toes was intact but reddened. The radiograph showed destructive changes at the proximal interphalangeal joint of the second toe. The base of the middle phalanx of this toe was slightly pointed. The lack of skin ulcerations makes it unlikely that the changes were caused by osteomyelitis, even though hematogeneous osteo-

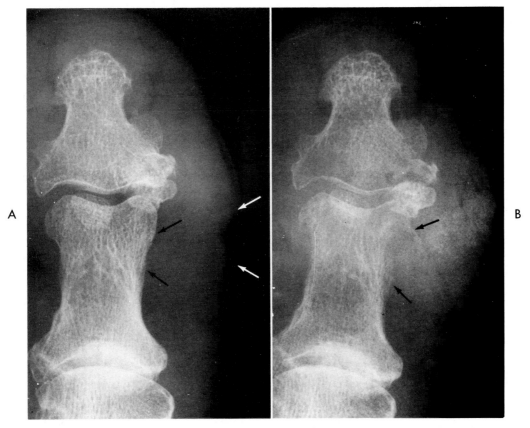

**FIG 16–9.**
Osteomyelitis. **A,** small soft tissue ulceration over medial aspect of proximal phalanx contains small erosion (*white arrows*). **B,** 3 weeks later, erosion of proximal phalanx has enlarged (*arrows*). Medial aspect of base of distal phalanx has also been destroyed. Soft tissue of toe is swollen.

myelitis cannot be entirely excluded. The lesion of this patient healed with bed rest and skin protection. He had no antibiotic therapy.

On the other hand, the 64-year-old woman whose toe is shown in Figure 16–9 had developed a skin ulceration of the medial aspect of her left great toe. A small erosion had developed in the cortex of the metaphysis of the proximal phalanx. Three weeks later this had progressed to a much deeper ulcer with severe bone destruction. These findings were consistent with osteomyelitis and were confirmed microscopically after amputation of the toe. Similar changes are seen in the heads of the third and fourth metatarsals in the patient in Figure 16–11. The erosive changes over the heads of the metatarsals, soft tissue ulceration, and swelling had developed in approximately 6 weeks.

Pathologic fractures through areas of osteomyelitis, often in the distal portions of the first or second proximal phalanges, may also occur in patients with diabetes. Frequently there is no history of significant trauma in these individuals.[37]

Soft tissue infection can be seen radiographically as edema, ulceration, or subcutaneous air collections. Edematous fluid separates the subcutaneous fat into lucent globules, producing a reticulated pattern and widening the subcutaneous tissues (Figs 16–10 and 16–11). Ulcerations are demonstrated radiographically as defects or irregularities in the skin surface and are usually visible on routine foot films (see Figs 16–6,A, 16–9,A, 16–11). Specific soft tissue technique films are unnecessary, bright lighting of the routine foot films will make the soft tissue radiographically apparent. When the skin is ulcerated, infection caused by gas-forming organisms may extend from the ulcer and produce subcutaneous air (see Figs 16–6,B, and 16–12).

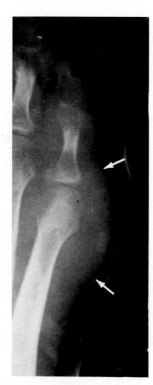

**FIG 16–10.**
Edema lateral to fifth metatarsal head. Soft tissue thickening is prominent.

**FIG 16–11.**
Soft tissue ulceration near head of fifth metatarsal (*white arrows*). Dense, slightly lobulated periosteal new bone formation about third and fourth metatarsal shaft is caused by chronic vascular insufficiency (*black arrows*).

The 64-year-old woman whose foot is shown in Figure 16–12 had a 15-year history of diabetes mellitus. Three weeks before seeing her physician she developed a painful, bleeding sore on her foot. On examination the medial plantar aspect of the red, swollen foot contained an ulcer from which anaerobic streptococci were cultured. Severe infection resulted in an above-knee amputation.

In the diabetic patient coliform organisms are the most common cause of subcutaneous air. In some patients the collection of gas may not be caused by infection but may be only air sucked in under the skin by movement of the part containing an ulceration. A localized area of destruction of bone directly adjacent to an ulceration of soft tissue may be caused by osteomyelitis or diabetic osteopathy. Radiographically this differentiation may be difficult, and a trial of conservative therapy should be made. Again, the degree of vascularization of the remaining part of the foot would be a consideration in the proper treatment of osteomyelitis.

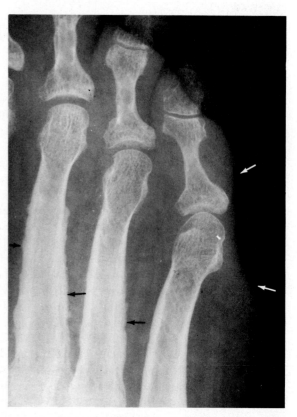

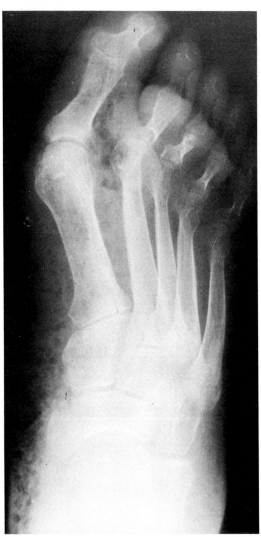

**FIG 16–12.**
Extensive subcutaneous air with infection about great toe, first metatarsal, and medial aspect of foot. *(Courtesy of Murray K. Dalinka, M.D., Jack Edeiken, M.D., Philadelphia.)*

## SPECIAL IMAGING METHODS

In the presence of active infection, the bone changes of osteomyelitis may not be apparent on radiographs for 10 to 14 days. Magnification radiography, scintigraphy, computed tomography (CT), and magnetic resonance imaging (MRI) are employed to increase the accuracy of imaging for the presence of infection.[65] The distinction between simple cellulitis and osteomyelitis is important for patient prognosis, as well as clinical management. With the use of MRI, diagnostic imaging cannot only distinguish between infected cellulitis and osteomyelitis but can detect focal abscess formation that would necessitate surgical drainage.

## Magnification Radiography

Direct radiographic magnification techniques have been improved by the development of microfocal spot x-ray tubes. A small (100–150 μm) focal spot produces a magnified image of unusual clarity and definition, particularly in delineating the fine detail of bone structures in which early osteomyelitis or, less commonly, neuropathic change is suspected.[33] They may prove useful in detecting focal areas of cortical erosion in an area of suspected osteomyelitis. However, the presence of focal cortical erosion is not specific, because early neuropathic change can have a similar appearance. Magnification radiographs can monitor response to therapy with healing periosteal reaction, reflecting a response to therapy (Fig 16–13). Magnification radiographs can also demonstrate otherwise subtle trabecular disruptions associated with insufficiency fracture.

Magnification radiography's imaging characteristics also enhance soft tissue detail. An image enlarged up to four times can be readily obtained on commercially available equipment.[18, 26] Direct radiographic magnification results in a fourfold increase in skin dose when compared with conventional radiographic techniques and therefore should be used in only carefully selected cases.[17] Although not a routine examination, the role of magnification radiography may be the evaluation of equivocal plain film findings. If there is a strong clinical suspicion of focal osteomyelitis underlying soft tissue ulceration, magnification radiographs may demonstrate focal cortical erosions or inflammatory periosteal changes.

## Radionuclide Imaging

Bone scintigraphy with technetium 99m phosphonates, leukocytes (white blood cells) labeled with indium 111, and gallium 67 citrate all have been reported as useful in the detection of acute osteomyelitis in the dia-

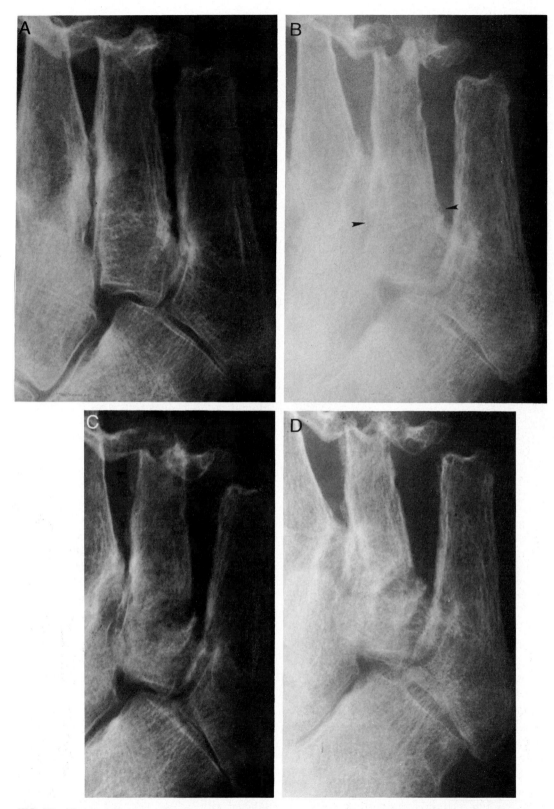

**FIG 16–13.**
Magnification radiographs in patient with foot ulcer over fourth metatarsal head. **A,** original examination with chronic metatarsal amputation defects. **B,** at 4 weeks, linear density seen in base of fourth metatarsal raises question of stress fracture. **C,** at 8 weeks, osteopenia in fourth metatarsal with resorption at suspected stress

betic foot.[14, 21, 29] In the patient with equivocal radiographs, bone scanning has been very helpful in identifying cases of subradiographic osteomyelitis (Fig 16–14).[46] These agents rely on tissue response to infection. In the diabetic patient, neuropathic osseous change, manifesting as increased uptake on both technetium and gallium scans, decreases the specificity of these examinations for the detection of osteomyelitis.

Technetium 99m is the most widely employed agent in scintigraphic imaging. It is ideally suited for clinical imaging, with a short half-life and an optimal photopeak for gamma cameras. Readily available portable molybdenum radioisotope generators provide a reliable source of $^{99m}$Tc. It is intravenously administered bound to either methylene diphosphonate or hydroxymethylene diphosphonate.

In a patient with suspected osteomyelitis, the standard $^{99m}$Tc bone scan examination is performed in three phases: flow, blood pool, and delayed. Dynamic flow phase imaging begins at the moment of intravenous radiopharmaceutical injection. A series of 5-second image acquisitions are obtained at the site of suspected osteomyelitis. Static blood pool images are obtained approximately 5 minutes after injection. Static delayed images are acquired approximately 3 to 4 hours after injection.

Technetium diphosphonate works by localizing in areas of increased bone metabolism, as well as regions of increased vascularity. Focally increased bone metabolism occurs in both diabetic neuropathy and osteomyelitis. Thus, bone scan images in a diabetic patient with cellulitis and neuropathic change will look similar to those of a diabetic patient with cellulitis and neuropathic change and superimposed osteomyelitis.

Processes that can demonstrate increased uptake on flow and pool images include cellulitis, septic synovitis, and abscess.[56, 63] In both soft tissue inflammation and osteomyelitis there is hyperemia demonstrated as increased radiopharmaceutical uptake on flow and blood pool images. In soft tissue processes, there is typically decreased soft tissue uptake on the delayed images with no focal bone uptake. In osteomyelitis, there is increased activity, localizable to bone on the delayed images. A four-phase scan involving additional imaging 24 hours after injection has been proposed.[2] It has been reported to raise the specificity of the examination in those patients with vascular insufficiency, including diabetics. In osteomyelitis there is further sequestration of activity on the delayed images. The use of four-phase bone scan does not seem to be widespread.[53]

In a review by Schauwecker,[53] the sensitivity of bone scans for osteomyelitis is 94%, and specificity 95%. However, in patients with complicating conditions, including diabetes, the specificity decreases to 33%. The sensitivity remains at 95%. The limitation of the bone scan occurs in a patient with neuropathic osseous change that demonstrates increased uptake on delayed images, the same appearance as osteomyelitis. The low specificity of $^{99m}$Tc for differentiation of neuropathic bone change from superimposed osteomyelitis limits the clinical usefulness of bone scan in the diabetic patient.

Gallium citrate has been employed in the imaging of acute osteomyelitis. The mechanism of Ga localization is by both granulocyte and bacteria uptake. However, Ga also localizes nonspecifically in areas of increased bone remodeling. Therefore it demonstrates the same lack of specificity as $^{99m}$Tc, accumulating nonspecifically in areas of diabetic osteoarthropathy. Some authors have reported increased specificity of Ga imaging by computer subtraction of concurrent $^{99m}$Tc imaging. Gallium uptake out of proportion to $^{99m}$Tc uptake supports the presence of infection.[19, 22, 24, 61] Some authors[2] have proposed a role for Ga in the imaging of chronic osteomyelitis.

Indium 111 WBC imaging relies on the localization of WBCs within areas of focal leu-

---

fracture. Periosteal reaction distally with focal erosion of stump. New periosteal reaction head of fifth metatarsal. Findings are suspicious for superimposed osteomyelitis at metatarsal head and possibly at fracture site. **D,** 4 months later after extended course of antibiotics. Periosteal changes have matured with overall increased ossification, indicating positive response to antibiotic with healing response.

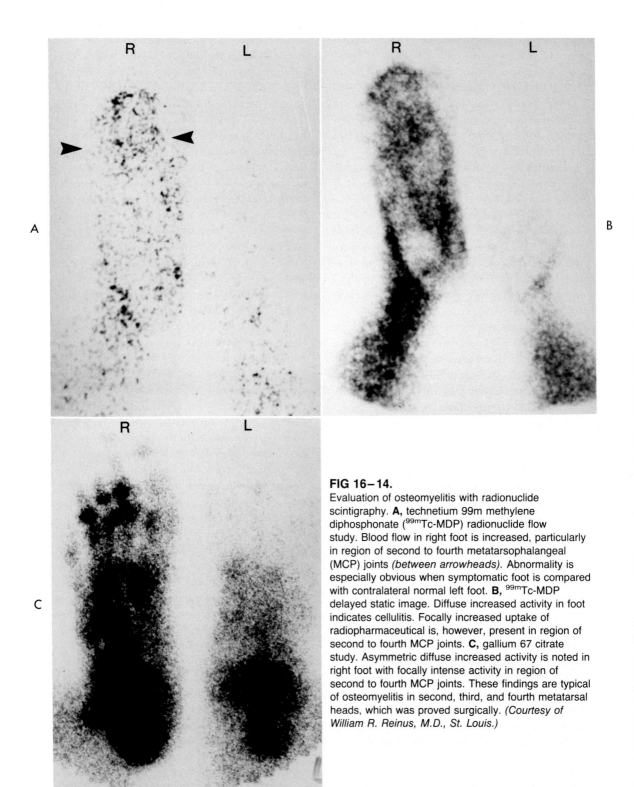

**FIG 16–14.**
Evaluation of osteomyelitis with radionuclide scintigraphy. **A,** technetium 99m methylene diphosphonate ($^{99m}$Tc-MDP) radionuclide flow study. Blood flow in right foot is increased, particularly in region of second to fourth metatarsophalangeal (MCP) joints *(between arrowheads)*. Abnormality is especially obvious when symptomatic foot is compared with contralateral normal left foot. **B,** $^{99m}$Tc-MDP delayed static image. Diffuse increased activity in foot indicates cellulitis. Focally increased uptake of radiopharmaceutical is, however, present in region of second to fourth MCP joints. **C,** gallium 67 citrate study. Asymmetric diffuse increased activity is noted in right foot with focally intense activity in region of second to fourth MCP joints. These findings are typical of osteomyelitis in second, third, and fourth metatarsal heads, which was proved surgically. *(Courtesy of William R. Reinus, M.D., St. Louis.)*

kocyte sequestration. Indium WBCs also normally localize to areas of active bone marrow. However, active bone marrow is not present in adult feet. Therefore, any sequestration of [111]In activity within the mature foot is indicative of infection.[3, 34, 38, 49]

Although [111]In is currently the most specific radiopharmaceutical agent for acute inflammation, the major disadvantage of [111]In scanning is the labor-intensive protocol that must be followed to label the leukocytes. For this reason, some centers rely on commercial laboratories to perform the labeling. The entire process is beyond the scope of these pages. In general, the labeling procedure involves drawing 50 mL of the patient's blood, followed by repeated centrifuging to isolate the WBC portion, which is tagged with [111]In and then reinjected into the patient. Routine [111]In imaging is performed 4 and 24 hours after injection. The labor-intensive labeling process and the costly cyclotron-produced In contribute to make [111]In WBCs one of the more expensive scintigraphic imaging procedures.

[111]In oxine is an agent that relies on sequestration of WBCs and does not respond to altered bone metabolism. In several studies, WBCs labeled with [111]In oxine have been demonstrated to be the radiopharmaceutical of choice for imaging suspected osteomyelitis in the diabetic patient.[29, 34, 54, 55] In these studies, sensitivity of [111]In WBC scanning for the detection of osteomyelitis was reported at 75% to 100%. The specificity ranged from 79% to 89%, which is an improvement compared with the [99m]Tc bone scan. The false positive results of [111]In scans have been noted in patients with rapidly progressive osteoarthropathy.[55]

Indium scans generally have poor spatial resolution. Although sensitive for infection, [111]In scanning may not allow the separation of soft tissue uptake from uptake in adjacent bone.[34, 35] This makes it difficult to distinguish cellulitis from osteomyelitis, thus resulting in false positive interpretation. To increase the anatomic sensitivity of the [111]In images, studies have performed concurrent [99mTc] and [111]In imaging. Computer image manipulation can provide better discrimination between soft tissue and bone uptake.[25, 54, 59] However, in one series, [111]In scanning alone was performed with similar specificity for distinguishing cellulitis from osteomyelitis as studies that employed both modalities.[29]

## Computed Tomography

The role of CT is to assess subtle plain film abnormalities such as periosteal or cortical erosion that may indicate underlying bone infection.[67] It can provide precise imaging of cortical articular surfaces.[57, 58] Computed tomography imaging should be directed to the area of specific clinical concern such as the area of bone scan abnormality or at the location of foot ulcer (Fig 16–15). The CT technique consists of thin-section, high-resolution images perpendicular to the bone cortex. This will provide the greatest sensitivity for subtle erosions, especially when they are not seen or are questionably seen on plain or magnified radiography. Computed tomography can show the presence of an abnormal medullary space and can show areas of soft tissue abnormality; however, MRI is generally more sensitive in showing these abnormalities.

The role of CT to provide detailed views of subtle erosions has been supplanted to a degree by MRI, especially because of the value of MRI to examine medullary spaces and soft tissues. In those patients who have a cardiac pacemaker or other contraindication to MRI, CT continues to serve as a primary cross-sectional imaging modality.

## Magnetic Resonance Imaging

Magnetic resonance imaging has quickly become incorporated into routine clinical management of many clinical problems, including the diabetic foot. It offers direct multiplanar imaging, and the ability to resolve soft tissue contrast provides detailed anatomic images superior to other imaging modalities.[7] The presence and extent of both bone marrow and soft tissue inflammatory processes can accurately be evaluated.[15, 39, 60]

For image contrast and detail, MRI relies on the amount of free protons in the tissues,

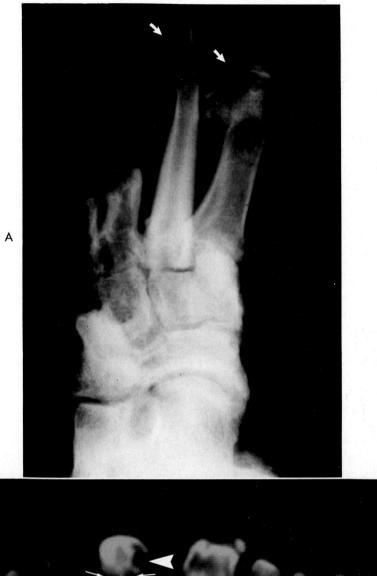

**FIG 16–15.**
Evaluation of osteomyelitis with CT. **A,** conventional radiography. Poorly marginated lucency is present at base of first and second proximal phalanges *(arrows)* consistent with diagnosis of osteomyelitis. Note previous partial third and fourth metatarsal and fourth proximal and middle phalangeal resections. First metatarsal head and adjacent sesamoid bones appear to be spared. **B,** transmetatarsal CT scan at level of first metatarsal head demonstrates unsuspected erosion of plantar *(arrows)* and medial cortical surfaces *(large arrowhead)* of first metatarsal head along with apposing articular surfaces of two adjacent sesamoid bones *(small arrowheads).* Contralateral first metatarsal head and sesamoid bones are normal. In this case CT demonstrates true extent of bony disease with greater accuracy than conventional radiography.

which, in general, is proportional to the tissue water content. Water demonstrates decreased signal on $T_1$-weighted images and increased signal on $T_2$-weighted images. Magnetic resonance images of the foot are usually acquired in the coronal and sagittal plane. Most MRI scanners employ the head surface coil for foot imaging. Spin echo images of $T_1$, proton density, and $T_2$ weighting are standard. With the clinical question of osteomyelitis, spin echo images are usually supplemented with short-tau inversion recovery (STIR) images. The STIR images null fat signal and as a result normal bone marrow is absent of signal.[68] Thus, these images are very sensitive to bone marrow edema (Fig 16–17).

On MRI images, the diagnosis of osteomyelitis is made by detection of focal bone marrow edema, which is an indication of osteomyelitis. Usual criteria for osteomyelitis are focally decreased signal on $T_1$-weighted images and focally increased marrow signal on STIR images.[68] $T_2$ images, although very sensitive for the presence of fluid, sometimes do not allow definite ana-

tomic distinction between soft tissue and marrow processes. This limits the specificity of $T_2$-weighted images to differentiate superficial cellulitis or edema from deeper extension into the bone marrow indicative of osteomyelitis.

The sensitivity of MRI for the presence of osteomyelitis has been reported between 90% and 100%, with a specificity of 80%.[62, 64, 68] The specificity decreases in the presence of septic arthritis, occult bone fracture, and recent surgery, including bone biopsy.[13] Rapidly progressive, noninfected, osteoarthropathy can demonstrate bone marrow edema on MR images. Therefore, as with [111]In WBC imaging, rapidly progressive noninfected neuropathic osteoarthropathy may be indistinguishable from osteomyelitis on MRI imaging.[55] This is disappointing, because these patients usually have a high clinical suspicion for osteomyelitis. In these patients, biopsy may be considered for diagnosis.

Focal edema localized to the soft tissues does not necessarily indicate cellulitis. Diffuse soft tissue edema, fluid in tendon sheaths, and joint effusions have been noted

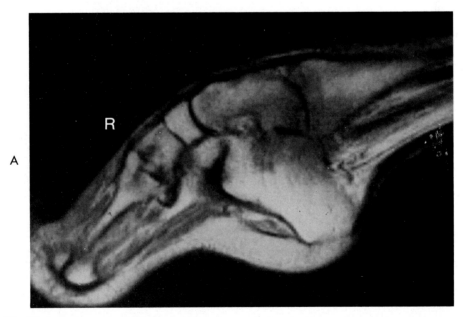

**FIG 16–16.**
Evaluation of osteomyelitis with MRI. **A,** $T_1$-weighted (600TR/35TE) sagittal image. Normal bright *(white)* marrow acitivity of distal tibia, posterior talus, and cranial calcaneus is replaced with abnormal lower intensity signal. **B,** $T_1$-weighted (600TR/45TE) sagittal image. Normal marrow signal in contralateral asymptomatic ankle region is homogeneous and bright. **C,** $T_2$-weighted (1500TR/120TE) sagittal image. Marrow signal in distal tibia, talus, and subarticular calcaneus is slightly brighter and less uniform *(arrows)* than that of lower-intensity normal navicular and first cuneiform bones and proximal metatarsal diaphysis included on the same image. Findings are characteristic of osteomyelitis. *(Courtesy of William R. Reinus, M.D., St. Louis.)* *(Continued.)*

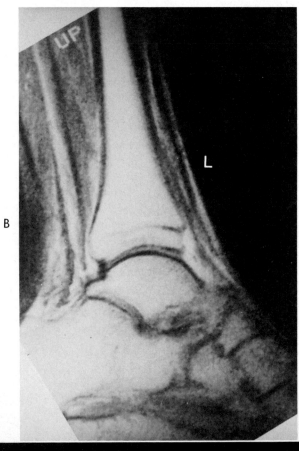

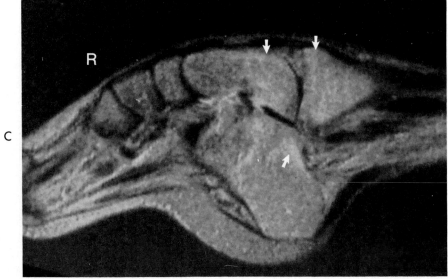

**FIG 16–16 (cont.).**

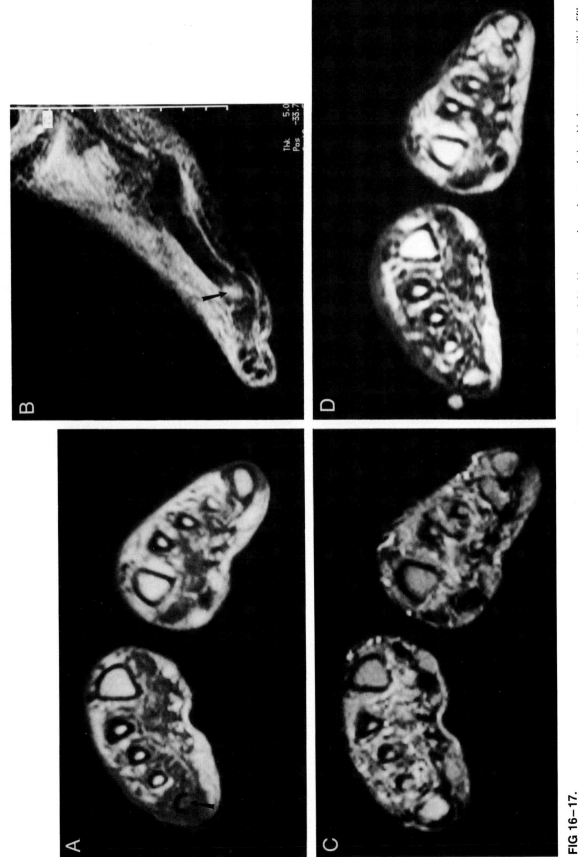

**FIG 16–17.**

Magnetic resonance imaging examination of 45-year-old man with foot ulcer adjacent to left fifth metatarsal. **A,** T$_1$-weighted images show decreased signal in bone marrow within fifth metatarsal head and within surrounding soft tissues. **B,** STIR image demonstrates focal increased signal within fifth metatarsal head. **C,** T$_2$-weighted image shows increased signal within bone marrow compared with opposite metatarsal. Note increased soft tissue of right foot compared with left. Findings on all pulse sequences are compatible with osteomyelitis. **D,** patient returned 4 months later for right foot ulcer, which demonstrates normal marrow signal in fifth metatarsal head (no edema), indicating healed infection.

with regularity in nonsymptomatic diabetic patients.[5, 40] Increased soft tissue fluid has been demonstrated secondary to neuropathic change. In selected patients, MRI can be useful for the noninvasive detection of focal abscess formation. This would be demonstrated by focal pockets of fluid within the soft tissues.[11] These abscesses could be treated with local incision and drainage, with the MRI providing anatomic information to focus the surgical incision.

Magnetic resonance imaging is the method of choice at many institutions for the detection of osteomyelitis. Its sensitivity and specificity are comparable with scintigraphic examination. The ability to clearly identify potentially surgically treatable soft tissue processes is advantageous. In recent years the availability of MRI has become widespread; however, it continues to be a relatively expensive examination. For this reason, [111]In could be considered as the more economical examination. However, when one considers the combined cost of an In and [99m]Tc bone scan, which are usually performed concurrently, the MRI is the economical imaging choice.

## SUMMARY

Examination of the diabetic foot has benefited through the use of advanced imaging. The presence of concurrent pathologic conditions continues to hamper consistently accurate diagnosis. The following algorithm for the diabetic patient with suspected osteomyelitis infection could serve as general guidelines, but individual institutions may have local factors that make global standardization impractical.

The work-up of the diabetic foot with suspected infection should begin with plain radiographs. This, if for no other reason, can establish a baseline for the patient. With unremarkable plain films, a [99m]Tc bone scan is probably the most appropriate and economical test. The bone scan's problem is not sensitivity but specificity. As previously noted, a negative bone scan essentially excludes acute or chronic osteomyelitis. With abnormal plain films the next best imaging test is controversial. Detailed views using CT, mag-

nification, or both may clarify cortical destruction. Magnetic resonance imaging and [111]In scanning have high sensitivity and similar specificity; MRI is preferred at some centers, given the ease of the procedure relative to the labor-intensive labeling protocol for [111]In scanning and the higher imaging resolution of MRI to differentiate between bone and soft tissue infection. With current imaging methods, it may be impossible to differentiate rapidly progressive osteoarthritis from acute osteomyelitis. Future comparative study may further define the specific role of these various important imaging modalities.

## REFERENCES

1. Alazraki N, Dries D, Datz F, et al: Value of 24-hour image (four phase bone scan) in assessing osteomyelitis in patients, *J Nucl Med* 125:17–24, 1988.

2. Alazraki N, Fierer J, Resnick D: Chronic osteomyelitis: monitoring by 99mTc phosphate and 67-gallium imaging, *AJR* 145:767–771, 1985.

3. Al-Sheikh W, Sfakianakis GN, Mnaymneh W, et al: Subacute and chronic bone infections: diagnosis using In-111, Ga-67, and Tc-99m MDP bone scintigraphy and radiography, *Radiology* 155:501–506, 1985.

4. Baldwin SC, Black JR: Pedal stress fracture associated with diabetic peripheral neuropathy, *J Am Podiatr Med Assoc* 76:30–32, 1986.

5. Beltran J, Campanini DS, Knight C, et al: The diabetic foot: magnetic resonance imaging evaluation, *Skeletal Radiol* 19:37–41, 1990.

6. Beltran J, McGhee RB, Schaffer PB, et al: Experimental infections of the musculoskeletal system: evaluation with MR imaging and TC-99m MDP and Ga-67 scintigraphy, *Radiology* 167:167–172, 1988.

7. Berquist TH, Brown ML, Fitzgerald RH, et al: Magnetic resonance imaging: application in musculoskeletal infection, *Magn Reson Imaging* 3:219–230, 1985.

8. Clouse ME, Gramm HF, Legg M, et al: Diabetic osteoarthropathy: clinical and roentgenographic observations in 90 cases, *AJR* 121:34, 1974.

9. Connolly JF, Jacobsen FS: Rapid bone destruction after a stress fracture in a diabetic (Charcot) foot, *Nebr Med J* 70:438–440, 1985.

10. Coventry MB, Rothacker GW Jr: Bilateral calcaneal fractures in a diabetic patient, *J Bone Joint Surg* 61A:462, 1979.

11. Durham JR, Lukens ML, Campanini DS, et al: Impact of magnetic resonance imaging on the man-

agement of diabetic foot infections, *Am J Surg* 162:150–153, 1991.

12. El-Khoury GY, Kathol MH: Neuropathic fractures in patients with diabetes mellitus, *Radiology* 134:313–316, 1980.

13. Erdman WA, Tamburro F, Jayson HT: Osteomyelitis: characteristics and pitfalls of diagnosis with MR imaging, *Radiology* 180:533–539, 1991.

14. Eymontt MJ, Alavi A, Dalinka MK, et al: Bone scintigraphy in diabetic osteoarthropathy, *Radiology* 140:475–477, 1991.

15. Fletcher BD, Scoles PV, Nelson AD: Osteomyelitis in children: detection by magnetic resonance, *Radiology* 150:57–60, 1984.

16. Forestier J, Lagier R: Ankylosing hyperostosis of the spine, *Clin Orthop* 74:65, 1971.

17. Genant HK: Magnification radiography, in Resnick D, Niwayama G, editors: *Diagnosis of bone and joint disorders*, Philadelphia, 1988, WB Saunders, pp 84–107.

18. Genant HK, Doi J, Mall JC: Optical versus radiographic magnification for fine detail skeletal radiology, *Invest Radiol* 2:160, 1975.

19. Gilday DL: Problems in the scintigraphic detection of osteomyelitis, *Radiology* 135:791, 1980.

20. Griffiths HJ: Diabetic osteopathy, *Orthopedics* 8:398–406, 1985.

21. Gupta NC, Prezio JA: Radionuclide imaging in osteomyelitis, *Semin Nucl Med* 18:287–299, 1988.

22. Handmaker H: Acute hematogenous osteomyelitis: has the bone scan betrayed us? *Radiology* 135:787–789, 1980.

23. Harris J, Carter AR, Glick EN, et al: Ankylosing hyperostosis: I, clinical and radiological features, *Ann Rheum Dis* 31:69, 1972.

24. Hetherington VJ: Technetium and combined gallium and technetium scans in the neurotrophic foot, *J Am Podiatr Assoc* 72:458–463, 1982.

25. Jacobson AF, Harley JD, Lipsky AF, et al: Diagnosis of osteomyelitis in the presence of soft tissue infection and radiologic evidence of osseous abnormalities: value of leukocyte scintigraphy, *AJR* 157:807–812, 1991.

26. Johnson JTH: Neuropathic fractures and joint injuries: pathogenesis and rationale of prevention and treatment, *J Bone Joint Surg* 49A:1–30, 1967.

27. Julkunen H, Karava R, Viljanen V: Hyperostosis of the spine in diabetes mellitus and acromegaly, *Diabetologia* 2:123, 1966.

28. Kathol MH, El-Khoury GY, Moore TE, et al: Calcaneal insufficiency avulsion fractures in patients with diabetes mellitus, *Radiology* 180:725–729, 1991.

29. Keenan AM, Tindel NL, Alavi A: Diagnosis of pedal osteomyelitis in diabetic patients using current scintigraphic techniques, *Arch Intern Med* 149:2262–2266, 1989.

30. Kraft E, Spyropoulos E, Finby N: Neurogenic disorders of the foot in diabetes mellitus, *AJR* 124:17–24, 1975.

31. Kristiansen B: Ankle and foot fractures in diabetics provoking neuropathic joint changes, *Acta Orthop Scand* 51:975–979, 1980.

32. Landon GC, Johnson KA, Dahlin DC: Subungual exostoses, *J Bone Joint Surg* 61A:256, 1979.

33. Lee SM, Lee RGL, Wilinsky J, et al: Magnification radiography in osteomyelitis, *Skeletal Radiol* 15:625–627, 1986.

34. Maurer AH, Millmond SH, Knight LC, et al: Infection in diabetic osteoarthropathy: use of Indium-labeled leukocytes for diagnosis, *Radiology* 161:221, 1986.

35. McCarthy K, Velchik MG, Mandell GA, et al: Indium-111-labeled white blood cells in the detection of osteomyelitis complicated by a pre-existing condition, *J Nucl Med* 29:1015–1021, 1988.

36. Meltzer AD, Skuersky N, Ostrum BJ: Radiographic evaluation of soft tissue necrosis in diabetics, *Radiology* 90:300, 1968.

37. Mendelson EB, Fisher MR, Deschler TW, et al: Osteomyelitis in diabetic foot: a difficult diagnostic challenge, *RadioGraphics* 3:248–261, 1983.

38. Merkel KD, Brown ML, Dewanjee MK, et al: Comparison of indium-labeled-leukocyte imaging with sequential technetium-gallium scanning in the diagnosis of low-grade musculoskeletal sepsis: a prospective study, *J Bone Joint Surg* 67A:465–476, 1985.

39. Modic MT, Feiglin DH, Piraino DW, et al: Vertebral osteomyelitis: assessment using MR, *Radiology* 157:157–166, 1985.

40. Moore TE, Yuh WTC, et al: Abnormalities of the foot in patients with diabetes mellitus: findings on MR imaging, *AJR* 157:813–816, 1991.

41. Murphy WA, Totty WG: Musculoskeletal magnetic resonance imaging, in *Magnetic resonance annual 1986*, New York, 1986, Raven Press, pp 1–35.

42. Newman JH: Non-infective disease of the diabetic foot, *J Bone Joint Surg* 63B:593–596, 1981.

43. Newman LG, Waller J, Palestro CJ, et al: Unsuspected osteomyelitis in diabetic foot ulcers: diagnosis and monitoring by leukocyte scanning with indium-111 oxyquinoline, *JAMA* 266:1245–1251, 1991.

44. Nguyen VD, Keh RA, Daehler RW: Freiberg's disease in diabetes mellitus, *Skeletal Radiol* 20:425–428, 1991.

45. Pambor M, Neubert H: Tumorartige begleitreaktionen der haut bei exostoses der zehenendphalangen, *Dermatol Monatsschr* 157:532, 1971.

46. Park H-M, Wheat LJ, Siddiqui AR, et al: Scintigraphic evaluation of diabetic osteomyelitis: concise communication, *J Nucl Med* 23:569–573, 1982.

47. Phemister DB: Lesions of bones and joints arising from interruption of circulation, *J Mt Sinai Hosp NY* 15:55, 1948.

48. Pogonowska MJ, Collins LC, Dobson HL: Diabetic osteopathy, *Radiology* 89:265, 1967.

49. Raptopoulos V, Doherty PW, Goss TP, et al: Acute osteomyelitis: advantage of white cells in early detection, *AJR* 139:1077–1082, 1982.

50. Reinhardt K: The radiological residua of healed diabetic arthropathies, *Skeletal Radiol* 7:167–172, 1981.

51. Resnick D: Disorders of other endocrine glands and of pregnancy, in Resnick D, Niwayama G, editors: *Diagnosis of bone and joint disorders*, Philadelphia, 1988, WB Saunders, pp 2286–2319.

52. Resnick D, Niwayama G: Diffuse idiopathic skeletal hyperostosis (DISH): ankylosing hyperostosis of Forestier and Rotes-querol, in Resnick D, Niwayama G, editors: *Diagnosis of bone and joint disorders*, Philadelphia, 1988, WB Saunders, pp 1562–1732.

53. Schauwecker DS: The scintigraphic diagnosis of osteomyelitis, *AJR* 158:9–18, 1992.

54. Schauwecker DS, Park HM, Burt RW, et al: Combined bone scintigraphy and indium-111 leukocyte scans in neuropathic foot disease, *J Nucl Med* 29:1651–1655, 1988.

55. Seabold JE, Flickinger FW, Kao SCS, et al: Indium-111-leukocyte/technitium-99m-MDP bone and magnetic resonance imaging: difficulty of diagnosing osteomyelitis in patients with neuropathic osteoarthropathy, *J Nucl Med* 31:539–556, 1990.

56. Seldin DW, Heiken JP, Alderson PO: Effect of soft-tissue pathology on detection of pedal osteomyelitis in diabetics, *J Nucl Med* 26:988–993, 1985.

57. Solomon MA, Gilula LA, Oloff LM, et al: CT scanning of the foot and ankle: part 1, normal anatomy, *AJR* 146:1192–1203, 1986.

58. Solomon MA, Gilula LA, Oloff LM, et al: CT scanning of the foot and ankle: part 2, clinical applica-

tions and review of the literature, *AJR* 146:1204–1214, 1986.

59. Splittgerber GF, Spiegelhoff DR, Buggy BP: Combined leukocyte and bone imaging used to evaluate diabetic osteoarthropathy and osteomyelitis, *Clin Nucl Med* 14:156–160, 1989.

60. Totty WG: Radiographic evaluation of osteomyelitis using magnetic resonance imaging, *Orthop Rev* 18:587–592, 1989.

61. Tumeh SS, Aliabadi P, Weissman BN, et al: Chronic osteomyelitis: bone and gallium scan patterns associated with active disease, *Radiology* 158:685–688, 1986.

62. Ulger E, Moldofsky P, Gatenby R, et al: Diagnosis of osteomyelitis by MR imaging, *AJR* 150:605–610, 1988.

63. Visser JH, Oloff L, Jacobs AM, et al: The use of differential scintigraphy in the clinical diagnosis of osseous and soft tissue changes affecting the diabetic foot, *J Foot Surg* 23:74–85, 1984.

64. Wang A, Weinstein D, Greenfield LM, et al: MRI and diabetic foot infections, *Magn reson imaging* 8:805–809, 1990.

65. Wegener WA, Alavi A: Diagnostic imaging of musculoskeletal infection, *Orthop Clin* 22:401–418, 1991.

66. Whitehouse FW: On diabetic osteopathy: a radiographic study of 21 patients, *Diabetes Care* 1:303, 1978.

67. Williamson BRJ, Treates CD, Phillips CD, et al: Computed tomography as a diagnostic aid in diabetic and other problem feet, *Clin Imaging* 13:159–163, 1989.

68. Yuh, W.T.C., Corson J.D., Baraniewski, H.M. et al: Osteomyelitis of the foot in diabetic patients: evaluation with plain film, 99m-Tc-MDP bone scintigraphy, and MR imaging, *AJR* 152:795–800, 1989.

# CHAPTER 17

# Radiologic Intervention in Diabetic Peripheral Vascular Disease

**Thomas M. Vesely, M.D.**

**Daniel Picus, M.D.**

**Louis A. Gilula, M.D.**

Vascular disease is a common complication of diabetes. Atherosclerosis occurs approximately 10 years earlier in diabetic than in nondiabetic patients, and the risk of symptomatic atherosclerotic disease in diabetics is increased twofold to threefold. Studies of large groups of patients with adult-onset diabetes show at the time of diagnosis that approximately 22% have radiographic evidence of arterial calcification, 13% lack one or more arterial pulses, and approximately 5% have a history of lower extremity claudication. Both infection and occlusive arterial disease contribute to the necrosis of tissue requiring amputation.

## PLAIN RADIOGRAPHY

Vascular calcifications occur in 16% to 25% of diabetic patients. Several different types of calcification in the vessels of the lower limb are readily apparent on radiographs. The type of calcification may be a clue to the degree of vascular occlusive disease. The atherosclerotic lesions found in diabetics occur in the intimal layer of the arterial wall. Calcification associated with atherosclerosis generally occurs near the internal elastic membrane. Radiographically, intimal calcifications are distributed in an irregular fashion along the vessel wall (Fig 17–1). Because this intimal calcification is superficial and closer to the lumen, stenosis, occlusion, or both are common. Such atherosclerotic intimal calcifications frequently extend from the iliac arteries peripherally.

## ANGIOGRAPHY

Arteriography remains the gold standard for evaluation of the vascular supply to the leg and foot. Noninvasive tests, including Doppler ultrasound, segmental pressures, and toe pressures, are safe and reliable methods but are limited in their anatomic definition. Intravascular ultrasound and angioscopy are new methods undergoing clinical investigation that may provide better characterization of specific atherosclerotic lesions, but their clinical utility remains unproved.

In younger patients with vascular insufficiency, a presumptive diagnosis of diabetes can be made when the arteriogram shows severe, diffuse, atherosclerotic disease involving the anterior and posterior tibial arteries, as well as the peroneal artery. The popliteal and superficial femoral arteries may show only minimum atheromatous changes, whereas the iliac arteries and aorta usually have no disease at all (Fig 17–2). This pattern is often obscured in older patients with diffuse atherosclerotic disease. The effects of infrapopliteal small-vessel dis-

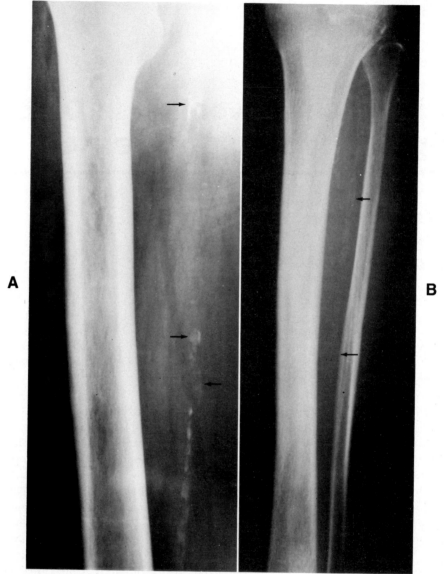

**FIG 17–1.**
Vascular calcification *(arrows)*. **A,** arteriosclerosis. Calcified atheromatous plaques throughout the superficial femoral artery. Calcification is coarse and unevenly distributed. **B,** arteriosclerosis of popliteal artery branches. Vessels lie in central portion of calf muscles near tibia and fibula.

ease may be aggravated by either segmental occlusion or stenosis of a major inflow vessel, beginning anywhere from the aorta through the popliteal artery trifurcation (Fig 17–3). The possibility of large-vessel stenosis or occlusion superimposed on distal diabetic vascular disease is the most important indication for angiography in diabetic patients. Percutaneous vascular interventions such as transluminal angioplasty, atherectomy, and vascular stents, as well as conventional surgical bypass procedures, will often improve inflow in these cases and prevent extension of gangrenous changes in the foot.

**FIG 17–2.**
Single arteriogram from patient with diabetic vascular disease. **A,** pelvic vessels show minimum atheromatous involvement. **B,** thigh vessels in same arteriogram show moderate arteriosclerosis. **C,** branches of popliteal artery in same arteriogram show diffuse, severe occlusive vascular disease.

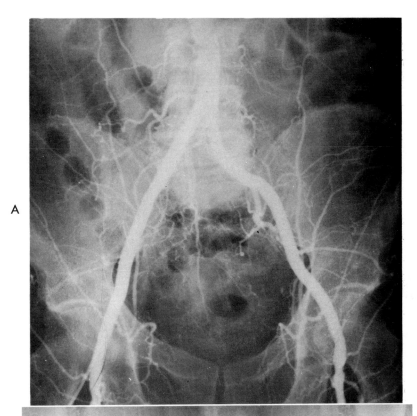

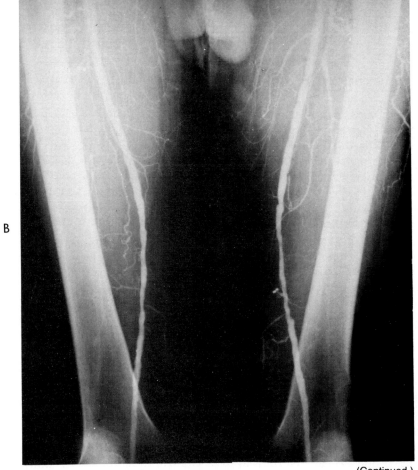

(Continued.)

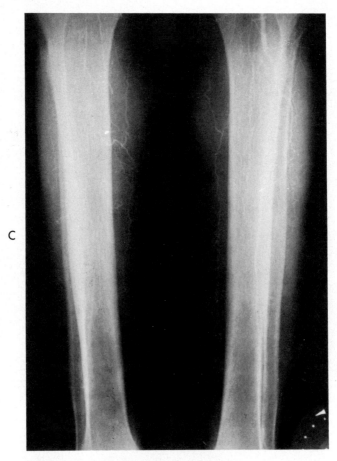

**FIG 17–2   (cont.).**

Therapeutic decisions therefore should not be made before angiography, because one cannot assume that small-vessel disease is the sole cause of vascular insufficiency in the lower limb.[3] Angiography should not, however, be done just for completeness of the work-up. For example, a patient with claudication for whom neither angioplasty nor surgery is otherwise contemplated does not require angiography. On the other hand, the limbs of some patients who are considered to be candidates only for an amputation may be salvaged with vascular surgery or percutaneous transluminal angioplasty, and in these patients angiography should be considered.

## PROCEDURE AND TECHNIQUE

The physician performing the arteriogram should visit the patient the day before the examination and explain the procedure

in detail. Because complications can occur with any angiographic procedure, informed, written consent is necessary. An intravenous (IV) line should be started, preferably the evening before the study, to allow for adequate hydration. Dehydration increases the risk of contrast material-induced renal failure.

Local lidocaine anesthesia and fluoroscopic guidance are used to pass an angiographic catheter percutaneously in a retrograde direction through one common femoral artery. The catheter tip is placed in the distal abdominal aorta. Sixty to 80 mL of contrast material is injected over 6 to 10 seconds. Films are obtained by having either the gantry or table top move while acquiring images along the extremities. This allows radiographic evaluation of the entire arterial supply to both lower extremities with one injection of contrast material.

The vessels of the lower limb must be studied from the aortic bifurcation to the

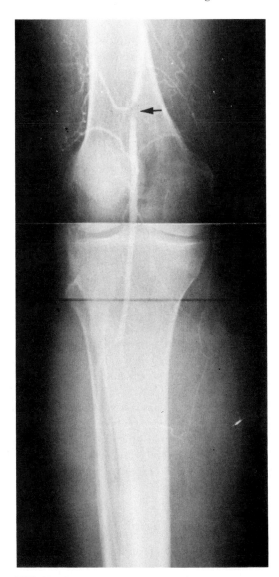

**FIG 17–3.**
Popliteal artery occlusion *(arrow)*. Recanalizing occluded segment can improve distal arterial inflow in many such diabetic patients.

foot. Both the common and external iliac arteries must be widely patent when bypass grafting of the superficial femoral artery is contemplated. All hemodynamically significant stenoses in the distal abdominal aorta and iliac arteries must be either repaired by percutaneous vascular interventions or bypassed before distal repair. A stenosis proximal to either a bypass graft or repaired stenotic segment will decrease inflow and may result in occlusion of the repaired segment. In other words, if flow is significantly diminished upstream, it cannot be improved

downstream, no matter how large the bypass or how successful the dilation.

In some circumstances, especially in patients with severe peripheral vascular disease, blood flow to the lower limbs is so slow that adequate evaluation of the calf artery branches is not possible with the standard technique. Usually this can be handled by filming at a much slower rate. Rarely, to visualize the popliteal artery branches more accurately, it may be necessary to deliver contrast material directly to the involved vessel. This can be done by passing a catheter from the contralateral common femoral artery across the aortic bifurcation and placing it into the ipsilateral common femoral artery. Alternatively, an antegrade puncture can be made into the ipsilateral common femoral artery and a catheter passed into the superficial femoral artery or popliteal artery (Fig 17–4).

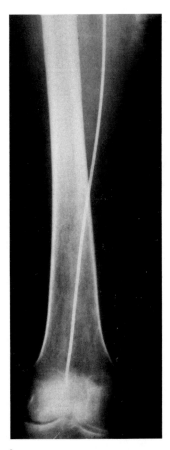

**FIG 17–4.**
Catheter positioned antegrade in superficial femoral artery with tip in popliteal artery to deliver contrast material directly to infrapopliteal vessels.

Several other maneuvers can be performed to improve visualization of peripheral blood flow.[12] Intra-arterial injection of tolazoline or nitroglycerin before the injection of contrast material produces arterial dilation and improves visualization of the popliteal artery branches in 20% to 40% of patients. Reactive hyperemia is also useful in demonstrating the distal leg vessels. This is produced by inflating a blood pressure cuff around the thigh to a level above systolic arterial pressure for 2 minutes. Contrast material is injected immediately after release of the blood pressure cuff.

Balloon occlusion angiography can help to visualize severely diseased vessels by eliminating the inflow of unopacified blood. A balloon occlusion catheter is placed into the external iliac artery and the balloon inflated. Contrast is injected through the catheter to opacify the distal vessels. This technique usually produces diagnostic images in patients with severe peripheral disease.

Intra-arterial pressure measurements are obtained across lesions suspected to be hemodynamically significant. Vasodilators such as tolazoline or nitroglycerin can be used to accentuate pressure gradients across stenoses.

## COMPLICATIONS

Local bleeding and hematoma formation are the most common complications of peripheral angiography, occurring in 5% of the cases. These are usually of only minimum significance when the femoral route is used. The axillary artery, however, may bleed more substantially than the femoral artery. This is because the axillary artery is difficult to compress and because there is relatively little surrounding tissue to tamponade a developing hematoma. Axillary hematomas may lead to significant brachial plexus nerve damage (0.6%).

Thrombosis is the other major local catheter-related complication. The primary factors influencing arterial thrombosis include the catheter size relative to the vessel size, the length of the procedure, and the degree of atherosclerotic disease in the vessel. Intra-arterial heparin is administered when a catheter traverses a severe stenosis and during prolonged interventional procedures. Facilities for surgical thrombectomy must be readily available in any setting where angiography is performed. With early recognition and treatment of thrombosis, the extremity should recover without any harmful sequelae.

Peripheral embolization is a rare complication of diagnostic angiography (<0.1%). Usually it is the result of catheter manipulation in a very atherosclerotic aorta, with subsequent showering of cholesterol material downstream. Thrombolytic infusions (e.g., urokinase) are rarely successful in reversing this type of embolization. With catheter manipulation in the abdominal aorta, the cholesterol crystals can also embolize into the renal and mesenteric arteries. This can have devastating results. Patients with widespread cholesterol embolization have a 70% to 80% mortality. The etiology of death is multifactorial but is commonly related to cardiac and renal embolization.

High doses of contrast material may reduce renal function, particularly in diabetic patients with renal insufficiency.[30] Frequently a transient elevation in serum creatinine level is seen after angiography. The creatinine level peaks approximately 3 days after administration of contrast and returns to baseline within 7 days in the majority of patients. Important factors determining the incidence of contrast-induced nephropathy include renal insufficiency, diabetes mellitus, multiple myeloma, and dehydration, as well as the type and total dose of contrast administered. Several studies suggest that newer, low osmolar contrast agents offer a decreased incidence of acute renal failure compared with ionic agents.[5, 19, 24] Diabetics with preexisting renal insufficiency are much more likely to develop significant contrast-induced nephropathy than diabetics with normal renal function.[5, 24] Among diabetics, several factors predispose to transient nephrotoxicity after angiography, including insulin-dependent diabetes, duration of diabetes greater than 10 years, and elevated serum creatinine levels.[5]

A fourth group of angiographic complications include so-called idiosyncratic, or allergic, reactions to contrast material. Minor reactions to contrast material are common and are self-limited. These include nausea, vomiting, and itching. More serious reactions include hypotension, laryngeal edema, and bronchospasm. These reactions are no more common in diabetic patients. If a patient has had a previous reaction to iodinated contrast material, premedication with prednisone (50 mg orally every 6 hours for 24 to 48 hours) and diphenhydramine (50 mg intramuscularly 1 hour before the study), may reduce the incidence and severity of these reactions.

Newer low osmolar contrast agents are frequently used for peripheral arteriography. Preliminary data suggest that these agents may have fewer undesirable side effects (e.g., allergic reactions, cardiovascular and renal dysfunction). Patients prefer low osmolar contrast because intra-arterial injections are less painful. However, these agents cost 10 to 15 times more than conventional contrast material. Until more convincing data are available, it is therefore difficult to recommend the widespread use of these newer agents. We are currently using these agents in patients with a history of contrast material reactions, compromised cardiovascular systems, or a generalized debilitated condition.

## Digital Subtraction Angiography

Digital subtraction angiography (DSA) has been shown to be useful in a wide variety of vascular applications. The DSA technique uses high-resolution fluoroscopy with computed image acquisition and processing to amplify the signal from iodinated contrast material. The first step is to obtain a fluoroscopic image of the area of interest before the arrival of the contrast agent. This image is stored in the computer in digital form. Subsequently, as the contrast agent passes through the region being studied, multiple images are made and digitally subtracted from the mask. The final subtracted images show the arteries without the overlying bone and soft tissue structures (Fig 17–5). Additional features such as roadmapping, last image freeze, and postprocessing of images enhance the usefulness of DSA, especially during complicated procedures.

Although some individuals advocate DSA for examining the arterial anatomy of the lower limbs, its primary role is as an adjunct to the conventional angiographic examination. The ability to obtain multiple images and projections rapidly is helpful in evaluating areas that are questionable on the conventional angiographic examination. In addition, delayed views of the infrapopliteal vessels can be obtained using very small amounts of contrast material. Digital subtraction angiography images can be obtained with dilute contrast material, which decreases the feeling of heat and pain often associated with conventional angiographic examinations.

The primary advantage of DSA in the diabetic patient is that only a very small amount of intra-arterial contrast material need be injected to obtain images. Because the incidence of contrast media–associated acute renal failure depends on the dose of contrast material used, this technique should decrease the incidence of these complications.

The major limitation of DSA for peripheral vascular disease is the small size of the image intensifier and therefore the small field of view available for each injection. Even with the use of a 14-in. image intensifier, an average of eight or nine injections are necessary to evaluate the entire lower limb blood supply. New technology may allow a single injection of contrast material to be used to view the entire arterial supply of the lower limbs with DSA.[13]

A second potential limitation of DSA is that the spatial resolution is less than that of conventional angiography. However, with the much improved contrast resolution of DSA, this is rarely a problem.

## PERCUTANEOUS TRANSLUMINAL ANGIOPLASTY

### Histologic and Pathologic Considerations

The initial speculation on the success of percutaneous transluminal angioplasty (PTA) has been replaced by experimental studies. Atheromatous plaque may be fibro-

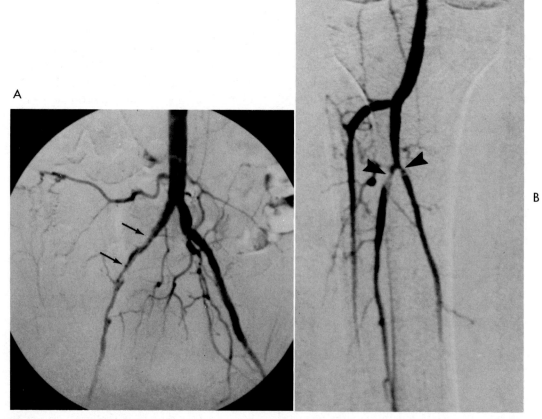

**FIG 17–5.**
Intra-arterial digital subtraction angiograms. **A,** anteroposterior view of pelvis shows severe disease in right common and external iliac arteries *(arrows).* Image obtained with injection of 12 mL 20% dilute contrast material into distal abdominal aorta. Commonly injection of 60 to 80 mL 60% contrast material is needed to produce such an image without DSA. **B,** anteroposterior view of popliteal trifurcation. Moderate stenoses are seen at origin of peroneal and posterior tibial arteries *(arrowheads).* Note how well vessels are seen when free from overlying bone.

muscular or complicated. In the former, the smooth muscle cells, collagen, and elastic fibrils proliferate in the intima. Fibromuscular plaque is converted into complicated plaque by central necrosis, lipid infiltration, hemorrhage, thrombosis, and calcification. When the plaque ruptures, a mural thrombus forms on its surface. If blood flow is restricted by the stenosis, the mural thrombus may extend to occlude the vessel. If sufficient flow remains, the mural thrombus may organize and become fibrous, enlarging the original plaque.

It was initially postulated that in a successful dilation, the dilating balloon compressed the atheroma against the vessel wall. However, it has now been shown that shearing of the plaque occurs when the

balloon is the same diameter as the vessel lumen.[6, 9] When the balloon is larger, the endothelial plaque is split, allowing a wider gap in the lumen. These findings explain the rough and ragged appearance of the vessel lumen immediately after dilation. Within 3 weeks, the plaque becomes smoother and retracts from the vessel lumen, producing a moderate increase in the vessel diameter. If the plaque endothelium has been split, greater retraction of the plaque occurs with healing, producing a larger lumen.

Because disruption of the intima produces platelet accumulation, antiplatelet medication given before and after angioplasty has proved effective. Increased blood flow over the injured intima also

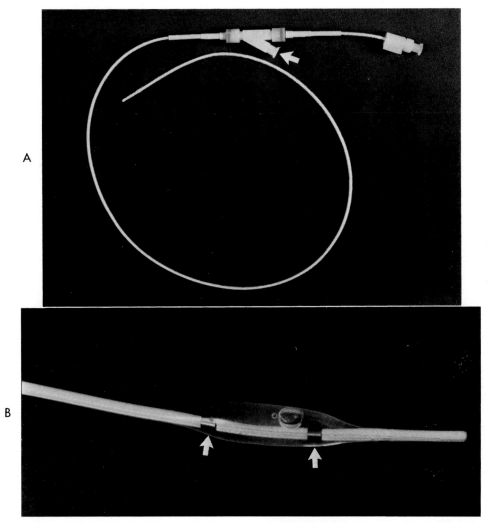

**FIG 17-6.**
**A,** double-lumen dilating catheter. End connector allows passage of guide wires and contrast material to opacify vessel lumen. Side connector *(arrow)* is used to inflate balloon with contrast agent. **B,** inflated balloon. Metal rings mark ends of balloon *(arrows)*. (See also Fig 17-7.)

reduces the potential for thrombus formation.

## Technique

Planning for angioplasty requires a detailed diagnostic angiogram to assess the patency of both the inflow and outflow vessels, as well as the length and degree of the stenosis or occlusion to be dilated. The radiologist, vascular surgeon, and attending physician all should agree on the treatment technique. In some instances, angioplasty alone is adequate for treatment, whereas in other cases, angioplasty of a stenosed iliac artery might precede a femoropopliteal bypass graft.

The arterial puncture site is prepared using sterile technique and infiltrated with a local anesthetic similar to preparing for angiography. Heparin and other pharmacologic adjuncts are administered (see later section). The angioplasty catheter is placed into the vessel in either an antegrade or a retrograde fashion, depending on the vessel to be dilated. Contrast material injected through the catheter lumen identifies the stenosis. The guidewire is manipulated through the stenosis, followed by the angioplasty catheter. The balloon straddles the stenosis, as indicated by the radiopaque markers identifying the balloon ends (Figs 17–6 and 17–7). The balloon is then inflated several times. After the dilation is completed, the catheter is pulled back from the stenosis, and contrast material is injected to evaluate the result. If the dilation is judged to be inadequate, immediate redilation can be performed with either the same or a larger balloon catheter. The dilated segment often has an irregular surface secondary to intimal disruption (Fig 17–8). This irregular surface will remodel and become smoother in the weeks after dilation.

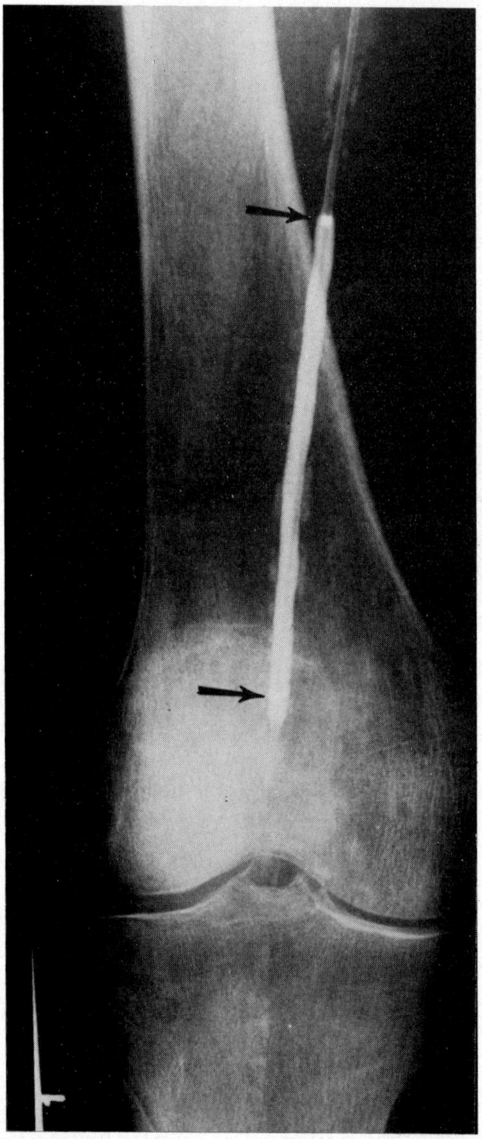

## Iliac Arteries

Solitary iliac artery stenoses, occurring most often near the aortic bifurcation, are short (see Fig 17–9). They usually occur in middle-aged patients and are ideal lesions for PTA. Most such stenoses of the common and proximal external iliac arteries are approached in a retrograde fashion from the ipsilateral side. A second angiographic catheter may be positioned from the contralateral femoral artery and used both to visualize the proximal end of the stenosis and to measure intra-arterial pressure within the aorta (Fig 17–10).

Chronic and acute iliac artery occlusions have been successfully recanalized. Careful pressure must be exerted in traversing these lesions, however, because the natural course of the occluded segment may be difficult to identify. Some authors have recommended short-term infusions of thrombolytic agents (urokinase) before attempting recanalization of occluded segments of the iliac artery. The rationale for the use of thrombolytic agents before angioplasty in an occluded iliac artery is that a large component of the occlusion usually represents thrombus. Lysing as much of the thrombus as possible before PTA should decrease the incidence of distal embolization after recanalization.

## Femoral Arteries

The distal external iliac and common femoral arteries are best approached by passing the catheter over the aortic bifurcation from the contralateral common femoral artery. Direct access from the ipsilateral side is usually not advisable because the puncture site would be too close to the diseased vessel.

Lesions of the superficial femoral artery, on the other hand, are approached in an antegrade fashion through an ipsilateral common femoral artery puncture (Fig 17–11). The catheter passage and dilation technique are similar to those used for the iliac artery, except smaller balloons are used. Contrary

**FIG 17–7.**
Percutaneous transluminal angioplasty balloon inflated in proximal popliteal artery. Metal markers define ends of balloon to facilitate positioning *(arrows)*.

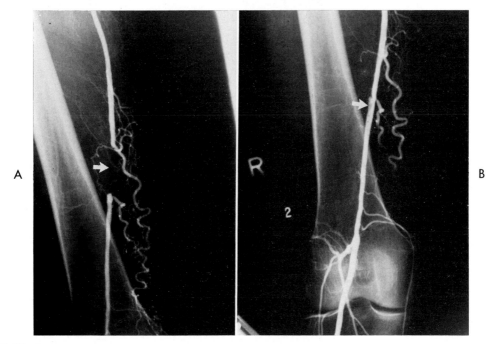

**FIG 17–8.**
Distal superficial femoral artery occlusion. **A,** predilation *(arrow)*. **B,** postdilation. Note resulting intimal irregularity *(arrow)*.

to the technique used in the iliac artery, more force can be exerted in passing catheters through a femoral artery stenosis because false aneurysms and hemorrhage are not as serious a problem in the thigh and can be readily controlled. Multiple stenoses in the same artery may be dilated in succession.

Occluded segments as long as 10 cm in the superficial femoral artery have been successfully recanalized and dilated, although the success rate rapidly diminishes when these occluded segments exceed 5 cm. Even though the lumen of an occluded segment cannot be seen radiographically, the guide wire usually passes directly through the occlusion and into the distal vessel. Attempting to pass a guide wire through an occluded segment may result in perforation of the vessel wall, but there is rarely any significant hematoma formation. It has even been possible to redirect the guide wire and successfully complete the dilation after such a perforation.

Stenoses of the deep femoral artery are easily treatable with PTA and approached from either the ipsilateral or contralateral side. Stenoses of femoropopliteal bypass graft anastomoses may also be dilated successfully in a similar manner.

## Popliteal Artery and Its Branches

The popliteal artery is approached in the same fashion as the superficial femoral artery (Fig 17–12). Recently balloon angioplasty of the infrapopliteal vessels has become possible. The technique is similar to that used for coronary angioplasty. Small balloon catheters, as well as extremely flexible steerable guide wires, are used. Generally only the proximal portions of these vessels are amenable to angioplasty. However, in selected circumstances dilation can be performed below the middle of the calf.

## Medications for Use Before, During, and After Percutaneous Transluminal Angioplasty

Medications used before, during, and after PTA are directed toward relief of pain and anxiety, prevention of arterial spasm, and prevention of thrombosis. Most proce-

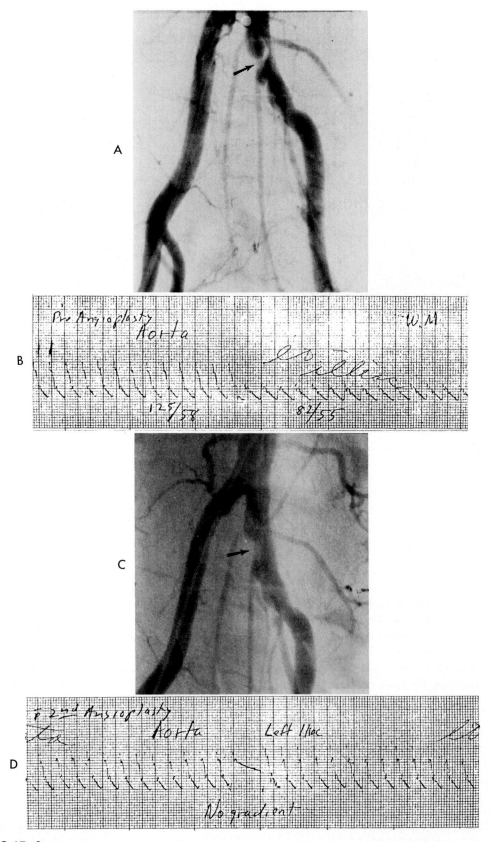

**FIG 17–9.**
Left common iliac artery dilation. **A,** stenosis *(arrow).* **B,** pressure measurements of aorta *(left)* and left common iliac artery distal to stenosis *(right).* Pressure gradient was 43 mm. **C,** partial dilation of stenosis *(arrow).* Pressure gradient decreased. **D,** final pressure recording after complete dilation. There was no gradient.

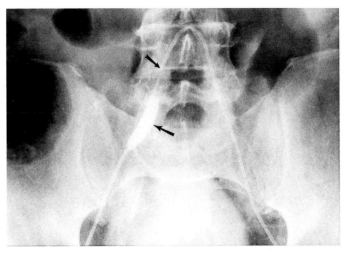

**FIG 17–10.**
Dilating balloon in right common iliac artery *(long arrow)*. Tip of catheter passed from contralateral iliac artery can be used to opacify stenosis and record pressures proximal to stenosis *(short arrow)*. Angioplasty catheter can be passed similarly over aortic bifurcation when distal external iliac and common femoral artery stenoses are treated.

dures are performed with IV analgesia appropriate to the patient's age and condition.

Arterial spasm is treated with intra-arterial administration of nitroglycerin in 100-μg aliquots. Nitroglycerin can be given freely as long as the patient's blood pressure remains stable. In addition, sublingual nifedipine (Procardia) (10 mg) has been found to be useful.

Thrombosis may be reduced by the use of intra-arterial heparin (1,500–5,000 units). It is usually given after crossing the stenosis, depending on the preference of the angiographer.

Considerable controversy exists among angiographers regarding medication after the procedure. Some advocate heparin immediately after the procedure, whereas oth-

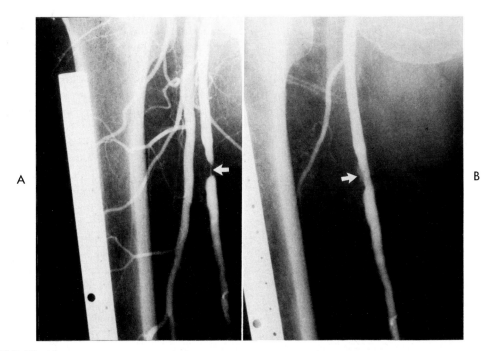

**FIG 17–11.**
Proximal superficial femoral artery stenosis *(arrow)*. **A**, predilation. **B**, postdilation. Shallow plaque remains.

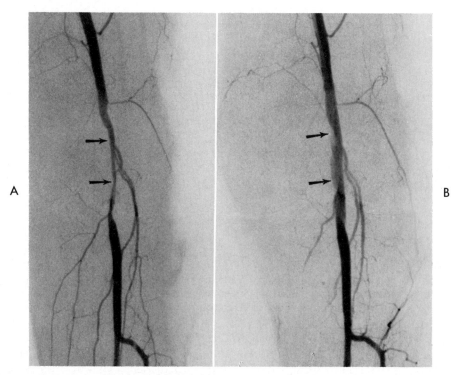

**FIG 17–12.**
Popliteal artery dilation. **A,** Predilation angiogram shows 3-cm stenosis *(arrows).* **B,** postdilation angiogram shows residual irregularity but widely patent vessel *(arrows).*

ers recommend no anticoagulants at all. There is almost uniform use of aspirin (300 mg/day) for all patients after angioplasty.

## COMPLICATIONS

About 5% of all angioplasty patients have some type of complication, most of which are reversible or correctable. The following list applies to all of the vessels discussed in this chapter; some specific situations are described:

1. Peripheral embolization, a much-feared complication, has, in fact, not been a frequent occurrence. Most such embolization is asymptomatic. Significant embolism is most likely to occur when dilation is attempted in a recently occluded vessel. In these instances, a trial of local catheter-directed thrombolytic therapy (urokinase) may be helpful before angioplasty.

2. Irregularity of the intima immediately after angioplasty is a normal, expected result of the procedure. Arteriograms taken

weeks or months later prove that remodeling smooths the intima.

3. Local dissection by the guide wire at the angioplasty site may occasionally lead to termination of the procedure, but often the true lumen can be renegotiated. The uplifted intima will then be pushed against the media and will be of no consequence. If a severe dissection occurs, vascular stents may be used but are approved for placement only within the iliac arteries.

4. Thrombosis of a dissection site will prevent further manipulation. Local infusion of urokinase should be considered. Surgical correction is also possible.

5. Vessel perforation may or may not be serious, depending on the site. Large retroperitoneal hematomas may follow an iliac artery perforation where local control is not easily obtained. Sometimes the catheter can be renegotiated into the vessel and the balloon inflated over the perforation to control the hemorrhage before surgical repair. Bleeding from femoral and popliteal artery perforations is rarely significant.

6. Vessel spasm after manipulation or

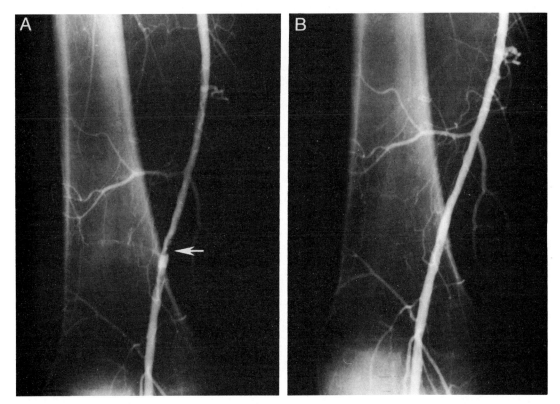

**FIG 17–13.**
Atherectomy. **A,** eccentric plaque in the proximal popliteal artery *(arrow)*. **B,** Postatherectomy. Restoration of original luminal diameter.

perforation is particularly prevalent in the popliteal and infrapopliteal vessels. Spasm may be controlled by intra-arterial administration of nitroglycerin, nifedipine, or both before and after entering these vessels.

7. Balloon rupture rarely produces arterial damage. Although extremely unusual, the frequency of balloon rupture can be reduced further by using a hand-held pressure gauge during inflation. Most balloons rupture longitudinally, and the catheter can still be removed easily. If the balloon ruptures circumferentially, it may buckle, preventing extraction of the catheter at the puncture site. Extraction through a sheath may be successful, but in extremely rare cases a surgical arteriotomy is necessary.

## RESULTS

The initial success in relieving stenoses and occlusions, as well as long-term patency after PTA, is best when the vessels are large and the stenoses short. Therefore, iliac ar-

tery PTAs have a greater success rate than femoral and popliteal artery procedures. Five-year patency rates of 70% to 80% are reported for iliac artery stenoses in both diabetic and nondiabetic patients.[4, 36] This rate compares well with the aortofemoral bypass graft patency rate of 80% to 90% at 3 to 5 years. Patency after superficial femoral artery angioplasty ranges from 60% to 70% at 5 years. In comparison, femoropopliteal bypass vein graft patency at 2 years is approximately 80% to 90% with good runoff and 60% to 70% with poor runoff. Patency rates drop significantly with the use of synthetic materials (e.g., Gore-Tex).

Long-term patency after PTA in the lower limbs is influenced by the severity of the peripheral vascular disease. Long stenoses (>10 cm) and heavily calcified stenoses have a significantly lower successful long-term patency rate. No significant difference in duration of patency between successfully treated stenoses and occlusions is noted. Several reports suggest that in the diabetic patient, PTA in the superficial femoral or popliteal arteries has a slightly poorer long-term patency rate than in the nondiabetic patient. This may be related to the severity of their vascular disease and not to the presence of diabetes per se.[36] Angioplasty results are comparable in diabetic and nondiabetic patients with a similar severity of peripheral vascular disease.

Little experience has been reported in dilations of the popliteal artery branches. This is a particular problem in diabetic patients in whom the tibial and peroneal arteries are often severely diseased. Angioplasty in this area in patients with diffuse disease is difficult and should be used only for potential limb salvage. Whether it will compare favorably with in situ vein bypass grafting remains to be seen.

Because PTA treats only segments of a vessel, recurrence of symptoms is often the result of new or increasing disease at a site proximal or distal to the dilation. In this regard, bypass grafts have an advantage, because even occlusion of the entire bypassed segments will not produce new ischemic symptoms.

Close follow-up with noninvasive hemodynamic testing should be done. This may show early recurrence before the onset of clinical symptoms. These noninvasive findings may prompt early retreatment when the stenoses are still amenable to PTA.

Angioplasty is successful in diabetic patients and can be used effectively to treat peripheral vascular disease in this patient population. Despite the small-vessel disease so common in diabetic patients, improvement in inflow (iliac and superficial femoral arteries) can lead to improved lower limb viability. Frequently this is sufficient to allow ulcers to heal and thus prevent amputation.

## NEW TECHNOLOGY

Recent advances in technology have added several new devices for the percutaneous treatment of peripheral vascular disease. These include lasers, atherectomy and other recanalization devices, vascular stents, and intravascular ultrasound.

Elastic recoil of the vessel wall and intimal hyperplasia induced by balloon dilatation can lead to restenosis after PTA. Patients with severe or diffuse atherosclerotic disease have an increased risk of restenosis after conventional angioplasty techniques. Progression of atherosclerotic disease can cause restenosis, as well as decrease the distal runoff accentuating more proximal lesions. For all of these reasons, new devices, or new applications of devices, have been developed. The primary goal is to improve long-term patency, either by removal of the plaque itself, or by placement of an intravascular stent that can oppose elastic recoil or support an intimal dissection.

Recently there have been numerous reports in medical journals and the general public press concerning the use of lasers for treatment of peripheral vascular disease. Since their early development, people seem to be inherently interested in lasers. With their new application toward vascular stenosis, there was a presumption that lasers would offer better results than conventional angioplasty.

Multiple different laser sources and delivery systems have been developed to ablate (vaporize) atherosclerotic plaque. Whereas angioplasty redistributes plaque, laser ablation removes it. Early laser systems were complicated by a high perforation rate. Newer systems, such as eximer lasers, are safer but are relatively large systems requiring special facilities. The true role of laser in the treatment of vascular disease has yet to be defined. The safer, newer laser systems are able to remove only a small amount of plaque. Most frequently, this ability is used to create an initial channel through occluded vessels. Once a "pilot hole" has been opened, conventional angioplasty techniques are utilized to further open the stenosis. Ongoing developments may allow laser vaporization of larger amounts of plaque without subsequent angioplasty. Currently laser is most often used to recanalize occlusions before standard balloon angioplasty. The question as to whether the use of lasers as an adjunct to standard angioplasty offers any advantage has yet to be answered. No randomized, prospective trials have compared the results of angioplasty with and without laser.

Atherectomy and mechanical recanalization devices are motor-driven tools that are also used to physically remove plaque. The Simpson directional atherectomy catheter allows excision and removal of atherosclerotic material (Fig 17–13). It is particularly useful in eccentric lesions and those resistant to angioplasty. Various other high- and low-speed mechanical recanalization catheters are available to create channels through occlusions before angioplasty. Most have rotating or pulsating components that cut or displace plaque. The channel size is only as large as the catheter, so subsequent angio-

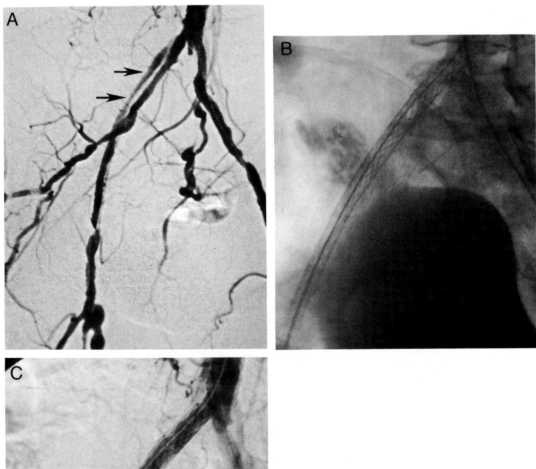

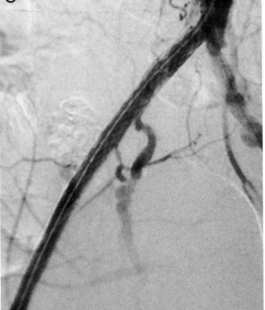

**FIG 17–14.**
Intravascular stents. **A,** iatrogenic dissection of common iliac artery with 45 mm Hg gradient. **B,** after placement of six stents in tandem. **C,** arteriogram shows patent vessel. No residual gradient.

plasty is necessary and no tissue is extracted. Although helpful in specific instances, these devices do not offer any major advantage over conventional techniques.

Several types of intravascular stents are undergoing clinical investigation. Currently, only the Palmaz stent is Food and Drug Administration approved, and only for placement in the iliac arteries. Indications for stent placement include suboptimal result after angioplasty, either a residual stenosis or persistent gradient; recurrent stenosis despite multiple angioplasties; or dissection of the iliac arteries after angioplasty or from guide wire manipulations. Vascular stents are extremely useful for the repair of suboptimal angioplasty or heavily calcified lesions (Fig 17–14). Although long-term clinical data have not been obtained, early data suggest a restenosis rate similar, or possibly better than, conventional angioplasty. Clinical trials are currently evaluating stents for use in femoral and renal arteries. Complication rates are somewhat higher during these intravascular stent procedures

(13%) related primarily to puncture site hematoma from the large size of the stent introducer.

Intravascular ultrasound (IVUS) has the capability of characterizing atherosclerotic lesions in a different way than arteriography (Fig 17–15). It allows a cross-sectional analysis of the three layers of the arterial wall. Atheroma, calcification, intimal hyperplasia and ulceration all can be visualized. An early lesion, the fatty streak, can be visualized by IVUS but is not detected by arteriography. Clinically, IVUS is helpful in evaluation of lesions after a percutaneous intervention such as angioplasty or atherectomy. The area of residual stenosis and flow velocities can be calculated. Balloon dilatation can cause breaks in the arterial wall and intimal flaps that cannot be visualized with arteriography. Intravascular ultrasound aids in recognizing these lesions that may increase the risk of restenosis at the site of angioplasty. Better characterization of atherosclerotic lesions may allow a more specific and effective treatment.

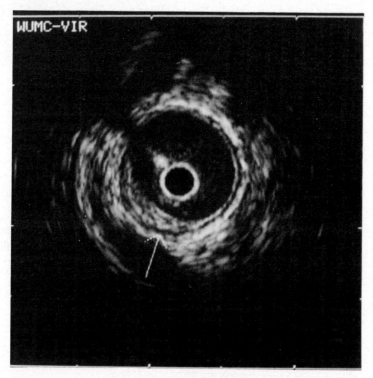

**FIG 17–15.**
Intravascular ultrasound. Ultrasound image obtained from a common iliac artery. Atheromatous plaque along the inferior wall *(arrow)*.

## CHOICE OF PATIENT AND PROCEDURE

The roles of surgery and PTA are in flux. The lesions most suitable for angioplasty are focal stenoses less than 5 cm and occlusions shorter than 10 cm, particularly in the superficial femoral and popliteal arteries. There is less agreement among authors regarding the desirability of dilating anterior and posterior tibial and peroneal arteries.

Percutaneous transluminal angioplasty provides a convenient means of relieving selected vascular stenoses and occlusions. It offers a considerably lessened hospital stay with relatively low morbidity. Patient stress is greatly reduced, and general anesthesia is not required. There is no question that angioplasty is an effective alternative to surgery when chosen and used properly as either a complementary or primary procedure. In addition, PTA does not interfere with subsequent surgical bypass procedures should they become necessary. The combination of PTA and bypass surgery may provide more years of leg use in a diabetic patient before an amputation may be eventually necessary. A cooperative assessment by the patient's physician, vascular surgeon, and radiologist should determine the appropriate therapy.

## REFERENCES

1. Abele JE: Balloon catheters and transluminal dilatation: technical considerations, *AJR* 135:901, 1980.
2. Alpert JR, Ring EJ, Freiman DB, et al: Balloon dilatation of iliac stenosis with distal arterial surgery, *Arch Surg* 115:715, 1980.
3. Andros G, Harris RW, Dulawa LB, et al: The need for arteriography in diabetic patients with gangrene and palpable foot pulses, *Arch Surg* 119:1260, 1984.
4. Becker GJ, Katsen BT, Dake MD: Noncoronary angioplasty, *Radiology* 170:921–940, 1989.
5. Billstrom A, Hietala SO, Lithner F, et al: Nephrotoxicity of contrast media in patients with diabetes mellitus, *Acta Radiol* 30:509–515, 1989.
6. Block PC, Fallon JT, Elmer L: Experimental angioplasty: lessons from the laboratory, *AJR* 135:907, 1980.
7. Burnett JR, Walsh JA, Howard PR, et al: Transluminal balloon angioplasty in diabetic peripheral vascular disease, *Aust J Surg* 57:307–309, 1987.
8. Bush WH, Swanson DP: Acute reactions to intravascular contrast media: types, risk factors, recognition, and specific treatment, *AJR* 157:1153–1161, 1991.
9. Castaneda-Zuniga WR, Formanek A, Tadavarthy M, et al: The mechanism of balloon angioplasty, *Radiology* 135:565, 1980.
10. Colapinto RF, Harries-Jones EP, Johnston KW: Percutaneous transluminal recanalization of complete iliac artery occlusions, *Arch Surg* 116:277, 1981.
11. Cragg AH, Gardiner GA, Smith TP: Vascular applications of laser, *Radiology* 172:925–935, 1989.
12. Darcy MD: Lower extremity arteriography: current approach and techniques, *Radiology* 178:615–621, 1991.
13. Engeler CE, Yedlicka JW, Letourneau JG, et al: Intravascular sonography in the detection of arteriosclerosis and evaluation of vascular interventional procedures, *AJR* 156:1087–1090, 1991.
14. Fallon JT: Pathology of arterial lesions amenable to percutaneous transluminal angioplasty, *AJR* 135:913, 1980.
15. Ford K, Braull SD, Moore AV, et al: Percutaneous transluminal angioplasty in diabetic patients: an effective treatment modality, *Cardiovasc Intervent Radiol* 7:204, 1984.
16. Gallino A, Mahler F, Probst P, et al: Percutaneous transluminal angioplasty of the arteries of the lower limbs: a 5-year follow-up, *Circulation* 70:619, 1984.
17. Gardiner GA, Meyerovitz MF, Stokes KR, et al: Complications of transluminal angioplasty, *Radiology* 159:201–208, 1986.
18. Garvey CJ, Wilkins RA, Lewis JD: Peripheral vascular disease: prospective study of intraarterial digital subtraction angiography using a 9-inch intensifier, *Radiology* 159:423, 1986.
19. Greenberger P, Patterson R, Kelly M, et al: Administration of radiographic contrast media in high risk patients, *Invest Radiol* 15(suppl):540, 1980.
20. Harris KG, Smith TP, Cragg AH, et al: Nephrotoxicity from contrast material in renal insufficiency: ionic versus nonionic agents, *Radiology* 179:849–852, 1991.
21. Horvath L: Percutaneous transluminal angioplasty: importance of anticoagulant and fibrinolytic drugs, *AJR* 135:951, 1980.
22. Jacobs JB, Hannafee WN: The use of priscoline in peripheral arteriography, *Radiology* 88:1957, 1967.
23. Kannel WB, McGee DL: Diabetes and vascular disease—the Framingham study, *JAMA* 241:2035, 1979.

24. Krepel VM, van Andel GJ, van Erp WFM, et al: Percutaneous transluminal angioplasty of the femoropopliteal artery: initial and longterm results, *Radiology* 156:325, 1985.

25. Lautin EM, Freeman NJ, Schoenfeld AH, et al: Radiocontrast associated renal dysfunction: incidence and risk factors, *AJR* 157:49–58, 1991.

26. Lautin EM, Freeman NJ, Schoenfeld AH, et al: Radiocontrast associated renal dysfunction: a comparison of lower osmolality and conventional high osmolality contrast media, *AJR* 157:59–65, 1991.

27. Lowman BG, Queral LA, Holbrook WA, et al: Transluminal angioplasty during vascular reconstructive procedures, *Arch Surg* 116:829, 1980.

28. Meema HE, Oreopoulos DG: Morphology, progression, and regression of arterial and periarterial calcifications in patients with end-stage renal disease, *Radiology* 158:671, 1986.

29. Motarjeme A, Keifer JW, Zuska AJ: Percutaneous transluminal angioplasty of the iliac arteries: 66 experiences, *AJR* 135:937, 1980.

30. Palmaz JC, Garcia OJ, Schatz RA, et al: Placement of balloon expandable intraluminal stents in iliac arteries: first 171 procedures, *Radiology* 174:969–975, 1990.

31. Parfrey PS, Griffiths SM, Barrett BJ, et al: Contrast material-induced renal failure in patients with diabetes mellitus, renal insufficiency, or both, *N Engl J Med* 320:143–149, 1989.

32. Picus D, Hicks ME, Darcy MD, et al: Comparison of nonsubtracted digital angiography and conventional film-screen angiography for the evaluation of patients with peripheral vascular disease, *J Vasc Intervent Radiol* 2:359–364, 1991.

33. Rhodes GR, Rollins D, Sidawy AN, et al: Popliteal-to-tibial in situ saphenous vein bypass for limb salvage in diabetic patients, *Am J Surg* 154:245–247, 1987.

34. Schoop W, Levy H, Cappius G, et al: Early and late results of PTA in iliac stenoses, in Zeitler E, Gruntzig A, Schoop W, editors: *Percutaneous vascular recanalization: techniques, applications, clinical results*, New York, 1978, Springer-Verlag.

35. Silver K, Sollitto RJ, Jamil Z: Digital subtraction angiography versus noninvasive testing in the vascular assessment of the ischemic foot, *J Foot Surg* 26:217–221, 1987.

36. Smith TP, Cragg AH, Berbaum KS, et al: Comparison of the efficacy of digital subtraction and film screen angiography of the lower limb: prospective study of 50 patients, *AJR* 158:431–436, 1992.

37. Stokes KR, Strunk HM, Campbell DR, et al: Five-year results of iliac and femoropopliteal angioplasty in diabetic patients, *Radiology* 174:977–982, 1990.

38. Tabbara M, White R, Cavaye D, et al: In vivo human comparison of intravascular ultrasonography and angiography, *J Vasc Surg* 14:496–504, 1991.

39. van Andel GJ, van Erp WFM, Krepel VM, et al: Percutaneous transluminal dilatation of the iliac artery: long-term results, *Radiology* 156:321, 1985.

40. Waltman AC: Percutaneous transluminal angioplasty: iliac and deep femoral arteries, *AJR* 135:921, 1980.

41. Widlus DM, Osterman FA: Evaluation and percutaneous management of atherosclerotic peripheral vascular disease, *JAMA* 261:3148–3154, 1989.

# CHAPTER 18

# Vascular Surgery

**Brent T. Allen, M.D.**
**Charles B. Anderson, M.D.**
**Willard B. Walker, M.D.**
**Gregorio A. Sicard, M.D.**

Diffuse vascular disease is the most important factor leading to the increased mortality and morbidity in patients with diabetes mellitus. Diabetes is the seventh leading cause of death in the United States and is the most frequent cause of nontraumatic amputations.[2] The vascular complications of diabetes mellitus can occur in multiple locations, including the coronary, cerebral, retinal, renal, and peripheral circulations. Patients with diabetes mellitus are two to four times more likely to die from heart disease and two to six times more likely to suffer a stroke. Diabetes is the leading cause of blindness between the ages of 25 to 74 years and accounts for more than 30% of the new cases of end-stage renal disease each year. Patients with diabetes are 15 times more likely to have peripheral vascular disease and 22 times more likely to have foot ulceration or gangrene than nondiabetics.[71]

Vascular disease in diabetics is a tremendous burden to the health care system. Diabetic complications account for 2% of all hospitalizations reviewed by the 1987 National Hospital Discharge Survey.[107] The total cost in this survey of in-hospital treatment for late complications of diabetes was estimated at $5091 million. Peripheral arterial diabetic complications accounted for $873 million (17%) of this total and ranked second only to heart disease as the most costly of diabetic complications requiring hospitalization. Peripheral vascular disease accounted for more in-hospital days (14.4) than any other complication of diabetes.[107]

## INCIDENCE

Diabetes affects as many as 14 million people in the United States, approximately 5% to 6% of the population. More than 725,000 new cases are diagnosed each year, and the incidence has increased during the 1980s. The prevalence tends to be slightly higher in women than in men, especially in black Americans.[2]

Melton et al.[105] found that the incidence of symptomatic occlusive arterial disease in 1,073 diabetic patients was 21.3 and 17.6 per 1,000 persons per year for men and women, respectively. The incidence of peripheral vascular disease increased with age and duration of the diabetes. Furthermore, approximately 20% of diabetics with occlusive arterial disease had experienced gangrene. The cumulative incidence of vascular disease in diabetics has been estimated to be 15% at 10 years after the initial diagnosis of the disease and 45% at 20 years. Uusitupa et al.[141] reported that the age adjusted incidence of claudication was significantly higher among middle-aged diabetic men and women than in nondiabetic persons (men 20.3% vs. 8.0%; women 21.8% vs. 4.2%, respectively). Janka et al.[72] estimated a 16% prevalence of peripheral vascular disease in

623 diabetic patients when patients with symptoms were screened with Doppler measurements of limb perfusion. There was a marked increase in peripheral vascular disease with age from 3.2% of those patients less than 50 years to 55% of those more than 80 years of age. Duration of diabetes and degree of hyperglycemia correlated with distal peripheral vascular disease but did not correlate with proximal arterial disease.

Diabetes appears to augment atherosclerosis, and it has its greatest impact in populations with other risk factors such as smoking and hypertension. Sternby[130] showed that diabetes is a strong risk factor for peripheral vascular disease involving the aorta, cerebral, femoral, and coronary arteries. The atherogenic effect of diabetes seems to be clinically more pronounced in the peripheral and coronary arteries than in the aorta or cerebral circulation, which may explain the absence of diabetes aggravated atherosclerosis in some animal models in which the aorta has been the vessel studied.

## PATHOGENESIS

Three factors combine to promote tissue necrosis in diabetic feet: (1) trauma, (2) neuropathy, and (3) ischemia. The relative contribution of each of these factors varies among patients. Trauma and neuropathy are interrelated. Patients with severe neuropathy are prone to traumatic ulceration because of alterations in weight-bearing forces producing pressure points and because of loss of protective sensation. If the traumatized tissue has adequate blood supply, patients often develop a chronic ulcer surrounded by hypertrophic callus that bleeds easily when debrided. A mal perforans ulcer on the plantar surface of the foot overlying the metatarsal heads is an example of this pathophysiology. Traumatized tissue in patients with arterial insufficiency lacks the blood supply to support healing mechanisms or resist infection. In this setting ischemic ulcerated tissue is likely to become septic and progressively enlarge, thus jeopardizing the foot. The initial and most important step in managing diabetic foot ulceration is to control sepsis in the foot with antibiotics and debridement of necrotic tissue. This is performed during the patient's initial management while the degree of arterial insufficiency is being assessed.

A common misconception is that diabetic ulceration is caused primarily by "microvascular" disease. This mechanism was first suggested by Goldenberg et al.[55] after retrospectively studying diabetic and nondiabetic amputation specimens with light microscopy. Histologic examination reportedly revealed a material that was positive on periodic acid–Schiff staining in the arterioles of diabetics. This material was thought to be the obstructing pathogenic lesion in diabetic vascular disease. However, subsequent prospective investigations have failed to confirm the presence of an obstructive arteriolar lesion in diabetics.[8, 70] Diabetic patients do have muscle capillary basement membrane thickening that may not involve all capillaries in all patients to the same degree. The thickened capillary basement membrane apparently does not represent a barrier to gas exchange in studies documenting no difference in transcutaneous oxygen tension in diabetic or nondiabetic patients with vascular disease of similar severity.[150]

Although diffusion of oxygen through diabetic capillaries does not appear impaired, an alteration in capillary blood and serum viscosity, as well as flow abnormalities in leukocytes, erythrocytes, platelets, and plasma proteins, has been reported.[43, 75, 104, 126] The hyperviscosity seen in diabetic patients stems from hyperglycemic glycosylation of the red blood cell membrane, leading to membrane stiffening and subsequent decreased red blood cell deformability and increased erythrocyte aggregation. Red blood cell membrane glycosylation is directly proportional to serum glucose levels. The hemoglobin molecule is also susceptible to glycosylation, a reaction that increases hemoglobin's affinity for oxygen and therefore may contribute to ischemia in affected tissues.[123]

Diabetics are unique in their propensity toward calcific obstructive atherosclerosis that is most prominent in the tibial arteries between the knee and ankle. The arterial lesions in this location are the most important reason for the increased risk of tissue necrosis and limb loss in the diabetic population. Commonly, the lower limb vessels proximal to the knee and in the foot are less diseased. The basis for the distribution of diabetic lower limb vascular disease is unknown. Fortunately, the frequent sparing of the proximal femoral and pedal arteries allows for femoropedal artery bypass and limb salvage in many cases.

Finally, diabetics are susceptible to the atherogenic factors common to nondiabetic patients such as smoking, family history, hypertension, and hyperlipidemia. Diabetes in patients with such risk factors seems to potentiate the risk of cardiovascular complications from atherosclerosis.

## CLINICAL MANIFESTATIONS

Patients consulting a vascular surgeon for evaluation of lower limb ischemia typically complain of muscle pain with ambulation (claudication), constant foot pain (rest pain), or tissue necrosis (ulceration or gangrene).

Lower limb claudication, the most common presenting symptom of patients with peripheral vascular disease, is a weakness, cramping or fatigue of exercised muscle groups associated with prompt relief by rest. Although usually very specific in its manifestation, occasionally it can be difficult to differentiate from "pseudoclaudication syndromes" such as degenerative arthritis of the spine, hips, or feet, neuritis, and venous claudication. In arterial claudication, the prompt relief by rest, the reproducibility of the symptoms during exercise, and the absence of symptoms at rest differentiates it from the pseudoclaudication syndromes. Patients with pseudoclaudication usually must sit or lie down to obtain relief, whereas in arterial claudication, cessation of the exercise is usually sufficient. The length of time for resolution of the pain is longer in pseudoclaudication than in arterial claudication, often requiring 20 to 30 minutes in the former and 2 to 3 minutes in the latter.

Generally the level of the vascular obstruction can be estimated by the muscle groups producing of the symptoms of claudication. Claudication in the buttocks indicates a blockage in the terminal aorta. Thigh claudication indicates disease in the iliac arteries, and calf claudication suggests obstruction in the superficial femoral arteries. Fatigue or paraesthesias in the foot is an uncommon symptom of claudication but may indicate obstructive disease of the vessels of the calf. Claudication alone, as is discussed later, is typically not associated with limb-threatening ischemia but may be severely disabling.

Claudication often slowly worsens and is accompanied by other symptoms of arterial insufficiency. As claudication progresses from walking three blocks to walking only one block, to walking from the bedroom to the bathroom, the patient may begin to complain of numbness of the foot, night pain, and, later, rest pain, ischemic ulcers, or gangrene.

Nighttime numbness and pain in the foot, termed rest pain, are frequently located on the forefoot and are prominent complaints in patients with limb-threatening ischemia. Sleeping supine eliminates gravity's contribution to arterial perfusion, and the blood pressure normally drops during sleep; hence, the foot becomes more ischemic as the flow through the collateral vessels decreases. Ischemic pain arouses the patient from sleep, who gets relief by walking a few steps. This presumably elevates the blood pressure, restores gravity's effect, and improves perfusion of the feet. Frequently patients with severe rest pain sleep in chairs with their feet in a dependent position to minimize discomfort. Rest pain, persistent numbness, painful ulcers, and frank gangrene are symptoms of limb-threatening ischemia and require prompt investigation.

### Diabetic Neuropathy

The symptoms of lower limb arterial insufficiency in diabetics are sometimes difficult to distinguish from neuropathy. Diabetic patients frequently are referred for vascular evaluation because of a constant burning pain or tingling sensation in the foot. These symptoms are typical of neuropathic pain; they are most severe at night and generally not relieved by position change. The pain usually circumferentially involves the entire foot or lower limb in a "stocking-glove" distribution and commonly is bilateral. This type of neuropathic pain is not caused by macrovascular disease and often is found in diabetic patients with normal limb perfusion. It may be present in patients with other symptoms of arterial insufficiency (e.g., claudication) but is not improved with revascularization.

Ulceration of the diabetic foot is another common stimulus for a vascular evaluation. Diabetic neuropathy may compromise protective sensation and predispose diabetics to ulceration. This may occur in spite of normal perfusion and lead to a chronic draining wound that will not heal until the source of trauma is eliminated. The classic example of this is the mal perforans ulcer that heals rapidly once traumatic ambulation is avoided.

Neuropathic ulceration may be the inciting event, leading to severe sepsis or gangrene in an ischemic diabetic foot. Once traumatic ulcers have developed in ischemic limbs, the blood flow may be insufficient to promote healing or resist infection. Septic necrosis (gangrene) may progress quickly, involving previously viable tissue and produce limb or life-threatening complications.

Diabetic neuropathy may delay the manifestation of patients with critical limb ischemia. Patients with severe neuropathy frequently do not experience ischemic rest pain as a warning sign of impending tissue necrosis. Hence, they seek medical attention only after a nonhealing ulcer or a gangrenous toe develops. Thomas et al.[139] noted less preoperative ischemic pain in diabetic vs. nondiabetic patients with limb-threatening arterial insufficiency (44% vs. 68%). The prevalence of tissue necrosis in diabetics compared with nondiabetic patients with peripheral vascular disease is illustrated by our experience at Barnes Hospital with 228 patients who required amputations in the foot (toe and transmetatarsal) for tissue necrosis. Diabetics accounted for 70% (160 patients) of this group.

## Physical Examination

Physical examination yields important clues to the degree of vascular impairment in the diabetic patient. Fundoscopic examination can sometimes provide important information regarding the severity and duration of the vascular involvement. Palpation and auscultation of the extracranial carotid artery may detect a thrill or bruit, which suggests the possibility of atherosclerotic narrowing at the carotid bifurcation and should be further evaluated with duplex sonography. Cardiac evaluation may detect arrhythmias or abnormal heart sounds indicative of ischemic heart disease. Examination of the abdomen may detect an asymptomatic abdominal aortic aneurysm or identify bruits associated with visceral, renal, or iliac artery occlusive disease.

Evaluation of the extremities in the diabetic patient is extremely important and can often pinpoint the level of arterial obstruction. An audible bruit or the absence of pulses in the groin indicates aortoiliac occlusive disease, which is less common than distal disease in diabetics. The palpation of popliteal, posterior tibial, and dorsalis pedis pulses helps to localize the site of infrainguinal occlusive disease. Although uncommon, occasionally a weak pedal pulse may be palpable in spite of an occluded superficial femoral artery, indicating extensive collateral blood flow from the deep femoral artery to the popliteal artery. Diminished hair growth, reduced perspiration, and decreased temperature in the lower limb all are suggestive of inadequate circulation.

In diabetics, careful inspection of the feet is important (see Chapter 2). Sensory changes (pain, light touch, position sense) should be noted. The presence of erythematous pressure points, ischemic ulcers, neuropathic ulcers ("mal perforans" ulcers), gangrenous toes, calluses, and hypertrophic nails may provide important information regarding the degree of vascular or neuropathic involvement of the extremity. Dependent cyanosis and rubor of the feet suggests arterial insufficiency, especially in patients who note relief of rest pain with foot dependency. Dependent rubor results from vasodilation secondary to ischemia and is more indicative of distal arterial obstruction. Cyanosis may be present because of venous insufficiency in patients with little or no arterial disease.

## DIAGNOSIS

### Noninvasive Vascular Diagnostic Techniques

The noninvasive vascular laboratory is a cornerstone in the objective evaluation of patients with vascular disease (see Chapter 15). The vascular laboratory can provide accurate information regarding the location and severity of occlusive disease and the need for angiography and establish a baseline for serial follow-up. These studies are well accepted by patients because they are noninvasive, inexpensive, and can be performed on an outpatient basis. The noninvasive vascular studies can help clarify the contribution of vascular disease to lower limb symptoms in diabetic patients with neuropathy.

Lower limb systolic Doppler arterial pressures and waveform analysis obtained at the proximal thigh, above-knee, below-knee, ankle, and toe levels have become the gold standard in the noninvasive evaluation of patients with peripheral vascular disease. This technique uses pneumatic cuffs to occlude vessels and depends on the compressibility of vessels. The blood pressure at the ankle in one of the pedal arteries is compared with the brachial artery pressure, and an ankle-brachial index (ABI) is calculated. However, peripheral arteries may be relatively incompressible secondary to marked medial calcification common in diabetics (Fig 18–1).[58, 109] Tenembaum et al.[138] demonstrated that the average foot pressure in the diabetic was 20 mm Hg greater than the pressure in nondiabetic controls. This complicates the use of segmental pressures alone for assessing lower limb perfusion. In extreme cases of arterial calcification, occlusive compression is not possible even at 300 mm Hg; thus, segmental pressures in such situations cannot assess arterial perfusion.

Because the ABI may not be reliable in some diabetic patients as a result of vessel incompressibility, a technique for the measurement of *digital* systolic pressures has been reported as being more informative regarding degree of distal macrovascular disease.[59, 90] This technique, expressed as a toe-brachial index (TBI), or, in certain cases, as a toe-ankle index (TAI), permits the evaluation of pressure proximal to the toes, as well as changes distal to the ankle. Some studies[91, 109] have demonstrated excellent correlation of TBI with angiographic findings. No difference in the TBIs of diabetic and nondiabetic groups among patients with claudication was reported by Vincent et al.[146] The use of toe pressures and TBIs for assessing healing potential has been previously described by various investigators. Barnes et al.[9] reported the healing of all foot amputations in diabetics if the toe pressures were greater than 25 mm Hg and greater than 10 mm Hg in nondiabetics. Ramsey et al.[116] reported healing of foot ulcers in diabetics if they had toe pressure of 30 mm Hg or more. Conversely, Boone and Pomajzl[18] reported that a minimal toe pressure of 45 mm Hg was required to assure healing of forefoot amputations. These data indicate that toe blood pressures in the range of 25 to 45 mm Hg are good indicators of healing potential of ulcers and amputations in the diabetic foot.

Arterial waveform analysis is an important component of the lower limb Doppler blood pressure evaluations, especially in diabetics with noncompressible vessels (Fig 18–2). This technique becomes especially useful for evaluation of disease in the femoral, popliteal, and tibial regions, where blunted monophasic waveforms suggest occlusive arterial disease even in the presence of normal Doppler pressures secondary to incompressible vessels. The routine evaluation of waveforms in conjunction with the segmental pressures and segmental indices increases the accuracy of Doppler testing.

The use of radioisotope clearance has been reported as a valuable technique in the evaluation of ischemic limbs and specifically for determining the proximal amputation site.[85, 92, 96] Malone et al.[96] demonstrated that 70 of 74 (95%) amputations with xenon 133 clearance of more than 2.2 mL/100 g of

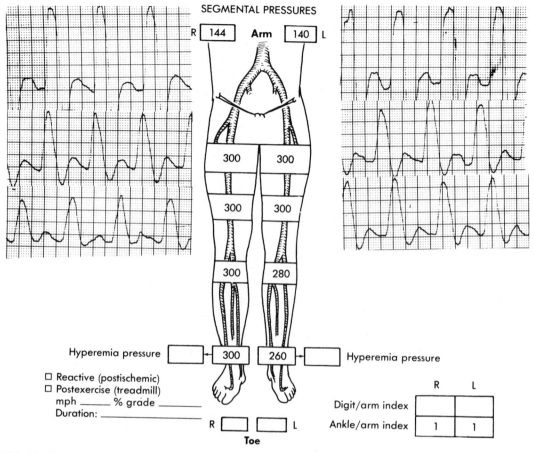

**FIG 18–1.**
Lower limb segmental pressures and waveforms in a diabetic patient. Note normal waveforms but falsely elevated segmental pressures from vessel incompressibility.

tissue per minute healed primarily. The presence of diabetes mellitus did not affect the incidence of primary healing when compared with nondiabetics. Another noninvasive technique is the transcutaneous oxygen tension measurement of ischemic extremities. Kram et al.[84] found that preoperative values for anterior and posterior calf transcutaneous oxygen tension were significantly lower in patients in whom a below-knee amputation failed to heal, compared with patients whose amputations healed. Successful amputation healing occurred in only 50% of patients with calf oxygen tensions less than 20 mm Hg, but healing occurred in 96% of patients with calf oxygen tensions greater than 20 mm Hg. Further investigation of this technique and its usefulness in diabetics with peripheral vascular disease remain to be determined.

## Radiographic Evaluation of Vascular Disease

A variety of radiographic techniques have been developed over the last 60 years to visualize large- and small-caliber vessels. Important modifications in contrast materials and the techniques of arteriography have occurred since the original description by Brooks[24] for lower extremity arteriography in 1924 and later for aortic visualization by Dos Santos et al.[44] in 1929.

Soft tissue radiographs are helpful in determining the extent of vascular calcifications (Figs 18–3 to 18–5). Twenty percent to 25% of patients with adult-onset diabetes have radiographic evidence of arterial calcification.[3, 54, 140] Interestingly, calcification of the media that is typically seen in diabetics is not commonly associated with complete vascular

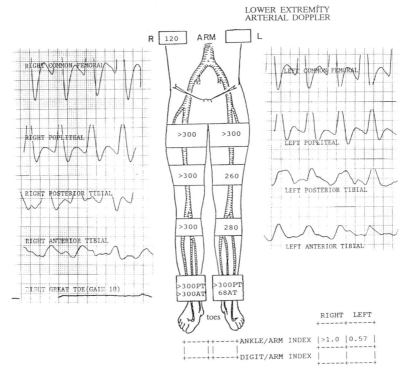

**FIG 18–2.**
Lower limb segmental pressures and waveforms in a diabetic patient with severe infrapopliteal occlusive disease. Note falsely elevated ankle pressures with abnormal waveforms.

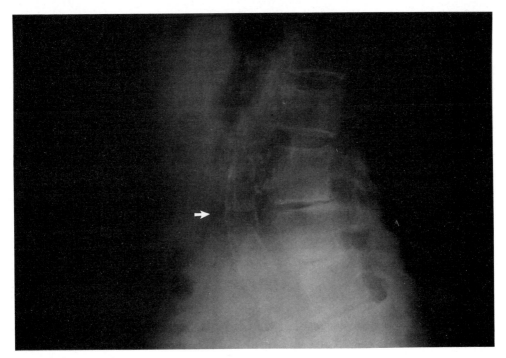

**FIG 18–3.**
Marked aortic calcification in a diabetic patient ("eggshell aorta").

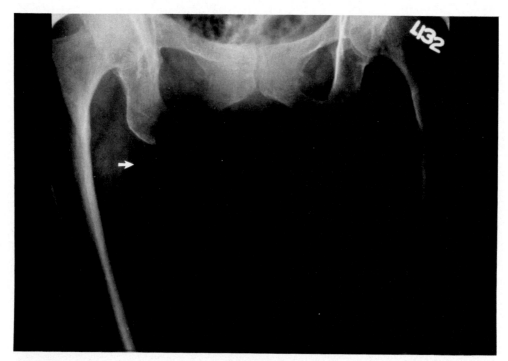

**FIG 18–4.**
Diffuse femoral artery calcification in a diabetic patient.

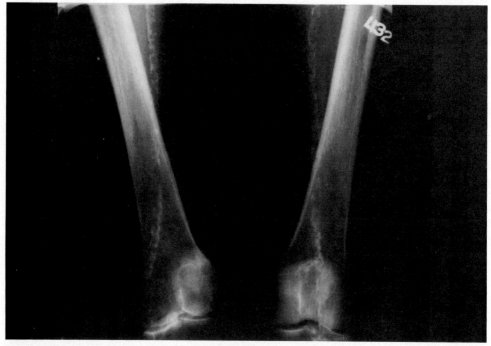

**FIG 18–5.**
Extensive superficial femoral and popliteal calcification in a diabetic patient.

occlusion. Correlation between sites of calcifications in patent vessels and the arteriogram can provide important information regarding the appropriate surgical procedure, especially because severe calcification indicates that a vascular anastomosis would be difficult or impossible to perform.

Transfemoral arteriography has become the routine approach for radiologic evaluation of the aortoiliac and leg vessels. This technique has been previously described by various authors.[78, 124, 148] Because of the increased incidence of renal impairment in the diabetic population, low-dose arteriography, combined with adequate hydration before and after the procedure, is mandatory. Eisenberg et al.[47] reported no acute renal failure in 537 patients who underwent adequate hydration before major angiography. In a study evaluating renal dysfunction after arteriography, Mason et al.[101] found no significant renal failure and a 25% decrease in glomerular filtration rates in only 18% of diabetics who were appropriately hydrated.

Harkonen and Kjellstrand[61] reported significant renal impairment in 76% after intravenous pyelography in diabetics with serum creatinine levels of 2 mg/dL or higher. Although in most patients the renal impairment is reversible, a high incidence of chronic renal failure is found, especially if the patients have serum creatinine levels higher than 5 mg/dL. Possible etiologic factors in dye induced renal impairment include (1) direct toxicity to tubules, (2) tubular plugging by proteinaceous casts, and (3) changes in renal hemodynamics causing cortical ischemia. Dehydration and a large contrast load seem to be aggravating factors. Most diabetics with peripheral vascular disease have significant occlusive disease in the distal popliteal artery or below the trifurcation; yet the aortoiliac and femoral vessels can be relatively disease free (Fig 18–6). In patients with unilateral leg ischemia and adequate femoral arterial inflow (determined by physical examination and noninvasive techniques), isolated angiography of the

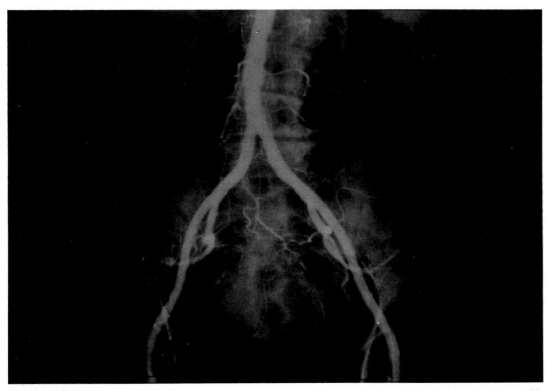

**FIG 18–6.**
Arteriogram in a diabetic patient with significant femoropopliteal occlusive disease but minimal aortic and iliac artery vascular disease.

symptomatic limb should be considered to decrease the contrast load. Adequate preangiography information to the radiologist regarding the presence or absence of a popliteal pulse, along with the noninvasive results, may avoid the excessive use of dye in an attempt to maximize visualization of the distal tibial and foot vessels. Close attention to postangiography urine output and serum creatinine levels for at least 4 days is important. Because of its potential complications, arteriography should be considered only in patients who are potential candidates for angioplasty, surgical revascularization, or both. The use of less nephrotoxic contrast agents, along with refinements in intra-arterial digital vascular imaging techniques, will reduce this complication.

The importance of visualizing the arterial anatomy of the foot and its direct correlation with patency of arterial bypass procedures has been described by O'Mara et al.[110] Similarly, Imparato et al.[69] also demonstrated the importance of visualizing the pedal arch and its relationship to graft patency. In their series of extended distal bypasses, 35 of 40 (87.5%) limbs with an intact primary or secondary arch demonstrated early graft patency, whereas only 2 of 16 limbs (12.5%) without a patent primary or secondary arch underwent successful revascularization.

Occasionally inadequate visualization of the subtrifurcation circulation by routine arteriography may lead to unnecessary amputation. If the Doppler examination suggests patent vessels in the distal leg, the use of preoperative or intraoperative downstream (antegrade) arteriography may enhance distal vessel visualization that could lead to a limb salvage procedure rather than amputation. The technique of intraoperative arteriography before the bypass as an antegrade injection with proximal inflow occlusion, as described by Flanigan et al.,[52] provides excellent visualization of the distal circulation in most patients.

Recent advances in computed radiology have opened new avenues in the field of arterial dye visualization. Digital vascular imaging (DVI) using an IV or intra-arterial bolus of contrast is an old concept[16, 128] that had to await the development of image-intensified television fluoroscopy systems that offer electronic subtraction. Venous injections were hoped to be an effective method of evaluating the arterial system.[118] However, they require relatively large contrast loads and produce poor-quality images. Digital imaging with intra-arterial injection requires only small volumes of contrast and produces high-quality images. Intra-arterial digital subtraction angiography is now state-of-the-art and is able to produce excellent angiograms even in the distal pedal circulation with a minimal amount of contrast.

## MANAGEMENT OF SYMPTOMATIC PERIPHERAL VASCULAR DISEASE

### Medical Management

Intermittent calf claudication is not a mandatory indication for operative intervention unless it becomes incapacitating. Boyd[19] in 1962 followed 1,440 patients with intermittent claudication and found an amputation rate of 7.2% at 5 years. Imparato et al.[68] followed 104 patients with intermittent claudication and found that 82 out of 104 (79%) improved or remained with stable claudication and only 6 of 104 (5.8%) required amputation at 2.5 years' follow-up. Therefore, claudication is not limb threatening and in most patients has a benign natural history. Diabetics, however, are a unique subset of patients with a prevalence of claudication four to six times higher than the nondiabetic population.[129] The natural history of claudication in diabetics appears less favorable in a study by Jonason and Ringqvist,[74] who noted the 6-year amputation rate in diabetic claudicants to be 12.8% vs. 0.5% in nondiabetics. McAllister[102] followed 100 consecutive claudicants for 1 to 18 years and noted progressive ischemia in 16 of the 87 nondiabetics (18%) and 6 of the 13 diabetics (46%), with an average follow-up of 6 years. Only one of the nondiabetics (1%) required amputation, whereas six of the diabetics (46%) underwent amputation during the study period. Thus, diabetics with moderate claudication and a history of significant disease progression in a short period of time should undergo prompt and aggressive evaluation and possible revascularization.[12]

Most patients with one or more block claudication or symptoms of mild coolness in the feet usually do not require reconstructive arterial surgery and are best treated by conservative means. Sometimes when claudication first appears, it is severe (less than one block) and is usually related to progression of stenosis to complete occlusion or to occlusion of an important collateral. These symptoms typically will improve with conservative therapy as collateral circulation increases. Recommendations for conservative therapy are as follows:

1. Discuss the entire vascular and foot condition with the patient, including advance notice that action must be taken if the symptoms should worsen.
2. Advise the patient to stop smoking.
3. Recommend leg exercises, especially walking, which can be useful in extending pain-free ambulation.
4. Emphasize the importance of foot care; the treatment of any mycotic infections, prevention of dryness and cracking of the feet, the wearing of comfortable shoes, good foot hygiene, and nail care.
5. Normalize the cholesterol and lipid levels to prevent progression of the disease.
6. Maintain diabetic control to help reduce neuropathy.
7. Consider pharmacologic therapy (see below).
8. Repeat vascular laboratory arterial studies in 6 months and every 12 months thereafter to better assess improvement, stabilization, or progression of disease.

## Pharmacologic Treatment

A variety of drugs have been used to treat symptomatic peripheral vascular disease including vasodilators, antiplatelet or anticoagulant drugs, hemorrheologic drugs, and metabolic agents. The rationale for pharmacologic intervention in lower limb ischemia is to increase oxygen delivery or improve utilization of oxygen in ischemic tissues.

The use of vasodilators in patients with lower limb ischemia has been advocated to improve blood flow by reducing vascular resistance. In patients with obstructive vascular disease, however, the main determinant of blood flow is the vascular stenosis not vascular tone. In addition, hypoxia has a potent vasodilator effect, and thus patients with lower limb ischemia are already maximally vasodilated.[144] Recent studies using the calcium channel blocker nifedipine as a vasodilator failed to improve walking ability in patients with claudication.[127] The calcium channel blockers produce vasodilatation by preventing the influx of calcium into smooth muscle cells. To date no vasodilator has been shown to be of benefit in patients with chronic lower limb ischemia.[33]

Antiplatelet agents, including aspirin, prostacyclin ($PGI_2$), ticlopidine, and thromboxane synthetase inhibitors, have been extensively studied because of the platelet's key role in arterial thrombosis and atherosclerosis. Aspirin, a cyclo-oxygenase inhibitor, when used in combination with dipyridamole, has been shown to reduce the risk of cardiac death in patients with atherosclerotic disease and reduce the incidence of combined stroke and transient ischemic attacks in patients with carotid artery stenosis.[30, 51] Importantly, aspirin and dipyridamole may prolong prosthetic graft patency in lower limb revascularization when started preoperatively,[31, 32] but aspirin with or without dipyridamole has not been shown to improve claudication.

Prostacyclin is a potent inhibitor of platelet aggregation and a vasodilator. It has been effective in relieving ischemic rest pain, healing ischemic ulcers, and improving claudication in some studies, but its use is limited by the requirement for IV administration, short duration of action, and side effects of nausea and hypotension.[11, 67, 93]

Ticlopidine, an inhibitor of adenosine diphosphate−induced platelet aggregation, has been evaluated in multicenter trials to demonstrate small improvements in ambulatory distance in patients with claudication.[4, 7] The modest improvement with ticlopidine in patients with claudication may be in part related to its anticoagulant effect and its ability to reduce blood viscosity and RBC deformability.[112] In summary, antiplatelet agents may slow the progression of atherosclerotic disease but do not seem to offer meaningful symptomatic improvement in claudication.

Anticoagulation may improve ambulatory walking distance in claudicants, as demonstrated by Dettori et al.[41] in a controlled study of 30 patients who demonstrated a 236% increase in pain-free walking over a 12-month period when treated with adenocumurol and pentoxifylline compared with a 149% increase in controls. Two (6.7%) major bleeding complications occurred, however, suggesting that the risk of anticoagulation does not justify its use in claudication.

Pentoxifylline, a hemorrheologic drug derived from methylxanthine, decreases erythrocyte membrane rigidity, plasma fibrinogen levels, blood viscosity, and platelet aggregation.[1, 120, 132] It enjoys distinction as being the only medication approved by the Food and Drug Administration in the United States for the treatment of ischemic claudication. Pentoxifylline has undergone extensive evaluation regarding its efficacy in the treatment of intermittent claudication.[81] Most investigations have concluded that it is moderately effective in increasing initial and absolute claudication distances as measured by the exercise treadmill test. In addition, patients with ischemic rest pain or paraesthesias may benefit from its use.[81] However, although pentoxifylline may improve ambulatory distance in claudication, the claudication does not usually resolve completely, and therefore the practical benefit its use confers is questionable. In addition, maximal therapeutic benefit requires several weeks of drug administration. The drug has approximately a 5% incidence of significant gastrointestinal side effects (nausea) that may require cessation of therapy.

Carnitine and naftidrofuryl are two agents that appear to increase the metabolic efficiency of ischemic muscle. Naftidrofuryl increases delivery of carbohydrate and fatty acids to muscle mitochondria, whereas carnitine is an important cofactor for skeletal muscle metabolism promoting pyruvate uptake into the Krebs cycle and transport of long-chain fatty acids into mitochondria, thus increasing the production of adenosine triphosphate and reducing the loss of pyruvate into the muscle.[20] Both agents have been shown to significantly increase ambulatory distances in patients with claudica-

tion.[21, 77] Neither drug is available for clinical use in the United States.

Perhaps one of the most effective nonoperative treatments for ischemic claudication is supervised treadmill exercise. Many studies have demonstrated an increase in treadmill exercise performance and a reduction in claudicatory symptoms with an exercise conditioning program.* In addition, there is essentially no morbidity or mortality from this supervised mode of treatment. A recent study[65] in controlled exercise conditioning at the University of Colorado demonstrated an increase in maximal walking time on a graded treadmill by 123% and in pain-free walking time by 165%. Peak systemic oxygen consumption improved by 30%, confirming that the exercise tolerance was increased. It appears that a dedicated supervised program of progressive walking exercise can improve exercise performance and reduce claudicatory pain in patients with lower limb ischemia.

## Interventional Radiology

Traditionally surgical therapy in the form of bypass or endarterectomy was the only treatment option available in severe lower limb ischemia. The last 30 years have witnessed an explosion in percutaneous radiographically monitored catheter techniques, collectively referred to as endovascular procedures, to treat vascular stenoses or, in some cases, occlusions. The most common of these catheter-based procedures is balloon dilatation angioplasty, a concept first introduced by Dotter and Judkins[45] in 1964 and later modified by Gruntzig and Hopff,[57] who brought it to its present level of technology. In addition to balloon angioplasty, a variety of other endovascular procedures are available, including laser angioplasty, mechanical atherectomy, and intravascular stents. Endovascular techniques are attractive because they are minimally invasive procedures well tolerated and well received by patients. However, there is an increasing amount of evidence that many endovascular treatments do not produce durable results in many pa-

*See references 34, 36, 37, 48, 49, 64, 86, 94, 95, 98, and 99.

tients with lower limb ischemia. Therefore, the indications for these new procedures are not well defined, and patients being treated with catheter-based interventions should be carefully selected and followed. The radiologist's role in the treatment of diabetic vascular disease is discussed further in Chapter 17.

## Surgical Management of Lower Limb Arterial Insufficiency in Diabetic Patients

Lower limb ischemia is classified according to the location of the arterial obstruction. Because ischemic symptoms can result from intra-abdominal vascular disease (aortic, common, or external iliac arteries) or vascular lesions in the thigh (common femoral artery or superficial femoral artery), the inguinal ligament serves as a useful landmark to stratify patients on initial examination. Patients with an obstructive intra-abdominal aortoiliac arterial pathologic condition (inflow disease) complain of

claudication that progresses proximally to involve the thigh and buttocks and have poor femoral pulses often associated with a thrill or bruit. Ischemic rest pain in patients with such proximal disease is relatively uncommon because of the extensive collateral network that develops.

Obstructive infrainguinal arterial lesions are further divided into femoral popliteal and more distal infrapopliteal (subtrifurcation) disease. These lesions typically produce calf claudication or, in more extensive cases, rest pain or tissue necrosis in the foot and have nonpalpable popliteal or pedal pulses. Combinations of abdominal inflow and an infrainguinal obstruction (multilevel disease) frequently occur and require careful investigation and judgment to determine if one or both levels of occlusive disease need to be corrected to alleviate ischemic symptoms.

Diabetics are unique in the propensity to develop severe infrainguinal disease with relative sparing of the aortoiliac inflow segment (Figs 18–6 and 18–7). The most se-

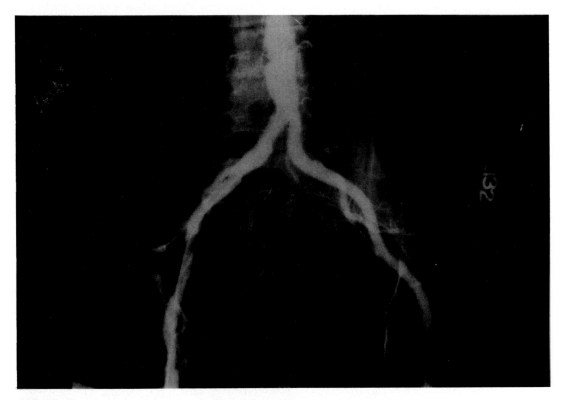

**FIG 18–7.**
Arteriogram in a diabetic patient shows moderate aortoiliac and right femoral artery vascular disease. Patient had marked distal disease.

verely affected vessels are often the subtrifurcation arteries: the anterior tibial,
posterior tibial, and peroneal vessels (Figs
18–8 and 18–9). The increased incidence of
distal lower limb vascular disease in diabetics is demonstrated by our experience at
Barnes Hospital in patients undergoing vascular reconstruction for various levels of arterial disease (Fig 18–10). Interestingly, no
significant difference of atherosclerotic renal
artery stenosis has been found between diabetics and nondiabetics.[100]

## AORTOILIAC OCCLUSIVE DISEASE

Although most diabetics do not have isolated aortoiliac occlusive disease, occasionally patients with occlusions below the inguinal ligament will have concomitant
aortoiliac obstructive disease (Fig 18–11).

**FIG 18–8.**
(Same patient as in Fig 18–7.) Arteriogram
demonstrates minimal popliteal vascular disease.

As mentioned, patients with aortoiliac occlusive disease usually do not have rest pain or
distal gangrene unless there are ulcerated
atherosclerotic plaques that embolize to the
foot or there are associated obstructive lesions in the femoropopliteal or infrapopliteal
arterial segments. Restoring adequate aortoiliac inflow usually relieves claudication
symptoms in both patients with isolated aortoiliac lesions and those with multilevel disease. However, in patients with multilevel
occlusive disease and distal tissue necrosis
or rest pain, a limb salvage rate of only 70%
to 85% should be expected with an inflow
procedure alone. Brewster et al.[22] reviewed
the results of aortofemoral reconstruction of
181 patients with multilevel occlusive disease. In their series, a limb salvage rate of
85% (80 of 94) was achieved in patients with
limb-threatening ischemia, but 29% of these
patients required both an inflow and in-

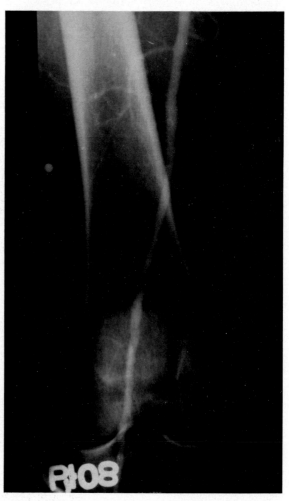

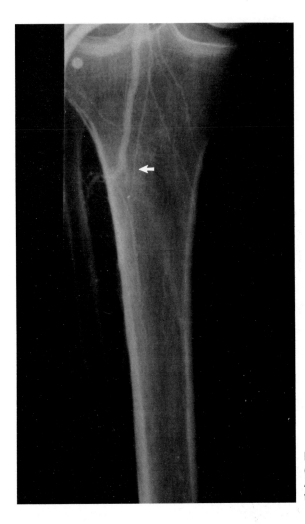

**FIG 18–9.**
(Same patient as in Figs 18–7 and 18–8.)
Arteriogram shows marked tibial and common
tibioperoneal trunk occlusive disease *(arrow)*.

frainguinal bypass to adequately revascularize the lower limbs. In patients with multilevel disease who were operated on for
claudication, both an inflow and infrainguinal bypass were required in 12 of 87
(10%) patients. More recently, Dalman et
al.[38] reported 62 patients undergoing simultaneous multilevel repair of lower limb occlusive disease. Tissue necrosis or rest pain
were present in 80%, and 48% were diabetic. The mortality rate (1.8%), morbidity
rate, and operative time in this group were
not significantly different from a nonran-
domized concurrent group of patients undergoing isolated inflow procedures. All patients with claudication were completely
relieved of symptoms, and the cumulative
limb salvage at 36 months of follow-up was
90.9%. Although numerous noninvasive
techniques have been described in an attempt to predict which patients will need a

distal bypass combined with inflow procedure, the reliability of these tests has not
been convincing.[17, 83, 107]

The options in surgical revascularization
in aortoiliac occlusive disease have remained
an area of controversy among vascular surgeons. Aortoiliac endarterectomy, bypass
grafting (aortoiliac or aortofemoral), and
extra-anatomic reconstructions (i.e., axillo-
femoral, femorofemoral) all have been reported to be effective. Most surgeons agree
that aortic reconstruction is best performed
with bypass grafts, although some cases
(i.e., localized aortoiliac disease, unilateral
iliac occlusive disease) can benefit from aortoiliac endarterectomy. The long-term success of unilateral iliofemoral endarterectomy
was emphasized in a report from van den
Dungen et al.,[143] who noted no deaths in 94
patients undergoing iliofemoral endarterectomy, with patency rates of 94%, 83%, and

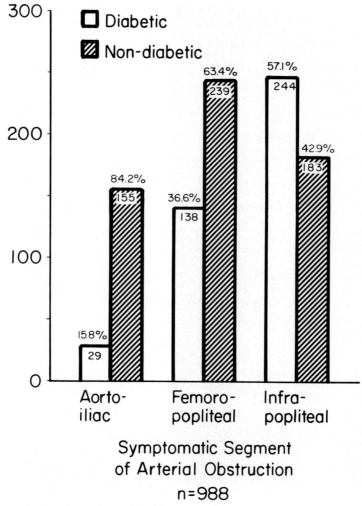

**FIG 18–10.**
Incidence of diabetes mellitus and the location of symptomatic arterial obstruction in 988 patients undergoing vascular reconstruction at Barnes Hospital, 1986–1991.

65% at 1 year, 5 years, and 10 years, respectively. In selected cases a familiarity with endarterectomy adds an important tool to the armamentarium of the vascular surgeon. A common technique of aortoiliac endarterectomy is depicted in Figure 18–12. An alternate novel technique of closed aortoiliac surgical endarterectomy using a "plaque cracker" instrument was originally described by LeVeen et al.[89] and is gaining popularity.[13, 149] It permits separation of the atherosclerotic plaque from the vessel wall without opening the vessel and subsequent extraction with a minimal number of arteriotomies (Fig 18–13). We have found this technique helpful, especially in unilateral iliac occlusive disease. Butcher and

Jaffe[27] reported their experience with aortoiliac endarterectomy in 94 patients from 1959 to 1970 at Barnes Hospital, St. Louis. The 5-year patency rate was 84% and 70% for nondiabetic and diabetic patients, respectively (Table 18–1).

The frequent presence of extensive disease involving both the aortoiliac and bilateral iliofemoral segments and the availability of durable and flexible synthetic grafts have made aortobifemoral grafting the procedure of choice for most patients with abdominal inflow arterial obstruction. Although some authors[111] prefer end-to-end aorta to graft proximal anastomosis, we have found the end-to-side graft to aorta anastomosis as effective. The most common techniques are

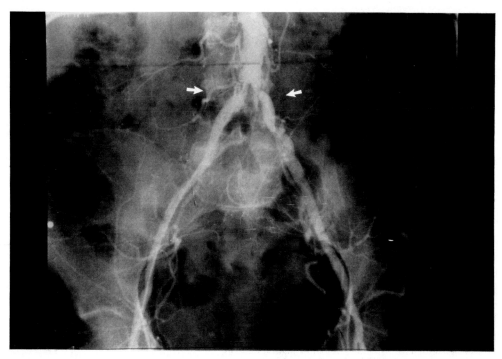

**FIG 18–11.**
Arteriogram in a diabetic patient with marked bilateral common iliac artery stenoses.

depicted in Figure 18–14. Most series indicate an early (30-day) graft patency rate of 95% to 99% and a 5-year patency from 74% to 88% (Table 18–2). Progression of atherosclerotic disease in the distal vessels accounts for the decrease in the 10-year patency rate to 62% to 77% in most series. Improvement in graft material, surgical techniques, and perioperative management have made this procedure successful and safe, with mortality rates less than 5% commonly reported.

The retroperitoneal approach to aortoiliac reconstruction may be better tolerated than the classic transperitoneal route by patients operated on for both aortoiliac occlusive and aneurysmal disease. A recent retrospective study reported by our group evaluating methods of aortoiliac reconstruction demonstrated a significant decrease in postoperative ileus, as well as hospitalization days, in patients operated on by the retroperitoneal approach when compared with the transabdominal approach.[125] A prospec-

**TABLE 18–1.**
Aortoiliac Endarterectomy (Barnes Hospital, 1959–1970)*

|  | No. of Patients | 5-yr Patency (%) | p Value |
|---|---|---|---|
| Diabetes |  |  |  |
|     Nondiabetic | 84 | 84 | NS |
|     Diabetic | 16 | 70 |  |
| Degree of ischemia |  |  |  |
|     Claudication alone | 73 | 83 | < 0.02 |
|     Rest pain, ulcer, gangrene | 26 | 70 |  |
| Femoral pulse |  |  |  |
|     Palpable | 53 | 92 | < 0.02 |
|     Absent | 108 | 78 |  |

*From Butcher H, Jaffe B: Ann Surg 173:925, 1971. Used by permission.

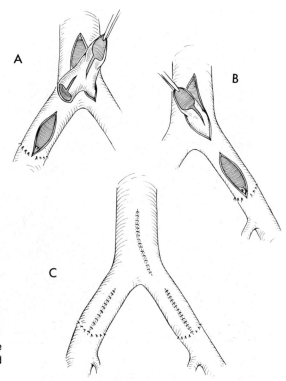

**FIG 18–12.**
Technique of aortoiliac endarterectomy. Note the importance of suturing down distal intima to avoid elevation of flap and thrombosis.

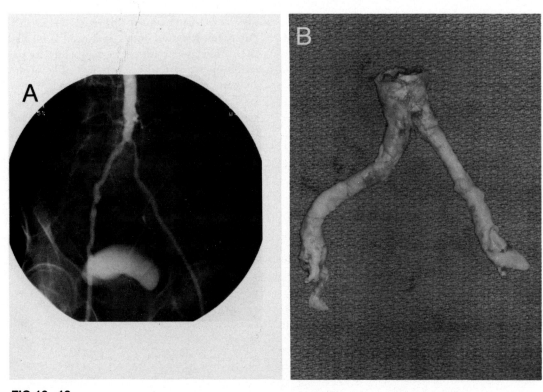

**FIG 18–13.**
Aortoiliac angiogram **(A)** and atherosclerotic plaque **(B)** in patient undergoing a bilateral aortoiliac endarterectomy using the "plaque cracker" technique.

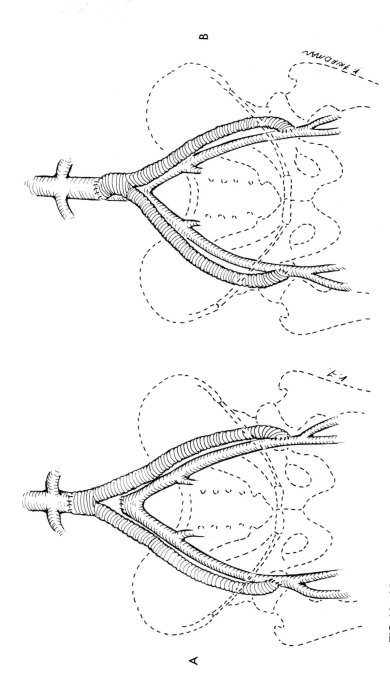

**FIG 18–14.**
Technique commonly used for aortofemoral bypass. **A,** end-to-end graft to aortic anastomosis. **B,** end-to-side graft-to-aortic anastomosis.

tive randomized comparison of these two approaches was subsequently done by Cambria et al.[28] and did not demonstrate significant differences between the two techniques. However, the retroperitoneal exposure is clearly advantageous in some patients (i.e., previous abdominal surgery, obesity, and cases requiring left renal artery reconstruction) and should be considered in selected patients. Our experience with these two approaches using endarterectomy or bypass in occlusive aortoiliac disease is shown in Table 18–3.

Some patients have aortoiliac disease that is not amenable to direct reconstruction. Such patients include those with cardiac disease that would not tolerate intraoperative aortic occlusion or those with previously failed aortic reconstruction. Lower limb revascularization in these cases can usually be achieved with an extra-anatomic bypass, a prosthetic bypass between a donor and recipient artery that is tunneled through a nonanatomic route. An example is a bypass from the axillary artery (donor vessel) to the femoral artery (recipient vessel) tunneled through the subcutaneous tissues along the lateral chest and abdominal wall to unilaterally revascularize the leg in a patient with an obstructed iliac artery. In the past this technique has had poor patency rates when used unilaterally compared with other forms of aortoiliac reconstruction. Recently better results have been noted when this type of bypass has been used for bilateral lower limb revascularization (axillobifemoral bypass). The addition of reenforcing plastic rings to these grafts prevents external compression in their subcutaneous location and has been another favorable modification. Harris et al.[62] noted a life table primary patency of 85% in 76 axillobifemoral bypass grafts performed with externally supported grafts and followed for an average of 28 months. Currently this technique is best suited for patients who are high operative risks for aortic cross-clamping or have aortoiliac disease not amenable to direct reconstruction.

## FEMORAL POPLITEAL OCCLUSIVE DISEASE

Arterial occlusive lesions in the femoropopliteal region can compromise the distal circulation of the lower limb, resulting in claudication, rest pain, tissue necrosis, or

**TABLE 18–2.**
Aortofemoral Graft Patency Rates

| Authors | No. of Patients | Patency | | Operative Mortality (%) |
|---|---|---|---|---|
| | | 5 Years | 10 Years | |
| Duncan et al.[46] | 87 | 74 | — | 2.3 |
| Malone et al.[97] | 180 | 82 | 66 | 2.5 |
| Brewster and Darling[22] | 406 | 88 | 74 | 1.1 |
| Nevelsteen et al.[108] | 352 | 80 | 62 | 5.1 |
| King et al.[80] | 79 | 79 | — | 4.8 |
| Szilagyi et al.[133] | 1,647 | 77 | 77 | 5.0 |

**TABLE 18–3.**
Elective Repair Aortoiliac Occlusive Disease (Barnes Hospital, 1985–1991)

| Procedure | Retroperitoneal | | Transperitoneal | | Total | |
|---|---|---|---|---|---|---|
| | n | % | n | % | n | % |
| Aortoiliac bypass | 20 | | 27 | | 47 | |
| Aortobifemoral bypass | 62 | | 72 | | 134 | |
| Endarterectomy | 7 | | 14 | | 21 | |
| Total | 89 | 44 | 113 | 56 | 202 | |
| Mortality | 1 | 1.1 | 2 | 1.8 | 3 | 1.5 |

combination thereof. Because mild claudication is associated with a low incidence of amputation as described by Boyd[19] and Imparato et al.,[68] most surgeons agree that the only absolute indications for femoral popliteal reconstruction should be disabling claudication or limb-threatening ischemia (rest pain, ischemic ulceration, and gangrene). Most series involving femoropopliteal reconstruction report an incidence of diabetes that ranges between 15% and 40% (see Fig 18–10). Unfortunately, most diabetics with arterial disease of the lower limb will have not only femoropopliteal lesions but concomitant trifurcation disease, which complicates revascularization procedures.

In patients with simple occlusion of the superficial femoral artery, the procedure of choice is a bypass from the common femoral artery to the popliteal artery (Fig 18–15). The distal anastomosis can be performed to the above-knee or below-knee segment of the popliteal artery, depending on which portion of the vessel is most suitable. An important consideration in femoropopliteal reconstruction is the type of vascular graft used in the bypass. All surgeons agree that the best graft material is autogenous saphenous vein. However, a number of patients will have had the vein used in a previous revascularization (e.g., coronary artery bypass), or less frequently it is inadequate for use as an arterial conduit. A variety of synthetic grafts are available in the absence of saphe-

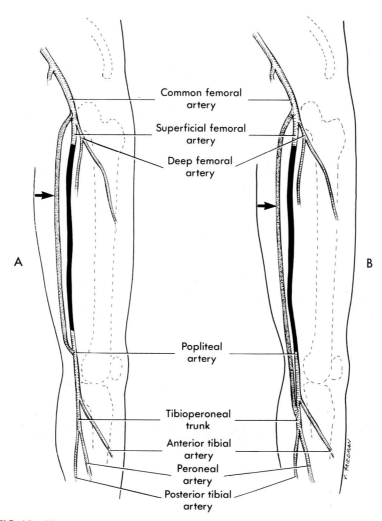

**FIG 18–15.**
Technique of above-knee **A,** and below-knee **B,** femoropopliteal bypass *(arrows).*

nous vein, but most vascular surgeons have used a graft constructed of polytetrafluoroethylene (PTFE) or less often a glutaraldehyde-tanned umbilical vein wrapped with a supporting Dacron mesh. We have preferred PTFE in this instance because of its attractive handling characteristics and performance.

The saphenous vein can be harvested for use as a "reversed" saphenous vein graft similar to the technique used in coronary artery bypass, or it can be prepared for use in situ by dividing the venous valves with an intraluminal valvulotome to permit proximal to distal flow and ligating the venous tributaries to prevent arteriovenous fistula formation. The proximal and distal ends of the vein are then anastomosed to the donor and recipient artery, respectively. Both of these techniques yield 5-year secondary patency rates (includes graft revisions) of 75% to 80% (Table 18–4). Many surgeons prefer the in situ method because of the better size match between the proximal and distal portions of the vein to the femoral and popliteal arteries.

When autologous vein is not available, a synthetic graft bypass to the popliteal artery is an acceptable alternative. Table 18–5 contains the primary patency rates for recent series of femoral popliteal bypass using PTFE to the above-knee or below-knee popliteal artery. The best patency rates are generally found when bypasses can be performed to the above-knee popliteal artery and in patients operated on for claudication. These patients typically have less severe vascular disease than patients with limb-threatening ischemia and therefore have better graft patency. The influence of disease distal to the popliteal artery (runoff) on patency was demonstrated by Prendiville et al.,[113] who noted in a series of 59 above-knee PTFE grafts with two or three patent runoff vessels from the popliteal artery a 4-year patency rate of 70% compared with 28% in grafts with poor runoff. Both cigarette smoking and diabetes adversely affected prosthetic graft patency. In contrast, Szilagyi et al.[134] found no difference in cumulative patency rates at 5 and 10 years between the diabetics and nondiabetics who underwent femoropopliteal and femoroinfrapopliteal bypass grafts. Similarly, Bergan et al.[14] could not demonstrate any difference in patency for all femoropopliteal grafts in

**TABLE 18–4.**

Recent Reports Containing 5-Year Patency for Infrainguinal Autogenous Vein Bypass*

| Study | Characteristics of Vein | No. of Cases | Distal Anastomosis† | Patency | | Bypass Done Because of Claudication (%) |
|---|---|---|---|---|---|---|
| | | | | Primary | Secondary | |
| Taylor et al.[137] | Reversed saphenous or alternative vein | 76 | AK popliteal | 76 | 76 | 20 |
| | | 199 | BK popliteal | 80 | 86 | |
| | | 241 | Infrapopliteal | 69 | 77 | |
| Leather et al.[87] | In situ | 304 | BK popliteal | 59 | 76 | 3 |
| | | 608 | Infrapopliteal | | | |
| Hobson et al.[66] | Reversed saphenous | 75 | BK popliteal | 74 | — | <14 |
| | | 50 | Infrapopliteal | 42 | — | |
| Berkowitz and Greenstein[15] | Reversed saphenous | 102 | Infrapopliteal | 47 | 70 | 14 |
| Kent et al.[79] | Reversed 80% In situ 20% | 87 | AK popliteal | 78 | — | 100 |
| | | 80 | BK popliteal | | | |
| Veith et al.[145] | Reversed saphenous | 98 | AK popliteal | 68 | — | 18 |
| | | 49 | BK popliteal | | | |
| Barnes et al.[10] | In situ 74%; nonreversed translocated 15%; reversed 11% | 150 | AK popliteal BK popliteal Infrapopliteal | 66 | — | 31‡ |

*From Curr Probl Surg 1991; 28:132.
†AK = above-knee; BK = below-knee.
‡Percent from series including 52 polytetrafluoroethylene grafts.

## TABLE 18–5.

Recent Reports Containing 5-Year Patency for Infrainguinal Polytetrafluoroethylene Bypass*

| Study | No. of Cases | Distal Anastomosis† | Primary Patency | Bypass Done Because of Claudication (%) |
|---|---|---|---|---|
| Prendiville et al.[113] | 114 | AK popliteal | 42 | 39 |
| Quinones-Baldrich et al.[115] | 101 | AK popliteal | 63 | 42 |
| | 45 | BK popliteal | 44 | |
| McAuley et al.[103] | 90 | AK popliteal | 40 | 30 |
| | 37 | BK popliteal | | |
| Sterpetti et al.[131] | 90 | AK popliteal | 58 | 46 |
| Ascer et al.[5] | 228 | AK popliteal | 55 | Limb salvage cases |
| | 199 | BK popliteal | | |
| Hobson et al.[66] | 80 | BK popliteal | 22 | <14 |
| | 41 | Infrapopliteal | 12 | |
| Kent et al.[79] | 63 | AK popliteal | 52 | 100 |
| | 19 | BK popliteal | | |
| Veith et al.[145] | 118 | AK popliteal | 38 | 11 |
| | 53 | BK popliteal | | |
| Barnes et al.[10] | 52 | AK popliteal | 46 | 31‡ |
| | | BK popliteal | | |
| | | Infrapopliteal | | |

*From Curr Probl Surg 1991; 28:135.
†AK = above-knee; BK = below-knee.
‡Percent from series also including 150 vein grafts.

diabetics compared with nondiabetics at 12 and 24 months, respectively. Cutler et al.[35] reported a 5-year patency rate of 70% in patients with diabetes mellitus compared with 75% in patients without diabetes mellitus.

An important consideration in selecting an autologous vein graft or synthetic graft for a femoral popliteal bypass is the patient's general health and the estimated chance that progressive vascular disease distal to the bypass will require further reconstruction in the future. Bergan et al.[14] demonstrated in a randomized prospective study that the patency rate at 2½ years was not significantly different between saphenous vein or PTFE grafts to the popliteal artery. Saphenous vein graft bypasses (reversed or in situ) generally require larger incisions and longer anesthesia times that may not be well tolerated by medically fragile patients. Therefore, a PTFE graft may be preferred over a saphenous vein graft in elderly patients with a limited life expectancy (<2 years) who have a popliteal artery with good runoff.

Catheter based procedures have not been very helpful in managing arterial lesions in the femoral popliteal segment. Jeans et al.[73] recently reported a 7-year prospective study of 370 patients undergoing 500 percutaneous transluminal angioplasties. The 5-year cumulative patency rate in patients with femoropopliteal lesions was 41%. As was found in the surgical treatment of this problem, the 3-year patency rate in patients with two- or three-vessel runoff was better (78%) than in those patients with one-vessel runoff (25%). The potential for improved results with the addition of laser-assisted balloon angioplasty has been much publicized. A 3-year prospective trial of 28 patients (27 with advanced disease) undergoing laser thermal-assisted angioplasty was recently reported by White et al.[147] They noted successful recanalization in 18 patients (67%). However, the cumulative patency for successful procedures by life table analysis was 55.5%, 38.8%, and 11.1% at 3, 6, and 12 months, respectively. Hence, laser-assisted angioplasty at the present level of development seems to be of limited use in patients with severe femoropopliteal disease. In general the addition of a laser energy to balloon angioplasty in the treatment of femoropopliteal lesions does not improve the results of balloon angioplasty alone and is associated with an increased complication rate.

We recommend an aggressive surgical approach to diabetic patients, especially those with significant lower limb vascular insufficiency with less than one block calf claudication. When obstructive lesions in the superficial femoral artery are found in a diabetic with *progressive* symptoms and an ankle-arm index by Doppler pressures of less than 0.30, revascularization (bypass or, rarely, angioplasty; see Chapter 17) should be considered based on the arteriographic findings. Although saphenous vein remains the conduit of choice for femoropopliteal bypass, PTFE grafts can provide an adequate alternative, especially at the above-knee level when autologous vein is not available.

## INFRAPOPLITEAL VASCULAR OCCLUSIVE DISEASE

The incidence of infrapopliteal vascular occlusive disease in the diabetic patient is higher than in the nondiabetic population and is the most important vascular factor in the propensity for diabetic patients to develop ischemic symptoms in the foot. The peroneal artery appears most susceptible to diabetic vascular disease as noted in a series by Dardik et al.,[39] in which diabetes mellitus occurred in 88% of the patients undergoing peroneal artery bypass and 66% of the patients requiring tibial artery bypass. Other studies have reported the incidence of diabetes mellitus in patients with infrapopliteal vascular disease to range from 47% to 88% (see Fig 18–10).[6] Occlusive vascular disease in the smaller muscular arteries of the leg in diabetic patients frequently requires an arterial bypass from the femoral artery in the groin to the tibial, peroneal, or dorsalis pedis arteries of the lower limb or foot for limb salvage. Preoperative angiography often with digital subtraction techniques is critical to determine which of these distal vessels are patent and in communication with the plantar arcades. The size of the vessel, amount of disease, and the runoff into the foot usually determines the site of the distal anastomosis. Saphenous vein bypass using the in situ technique currently is the most common method of revascularization in infrapopliteal disease. This technique

minimizes trauma and warm ischemia to the vein graft. In addition, the vasa vasorum that supply nutrients to the vessel are preserved over the majority of the vein's length. Meticulous technique, including careful dissection of the vessel, preservation of tributaries, and the use of magnifying loops to assure a properly constructed anastomosis, is important in the success of these distal procedures. The propensity for diabetic vessels to develop medial calcification can make these procedures especially challenging. Most vascular surgeons advise an intraoperative completion arteriogram to ascertain the lack of technical errors, the absence of clot formation at the distal anastomosis, and the integrity of the distal vessels communicating with the plantar arterial arch.

A common misconception is that the results of distal vascular reconstruction are worse in diabetics than nondiabetics. It is important to emphasize that distal vascular reconstruction is at least as successful if not more successful in the diabetic population when compared with nondiabetics. The findings of Rosenblatt et al.[119] support this observation (Fig 18–16). They noted in diabetics undergoing distal arterial reconstruction a cumulative 1- and 4-year patency rate of 95% and 89%, respectively, whereas the rates in nondiabetics were 85% and 80%, respectively. The 1-year patency rate in diabetic vs. nondiabetic patients undergoing revascularization for threatened limb loss approached statistical significance ($P = 0.056$) in favor of diabetics. Therefore, distal vascular reconstruction should not be categorically withheld from diabetic patients because of anticipated poor results.

An important element in the long-term success of infrapopliteal bypass is the availability and quality of an autogenous vein graft. The patency rates for PTFE placed to the infrapopliteal vessels has been disappointing—approximately 40% at 1 year and 10% at 5 years. Bergan et al.[14] reported a 2-year patency rate of 77% for infrapopliteal autogenous vein bypass grafts, and 34% when PTFE grafts were used. Similarly, Ricco et al.[117] demonstrated a 20% 2-year patency rate in PTFE grafts compared with a 62% 2-year patency rate for

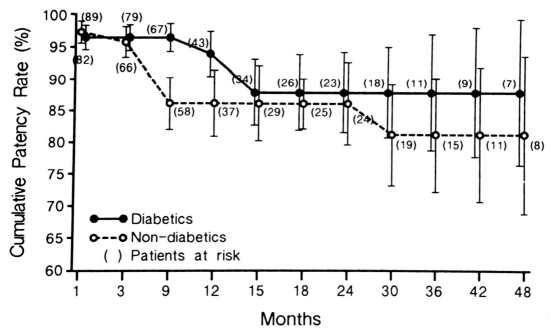

**FIG 18–16.**
Forty-eight-month cumulative patency in diabetics and nondiabetics undergoing distal arterial reconstruction. *(From Rosenblatt MS, Quist WC, Sidawy AN, et al: Surg Gynecol Obstet 171:331–335, 1990. Used by permission.*

autogenous grafts when used in the infrapopliteal position.[53] Flinn et al.[53] have noted modest improvement in infrapopliteal prosthetic graft patency through the use of long-term anticoagulation. The 2- and 4-year cumulative patency rate was 45% and 37%, respectively, in a series of 75 infrapopliteal PTFE grafts maintained initially on heparin and then long-term warfarin. A slight increase in bleeding complications (17%) was noted.

The lesser saphenous vein or arm veins are important alternate sources of autologous vein grafts when the ipsilateral or contralateral greater saphenous vein is unavailable. Although the harvesting of these grafts requires multiple incisions and frequently short segments of vein must be anastomosed to achieve adequate lengths, the long-term patency is clearly better than prosthetic material when one is bypassing to the infrapopliteal arteries, as demonstrated by Harris et al.[63] They reported patency rates at 1, 3, and 5 years in 67 patients undergoing 70 cephalic vein bypasses of 85%, 72%, and 68%, respectively. Overall limb salvage was 85% at 5 years in these patients, 90% of

whom required construction of the distal anastomosis at the infrapopliteal level.

Although most reports dealing with infrapopliteal bypass grafts describe the common femoral artery as the donor site for the inflow, various reports have documented the suitability of the popliteal artery as an adequate inflow site in those patients without significant superficial femoral artery disease, as commonly found in diabetics.[50] In diabetic patients with good inflow to the popliteal artery, a popliteal to distal bypass allows the use of a shorter saphenous vein or other autologous vein and can be extended to pedal arteries with good results.[25, 26] In a series reported by Schuler et al.,[121] 23 out of 29 (79%) patients with popliteal to infrapopliteal bypass for limb salvage were diabetics. He reported an 84% graft patency rate at 31 months. The limb salvage rate in this study was lower (70% vs. 84%) than the cumulative graft patency rate, which differs from the reports of DeWeese and Rob[42] and, more recently, Bergan et al.,[14] which demonstrate that limb salvage exceeds long-term graft patency by as much as 20%.

The fact that the rate of limb salvage is

typically higher than patency rate after lower limb vascular bypass is an important concept to emphasize. Many diabetic patients have marginal perfusion in an otherwise normal-appearing foot. Minor trauma can damage the skin and lead to nonhealing ulcers or infection because of the minimal blood supply. These injuries may progress and ultimately destroy the foot, resulting in an amputation. Revascularization of the leg can promote healing of the ulcer and restore foot viability. Once the ulcer is healed, graft thrombosis most frequently causes the limb to revert to its pre-bypass level of marginal but adequate perfusion; hence, limb salvage is greater than graft patency.

Although the limb salvage rate seems to be higher for the femorotibial than the femoral peroneal bypass graft, the results with a peroneal bypass in the presence of a patent pedal arch are acceptable. Furthermore, the use of the in situ technique has provided excellent results for peroneal artery bypass.[76] Dardik et al.[39] demonstrated a cumulative patency rate of 50% at 12 months in diabetics who underwent femoral peroneal bypass graft. In this report the cumulative limb salvage rate of 79% at 30 months for the peroneal groups makes this reconstruction worthwhile, especially in selected cases with a patent pedal arch (Fig 18–17). Occasionally there is not a suitable artery to bypass to above the ankle, but a dorsalis pedis artery, posterior tibial artery, or plantar artery reconstitutes in the foot. In other cases, none of the distal vessels is seen at angiography but a Doppler signal is audible in the dorsalis pedis or posterior tibial areas. In this group of patients, if amputation is inevitable, an exploration of the pedal vessels is indicated and can lead to successful revascularization (Fig 18–18). Auer et al.[6] demon-

**FIG 18–17.**
Intraoperative arteriogram of a femoroperoneal in situ saphenous vein bypass in a diabetic patient. Note posterior perforating branch from peroneal artery filling posterior tibial artery and plantar arch.

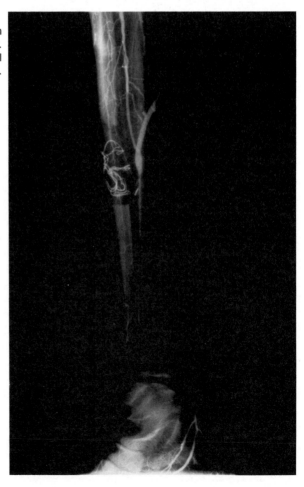

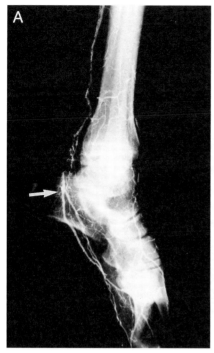
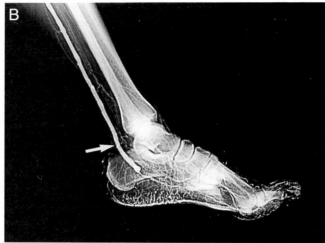

**FIG 18–18.**
**A,** preoperative arteriogram in a diabetic patient with gangrene of the fourth and fifth toes shows no suitable recipient vessel for distal bypass above ankle. Plantar arteries *(arrow)* reconstitute in foot and are minimally diseased. **B,** intraoperative angiogram demonstrates revascularization of common plantar artery with a saphenous vein graft *(arrow)* originating from the popliteal artery.

strated a 62% 5-year patency in dorsalis pedis bypass grafts in 29 patients. Common procedures done to the infrapopliteal and pedal vessels are shown in Figure 18–19. Routine use of intraoperative post-bypass arteriography, especially in distal tibial, peroneal bypass, or pedal, provides information regarding the presence or absence of technical errors (Fig 18–20) or thrombi (Fig 18–21) and a better visualization of the vasculature distal to the bypass.

## LIMB SALVAGE WITH TISSUE TRANSFER

The application of tissue transfer procedures to diabetic foot ulcers has enhanced our ability to avoid amputation in patients with extensive tissue loss. This technique is frequently performed by vascular and plastic surgeons working together. Healthy muscle with or without overlying skin is harvested from distant sites (latissimus dorsi, serratus anterior, rectus abdominous, or forearm muscle flaps based on the radial artery) with preservation of the artery and vein supplying the tissue. The flap is placed in the wound and locally revascularized, often from a femoropedal vessel saphenous vein graft (Fig 18–22). Limb salvage rates of 75% to 80%, as well as ambulation in the majority of patients, can be expected.[29, 56]

### Lumbar Sympathectomy

The benefit of lumbar sympathectomy in the treatment of occlusive arterial disease remains controversial.[88, 135] In diabetic patients, the benefit of this procedure is more disputed because of the common occurrence of autosympathectomy as a result of the associated neuropathy.[82, 114] Our opinion is that sympathectomy in the diabetic patient is of little benefit and its use is not warranted.

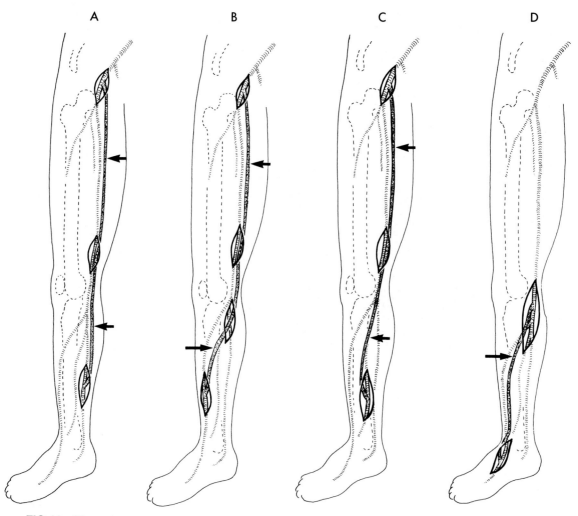

**FIG 18–19.**
Technique for femoral posterior tibial bypass **(A)**, femoral anterior tibial bypass **(B)** *(arrows)*, femoral peroneal bypass **(C)**, and popliteal to dorsalis pedis bypass *(arrows)*.

## Postoperative Follow-up

Atherosclerotic vascular disease is a progressive systemic condition, especially in patients with associated risk factors (e.g., diabetes, smoking, hypertension, hyperlipidemia). The most common causes of postoperative or long-term death in the patient with reconstructive vascular surgery are myocardial infarction and stroke. Moreover, patients with reconstructive vascular surgery tend to develop progression of vascular disease in the bypass graft or the distal arteries. Cessation of smoking, tight control of hypertension and hyperglycemia, and weight control are impor-

tant components of the follow-up in diabetics with reconstructive vascular procedures. Furthermore, frequent (every 6–12 months) evaluation in the noninvasive vascular laboratory may detect stenosis in the vascular graft or progression of disease distal to the graft. Early detection of a stenosis in the bypass graft (Fig 18–23) or distal to the graft may allow for salvage of the conduit prior to thrombosis by either percutaneous angioplasty or reoperation.

Occasionally acute occlusion of chronically implanted grafts will result in recurrence of pre-bypass symptoms or more severe limb ischemia. Limb-threatening isch-

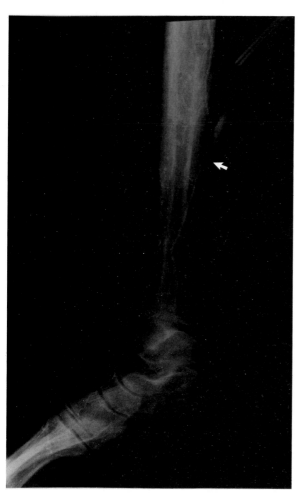

**FIG 18–20.**
Intraoperative arteriogram of a femoral posterior tibial bypass in a diabetic patient. Note obstruction in anastomotic area *(arrow)* secondary to thrombus, which required postangiography embolectomy.

emia should be evaluated by angiography to define the anatomy and assess progression of disease since the revascularization procedure. Further options in reconstruction will depend on the arteriographic findings.

Thrombolytic therapy has gained popularity in the nonoperative management of thrombosed vascular grafts or thrombosis proximal to a stenosis in a native vessel. Although systemic heparinization can be of help in acute arterial thrombosis, it will benefit only those patients with adequate collateral flow distal to the acute occlusion.[40, 60] Most radiologists and vascular surgeons agree that systemic thrombolytic therapy administered intravenously for graft thrombolysis is contraindicated because of the significant hemorrhagic complications associated with a systemic lytic

state. The best method of thrombolytic therapy for arterial or graft thrombosis is that of low-dose local therapy administered directly into the thrombus, because it is associated with fewer systemic complications.[142] The basic technique requires percutaneous placement of an intra-arterial catheter directly into the clot or just proximal to it. Patients are started on a thrombolytic agent (urokinase, streptokinase or tissue plasminogen activator) regimen administered through the catheter into the thrombus. Preinfusion and coagulation studies every 4 hours are performed to avoid systemic thrombolysis. Distal perfusion and potential bleeding sites are monitored carefully, and progress is monitored angiographically every 4 to 12 hours. If ischemic symptoms progress or bleeding complications occur, the thrombolytic agent

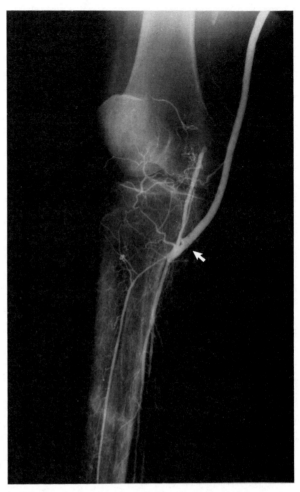

**FIG 18–21.**
Intraoperative arteriogram after thrombectomy of
PTFE femoropopliteal bypass. Note irregularity in
distal PTFE graft *(arrow)* secondary to intimal
hyperplasia. This was resolved by endarterectomy
and patch angioplasty.

is discontinued and surgical thrombectomy
performed. A favorable experience with
thrombolytic salvage of 30 thrombosed
lower limb vascular grafts was reported
recently by Seabrook et al.[122] Patency was
initially restored to all bypasses. However,
adjunctive surgical thrombectomy was
necessary to remove persistent thrombus
after thrombolytic infusion in six cases.
Underlying morphologic defects (intimal
hyperplasia) were noted in 15 grafts—7
connected with balloon angioplasty and
8 with surgery. Five (33%) significant
hemorrhagic complications occurred, one
of which resulted in a lethal myocardial
infarction. Thrombolytic therapy is an important consideration in the initial management of acute vascular graft thrombosis. Caution must be exercised, however,
in choosing thrombolytic treatment, which

often takes several hours or days to complete. Thrombolysis should be avoided in
favor of surgical thrombectomy in critically
ischemic limbs that are immediately threatened.

## UPPER LIMB COMPLICATIONS IN DIABETICS

Occlusive arterial lesions of the upper
limb are much less common than in the
lower limb and may be associated with thoracic outlet syndrome or collagen vascular
disorders. It has been estimated that two
thirds of patients with localized finger gangrene have large artery proximal obstruction, and the remaining one third have systemic diseases associated with diffuse

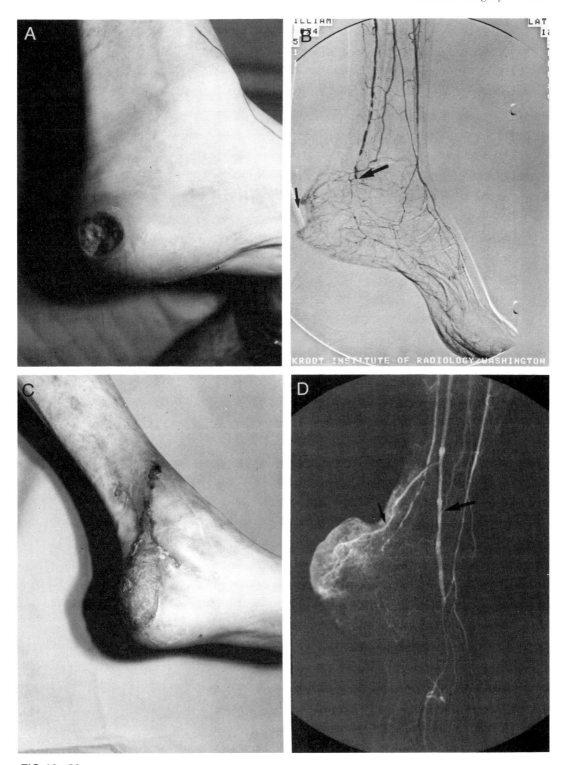

**FIG 18–22.**
**A,** chronic left heel ulcer in diabetic patient at prolonged bed rest because of hip fracture. **B,** preoperative angiogram demonstrates poor perfusion to ulcer *(small arrow)* secondary to occlusion of posterior tibial artery *(large arrow).* **C,** ulcer healed 6 weeks after serratus anterior muscle free flap and skin graft revascularized from popliteal to dorsalis pedis reversed saphenous vein bypass. **D,** postoperative angiogram demonstrates revascularization of free flap. Popliteal to dorsalis pedis reversed saphenous vein graft *(large arrow).* Artery to free flap *(small arrow).*

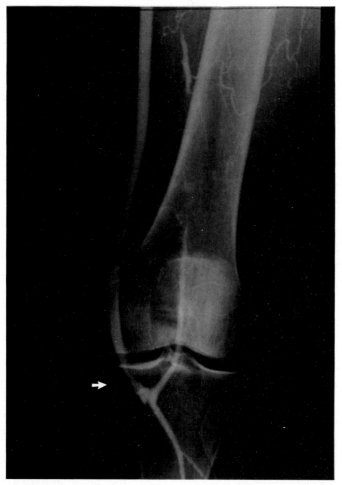

**FIG 18–23.**
Femoral arteriogram obtained 20 months after a PTFE femoropopliteal bypass. Note marked stenosis in distal graft *(arrow).* Arterial noninvasive studies demonstrated a diminished ankle-arm index, which suggested a stenosis despite a patent graft. Patient underwent successful endarterectomy and patch angioplasty.

occlusions of palmar and digital arteries.[136] In the latter group, collagen vascular disorders such as hypersensitivity angiitis, scleroderma and systemic lupus erythematosus are the main causative factor.

Diabetes mellitus, although not commonly associated with upper limb gangrene, can occasionally lead to severe finger ischemia, especially in the dialysis or postrenal transplant patient. The decreased blood flow to the digits secondary to vascular access procedures, along with the digital arterial occlusive disease and the common practice of glucose monitoring with blood obtained from

finger sticks, makes the uremic patient at risk for hand ischemia and gangrene (Fig 18–24). These factors are responsible for the increased incidence of upper or lower limb loss. In the series reported by Mitchell[106] of 16 diabetic patients with successful renal allografts, 8 (50%) required one or more amputations, and 4 had amputations of two or more limbs, including the upper limb. Careful selection of vascular access sites, good hand care, and intentional interruption of the vascular access after successful allograft may decrease this complication.

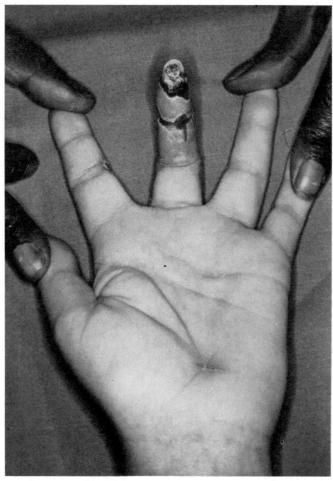

**FIG 18–24.**
Gangrene in the middle finger in a diabetic patient receiving corticosteroid therapy after renal transplant.

# REFERENCES

1. Ambrus JL, Ambrus CM, Taheri SA, et al: Red cell flexibility and platelet aggregation in patients with chronic obstructive vascular disease (CAOD) and study of therapeutic approaches, *Angiology* 35:418–426, 1984.

2. American Diabetes Association: *Diabetes facts*, 1991, American Diabetes Association.

3. Ansell G, Tweedie MCK, West CR, et al: The current status of reactions to intravenous contrast media, *Invest Radiol* 15(suppl 6):532, 1980.

4. Arian JC, Blancharg J, Boissel JP, et al: Multicenter double-blind trial of ticlopidine in the treatment of intermittent claudication and the prevention of its complications, *Angiology* 39:802–811, 1988.

5. Ascer E, Veith FJ, Gupta SK, et al: Six year experience with expanded polytetrafluoroethylene arterial grafts for limb salvage, *J Cardiovasc Surg* 26:468–472, 1985.

6. Auer AJ, Hurley JJ, Binnington HB, et al: Distal tibial vein grafts for limb salvage, *Arch Surg* 118:597, 1983.

7. Balsano F, Coicheri S, Libretti A, et al: Ticlopidine in the treatment of intermittent claudication: a 21 month double-blind trial, *J Lab Clin Med* 114:84–91, 1989.

8. Barner HB, Kaiser GC, Willman VL: Blood flow in the diabetic leg, *Circulation* 43:391–394, 1971.

9. Barnes RW, Shanik GD, Slaymaker EE: An index of healing in below-knee amputation: leg blood pressure by Doppler ultrasound, *Surgery* 79:13, 1976.

10. Barnes RW, Thompson BW, MacDonald CM, et al: Serial noninvasive studies do not herald postoperative failure of femoropopliteal or femorotibial bypass grafts, *Ann Surg* 210:486–494, 1989.

11. Belch JJP, Drury JK, Capell H, et al: Intermittent epoprostenol (prostacyclin) infusion in pa-

tients with Raynaud's syndrome: a double-blind controlled trial, *Lancet* 1:313–315, 1983.

12. Bendick PJ, Glover JL, Kuebler TW, et al: Progression of atherosclerosis in diabetics, *Surgery* 93:834, 1983.

13. Bengoechea E, Cuesta MA, Doblas M: Extensive endarterectomy of the aorta, common and external iliac arteries and common femoral arteries by a modified LeVeen method, *Surgery* 99:537, 1986.

14. Bergan JJ, Veith FJ, Banhard VM, et al: Randomization of autogenous vein and polytetrafluoroethylene grafts in femoral-distal reconstruction, *Surgery* 92:921, 1982.

15. Berkowitz HD, Greenstein SM: Improved patency in reversed femoral-infrapopliteal autogenous vein grafts by early detection and treatment of the failing graft, *J Vasc Surg* 5:755–761, 1987.

16. Bernstein EF, Greenspan RH, Loken MK: Intravenous abdominal aortography: a preliminary report, *Surgery* 44:529, 1958.

17. Bernstein EF, Rhodes GA, Stuart SH, et al: Toe pulse reappearance time in prediction of aortofemoral bypass success, *Ann Surg* 193:201, 1981.

18. Boone GE, Pomajzl JM: Toe blood pressure by photoplethysmography: an index of healing in forefoot amputation, *Surgery* 89:569, 1981.

19. Boyd AM: The natural course of arteriosclerosis of the lower extremities, *Proc R Soc Med* 55:591, 1962.

20. Bremner J: Carnitine metabolism and function, *Physiol Rev* 63:1420–1480, 1983.

21. Brevetti G, Chiariello M, Ferulano G, et al: Increases in walking distance in patients with peripheral vascular disease treated with L-carnitine: a double-blind, cross-over study, *Circulation* 77:767–773, 1988.

22. Brewster DC, Darling CR: Optimal methods of aortoiliac reconstruction, *Surgery* 84:739, 1978.

23. Brewster DC, Perler BA, Robinson JG, et al: Aortofemoral graft for multilevel occlusive disease predictors of success and need for distal bypass, *Arch Surg* 117:1593, 1982.

24. Brooks B: Intra-arterial injection of sodium iodide, *JAMA* 82:1016, 1924.

25. Buchbinder D, Pasch AR, Rollins DL, et al: Results of arterial reconstruction of the foot, *Arch Surg* 121:673, 1986.

26. Buchbinder D, Pasch AR, Verta MJ: Ankle bypass: "Should we go the distance?" *Am J Surg* 150:216, 1985.

27. Butcher HR, Jaffe BM: Treatment of aortoiliac occlusive disease by endarterectomy, *Ann Surg* 173:925, 1971.

28. Cambria RP, Brewster DC, Abbott WM, et al: Transperitoneal versus retroperitoneal approach for aortic reconstruction: A randomized prospective study, *J Vasc Surg* 11:314–325, 1990.

29. Chowdary RP, Celani VJ, Goodreau JJ, et al: Free tissue transfers for limb salvage utilizing in situ saphenous vein bypass conduit as the inflow, *Plast Reconstr Surg* 87:529–535, 1991.

30. Canadian Cooperative Study Group: A randomised trial of aspirin and sulfinpyrazone in threatened stroke, *N Engl J Med* 297:53–59, 1978.

31. Clagett GP, Genton E, Salzman EW: Antithrombotic therapy in peripheral vascular disease, *Chest* 95(suppl):128–139, 1989.

32. Clyne CAC, Archer TJ, Atuhaire LX, et al: Random control trial of a short course of aspirin and dipyridamole (Persantin) for femorodistal grafts, *Br J Surg* 74:246–248, 1987.

33. Coffman JD: Vasodilator drugs in peripheral vascular disease, *N Engl J Med* 300:713–717, 1979.

34. Creasy TS, McMillan PJ, Fletcher EWL, et al: Is percutaneous transluminal angioplasty better than exercise for claudication?: preliminary results from a prospective randomised trial, *Eur J Vasc Surg* 4:135–140, 1990.

35. Cutler BS, Thompson JE, Kleinsasser LJ, et al: Autologous saphenous vein femoropopliteal bypass: analysis of 298 cases, *Surgery* 79:325, 1976.

36. Dahllof A, Bjorntorp P, Holm J, et al: Metabolic activity of skeletal muscle in patients with peripheral arterial insufficiency: effect of physical training, *Eur J Clin Invest* 4:9–15, 1974.

37. Dahllof A, Holm J, Schersten T, et al: Peripheral arterial insufficiency: effect of physical training on walking tolerance, calf blood flow, and blood flow resistance, *Scand J Rehabil Med* 8:19–26, 1976.

38. Dalman RL, Taylor LM Jr, Moneta GL, et al: Simultaneous operative repair of multilevel lower extremity occlusive disease, *J Vasc Surg* 13:211–221, 1991.

39. Dardik H, Ibrahim IM, Dardik II: The role of the peroneal artery for limb salvage, *Ann Surg* 189:189, 1979.

40. Dardik H, Sussman BC, Kahn M, et al: Lysis of arterial clot by intravenous or intra-arterial administration of streptokinase, *Surg Gynecol Obstet* 158:137, 1984.

41. Dettori AG, Pini M, Morrati A, et al: Adenocoumarol and pentoxifylline in intermittent claudication: a controlled clinical study, the APIC study group, *Angiology* 40:237–248, 1989.

42. DeWeese JA, Rob CG: Autogenous venous grafts ten years later, *Surgery* 82:775, 1977.

43. Dintenfass L: Blood viscosity factors in severe nondiabetic and diabetic retinopathy, *Biorheology* 14:151, 1977.

44. Dos Santos R, Lamas A, Pereira C: Arteriografia

da aorta e dos vasos abdominas, *Med Contemp* 47:93, 1929.

45. Dotter C, Judkins M: Transluminal treatment of arteriosclerotic obstructions: description of a new technique and a preliminary report of its application, *Circulation* 30:654, 1964.

46. Duncan WC, Linton RR, Darling RC: Aortoiliofemoral atherosclerotic occlusive disease: comparative results of endarterectomy and Dacron bypass grafts, *Surgery* 70:974, 1971.

47. Eisenberg RC, Bank WO, Hedgecock MW: Renal failure after major angiography, *AJR* 136:859, 1981.

48. Ericsson B, Haeger K, Lindell SE: Effect of physical training on intermittent claudication, *Angiology* 21:188–192, 1970.

49. Ernst EEW, Matrai A: Intermittent claudication, exercise, and blood rheology, *Circulation* 76:1110–1114, 1987.

50. Feldman AJ, Nevonen M, Berguer R: Experience with popliteal-infrapopliteal bypass grafting, *Surg Gynecol Obstet* 135:219, 1972.

51. Fields WS, Lemark NA, Frankowski RF: Controlled trial of aspirin in cerebral ischemia, *Stroke* 8:301–314, 1977.

52. Flanigan DP, Williams LR, Keifer T, et al: Prebypass operative arteriography, *Surgery* 92:627, 1982.

53. Flinn WR, Rohrer MJ, Yao JST, et al: Improved long term patency of infragenicular polytetrafluoroethylene grafts, *J Vasc Surg* 7:685–690, 1988.

54. Geoffrey J, et al: Osteo articular lesions of the foot in diabetic patients, *J Radiol* 59:557, 1978.

55. Goldenberg SG, Alex M, Joshi RA, et al: Nonatheromatous peripheral vascular disease of the lower extremity in diabetes mellitus, *Diabetes* 8:261–273, 1959.

56. Greenwald LL, Comerota AJ, Mitra A, et al: Free vascularized tissue transfer for limb salvage in peripheral vascular disease, *Ann Vasc Surg* 4:244–254, 1990.

57. Gruntzig A, Hopff H: Perkutane rekanalisation chronischer arterieller verschlusse miteinem neuen dilatationskatheten: modifikation der dotter technik, *Dtsch Med Wochenschr* 99:2502, 1974.

58. Guggenheim W, Kach G, Adams AP, et al: Femoral and popliteal occlusive vascular disease, *Diabetes* 18:428, 1969.

59. Gundersen J: Segmental measurements of systolic blood pressure in the extremities including the thumb and great toe, *Acta Chir Scand* 426(suppl):1, 1972.

60. Hargrove WC, Berkowitz HD, Freiman DB, et al: Recanalization of totally occluded femoropopliteal vein grafts with low-dose streptokinase infusion, *Surgery* 92:890, 1982.

61. Harkonen S, Kjellstrand CM: Exacerbation of diabetic renal failure following intravenous pyelography, *Am J Med* 63:939, 1977.

62. Harris EJ Jr, Taylor LM Jr, McConnell DB, et al: Clinical results of axillobifemoral bypass using externally supported polytetrafluoroethylene, *J Vasc Surg* 12:416–421, 1990.

63. Harris RW, Andros G, Dulawa LB, et al: Successful long term limb salvage using cephalic vein bypass grafts, *Ann Surg* 200:785–792, 1984.

64. Hedberg B, Langstrom M, Angquist KA, et al: Isokinetic plantar flexor performance and fatigability in peripheral arterial insufficiency, *Acta Chir Scand* 154:363–369, 1988.

65. Hiatt WR, Regensteiner JG, Hargarten ME, et al: Benefit of exercise conditioning for patients with peripheral arterial disease, *Circulation* 81:602–609, 1990.

66. Hobson RW II, Lynch TG, Jamil Z, et al: Results of revascularization and amputation in severe lower extremity ischemia: a five-year clinical experience, *J Vasc Surg* 2:174–185, 1985.

67. Hossman V, Auel H, Rucker W, et al: Prolonged infusion of prostacyclin in patients with advanced states of peripheral vascular disease: a placebo-controlled cross-over study, *Klin Wochenschr* 62:1108–1114, 1984.

68. Imparato AM, Kim GE, Davidson T, et al: Intermittent claudication: its natural course, *Surgery* 78:795, 1975.

69. Imparato AM, Kim GE, Madayag M, et al: Angiographic criteria for successful tibial arterial reconstruction, *Surgery* 74:830, 1973.

70. Irwin ST, Gilmore J, et al: Blood flow in diabetics with foot lesions due to "small vessel disease," *Br J Surg* 75:1201–1206, 1988.

71. Jacobs J, Sena M, Fox N: The cost of hospitalization for the late complications of diabetes in the United States, *Diabetic Med* 8 Symposium: S23-S29, 1991.

72. Janka HV, Standl E, Mehnert H: Peripheral vascular disease in diabetes mellitus and its relation to cardiovascular role factors: screening with the Doppler ultrasonic technique, *Diabetes Care* 3:207, 1980.

73. Jeans WD, Armstrong S, Cole SEA, et al: Fate of patients undergoing transluminal angioplasty for lower-limb ischemia, *Radiology* 177:559–564, 1990.

74. Jonason T, Ringqvist I: Diabetes mellitus and intermittent claudication, *Acta Med Scand* 218:217–221, 1985.

75. Jones RL, Peterson CM: Hematologic alterations in diabetes mellitus, *Am J Med* 70:339, 1981.

76. Karmody AM, Leather RP, Shah DM, et al: Peroneal artery bypass: a reappraisal of its value in limb salvage, *J Vasc Surg* 1:809, 1984.

77. Karnik R, Valentin A, Strollberger C, et al: Effects of naftidrofuryl in patients with intermittent claudication, *Angiology* 39:234–240, 1988.

78. Katzen BT: Angiography of the abdominal aorta and its branches, in *Interventional diagnostic and therapeutic procedures*, New York, 1980, Springer-Verlag.

79. Kent KC, Donaldson MC, Attinger CE, et al: Femoropopliteal reconstruction for claudication: the risk to life and limb, *Arch Surg* 123:1196–1198, 1988.

80. King RB, Myers KA, Scott DF, et al: The choice of operation in aortoiliac reconstructions for intermittent claudication, *World J Surg* 7:334, 1983.

81. Kokesh J, Kazmers A, Zierler RE: Pentoxifylline in the nonoperative management of intermittent claudication, *Ann Vasc Surg* 5:66–70, 1991.

82. Kott I, Urca I, Sanbank U: Lumbar sympathetic ganglia in atherosclerotic patients diabetic and nondiabetics, *Arch Surg* 109:787, 1974.

83. Kozloff L, Collins GJ Jr, Rich NM, et al: Fallibility of postoperative Doppler ankle pressures in determining the adequacy of proximal arterial revascularization, *Am J Surg* 139:326, 1980.

84. Kram HB, Appel PL, Shoemaker WC: Multisensor transcutaneous oximetric mapping to predict below-knee amputation wound healing: use of a critical $PO_2$, *J Vasc Surg* 9:796–800, 1989.

85. Lansen NA, Holstein P: Use of radioisotopes in assessment of distal blood flow and distal blood pressure in arterial insufficiency, *Surg Clin North Am* 54:39, 1974.

86. Larsen OA, Lassen NA: Effect of daily muscular exercise in patients with intermittent claudication, *Lancet* 2:1093–1096, 1966.

87. Leather RP, Shah DM, Chang BB, et al: Resurrection of the in situ saphenous vein bypass: 1000 cases later, *Ann Surg* 208:435–442, 1988.

88. Lee BY, LaPointe DG, Madden JL: Evaluation of lumbar sympathectomy by quantification of arterial pulsatile wave form, *Vasc Surg* 5:61, 1971.

89. LeVeen HH, Diaz C, Ip MW: Extraperitoneal aortoiliac disobliteration with plaque cracker, *Am J Surg* 136:221, 1978.

90. Lezack JD, Carter SA: Systolic pressures in the extremities of man with special reference to the toes, *Can J Physiol Pharm* 48:469, 1970.

91. Lezack JD, Carter SA: The relationship of distal systolic pressures to the clinical and angiographic findings in limbs with arterial occlusive disease, *Scand J Clin Lab Invest* 31(suppl 128):97, 1973.

92. Lindbjerg IF: Diagnostic application of the Xenon-133 method in peripheral arterial disease, *Scand J Clin Lab Invest* 17:589, 1965.

93. Linet OI, Mohberg NR, Sinzinger H, et al: Cycloprostin (epoprostenol) is effective in peripheral vascular disease. Paper presented at the Cardiovascular Pharmacotherapy International Symposium 1985, Geneva, April 22–26, 1985.

94. Lundgren F, Dahllof A, Lundholm K, et al: Intermittent claudication—surgical reconstruction or physical training?: a prospective randomized trial of treatment efficiency, *Ann Surg* 209:346–355, 1989.

95. Lundgren F, Dahllof AG, Schersten T, et al: Muscle enzyme adaptation in patients with peripheral arterial insufficiency: spontaneous adaptation, effect of different treatments and consequences on walking performance, *Clin Sci* 77:485–493, 1989.

96. Malone JM, Leal JM, Moore WS, et al: The "gold standard" for amputation level selection: xenon-133 clearance, *J Surg Res* 39:449, 1981.

97. Malone J, Moore WS, Goldstone J: The natural history of bilateral aortofemoral bypass grafts for ischemia of the lower extremities, *Arch Surg* 110:1300, 1975.

98. Mannarino E, Pasqualini L, Innocente S, et al: Physical training and antiplatelet treatment in stage II peripheral arterial occlusive disease: alone or combined? *Angiology* 42:513–521, 1991.

99. Mannarino E, Pasqualini L, Menna M, et al: Effects of physical training on peripheral vascular disease: a controlled study, *Angiology* 40:5–10, 1989.

100. Manuchoodapa C, D'Elia TA, Libertino JA, et al: Renal artery stenosis in hypertensive diabetics, *J Urol* 121:555, 1979.

101. Mason RA, Arbert LA, Giron F: Renal dysfunction after arteriography, *JAMA* 253:1001, 1985.

102. McAllister FF: The fate of patients with intermittent claudication managed nonoperatively, *Am J Surg* 132:593–595, 1976.

103. McAuley CE, Steed DL, Webster MW: Seven-year follow-up of expanded polytetrafluoroethylene (PTFE) femoropopliteal bypass grafts, *Ann Surg* 199:57–60, 1984.

104. McMillen DE, Gion KM: Glycosylated hemoglobin and reduced erythrocyte deformity in diabetes, in Strandl E, Mehrent H, editors: *Pathogenic concepts of diabetic microangiopathy*, New York, 1981, Thieme-Stratton.

105. Melton LJ, Macken KM, Palumbo PJ, et al: Incidence and prevalence of clinical peripheral vascular disease in a population based cohort of diabetic patients, *Diabetes Care* 3:650, 1980.

106. Mitchell JC: End stage renal failure in juvenile diabetes mellitus, *Mayo Clin Proc* 52:281, 1977.

107. National Center for Health Statistics: *National hospital discharge survey 1987*, Hyattsville Md, 1989, National Center for Health Statistics.

108. Nevelsteen A, Suy R, Daenen W, et al: Aortofemoral grafting: factors influencing late results, *Surgery* 88:642, 1980.

109. Nielsen PE, Rasmussen SM: Indirect measurement of systolic blood pressure by strain gauge technique at finger, ankle and toe in diabetic patients without symptoms of occlusive arterial disease, *Diabetologia* 9:25, 1973.

110. O'Mara CS, Flinn WR, Neiman HL, et al: Correlation of foot arterial anatomy with early tibial bypass patency, *Surgery* 89:743, 1981.

111. Pierce GE, Turrentine M, Stringfield S, et al: Evaluation of end-to-side v. end-to-end proximal anastomosis in aortobifemoral bypass, *Arch Surg* 117:1580, 1982.

112. Porter JM: *Curr Probl Surg* 28(1), January 1991.

113. Prendiville EJ, Yeager A, O'Donnell TF Jr, et al: Long term results with the above-knee popliteal expanded polytetrafluoroethylene graft, *J Vasc Surg* 11:517–524, 1990.

114. Quayle JB: Diabetic autonomic neuropathy in patients with vascular disease, *Br J Surg* 65:305, 1978.

115. Quinones-Baldrich WJ, Busuttil RW, Baker JD, et al: Is the preferential use of polytetrafluoroethylene grafts for femoropopliteal bypass justified? *J Vasc Surg* 8:219–228, 1988.

116. Ramsey DE, Manke DA, Sumner DS: Toe blood pressure: a valuable adjunct to ankle pressure measurement for assessing peripheral arterial disease, *J Cardiovasc Surg* 24:43, 1983.

117. Ricco JB, Flinn WR, McDaniel MD, et al: Objective analysis of factors contributing to failure of tibial bypass grafts, *World J Surg* 7:347, 1983.

118. Rosen RJ, Roven SJ, Taylor RF, et al: Evaluation of aorto-iliac occlusive disease by intravenous digital subtraction angiography, *Radiology* 148:7, 1983.

119. Rosenblatt MS, Quist WC, Sidawy AN, et al: Results of vein graft reconstruction of the lower extremity in diabetic and nondiabetic patients, *Surg Gynecol Obstet* 171:331–335, 1990.

120. Schroer R: Antithrombotic potential of pentoxifylline: a hemorrheological active drug, *Angiology* 36:387–398, 1985.

121. Schuler JJ, Flanigan P, Williams LR, et al: Early experience with popliteal to infrapopliteal bypass for limb salvage, *Arch Surg* 118:472, 1983.

122. Seabrook GR, Mewissen MW, Schmitt DD, et al: Percutaneous intraarterial thrombolysis in the treatment of thrombosis of lower extremity arterial reconstructions, *J Vasc Surg* 13:646–651, 1991.

123. Searles JM Jr, Colen LB: Foot reconstruction in diabetes mellitus and peripheral vascular insufficiency, *Clin Plast Surg* 18:467–483, 1991.

124. Seldinger SI: AIF techniques: catheter replacement of needle in percutaneous arteriography: new technique. *Acta Radiol* 39:368, 1953.

125. Sicard GA, Greeman MB, VanderWoude JC, et al: Comparison between the transabdominal and retroperitoneal approach for reconstruction of the infrarenal abdominal aorta, *J Vasc Surg* 5:19–26, 1987.

126. Skoorg F, Nielsen AV, Schlichtkull J, et al: Blood viscosity in diabetic patients, *Lancet* 1:129, 1966.

127. Solomon SA, Ramsay LE, Yeo WW, et al: B blockade and intermittent claudication: placebo controlled trial of atenolol and nifedipine and their combination, *Br Med J* 303:1100–1104, 1991.

128. Steinberg I, Finby N, Evans JA: A safe and practical intravenous method for abdominal aortography, peripheral arteriography and cerebral angiography, *AJR* 82:758, 1959.

129. Stemmer EA: Influence of diabetes on patterns of peripheral vascular disease, *Surg Rounds*, Jan 1990, pp. 43–53.

130. Sternby NH: Atherosclerosis and diabetes mellitus, *Acta Pathol Microbiol Scand* 194(suppl):152, 1968.

131. Sterpetti AV, Schultz RD, Feldhaus RJ, et al: Seven-year experience with polytetrafluoroethylene as above-knee femoropopliteal bypass graft: Is it worthwhile to preserve the autologous saphenous vein? *J Vasc Surg* 2:907–912, 1985.

132. Strano A, Davig, Avellone G, et al: Double-blind, crossover study of the clinical efficacy and hemorrheological effects of pentoxifylline in patients with occlusive arterial disease of the lower limbs, *Angiology* 35:459–466, 1984.

133. Szilagyi DE, Elliot JP, Smith RF, et al: A thirty-year survey of the reconstructive surgical treatment of aortoiliac occlusive disease, *Surgery* 3:421, 1986.

134. Szilagyi DE, Hageman JH, Smith RF, et al: Autogenous vein grafting in femoropopliteal atherosclerosis: the limits of its effectiveness, *Surgery* 86:836, 1979.

135. Szilagyi DE, Smith RF, Scerpella JR, et al: Lumbar sympathectomy, current role in treatment of atherosclerotic occlusive disease, *Arch Surg* 95:753, 1967.

136. Taylor LM, Baur GM, Porter JM: Finger gangrene caused by small artery occlusive disease, *Ann Surg* 193:453, 1981.

137. Taylor LM, Edwards JM, Porter JM: Present status of reversed vein bypass: five year results of a modern series, *J Vasc Surg* 11:193–206, 1990.

138. Tenembaum MM, Rayfield E, Junior J, et al: Altered pressure flow relationship in the diabetic foot, *J Surg Res* 31:307, 1981.

139. Thomas JH, Steers JL, Keushkerian SM, et al: A comparison of diabetics and nondiabetics with threatened limb loss, *Am J Surg* 156:481–483, 1988.

140. University Group Diabetes Program: A study of the effects of hypoglycemic agents on vascular complications in patients with adult-onset diabetes: I, design methods, and baseline results, *Diabetes* 19(suppl 2):747, 1970.

141. Uusitupa MIJ, Niskanen LK, Siitonen O, et al: 5-year incidence of atherosclerotic vascular disease in relation to general risk factors, insulin level, and abnormalities in lipoprotein composition in non-insulin-dependent diabetic and nondiabetic subjects, *Circulation* 82:27–36, 1990.

142. van Breda A, Katzen BT: Radiologic aspects of intra-arterial thrombolytic therapy, in Comerota AJ, editor: *Thrombolytic therapy*, Orlando, Fla, 1988, Grune & Stratton, pp 99–124.

143. van den Dungen JJ, Boontje AH, Kropveld A: Unilateral iliofemoral occlusive disease: long term results of the semiclosed endarterectomy with the ringstripper, *J Vasc Surg* 14:673–677, 1991.

144. Vanhoute PM: Endothelium and the control of vascular tissue, *News Phisiol Sci* 2:18–22, 1987.

145. Veith FJ, Gupta SK, Ascer E, et al: Six year prospective multicenter randomized comparison of autologous saphenous vein and expanded polytetrafluoroethylene grafts in infrainguinal arterial reconstructions, *J Vasc Surg* 3:104–114, 1986.

146. Vincent DG, Salles-Cunha SX, Bernhard VM, et al: Noninvasive assessment of toe systolic pressures with special reference to diabetes mellitus, *J Cardiovasc Surg* 24:22, 1983.

147. White RA, White GH, Mehringer MC, et al: A clinical trial of laser thermal angioplasty in patients with advanced peripheral vascular disease, *Ann Surg* 212:257–265, 1990.

148. White RI Jr: Principles of percutaneous catheterization, in *Fundamentals of vascular radiology*, Philadelphia, 1976, Lea & Febiger.

149. Widdershoven RMH, LeVeen HH: Closed endarterectomy: preferred operation for aortoiliac occlusive disease, *Arch Surg* 124:986–990, 1989.

150. Wyss CR, Matsen FA III, Simmons CW, et al: Transcutaneous oxygen tension measurements on limbs of diabetic and nondiabetic patients with peripheral vascular disease, *Surgery* 95:339–346, 1984.

# CHAPTER 19

# Medical Management of Surgical Patients With Diabetes

**Irl B. Hirsch, M.D.**

**Paul F. White, M.D., Ph.D.**

There are no recent studies assessing the frequency of surgery in diabetic patients. The most quoted evaluation was during the 1960s when it was estimated that diabetic patients had a 50% chance of undergoing surgery at least sometime during their life.[28] More recent statistics show that as many as 14 million Americans have diabetes.[4] Furthermore, mortality rates for diabetes-related deaths have decreased over the past 20 years.[4] If one considers all of the operations a patient with diabetes may need over the course of a lifetime related to one of the microvascular or macrovascular complications (in addition to non-diabetes-related surgery), the chance for surgery in a diabetic individual is likely much higher than 50%.

The prevalence of peripheral vascular disease (PVD) and distal symmetric polyneuropathy with diabetes is important to appreciate. Although the overall prevalence of PVD in diabetic populations is only 10%, after 20 years of diabetes the prevalence increases to 45%. Neuropathy is present in 8% of diabetic patients at diagnosis, but after 25 years one half of the patients with diabetes have developed symptoms of neuropathy.[4] Therefore, if only one half of the 14 million people in the United States with diabetes live 20 years (a conservative estimate), there would be approximately 3 million diabetic individuals with PVD and neuropathy. This is consistent with the estimate

that 25% of diabetic patients will eventually develop foot or leg problems.[34] It is therefore not surprising that lower limb surgery is responsible for more than one half of hospital admissions for all types of surgery in diabetic patients.[34]

Thus it is important for all health care professionals to be familiar with the medical management of the diabetic patient having surgery. There still is controversy regarding both the degree of metabolic control required during the perioperative period and the medical regimen that would be best suited for a specific situation. In terms of metabolic control, experimental data suggest plasma glucose concentrations greater than 200 mg/dL impair wound strength and wound healing, interfere with leukocyte function, and exacerbate ischemic brain damage.[13] However, there are no controlled clinical studies to show that uncontrolled diabetes results in an inferior outcome in terms of these endpoints or prolonged hospital stay. Few would argue that acute complications of uncontrolled diabetes may be avoided by providing adequate attention to the various metabolic parameters.

Because of a lack of controlled studies, there is no consensus on the optimum manner in which to manage the metabolic changes in patients with diabetes that occur during the perioperative period. However, if certain fundamental principles (e.g., the metabolic effects of anesthesia, the pharmacokinetics and dynamics of subcutaneous and intravenous insulin, and glucose requirements during the perioperative period) are better understood, a more rational approach to the perioperative management of patients with diabetes could be developed.

## METABOLIC RESPONSE TO SURGERY AND ANESTHESIA

Hyperglycemia is not uncommon during the perioperative period in the *nondiabetic* patient. Elevated blood glucose levels are caused by both (relative) insulin deficiency and insulin resistance.[13] Insulin secretion has consistently been found to be blunted with general anesthesia, and the increase in insulin resistance is presumed to be secondary to elevated counterregulatory hormone levels. The exact stress response is a function of the degree of trauma and can be modified by anesthesia. Therefore, declaring that surgery causes an increase in the four principal counterregulatory hormones (glucagon, the catecholamines epinephrine and norepinephrine, growth hormone, and cortisol) is an oversimplification of a complex metabolic process. Studies to date have shown remarkable variations in the individual counterregulatory hormone response to surgery,[13, 23] and this is likely the result of variations in surgical procedure, surgical technique, and type of anesthesia used.

The individual effects of the counterregulatory hormones include the following: (1) glucagon and epinephrine both stimulate gluconeogenesis and glycogenolysis (because epinephrine also inhibits pancreatic insulin secretion, there is decreased peripheral glucose uptake with catecholamine hypersecretion); (2) cortisol increases both gluconeogenesis and the resistance to glucose uptake by muscle; and (3) growth hormone secretion is somewhat more complicated, because it exerts both insulin-like and insulin-antagonistic effects. The former effect is weak and of minor importance, whereas the latter becomes evident after a lag period of 2 to 3 hours and induces insulin resistance in both the liver and peripheral tissues.[9, 19]

Another important aspect of the counterregulatory hormones are their effects on fat metabolism. Epinephrine, cortisol, and growth hormone all stimulate lipolysis, whereas glucagon has little, if any, effect on fat catabolism.[17] Insulin is the only antilipolytic hormone. The combination of absolute insulin deficiency, as seen in type I diabetes, and generalized counterregulatory hormone excess can potentially lead to metabolic decompensation with unrestrained lipolysis and ketoacidosis. It is therefore not surprising that if sufficient fluids are administered to the patient with type I diabetes (with normal renal function), significant ketosis may occur without the typical elevations in plasma glucose concentrations. This condition, called "euglycemic diabetic ketoacidosis," may account for up to 17% of all episodes of diabetic ketoacidosis.[24]

## PREOPERATIVE CONSIDERATIONS

Preoperative issues may be separated into two categories: (1) the assessment of the acute metabolic status and (2) the evaluation of the chronic complications of diabetes that may affect the surgical outcome. With regard to the former issue, because of the potential deleterious metabolic effects of surgery, significant preoperative hyperglycemia and electrolyte abnormalities should be corrected. Therefore, preoperative plasma glucose level and electrolyte concentrations, in addition to urinary ketone levels, should be measured *on the day of surgery*. Previous authors have suggested admitting diabetic patients 24 to 72 hours before surgery to improve metabolic control.[2, 30] This recommendation is not usually possible in today's world of same-day admissions and diagnosis-related groups. On the other hand, significant metabolic instability (e.g., ketosis, blood glucose levels > 400 mg/dL, hypokalemia) will require admission before elective surgery.

The complete assessment of the various chronic complications should ideally be completed before admission. Perhaps the most important of these is cardiovascular disease. Patients with diabetes are one and one-half to two times as likely to report having heart disease than their nondiabetic counterparts, and about two thirds of deaths in people with diabetes are caused by cardiovascular disease.[4] Evidence has also accumulated for the existence of a specific "diabetic cardiomyopathy," which is yet another potential perioperative risk.[35] The optimum preoperative cardiovascular assessment is controversial,[11, 20] in part because of the high frequency of asymptomatic myocardial ischemia in this population,[18] but also because of the relatively low predictive value of routine cardiovascular evaluation, especially in patients with renal disease.[15]

Preoperative evaluation also requires the assessment of diabetic nephropathy. A serum creatinine concentration is not a sufficient indicator for renal disease in diabetic patients because its level usually remains normal until the nephropathy is advanced.[27] Because the first harbinger of diabetic nephropathy is proteinuria, dipstick for urinary protein should be included in the minimum assessment of renal disease. It is now well established that persistent proteinuria with as little as 30 mg/24 hours is a strong predictor of nephropathy in patients with type I and II diabetes.[32] Albumin excretion rates between 30 and 300 mg/24 hours are called "microalbuminuria." Unfortunately, dipstick-positive proteinuria does not usually occur until urinary albumin excretion exceeds 250 to 300 mg/24 hours. Therefore, the American Diabetes Association now recommends yearly 24-hour urine collections for microalbuminuria for all patients with diabetes.[5] The preoperative assessment of proteinuria is important for two reasons. First, any potential nephrotoxic agent should be avoided for the patient with proteinuria. In addition, proteinuria is a predictor of mortality (mainly cardiovascular) in patients with type II diabetes.[22]

Autonomic neuropathy should also be assessed before surgery. A recent report showed that diabetic patients with autonomic dysfunction had an increased risk of perioperative hypotension.[6] Therefore, routine preoperative history should include questioning about the typical symptoms of autonomic dysfunction (resting tachycardia, early satiety, abdominal bloating and pain, gustatory sweating, diarrhea [often nocturnal] alternating with constipation and orthostatic hypotension). Autonomic dysfunction may be measured with much greater sensitivity by measuring variation in RR (interval between QRS complexes on electrocardiogram) during deep breathing, heart rate response to Valsalva's maneuver, as well as the blood pressure and heart rate response to standing.[10]

The need for medical consultation will vary depending on the surgeon's comfort with the various preoperative issues. Because of the complexity of medical problems, many of these patients should be followed by their family practitioner, internist, or endocrinologist during the perioperative period. Surgery in patients with diabetes is another situation that requires a team approach for the optimum care. Indeed, more hospitals are now using a diabetes clinical nurse specialist to consult with all patients admitted with diabetes.

## ANESTHESIA AND HYPOGLYCEMIA

Selection of the anesthetic modality is the prerogative of the anesthesiologist and is based on the type of surgery, the medical and surgical risks, and individual preferences without primary consideration of the presence of diabetes. Modern inhalation anesthesia has relatively little effect on metabolic regulation; spinal, epidural, and peripheral nerve blocks produce the least disturbance in glycemic control.[13] Ankle block is preferred for most patients requiring foot surgery. The prudent use of preoperative medication, including sedation and muscle relaxants, facilitates the anesthetic induction. These agents should be carefully titrated in elderly patients.

Any type of sedation may also impair symptom recognition of hypoglycemia. It is well documented that asymptomatic hypoglycemia is a common event in diabetic patients who are not receiving central nervous system depressants. One study documented a 29% incidence (each night) of asymptomatic nocturnal hypoglycemia (defined as plasma glucose concentration $< 55$ mg/dL).[26] The Diabetes Control and Complications Trial (DCCT) has described their experience with 817 subjects spanning 21 months for severe hypoglycemia (an event with symptoms consistent with hypoglycemia in which the patient required the assistance of another person).[7] These authors reported that nocturnal hypoglycemia and asymptomatic hypoglycemia while awake were responsible for 43% and 51%, respectively, of all episodes of severe hypoglycemia.[7] There are little published data for perioperative hypoglycemia. One review[14] has found a 13% incidence of perioperative hypoglycemia (blood glucose level $< 60$ mg/dL) in a group of 85 patients with type I diabetes. Therefore, any patient receiving a glucose-lowering agent and *any sedation* requires regular blood glucose monitoring.

## INSULIN-DEPENDENT DIABETES MELLITUS (TYPE I DIABETES)

Most diabetic patients requiring lower extremity surgery will have non-insulin-dependent diabetes (type II diabetes), albeit many will be insulin requiring. It is important for the health care provider to make the distinction between *insulin-dependent* diabetes (type I) and *insulin-requiring* diabetes (type II). Without insulin, patients with the former condition will develop ketosis, whereas patients with the latter will usually have more significant hyperglycemia.

There is general agreement that patients with type I diabetes receiving general anesthesia should receive their insulin as a continuous IV infusion[1, 13] because insulin availability after subcutaneous insulin injections is unpredictable in the usual outpatient setting.[12] The pharmacokinetics of subcutaneous insulin administered before or during surgery have never been studied. Intravenous insulin infusions have been shown to be safe and provide improved metabolic control compared with perioperative subcutaneous insulin injections.[3, 16, 25, 33] Hypoglycemia also tends to be less of a problem with the use of an IV infusion because the more pre-dictable and instantaneous insulin availability diminishes the risk of delivering an excessive amount of hormone.

Despite the agreement that patients with type I diabetes receiving general anesthesia should be administered insulin by IV infusion, subcutaneous insulin is still widely used.[14] Probably the primary reason for this is simply custom.[1] Anesthesiologists frequently administer large IV boluses of insulin during the intraoperative period.[14] Because the half-life of IV insulin is only 4 to 5 minutes, and the biologic half-life is less than 20 minutes,[31] this practice is not recommended.

The IV insulin infusion for an elective procedure with the patient under general anesthesia may be started on the morning of surgery. It is inappropriate to withhold insulin in the patient with type I diabetes. When serum insulin levels decline below a critical level, unrestrained hepatic lipolysis and ketogenesis may quickly develop into ketoacidosis. Basal insulin administration is required for patients with type I diabetes who are not eating. Because of its relatively short duration, subcutaneous regular insulin ("bolus insulin") is best suited for anticipatory mealtime glycemic excursions. Therefore, if the operation is scheduled for late morning or during the afternoon, it is less cumbersome to initiate the basal insulin with an IV insulin infusion than to administer subcutaneous insulin. If the blood glucose concentration is less than 120 mg/dL, the insulin infusion should be delayed until it rises above this level.

There are two general strategies for the IV insulin infusion. We prefer the variable rate insulin infusion (Table 19–1). With this, most authors suggest initiating the infusion at 1.0 U/hr; however, we recommend beginning at 0.5 U/hr in thin women, who tend to be more insulin sensitive. To avoid any problems with insulin adsorption to the plastic, 50 mL of the infusion mixture should be flushed through the tubing before it is connected to the patient. The algorithm in Table 19–1 is a guide that we have found to be quite effective, but extremely high or low blood glucose levels will require adjustments. The other option, the glucose-insulin-

**TABLE 19–1.**

Variable Rate Intravenous Insulin Infusion

1. Mix 25 U regular human insulin into 250 mL normal saline solution (0.1 U/mL).
2. Flush 50 mL of the infusion mixture through the tubing.
3. Do not start insulin until blood glucose level is >120 mg/dL.
4. General guidelines for initial dose for patients with type I diabetes:  men— 1.0 U/hr, women 0.5 U/hr; for patients with type II diabetes: 1.0 U/hr for all patients.
5. Blood glucose levels should be measured hourly during and immediately after surgery.
6. Insulin algorithm (may need to be altered depending on situation):

**Blood Glucose**
   (mg/dL)

| Blood Glucose (mg/dL) | |
| --- | --- |
| <70 | Turn infusion off × 15 min. Administer 10 g glucose.* |
| 70–120 | Decrease infusion by 3 mL/hr (0.3 U/hr) |
| 121–180 | No change in infusion rate |
| 181–240 | Increase infusion by 3 mL/hr (0.3 U/hr) |
| 241–300 | Increase infusion by 6 mL/hr (0.6 U/hr) |
| >300 | Increase infusion by 10 mL/hr (1.0 U/hr) |

*Restart infusion at 3 mL/hr (0.3 U/hr) after blood glucose level is >100 mg/dL (should be remeasured 15 min after turning off insulin infusion); if blood glucose is still <100 mg/dL, may wait another 15 min.

7. Do not stop insulin infusion until patient able to tolerate food orally; at that time, may give usual dose of premeal regular insulin (may give 4–8 U SC regular insulin before lunch meal if insulin is not usually given then).

potassium (GIK) infusion, has a fixed amount of glucose, insulin, and potassium in each bag of fluid (Table 19–2). Although this has been shown to be quite effective, it has the disadvantage of having to change the entire bag whenever the blood glucose level is outside of targeted values. Alternatively, insulin may be added to the bag. The major advantage of the GIK infusion is that if there is any variation in the rate of flow of the infusion, insulin and glucose delivery are affected equally. There are no studies di-

**TABLE 19–2.**

Glucose-Insulin-Potassium Infusion Protocol*

1. Based on 10% glucose: 32 U regular human insulin + 20 mEq KCl in 1 L 10% dextrose in 0.45% saline solution. Infuse at 100 mL/hr (0.32 U insulin/g glucose/hr).
2. Based on 5% glucose: 16 U regular human insulin + 20 mEq KCl in 1 L 5% dextrose in 0.45% saline solution. Infuse at 100 mL/hr (0.32 U/g/hr).
3. Measure blood glucose every hour during surgery, and every 1 to 2 hours thereafter.

| Blood glucose (mg/dL) | | Insulin Dose† | | |
| --- | --- | --- | --- | --- |
| | | 10% Glucose (U/L) | 5% Glucose (U/L) | U • g$^{-1}$ • hr$^{-1}$ |
| <80 | Reduce to | 24 | 12 | 0.24 |
| 81–120 | Reduce to | 28 | 14 | 0.28 |
| 120–180 | | No change | No change | 0.32 |
| 180–250 | Increase to | 36 | 18 | 0.36 |
| >250 | Increase to | 40 | 20 | 0.40 |

*Insulin may be mixed in 500-mL bags with half of doses of insulin noted above.
†Insulin content may need to be increased if excessive insulin resistance is present (e.g., infection).

rectly comparing the two different insulin infusion strategies, although some believe that the GIK infusion is safer for nonspecialized hospitals.[1]

The targeted blood glucose concentration is controversial. We strive for blood glucose levels between 120 and 180 mg/dL, but slightly higher targets (e.g., 150–200 mg/dL) are also acceptable. These values are chosen to minimize the risk of hypoglycemia and also to decrease the risk of excessive catabolism from hyperglycemia. Maintaining blood glucose levels less than 200 mg/dL will also diminish the deleterious effects of hyperglycemia, namely, impaired wound healing and strength, impaired phagocyte function, exacerbation of ischemic brain damage, and hyperosmolarity.

As a general guideline, most patients will require between 0.3 and 0.4 U of insulin/g of glucose per hour to achieve targeted glucose goals.[2] Patients with foot infections often require 0.6 to 0.8 U/g per hour. With a variable rate insulin infusion, the rate may be increased or decreased, and targeted blood glucose levels can rapidly be achieved. The glucose is typically administered as a constant infusion with 0.45% saline solution. With the GIK infusion, insulin may be added to the bag, or the bag may be reconstituted to achieve the appropriate mixture.

Another virtue of the variable rate insulin infusion or GIK infusion is the ease of managing the diabetes with postoperative vomiting. Vomiting may be related to anesthesia and surgery alone or to gastroparesis from the diabetes. If food is not tolerated, blood glucose levels may be easily managed without the guesswork involved with subcutaneous insulin. Because metoclopramide is the only antiemetic approved in the United States for the treatment of gastroparesis, it should be considered the drug of choice for the treatment of postoperative vomiting in diabetic patients.

Another controversial issue regards the required frequency of metabolic monitoring. Most authors agree that with general anesthesia blood glucose and electrolyte levels should be measured just before and after surgery. While the patient is receiving the IV insulin infusion, we prefer to obtain bed-side glucose determinations every hour during and immediately after surgery, and every 2 hours after that if there are no problems. Others believe it is safe to monitor less frequently.[1] There are no data investigating the optimum frequency of perioperative blood glucose monitoring. Urinary ketone levels should also be routinely measured in patients with type I diabetes. For patients who are not eating, urinary ketones should be measured daily until food is tolerated. This will identify any patient with early ketosis that may be exacerbated by starvation.

Sufficient glucose is required during the perioperative period both for basal energy requirements and for the prevention of hypoglycemia. Again, there are no data regarding the optimum quantity of glucose in diabetic patients. Most authors give 5 or 10 g of glucose each hour.[1, 2, 13, 29] The larger glucose infusion rate is preferred by some because of the greater energy provided in addition to a more anabolic quantity of insulin required. If 5 g of glucose are administered each hour in the presence of ketonuria, even if blood glucose levels are at or near target values, the glucose infusion should be increased to 10 g/hour. The ketonuria in this situation is likely caused by a lack of glucose.

Recommendations for the perioperative management for the patient with type I diabetes having local anesthesia are less clear. In one of their early studies, Alberti and Thomas[3] showed superiority with the GIK infusion compared to subcutaneous insulin for this situation. Most authors recommend IV insulin infusion in patients with type I diabetes when general anesthesia is not used; however, data are limited in this setting. For patients receiving ultralente insulin as their basal insulin or those using subcutaneous insulin infusion pumps, we find it easiest to continue with the home regimen during procedures requiring local anesthesia. We prefer the use of the IV insulin infusion for patients who receive neutral protamine Hagedorn (NPH) or lente with regular insulin at home. If subcutaneous insulin is used, a fraction of the usual morning dose may be given at the usual time (e.g., one-third to one-half the usual dose of intermediate and short-acting insulin), a glucose infusion should be initiated and bedside glucose levels should be monitored every hour during and immediately after the procedure.

## NON-INSULIN-DEPENDENT DIABETES MELLITUS (TYPE II DIABETES)

Patients with type II diabetes comprise the majority of individuals requiring lower limb surgery. However, the same basic principles of management apply to these patients as those with type I diabetes.

For procedures requiring general anesthesia, most authors agree that special treatment other than close blood glucose monitoring (hourly during surgery) is not required for patients whose diabetes is well controlled by diet therapy alone.[1, 2, 13, 29] Because of the overall hyperglycemic response to the surgery, the presence of a preexisting lower limb infection will contribute to insulin resistance, and therefore, many of these patients will require insulin to control their hyperglycemia. As mentioned previously, the insulin should be administered with either a variable rate IV insulin or GIK infusion. Targeted blood glucose concentrations are identical to those for patients with type I diabetes, and thus we suggest initiating insulin when the blood glucose level exceeds 200 mg/dL. This value is also chosen because fasting blood glucose levels greater than this manifest absolute deficiency with respect to insulin secretion.[8]

There is some disagreement regarding management strategies for patients requiring general anesthesia whose diabetes is well controlled with sulfonylureas. For patients who receive chlorpropamide at home, some have recommended stopping this longer-acting oral hypoglycemic agent several days before surgery and substituting a shorter-acting drug, such as tolbutamide.[2] Theoretically this practice, which has never been tested, should diminish the risk of sulfonylurea-induced hypoglycemia. This is particularly pertinent with local procedures that do not result in an exaggerated counterregulatory response. Alberti[1] recommends withholding all oral agents on the morning of surgery for procedures requiring either general or local anesthesia, because with the former, an insulin infusion will likely be required to control the hyperglycemia. If insulin is not instituted at the beginning of the procedure, it should be initiated when the blood glucose level exceeds 200 mg/dL. As a general rule, subcutaneous insulin should not be used for any patient receiving general anesthesia.[1, 13]

Treatment decisions for patients with type II diabetes receiving local anesthesia are similar, except that patients with *well-controlled* diabetes who are treated with diet alone or diet with oral agents likely will not require additional insulin. One study showed that 93% of patients with type II diabetes (fasting blood glucose levels 133 ± 36 mg/dL [mean ± standard error]) can achieve acceptable blood glucose control without insulin.[16] Therefore, unless blood glucose levels rise above the targeted values, no further specific therapy will be required, and the sulfonylureas may be safely omitted for that day. If insulin is required, there is no particular advantage of IV insulin over subcutaneous insulin in this population.[21] If subcutaneous insulin is used, we suggest starting with 4 to 6 units of regular insulin every 4 hours.

Patients whose diabetes is *poorly controlled* before their admission using sulfonylureas will require insulin to stay in the targeted blood glucose goals. Therefore, there are no situations in which it would be appropriate to administer the oral hypoglycemic agent before surgery with either general or local anesthesia. In addition, administering these agents could be potentially dangerous in the patient with well-controlled diabetes if enough calories were not provided.

Insulin-requiring patients with type II diabetes receiving local anesthesia should be managed similarly to patients with type I diabetes. Many of these patients are insulinopenic and thus behave metabolically like those with type I diabetes. Therefore, we also recommend the use of the variable rate insulin infusion or the GIK infusion in this population, although subcutaneous insulin is acceptable.

## POSTOPERATIVE TREATMENT

Because any diabetic patient requiring general anesthesia should be receiving a variable rate insulin or GIK infusion (except the rare patient with type II diabetes whose blood glucose concentrations do not exceed 200 mg/dL), postoperative management is simple. If the patient cannot tolerate food and blood glucose levels remain in the targeted range after 12 hours, the frequency of blood glucose monitoring often can be decreased to every 2 to 4 hours, although if any changes in the insulin dose are required, blood glucose measurements must be made more frequently. We measure urinary ketone levels daily because the presence of ketonuria in the presence of well-controlled glycemia indicates the need for greater quantities of glucose (starvation ketosis). Alternatively, ketonuria with unexplained hyperglycemia could represent one of a variety of problems, including sepsis, myocardial infarction, or even a pharmacy error with the insulin mixture. Finally, serum electrolyte levels should be measured immediately after surgery for all diabetic patients and on a daily basis for those receiving an insulin infusion.

We have found it easiest to continue the insulin infusion until solid food is tolerated. Thus, if nausea and vomiting are present, there will be no interruption of glucose and insulin therapy. If solid food is permitted for the lunch or supper meal on the day of surgery, the regular home dose of insulin may be administered 20 to 30 minutes before the meal and the insulin (and glucose) infusion stopped just before the meal. If regular insulin is not usually given before the lunch meal, 4 to 6 units of regular insulin (subcutaneous) may be given. If the patient will be spending the night in the hospital, it is sometimes easier to continue with the insulin infusion until the next morning to ensure that the morning meal is well tolerated.

Patients with type I diabetes receiving local anesthesia and an insulin infusion may be managed similarly after surgery. Patients using ultralente insulin or an insulin pump at home should continue with their usual doses of "basal" insulin, and supplemental regular insulin may be administered subcutaneously as needed every 4 hours. Because of the guess work involved when NPH and lente preparations are administered, recommendations are difficult if one decides to administer these insulins to this population or patients with type II diabetes who require insulin. If food is tolerated immediately after surgery, regular insulin may or may not be required, depending on the time of the day in relation to the "peaking" intermediate insulin. This problem is eliminated if an insulin infusion is used.

With the increasing emphasis on outpatient procedures, it is imperative that patients with diabetes are instructed how to manage their diabetes after discharge. Blood glucose monitoring should be continued every 1 to 2 hours after the patient returns home. For patients receiving insulin, a predetermined plan for insulin supplements should be created before discharge from the hospital. For those diet controlled or receiving a sulfonylurea, the patient should be instructed to contact the health care provider should the blood glucose concentration exceed a certain level. We would not encourage sending patients home if there are any problems with postoperative nausea and vomiting. However, should this develop after discharge, the patient should call the provider for further instructions. Patients with type I diabetes should always have the ability to measure urinary ketone levels at home, and any diabetic patient with nausea and vomiting should be screened for ketonuria. Most important, all patients should have specific guidelines as to when their providers should be contacted.

## SUMMARY

Lower limb surgery is a common occurrence for patients with diabetes, but large trials examining the optimal medical management and its relationship to surgical outcome of these patients are lacking. Although there is some disagreement about the perioperative management of these patients, there is general consensus about how these patients should be managed (Table 19–3).

**TABLE 19–3.**

Summary of Insulin Strategies for Perioperative Management in Diabetic Patient

|  | General Anesthesia | Local Anesthesia |
| --- | --- | --- |
| Type I diabetes | Insulin infusion* | Insulin Infusion† |
| Type II diabetes | Insulin infusion | Insulin infusion or subcutaneous Insulin‡ |

*Variable rate insulin infusion or glucose-insulin-potassium infusion.
†Patients receiving basal ultralente or a continuous subcutaneous insulin infusion may continue to receive basal subcutaneous insulin delivery.
‡Patients with well-controlled diabetes often will not require supplemental insulin.

Blood glucose levels should be maintained at less than 200 mg/dL but while avoiding hypoglycemia. All insulin-requiring patients who are receiving general anesthesia should be administered an insulin infusion, either variable rate insulin or a GIK infusion. Patients with type I diabetes who are administered local anesthesia are best managed with an insulin infusion, except those patients who receive basal insulin with ultralente insulin or an insulin pump, in which case they do well with subcutaneous insulin during and after surgery. However, there is the least amount of information about the most common situation, the poorly controlled patient with type II diabetes receiving local anesthesia. For these patients, there is probably no advantage in using IV insulin compared with subcutaneous insulin. There are no data to support the use of sulfonylureas on the day of surgery for patients with type II diabetes. Consideration should be given to stopping long-acting oral hypoglycemic agents, such as chlorpropamide, several days before surgery.

# REFERENCES

1. Alberti KGMM: Diabetes and surgery [editorial], *Anesthesiology* 74:209, 1991.

2. Alberti KGMM, Gill GV, Elliot MJ: Insulin delivery during surgery in the diabetic patient, *Diabetes Care* 5(suppl 5):65, 1982.

3. Alberti KGMM, Thomas DJB: The management of diabetes during surgery, *Br J Anaesth* 51:693, 1979.

4. Diabetes: 1991 vital statistics, American Diabetes Association: Alexandria, Va, 1991.

5. American Diabetes Association; Clinical Practice Recommendations: Standards of medical care for patients with diabetes, *Diabetes Care* 14(suppl 2):10, 1991.

6. Burgos LG, Ebert TJ, Asiddao C, et al: Increased intraoperative cardiovascular morbidity in diabetes with autonomic neuropathy, *Anesthesiology* 70:591, 1989.

7. DCCT Research Group: Epidemiology of severe hypoglycemia in the Diabetes Control and Complications Trial, *Am J Med* 90:450, 1991.

8. DeFronzo RA, Ferrannini E, Kovisto V: New concepts in the pathogenesis and treatment of non-insulin-dependent diabetes mellitus, *Am J Med* 74(suppl 1A):52, 1983.

9. Domalik LJ, Feldman JM: Carbohydrate metabolism and surgery, in Bergman M, Sicard GA, editors: *Surgical management of the diabetic patient*, New York, 1991, Raven Press, Chapter 2.

10. Ewing DJ, Clarke BF: Diagnosis and management of diabetic autonomic neuropathy, *Br Med J* 285:916, 1982.

11. Freeman WK, Gibbons RJ, Shub C: Preoperative assessment of the cardiac patients undergoing noncardiac surgical procedures, *Mayo Clin Proc* 64:1105, 1989.

12. Hirsch IB, Farkas-Hirsch R, Skyler JS: Intensive insulin therapy for type I diabetes, *Diabetes Care* 13:1265, 1990.

13. Hirsch IB, McGill JB, Cryer PE, et al: Perioperative management of surgical patients with diabetes mellitus, *Anesthesiology* 74:346, 1991.

14. Hirsch IB, White PF: A retrospective review of the perioperative management of IDDM during surgery, *Anesth Rev* (in press).

15. Holley JL, Fenton RA, Arthur RS: Thallium stress testing does not predict cardiovascular risk in diabetic patients with end-stage renal disease undergoing cadaveric renal transplantation, *Am J Med* 90:563, 1991.

16. Husband DJ, Thai AC, Alberti KGMM: Management of diabetes during surgery with glucose-insulin-potassium infusion, *Diabetic Med* 3:69, 1986.

17. Jensen, MD, Heiling, VJ, Miles JM: Effects of glucagon on free fatty acid metabolism in humans, *J Clin Endocrinol Metab* 72:308, 1991.

18. Koistinen MJ: Prevalence of asymptomatic myocardial ischaemia in diabetic subjects, *Br Med J* 301:92, 1990.

19. Lager I: The insulin-antagonistic effect of the counterregulatory hormones, *J Intern Med* 229(suppl 2):41, 1991.

20. Leppo J, Plaja J, Gionet M, et al: Noninvasive evaluation of cardiac risk before elective vascular surgery, *J Am Coll Cardiol* 9:269, 1987.

21. Malling G, Knudsen L, Christiansen BA, et al: Insulin treatment in non-insulin-dependent diabetic patients undergoing minor surgery, *Diabetes Nutr Metab* 2:125, 1989.

22. Mogensen CE: Microalbuminuria predicts clinical proteinuria and early mortality in maturity onset diabetes, *N Engl J Med* 310:356, 1984.

23. Monk TG, Mueller M, White PF: Treatment of stress response during balanced anesthesia, *Anesthesiology* 76:39, 1992.

24. Monro JF, Campbell IW, McCuish AG, et al: Euglycemic diabetic ketoacidosis, *Br Med J* 2:578, 1973.

25. Pezzarossa A, Taddei F, Cimicchi MG, et al: Perioperative management of diabetic subjects: subcutaneous vs intravenous insulin administration during glucose-potassium infusion, *Diabetes Care* 11:52, 1988.

26. Pramming S, Thorsteinsson B, Bendtson I, et al: Nocturnal hypoglycemia in patients receiving conventional treatment with insulin, *Br Med J* 291:376, 1985.

27. Reddi AS, Camerini-Davalos RA: Diabetic nephropathy: an update, *Arch Intern Med* 150:31, 1990.

28. Root HF: Pre-operative care of the diabetic patient, *Postgrad Med* 40:439, 1989.

29. Schade DS: Surgery and diabetes, *Med Clin North Am* 72:1531, 1988.

30. Shuman CR: Medical management of the surgical diabetic patient, in Levin ME, O'Neal LW, editors: *The diabetic foot*, ed 4, St Louis, 1988, Mosby-Year Book, p 333.

31. Turner RC, Grayburn JA, Newman GB, et al: Measurement of the insulin delivery rate in man, *J Clin Endocrinol* 33:279, 1971.

32. Tuttle KR, Stein JH, DeFronzo RA: The natural history of diabetic nephropathy, *Semin Nephrol* 10:184, 1990.

33. Watts NB, Gebhart SP, Clark RV, et al: Perioperative management of diabetes mellitus: steady-state glucose control with bedside algorithm for insulin adjustment, *Diabetes Care* 10:722, 1987.

34. Wheelock, FC Jr, Gibbons GW, Marble A: Surgery in diabetes, in Marble A, Kroll LP, Bradley RF, et al, editors: *Joslin's diabetes mellitus*, ed 12, Philadelphia 1985, Lea & Febiger, Chapter 34.

35. Zarich SW, Nesto RW: Diabetic cardiomyopathy, *Am Heart J* 118:1000, 1989.

# CHAPTER 20

# Role of Lower Limb Amputation in Diabetes Mellitus

## John H. Bowker, M.D.

Because of the finality of amputation in both a physical and psychologic sense, it seems appropriate to present in a book on diabetic foot care current thought and available options regarding limb amputation, especially its mitigation by the selection of prophylactic surgery or minor ablations whenever possible.

In recent decades, the percentage of lower limb amputations in diabetics has been growing. In 17 studies published between 1961 and 1968, 52% of patients, on average, had diabetes mellitus as the primary causal factor in amputation. The percentage of diabetics in these studies ranged from 30% to 75%.* This contrasts sharply with an earlier study by Kendrick[27] in 1956 which reported a diabetic population of only 16%.

Although good amputation surgery today includes the conservation of all viable, uninfected tissue, this was not always the case. It was a maxim for many years that diabetics with a gangrenous foot lesion should have a primary amputation at the transfemoral (above-knee) level because of their supposed inability to heal more distal amputation levels. That this is not true was strikingly shown by four series that compared the healing rates of transtibial (below-knee) amputations in diabetics to those with purely ischemic disease. Of 194 diabetics, 92%

healed their wounds. In contrast, only 75% of 188 patients with purely ischemic disease achieved healing.[14, 25, 29, 42] Two other reported series, each with 100 diabetics, reported transtibial healing rates of 99% and 90%, respectively.[19, 24] It seems clear, therefore, that the notion that diabetics should have a transfemoral amputation for foot lesions should be discarded.

Now that rehabilitation has been added to the two previous traditional stages of amputation, namely, ablation and reconstruction, preservation of ambulatory function has become a major goal. Comparative reports on prosthesis usage for transfemoral and transtibial levels have become of major interest. Average transfemoral prosthesis usage has been reported to average only 26.5% in a series of four papers published from 1943 through 1983.[3, 5, 34, 44] This contrasts sharply with an average 73.5% transtibial prosthesis usage rate reported in 13 papers from 1943 to 1987.*

As information on both the acceptable healing rates and physiologic efficacy[47] of transtibial amputation accumulated, reported ratios of transtibial/transfemoral amputation have changed to favor the transtibial level. Two studies covering the 1930s through the 1950s had an average transtibial/transfemoral ratio of 1:2.6.[5, 16] In contrast, data from six papers written between

---

*See references 1, 2, 7, 12–15, 21, 22, 31, 32, 34, 36, 38, 40, 42, and 44.

*See references 3, 5, 6, 13, 15, 24, 29, 31, 33, 36, 40, 42, and 43.

1970 and 1983 showed a definite reversal to an average transtibial/transfemoral ratio of 2:1.[7, 19, 21, 25, 26, 39]

Wagner[45] has led the way in demonstrating the efficacy of ever more distal amputations based on a foot lesion grading system with therapeutic significance (Fig 20–1). He has also promoted an evaluation of circulatory competence that is inexpensive and readily available, the Doppler segmental systolic blood pressure method. Utilizing this approach, Wagner[45] has achieved wound healing in more than 90% of diabetic patients who met the criteria for blood flow and whose limbs were amputated at the indicated level. In brief, the criteria are systolic pressure at the proposed amputation site at least 45% of brachial pressure and absolute systolic pressure of 70 mm Hg or higher at the site. All pressures are determined with the patient supine.

If severe calcification of distal vessels has resulted in systolic pressure readings far above normal, transcutaneous oxygen readings may be helpful. If Doppler-derived pressures are well below the level required, a vascular surgeon should be consulted re-

garding reconstruction. In regard to any type of level selection, no matter how sophisticated the laboratory examination, it is important to realize that no method has yet been devised that is totally effective in predicting failure of amputation healing at any particular level.

When a patient presents with an unremitting or recurrent ulcer, grade 1 or 2, over a bony prominence, consideration should be given to reduction of the bony prominence by ostectomy through an incision that preferably does not impinge on the weight-bearing surface of the foot. This is best done once the ulcer has at least temporarily healed but has been successfully accomplished in many cases while the lesion was present as long as it was not acutely inflamed or infected. The situation arises especially in cases of bony prominences in the plantar aspect of the foot, which are residual to Charcot collapse of the midfoot. Other situations that may benefit from prophylactic reduction of bony prominences include bunions, hammer toes, and extremely prominent metatarsal heads. It is preferable, however, to attempt to control these sit-

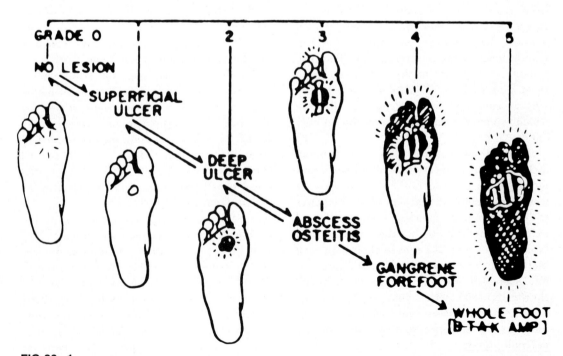

**FIG 20–1.**
Meggitt-Wagner diabetic foot lesion grading system. *(From* Resident training manual, *Ranchos Los Amigos Medical Center, Downey, Calif. Used by permission.)*

uations with proper shoewear. If this is not possible, careful vascular evaluation should be carried out preoperatively to give reasonable assurance that healing will occur.

## PREOPERATIVE CARE

In dealing with diabetic patients, with or without elements of peripheral vascular disease, the surgeon must assume that associated disease is present.[3, 40, 43] Special attention must be directed to control of arrhythmias, congestive heart failure, dehydration, electrolyte imbalance, hypertension, and bronchitis, as well as the diabetes itself. The emphasis should be on rapid preoperative treatment.

The infection that has led to the need for amputation may have totally disrupted regulation of the diabetic state. Because the control of hyperglycemia and infection are interdependent, they must be approached at the same time for optimum results (see Chapter 2). Broad-spectrum antibiotics should be started after aerobic and anaerobic wound cultures, pending bacterial sensitivity studies. Nephrotoxic drugs should be avoided if possible, but if needed, renal function must be closely monitored. To assist the surgeon in controlling these problems, a diabetologist, as well as an infection disease specialist, have much to offer both preoperatively and postoperatively (see Chapters 2 and 8).

Assessments of wound healing potential should include serum albumin levels as an indicator of nutritional status (normal ≥ 3.5 g/dL) and total lymphocyte count as a measure of immunocompetence (at least 1,500/mm³). If these are deficient, difficulty with primary wound healing may be expected.[18] Reversal of the catabolic state associated with severe infection should be initiated preoperatively. This is best done by oral hyperalimentation with the addition of nutritional supplements such as ascorbic acid, zinc, and ferrous sulfate. Significant increases in caloric intake, in an attempt to raise serum albumin levels, will require matching increases in insulin or other hypoglycemic agents.

At this juncture, a unique opportunity exists for the amputation surgeon to influence the surgical and prosthetic outcome insofar as patient compliance is concerned. To allay anxiety, the surgeon should outline a reasonably detailed account of the expected course, including prosthetic fitting. This is also an ideal opportunity for the surgeon to promote wound healing by strongly discouraging smoking both preoperatively and postoperatively.[40] A landmark Danish study showed a 50% increase in both wound infection and reamputation rates in cigarette-smoking lower limb amputees.[30]

If the patient's condition and time allow, the patient should meet the team members who will be caring for him or her postoperatively. Ideally the physical therapist can initiate a preoperative program to condition the entire body, prevent joint contractures, and teach safe ambulation with a walker or crutches.[12, 41] A preoperative visit by a trained amputee peer counselor matched with the patient by level of amputation, age, and sex can be very beneficial. A psychologist experienced in working with amputees can encourage them to express their anxieties regarding the surgical and prosthetic phases of care.

## QUALITIES OF GOOD AMPUTATIONS

Good amputation surgery includes the conservation of all tissue commensurate with the diagnosis. Any amputation must, of course, be done above the level of gangrenous tissue. Once this basic requirement has been met, an effort should be made to save maximum length to enhance future prosthetic usage.[8]

The next consideration is the provision of an adequate soft tissue envelope, consisting of skin, subcutaneous tissue, investing fascia and muscle, which will move easily over the enclosed bone and absorb shear forces at the limb-shoe or limb-prosthesis interface. Myoplasty (the suturing of muscles over the bone end) or, preferably, myodesis (the suturing of muscle to bone) will obviate the direct scarring of skin to bone. If not prevented, the adherent scar is likely to ulcerate, resulting in frequent interruptions of prosthesis use. Proper contouring of cut bone shafts is also very important to prevent soft tissue envelope damage from within as the bone compresses soft tissues between itself and the hard prosthetic socket or shoe.

Retention of a full range of proximal joint motion is another hallmark of a good amputation. This begins at surgery with correct muscle tensioning during myoplasty or myodesis and is enhanced by short-term rigid immobilization of joints during the painful postoperative phase. Thereafter, active range of motion exercises should suffice to prevent contractures.

There are several advantages in retaining maximum length of residual limb. A number of studies have shown that oxygen consumed per meter walked increases as the level of amputation rises, whereas gait cadence and velocity decrease (Fig 20–2).[4, 20, 47] Levels of amputation in the forefoot should require

the least increase in energy consumption, as well as the least alteration of body image. With less energy output, there is less cardiopulmonary stress, an important factor when one is dealing with diabetic dysvascular persons. The more distal the amputation, the better the opportunity to mask the physical loss and its accompanying impairment through retention of a more normal gait pattern.

## PARTIAL FOOT AMPUTATION

Until the middle of this century partial foot amputations were done almost exclusively after trauma. Both dry and wet gangrene were commonly treated by transfemoral and, later, transtibial amputation, the choice often being idiosyncratic based on the attitudes and prejudices of the surgeon and the prosthetist regarding a given level.

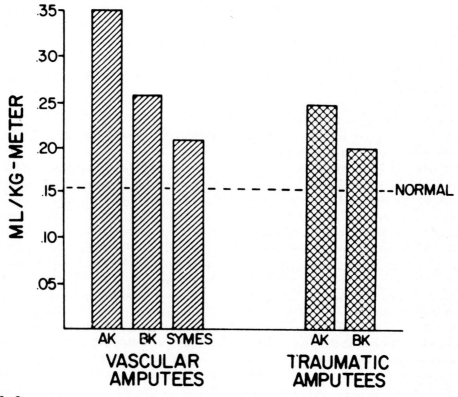

**FIG 20–2.**
Oxygen consumed per meter traveled in dysvascular and traumatic amputees at selected levels compared with normal. *(From Waters, RL, Perry J, Antonelli D, et al:* J Bone Joint Surg [Am] *58A:42–46, 1976. Used by permission.)*

At the present time, with confidence bolstered by better methods of level selection based on vascular and nutritional evaluations, a growing number of partial foot amputations are being done in cases of diabetes mellitus.

The partial foot amputee will continue to bear weight on the remaining foot in an approximately normal manner because of retention of most of the usual proprioceptive channels as opposed to the transtibial level in which an entirely new feedback pattern must be interpreted. After partial foot amputations, the heel lever is intact, and a variable portion of the forefoot (toe) lever remains. This ranges from full length in the case of a ray (toe and metatarsal) amputation to virtually none in the case of a midtarsal (Chopart) amputation. The degree of normality of the gait pattern depends largely on the length of the residual forefoot lever. Therefore forefoot lever length should be preserved whenever possible by election of a longitudinal (ray) amputation rather than a transverse level (transmetatarsal), tarsometatarsal (Lisfranc) or midtarsal (Chopart). One major advantage that all partial foot amputees share, however, is independence of a prosthesis in an emergency situation.

## Toes

In all partial foot amputations, the first step is debridement of all necrotic and infected tissue, including bone. All visually uninvolved tissue should be preserved for reconstruction. It follows that the flaps preserved for closure are frequently nonstandard in configuration. Primary wound closure can often be accomplished according to criteria discussed later. In the case of osteomyelitis of the distal phalanx of the great toe, if sufficient skin can be salvaged to cover the proximal phalanx, the resulting gait will be better than that after ablation at the metatarsophalangeal joint (Fig 20–3). Infection of the distal phalanx of the lesser toes, often seen with fixed mallet toe, can also be treated by removing only that phalanx (Fig 20–4). Removing the second toe alone removes the lateral support required by the hallux to prevent valgus (bunion) deformity (Fig 20–5). Because this results in greater bony prominence, it is better in this case to remove the second metatarsal at its proximal metaphysis along with the toe. The foot can then narrow, resulting in a good cosmetic and functional result (Fig 20–6). If toes 3 or 4 alone are removed, the

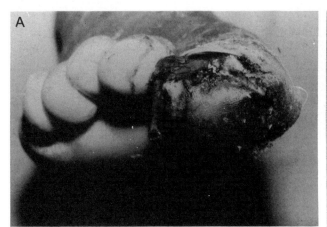
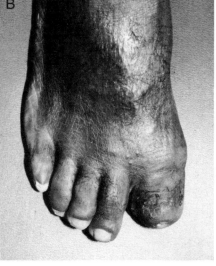

**FIG 20–3.**
**A,** 49-year-old diabetic with necrosis of the great toe and adequate web-space Doppler systolic pressures. **B,** same case showing interphalangeal amputation resulting from conservative debridement and closure over Kritter irrigation system. *(From Bowker JH:* AAOS Instructional Course Lecture *39:355–360, 1990. Used by permission.)*

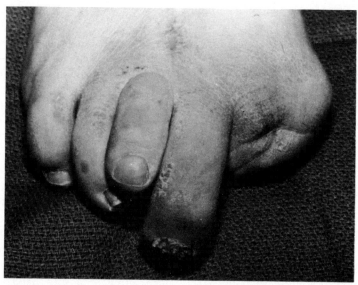

**FIG 20–4.**
Osteomyelitis in distal phalanx of the right second toe with mallet deformity at the distal interphalangeal joint. Long second metatarsal, as well as absence of great toe, combined to produce a toe at risk in this insensate foot. Excision of the distal phalanx with primary closure was curative.

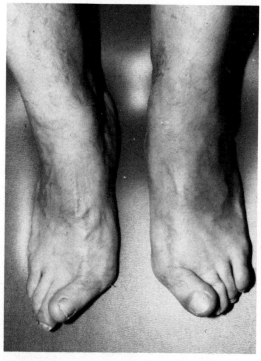

**FIG 20–5.**
Amputation of infected second toes with retention of second metatarsals has resulted in bilateral hallux valgus (bunion deformity) because of loss of lateral support of the great toes by the second toes. *Reprinted with permission (From Bowker JH. Atlas of limb prosthetics, ed 2, St Louis, 1992, Mosby Year Book, Chapter 2D.)*

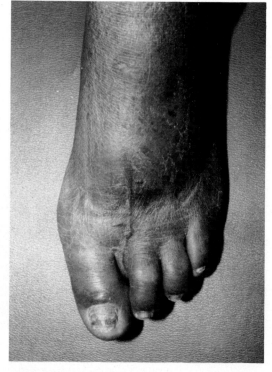

**FIG 20–6.**
Left foot with second ray resection for diabetic infection shows no significant hallux valgus because of lateral support provided by third toe after postoperative forefoot narrowing. *(From Bowker JH: Atlas of limb prosthetics, ed 2, St Louis, 1992, Mosby Year Book, Chapter 2D.)*

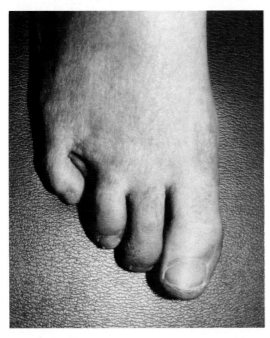

**FIG 20–7.**
Medial shift of right fifth toe to fill gap left by amputation of fourth toe tends to restore contour of distal forefoot. Fifth toe has developed no ulcerations since amputation 8½ years ago.

adjacent ones will tend to shift and fill in the gap (Fig 20–7). Leaving a lesser toe isolated should not be done because of its increased susceptibility to injury (Fig 20–8).

## Ray Resections

Ray resections are excellent examples of conservative forefoot ablations. The best of these, from both the functional and cosmetic points of view, are those of single lesser rays. In this case, only the width of the forefoot lever is affected, but rollover function and overall foot balance during terminal stance is not (Fig 20–9). Removal of the first ray is devastating to both stance and gait because an intact medial column is essential to proper forward progression (Fig 20–10). Because most infections of the first metatar-

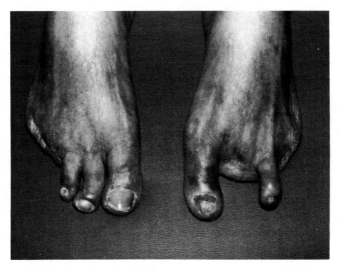

**FIG 20–8.**
Note striking difference in distal forefoot contours of right and left feet. On the right, the remaining lesser toes are protected by the great toe. On the left, the fourth toe is constantly exposed to minor trauma and should have been removed with the other lesser toes.

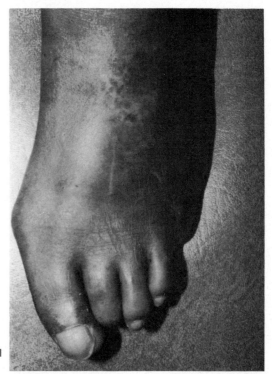

**FIG 20–9.**
Narrowing of forefoot after fifth ray amputation is
easily compensated by soft shoe insert with lateral
filler.

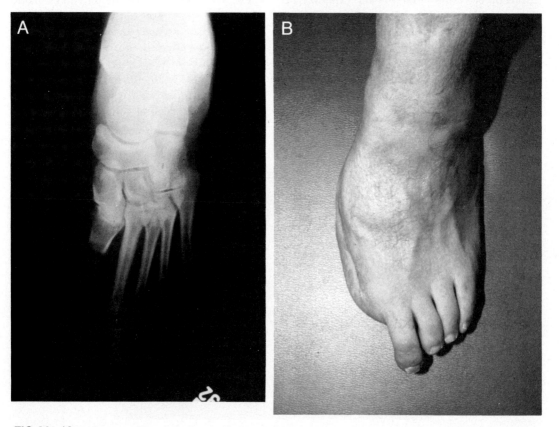

**FIG 20–10.**
**A,** radiograph of left foot after radical first ray amputation for a diabetic infection. There is insufficient metatarsal
shaft remaining to allow effective orthotic support. **B,** note planovalgus of foot secondary to loss of medial column
support. *(From Bowker JH:* J Prosthet Orthot *4:23–30, 1991. Used by permission.)*

sal involve only its head, as well as the hallux, it is usually feasible to save most of the metatarsal shaft. With this approach, a custom-molded shoe insert can be made that will support the medial arch of the foot in appropriate shoewear (see Chapters 24 and 25). The removal of two or more central rays is a poor choice both functionally and cosmetically (Fig 20–11). In contrast, all lateral toes and portions of their metatarsals can be removed in an oblique fashion with a good functional result once shod, providing the first ray remains intact (Fig 20–12).[9]

## Transmetatarsal Amputation

Transmetatarsal amputation is a viable option when all of the distal forefoot is involved transversely or if there is sufficient loss of the first and second rays to seriously disturb the balance of the forefoot. Blood flow studies at the metatarsal head level should be done to ensure that there is sufficient circulation to the distal plantar skin to support the flap (Fig 20–13). The longer the forefoot lever remaining, the better. To avoid removing excess metatarsal length, the surgeon should start the cuts on the medial side of the foot. Often just a partial removal of the first metatarsal head can be done, which will then allow relatively distal transections of the lesser metatarsals in a line parallel to the metatarsophalangeal toe break as the surgeon proceeds across the foot. The shafts should be contoured (beveled) on the plantar side to protect the plantar skin during gait. Sufficient intact skin should be present to cover the plantar and distal aspects of the metatarsal shafts (Fig 20–14). Any skin missing on the dorsum of

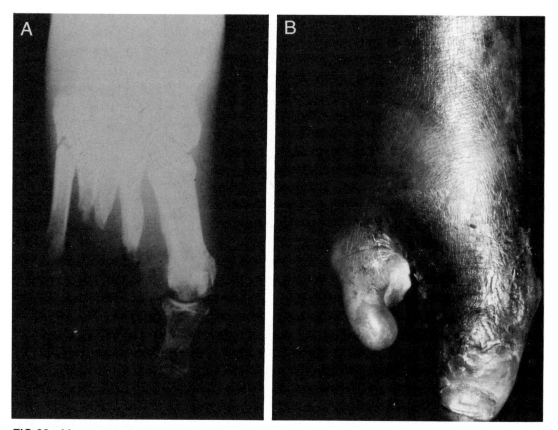

**FIG 20–11.**
**A,** radiograph of right foot after excision of three central rays for diabetic abscess. **B**, note poor cosmetic and functional result. The patient required a transmetatarsal amputation to correct continual plantar soft tissue ulceration. An oblique removal of all lateral rays might have averted this outcome. **(B** *from Bowker JH:* J Prosthet Orthot *4:23–30, 1991. Used by permission.)*

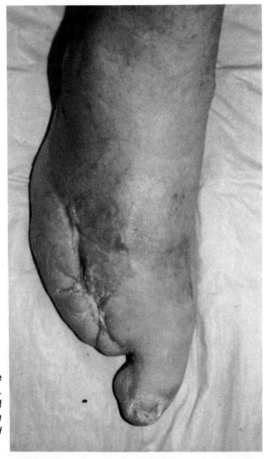

**FIG 20–12.**
The four lateral rays have been excised in an oblique fashion for severe abscess, leaving the first ray intact. Walking with shoes remained excellent because of preservation of medial arch and foot length. *(From Bowker JH: J Prosthet Orthot 4:23–30. 1991. Used by permission.)*

the foot can be easily replaced with split skin graft, but this is not advisable on the distal end of the residual foot if ulcerative breakdown is to be avoided.

## Tarsometatarsal (Lisfranc) and Midtarsal (Chopart) Amputation

There is a major caveat regarding these levels of amputation. If they are attempted in infected cases and fail, it may be very difficult to salvage a Syme ankle disarticulation because of the proximity of necrotic or infected tissue to the heel pad. At the tarsometatarsal level, great care must be taken to *preserve* the insertions of the forefoot extrinsic muscles. At the midtarsal level, the extrinsic muscles should be carefully dissected out and reattached to the talus (Fig 20–15).[46] Otherwise, severe muscle imbalance will occur. A percutaneous fractional heel cord lengthening is also strongly recom-

mended at these levels to weaken the triceps surae to further help prevent an equinus deformity (Fig 20–16). At either level, contracture can be discouraged and further triceps surae weakness induced by use of a postoperative cast for several weeks with the residual foot in a plantigrade position.

## Primary Closure Vs. Open Packing of Partial Foot Amputation Wounds

Prior to the pioneering work of Kritter,[28] partial amputations of the foot in diabetics were invariably left open. His studies led to a revolution in the closed management of these amputations. If his principles for closure are followed, primary healing can be achieved in 3 to 4 weeks in most cases. This avoids healing by secondary intention, which often takes 4 to 6 months. It may be used in any case in which pus in the presenting wound is either absent or minimal. With

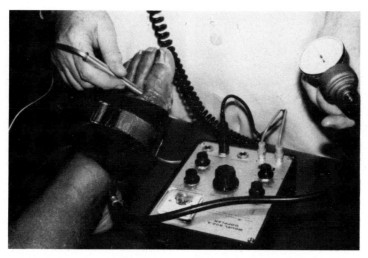

**FIG 20–13.**
Determination of systolic blood pressure at level of metatarsal necks by use of Doppler effect. Note placement of child-sized cuff on the midfoot. *(From Bowker JH:* Atlas of limb prosthetics, *ed 2, St Louis, 1992, Mosby Year Book, Chapter 2D.)*

the completion of debridement, the wound should appear clean with minimal inflammation of the remaining tissues. The methodology is quite simple. A 14- or 16-gauge polyethylene intravenous (IV) catheter with insertion needle is passed through the skin into the depths of the wound. The needle is withdrawn, the catheter trimmed to length, and the catheter hub sutured in place to the skin. A bag of normal saline solution is attached and run slowly into the wound. Once the system has been noted to be running well, the wound is closed loosely with a few widely spaced simple cutaneous sutures (Fig 20–17). The fluid escapes from the wound between the sutures and is absorbed by a soft dressing (Fig 20–18). Its outer portion is changed every 4 hours. The irrigation

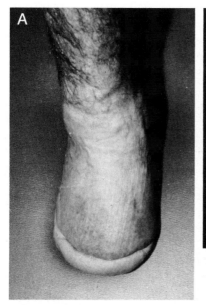
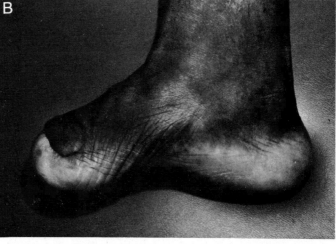

**FIG 20–14.**
Adequate transmetatarsal amputation . **A,** dorsal view. **B,** medial view. Note placement of distal plantar skin flap, overall length of residual forefoot, maintenance of medial arch, and absence of equinus deformity.

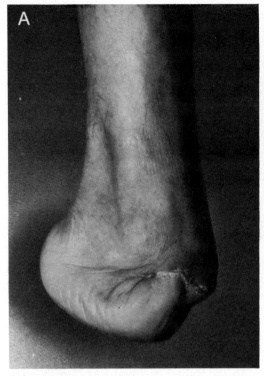
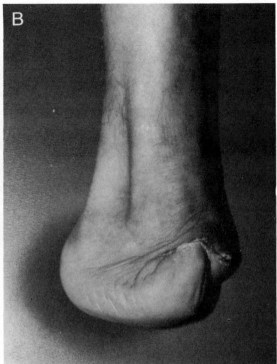

**FIG 20–15.**
Midtarsal (Chopart's) amputation. **A,** plantar flexed by intact triceps surae. **B,** dorsiflexed to neutral position by anterior tibial muscle attached to talus at time of reconstruction.

continues for 3 days at a rate of 1 L every 24 hours. Appropriate IV antibiotics are given concomitantly. If there is any evidence of purulence at the end of the irrigation period, the wound can simply be opened and packed at the bedside. With strict adherence to the criteria, however, this rarely occurs.

## SYME ANKLE DISARTICULATION

The advantage of the Syme ankle disarticulation over the transtibial level is end weight–bearing on the heel pad with normally channeled proprioceptive feedback (Figs 20–19 and 20–20). There are three

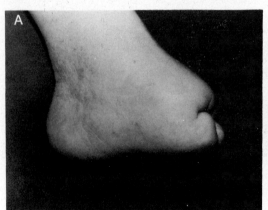
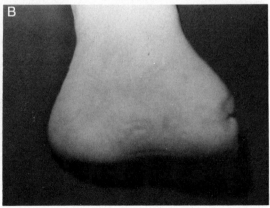

**FIG 20–16.**
Tarsometatarsal (Lisfranc's) amputation. **A,** 73-year-old diabetic woman in nursing home unable to walk in low partial foot prosthesis and shoe because of fixed equinus deformity. **B,** medial view of foot after percutaneous fractional heel cord lengthening. She attained adequate household ambulation status.

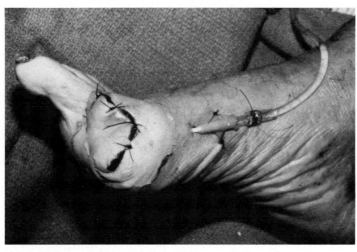

**FIG 20–17.**
Disarticulation of right great toe for diabetic gangrene with closure using flap salvaged from lateral aspect of toe. Note Kritter flow-through irrigation system. Sutures are widely spaced to permit egress of irrigation fluid. *(From Bowker JH: Atlas of limb prosthetics, ed 2, St Louis, 1992, Mosby Year Book, Chapter 2D.)*

criteris for success in this procedure. The first is selection of the proper candidate. Because the heel pad depends on the posterior tibial artery for its blood supply, preoperative evaluation of heel pad circulation is strongly recommended. Healing in malnourished persons or in those on renal dialysis is unreliable, although those with renal transplants will heal, albeit slowly. The key is a normal serum albumin level. A totally noncompliant patient is generally not a good candidate for this procedure.

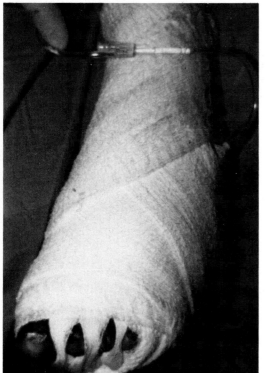

**FIG 20–18.**
Kritter irrigation system installed in left second ray amputation. Note the bulky bandage used to absorb irrigation fluid. The outer of three rolls is replaced every few hours. *(From Bowker JH: Atlas of limb prosthetics, ed 2, St Louis, 1992, Mosby Year Book, Chapter 2D.)*

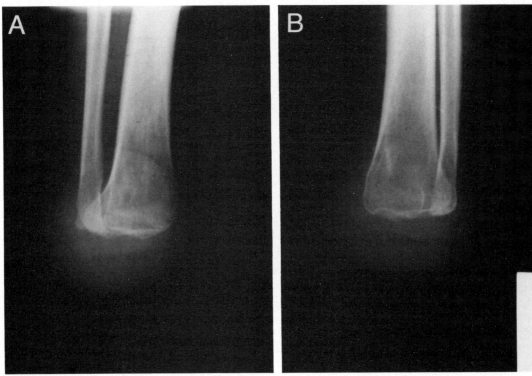

**FIG 20–19.**
**A,** lateral and, **B,** anteroposterior radiographs of a Syme ankle disarticulation. Note symmetric placement of thick fatty heel pad beneath tibia and fibula. The malleoli have been trimmed distally and laterally to reduce distal stump bulkiness.

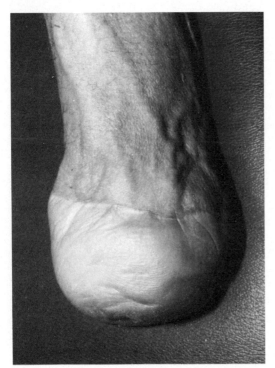

**FIG 20–20.**
Left Syme ankle disarticulation in 37-year-old type I diabetic woman 8 years after surgery. Although insensate to knee, she actively wears her prosthesis 14 to 16 hours daily.

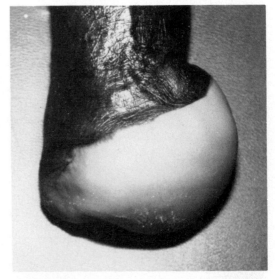

**FIG 20–21.**
Right Syme ankle disarticulation with fixed medial displacement of heel pad from walking without prosthesis. Ulcer is present distal to lateral malleolus made prominent by pad shift. Reduction required removal of 1.5 cm of distal tibia and fibula and resection of medial scar tissue. *(From Bowker JH, et al: Atlas of limb prosthetics, 1992, St Louis, Mosby Year Book, Chapter 25.)*

The second criterion is meticulous surgical technique. This is required throughout the procedure to avoid damage to the posterior tibial artery and to the vertically oriented, fat-filled chambers of the heel pad that provide cushioning for comfortable and long-lasting end bearing.[23] The heel pad flap must be meticulously designed and fitted to avoid both tissue redundancy or closure under tension. Either error can lead to failure of the procedure. Suturing of the deep fascial tissues of the heel pad to the anterior tibial cortex through drill holes is recommended to hold it firmly in place.

The third criterion is maintenance of the heel pad in a central position beneath the distal tibia. Postoperative application of a carefully padded lightweight cast of plaster of Paris or fiberglass will prevent pad shift during the first few weeks of healing. Once the pad is secure at 4 to 5 weeks, a walking cast can be applied. Regular cast changes are required as volume reduction occurs. Once the prosthesis is fit, minimal training is required for walking. Centralization of the heel pad is maintained as a function of a carefully maintained prosthesis. Patients are cautioned to avoid weight bearing without the prosthesis to prevent heel pad shift (Fig 20–21).

## TRANSTIBIAL (BELOW-KNEE) AMPUTATION

Because of preservation of the knee joint, this is the most proximal level at which near-normal function is available to the lower limb amputee.[10] Once it has been determined that the proximal extent of infection along tissue planes has precluded the choice of a partial foot amputation or Syme ankle disarticulation, transtibial amputation should be strongly considered rather than a transfemoral level.

If the patient has a severely abscessed foot, an open ankle disarticulation can be carried out in a very few minutes with the patient under local anesthesia (Fig 20–22). This will allow rapid reversal of the infection, enhancing control of the blood glucose

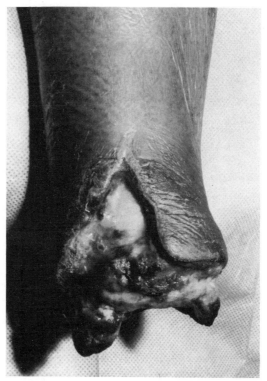

**FIG 20–22.**
Open ankle disarticulation for severe diabetic infection of entire foot. Note debridement of necrotic skin and distal tendons. *(From Bowker JH:* AAOS Instructional Course Lectures 39:355–360, 1990. *Used by permission.)*

level. This is far preferable to freezing procedures for control of severe foot infection, which are likely to cause thermal necrosis of normal calf tissues, leading to a transfemoral amputation.[35] If pus has tracked along musculotendinous planes, incisions can be extended proximally along the medial and lateral sides of the leg as necessary to drain and debride all involved compartments of infected and necrotic tissue (Fig 20–23,A and B). This technique will help preserve length for better limb-socket weight distribution and prosthetic function (Fig 20–23,C). The alternative to this approach is an initial short transtibial amputation well above any obvious infection if primary closure disregarding optimum function is the goal of the surgeon.

The only absolute contraindication to transtibial amputation is inadequate vascularity at amputation sites between the knee

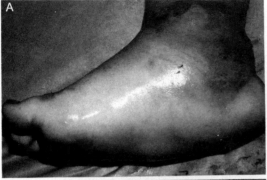

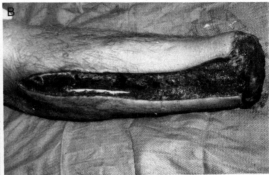

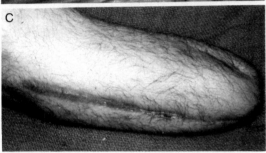

**FIG 20–23.**
**A,** severely abscessed right foot of 43-year-old insulin-dependent diabetic before supramalleolar amputation and wide debridement of all crural compartments for ascending infection. **B,** 17 days later. Anterior compartment wound is well granulated at time of partial closure. **C,** 3 months after initial open amputation. The residual limb is ready for prosthetic fitting. *(From Bowker JH, et al: Atlas of limb prosthetics, ed 2, St Louis, 1992, Mosby Year Book, Chapter 18A.)*

and ankle. With popliteal Doppler segmental systolic pressures at 50 mm Hg or more, healing is likely to occur. In the absence of detectable popliteal flow, a transfemoral amputation is suggested.[17] There are also conditions mistakenly thought of as contraindications. Loss of sensation at levels below the knee because of diabetic neuropathy does not represent a contraindication. With good prosthetic fitting and regular observation of the skin for areas of undue pressure, the amputee should do well. Even selected hemiparetic patients can become household ambulators with a transtibial prosthesis, provided that flexion or extension patterning is not extreme and that they develop reasonable balance and retain the ability to comprehend instructions (Fig 20–24). Some patients who are not prosthetic candidates will have sitting, turning, and kneeling abilities enhanced by leaving as much of the leg below the knee as possible.

Currently the most popular method of transtibial amputation utilizes a long posterior myofasciocutaneous flap, as introduced by Bickel[5] in 1943 and widely popularized by the educational efforts of Burgess.[11] The technique for long transtibial amputation that I use is described in detail elsewhere (Fig 20–25).[10] This method works equally

well whether the amputation is primary, above the level of distal gangrenous changes, or is a secondary procedure after initial fasciotomy or debridement of an infected leg. In this case, the medial and lateral debridement incisions on the leg fit very well into the final closure pattern (Fig 20–26).[10]

In either case, the provision of an adequate soft tissue envelope for the residual limb is paramount. A good posterior myofasciocutaneous flap can be formed down to the distal extent of the soleus muscle, with the technique becoming progressively easier as the amputation becomes more distal. There are several anatomic reasons for this. With distal tapering of the calf, the cross-sectional area of the leg progressively decreases, resulting in a much shorter and wider-based flap (Fig 20–27). Because posterior muscle bulk distally is less than in proximal areas of the leg, there is much less muscle excision required, less tendency for "dog-ear" formation, and far fewer venous complexes to ligate.

The end of the tibia and fibula are enclosed in muscle tissue, preferably by myodesis of the muscle to the tibia through drill holes (Fig 20–28). The present availability of strong absorbable suture materials obviates the need for permanent sutures. Subcu-

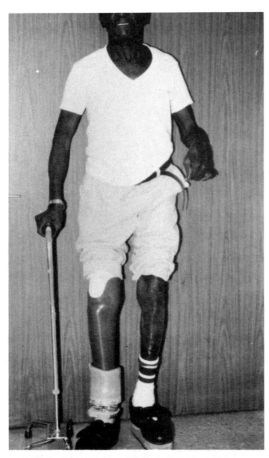

**FIG 20–24.**
Seventy-three-year-old diabetic with left hemiparesis after a cerebrovascular accident and a right transtibial amputation. He required a temporary shoe lift on the left until the prosthetic alignment device was removed with completion of the prosthesis. *(From Bowker JH, et al: Atlas of limb prosthetics, ed 2, St Louis, 1992, Mosby Year Book, Chapter 18A.)*

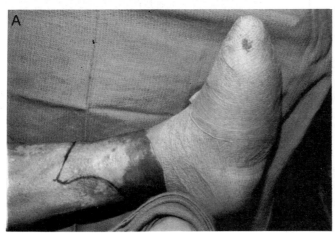

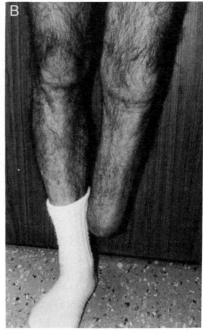

**FIG 20–25.**
**A,** lateral view of right leg and foot showing outline of a very short anterior flap and a long posterior flap adapted from FW Wagner, Jr., for use in long transtibial amputation. **B,** length comparison in 51-year-old diabetic between long transtibial amputation and intact lower limb. With a residual limb of this length, energy consumption for prosthetic ambulation is close to normal. *(**A** from Bowker JH, et al: Atlas of limb prosthetics, ed 2, St Louis, 1992, Mosby Year Book, Chapter 18A.)*

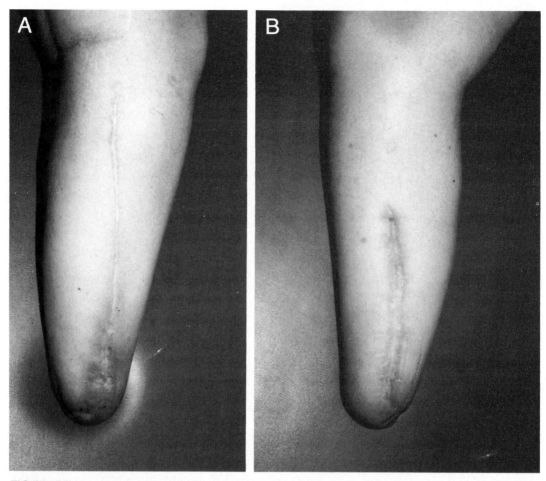

**FIG 20–26.**
**A,** lateral and, **B,** medial views of long transtibial amputation salvaged in case with infection ascending from abscessed foot. Complete debridement of lateral and posterior compartments was followed 2 weeks later by excision of clean granulation wounds and closure. *(**A** from Bowker JH:* AAOS Instructional Course Lectures *39:355–360, 1990. Used by permission.)*

taneous sutures are not necessary. During closure the skin is manipulated with gloved fingers and needle only, not contused with forceps. Widely spaced simple skin sutures are supplemented with adhesive paper strips (Fig 20–29).

The ideal cylindrical shape of a long transtibial amputation is enhanced by transecting the fibula only 0.5 to 1.0 cm shorter than the tibia (Fig 20–30). Bone wax should never be used in amputation surgery, because it interferes with secure healing of the deep soft tissues to the bone. Postoperative complications of edema, wound trauma, and knee flexion contracture are prevented by applying a very light and well-padded plaster or fiberglass cast with the knee in full extension (Fig 20–31). It is worn for 3 weeks,

with weekly changes for wound inspection and knee range of motion.

## KNEE DISARTICULATION

There are specific, limited indications for a knee disarticulation in the diabetic. If the patient has a knee flexion contracture severe enough to prevent use of a transtibial prosthesis, a knee disarticulation will provide the possibility of functional gait, although at a greater energy cost than required at the transtibial level. A relative indication for knee disarticulation is prolonged nonambulatory status. The frequent outcome of a transtibial amputation in the bed-bound, noncooperative patient is a knee flexion con-

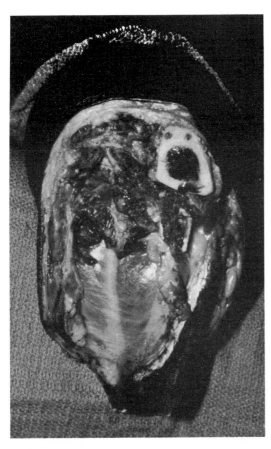

**FIG 20–27.**
Intraoperative view of a long transtibial amputation.
The deep posterior calf muscles have been excised
before myodesis to reduce distal bulkiness of the
stump. The gastrosoleus muscle provides good distal
padding. Note the drill holes placed in the tibia for
myodesis. *(From Bowker JH, et al:* Atlas of limb
prosthetics, *ed 2, St Louis, 1992, Mosby Year Book,
Chapter 25.)*

tracture with development of a pressure ulcer at the end (Fig 20–32). A knee disarticulation in such a situation will provide much
better sitting balance than a transfemoral
residual limb (Fig 20–33).[37] The knee disarticulation provides a muscle balanced residual limb with excellent end weight–bearing
capabilities. If the patient's mental and
physical status improve sufficiently, ambulation can then be attempted.

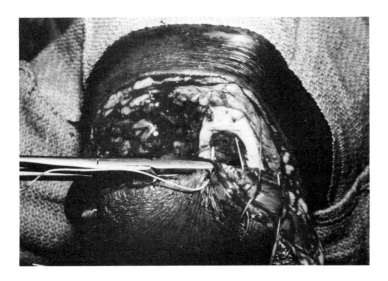

**FIG 20–28.**
Intraoperative view of myodesis in which the posterior myofascia and posterior and anterior investing fascia are
sutured to the tibia through drill holes. *(From Bowker JH, et al:* Atlas of limb prosthetics, *ed 2, St Louis, 1992,
Mosby Year Book, Chapter 25.)*

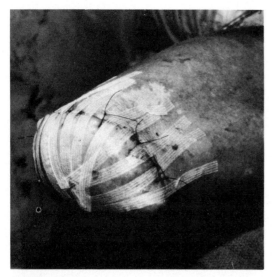

**FIG 20–29.**
Transtibial amputation wound loosely closed with a few widely spaced skin sutures reinforced with adhesive paper strips. In this way constriction of skin flaps is minimized. *(From Bowker JH, et al: Atlas of limb prosthetics, ed 2, St Louis, 1992, Mosby Year Book, Chapter 18A.)*

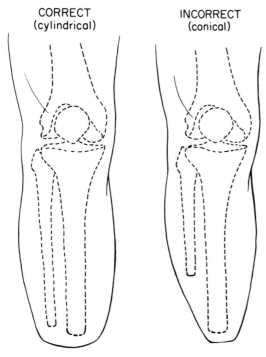

**FIG 20–30.**
A cylindrical residual limb results from cutting the fibula only minimally shorter than the tibia. This is preferable to a conical shape, which is produced by cutting the fibula too short, which makes the distal portion of the tibia unduly prominent. *(From Moore WS, Malone JM, editors: Lower extremity amputation, Philadelphia, 1989, WB Saunders. Used by permission.)*

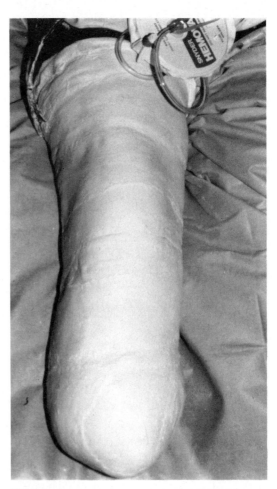

**FIG 20–31.**
Plaster of paris cast applied to long transtibial amputation with knee in full extension to prevent knee flexion contracture. The patella is heavily padded to prevent a pressure sore. Note drain tube exiting proximal end of cast for easy removal without disturbing cast. *(From Bowker JH, et al: Atlas of limb prosthetics, ed 2, St Louis, 1992, Mosby Year Book, Chapter 18A.)*

## TRANSFEMORAL (ABOVE-KNEE) AMPUTATION

There are very few indications for primary transfemoral amputation in the diabetic. One is aggressive, neglected infection that has moved along tissue planes proximal to the knee. Another is severe dysvascularity associated with diabetes in which no viable tissue distal to the knee remains. In cases of infection, a primary open amputation is mandatory. After resolution of the infection, the wound may be closed. If muscles are sufficiently viable to tolerate moderate tension,

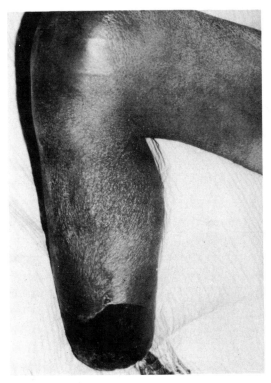

**FIG 20–32.**
Transtibial amputation in bed-bound diabetic. Note severe knee flexion contracture and necrotic distal end from excessive pressure. In retrospect, a primary knee disarticulation would have better served this patient.

a myodesis to the femur should be carried out; otherwise, a myoplasty can be done. The transfemoral level should be the last considered as the chances of an older patient becoming a functional walker are minimal.[3, 5, 34, 43]

## SUMMARY

Major amputation surgery in the diabetic is to be avoided if at all possible. Significant advances in blood flow determination, nutritional evaluation, antibiotic regimens, and techniques for salvage of the diabetic foot have occurred in recent years, making limb salvage rather than amputation the goal. This is provided that the salvaged limb will be functionally better than its prosthetic counterpart, keeping in mind that prosthetic replacement after amputation continues to fall far short in restoration of lost motor and sensory function.

The modern premise is that amputation is no longer considered simply the ablation of a useless or debilitating part but a reconstructive procedure to restore independent ambulation. To achieve optimal function, both the surgeon and patient must be willing to proceed with staged procedures, if necessary, to achieve the ultimate goal of a residual limb that will interface well with modified footwear or a prosthesis. To achieve this goal, an experienced surgeon should perform or directly oversee the amputation; it should not be delegated to the least experienced surgeon in training to do unsupervised.

After the proper selection of level for amputation, the most important criteria for successful surgery are the gentle handling of tissues and their proper technical management during the procedure. Tissue envelope flaps must be accurately related to the cross section of the limb at the bony level selected. This will eliminate the need for bone shortening to avoid closure under tension or the problems inherent in fitting limbs with redundant soft tissue. Although incision placement can be crucial in partial foot amputations, a variety of flap configurations in transtibial and transfemoral procedures have shown that incision site is not important as long as an adequate soft tissue envelope prevents incision scar adherence to underlying bone. It cannot be emphasized enough that the attitude of the surgeon toward amputation as a therapeutic modality affects the manner in which the amputation is performed, as well as the way in which postoperative management, including prosthetic care, is handled.

The prevention of lower limb amputation by salvage of all or most of the foot in patients with diabetic foot infections has become a reality. Success depends on timely presentation of the patient and control of hyperglycemia and infection by a combination of early and complete debridement, appropriate antibiotics, insulin, and nutritional enhancement. In cases of dry gangrene, a vascular surgeon should be consulted regarding the feasibility of vessel recanalization or reconstruction. Once healing has been achieved, the amputee must remain

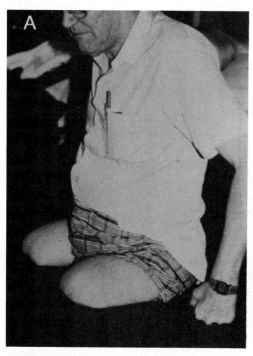
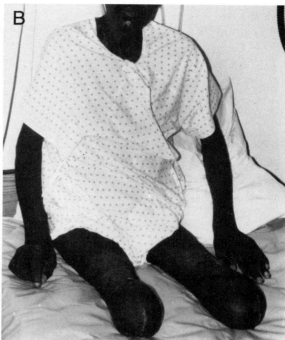

**FIG 20–33.**
**A,** bilateral transfemoral amputee with precarious sitting balance on short residual limbs. **B,** bilateral knee disarticulate showing good sitting balance because of large posterior thigh supporting surface. *(From Pinzur MS:* Atlas of limb prosthetics, *ed 2, St Louis, 1992, Mosby Year Book, Chapter 19A.)*

actively engaged on a life-long basis in a program devoted to prevention of further skin breakdown by use of appropriate footwear, tight control of diabetes, and education in foot care with emphasis on assumption of responsibility for self-care.

# REFERENCES

1. Alter AH, Moshein J, Elconin KB, et al: Below-knee amputation using the sagittal technique: a comparison with the coronal amputation, *Clin Orthop* 131:195–201, 1978.

2. Baker WH, Barnes RW, Shurr DG: The healing of below-knee amputations: a comparison of soft and plaster dressings, *Am J Surg* 133:716–718, 1977.

3. Barber GG, McPhail NV, Scobie TK, et al: A prospective study of lower limb amputations, *Can J Surg* 26:339–341, 1983.

4. Bard G, Ralston HJ: Measurement of energy expenditure during ambulation, with special reference to evaluation of assistive devices, *Arch Phys Med Rehabil* 40:415–420, 1959.

5. Bickel WH: Amputations below-the-knee in occlusive arterial diseases, *Surg Clin North Am* 23:982–994, 1943.

6. Block MA, Whitehouse FW: Below-knee amputation in patients with diabetes mellitus, *Arch Surg* 87:682–689, 1963.

7. Boontje AH: Major amputations of the lower extremity for vascular disease, *Prosthet Orthot Int* 4:87–89, 1980.

8. Bowker JH: Surgical techniques for conserving tissue and function in lower limb amputation for trauma, infection and vascular disease, *AAOS Instructional Course Lectures* 39:355–360, 1990.

9. Bowker JH: Medical and surgical considerations in the care of patients with insensate dysvascular feet, *J Prosthet Orthot* 4:23–30, 1991.

10. Bowker JH, Goldberg B, Poonekar PD: Transtibial amputation: surgical procedures and immediate postsurgical management, in Bowker JH, Michael JW, editors: *Atlas of limb prosthetics: surgical, prosthetic and rehabilitation principles*, ed 2, St Louis, 1992, Mosby-Year Book, Chapter 18A.

11. Burgess EM: The below-knee amputation, *Bull Prosthet Res* 10:19–25, 1968.

12. Castronuovo JJ, Deane LJ, Deterling RA, et al: Below-knee amputation: is the effort to preserve the knee joint justified? *Arch Surg* 115:1184–1187, 1980.

13. Chilvers AS, Briggs J, Browse NL, et al: Below- and through-knee amputations in ischaemic disease, *Br J Surg* 58:824–826, 1971.

14. Cranley JJ, Krause RJ, Strasser RS, et al: Below-the-knee amputation for arteriosclerosis obliterans, *Arch Surg* 98:77–80, 1969.

15. Cumming JGR, Jain AS, Walker WF, et al: Fate of the vascular patient after below-knee amputation, *Lancet* 2:613–615, 1987.

16. Dale WA, Capps W: Major leg and thigh amputations, *Surgery* 46:333–342, 1959.

17. Dean FH, Yao JST, Thompson RG, et al: Predictive value of ultrasonically-derived arterial pressure in determination of amputation level, *Am Surg* 41:731–737, 1975.

18. Dickhaut SC, DeLee JC, Page CP: Nutritional status: importance in predicting wound-healing after amputation, *J Bone Joint Surg (Am)* 66A:71–75, 1984.

19. Fearon J, Campbell DR, Hoar CS, et al: Improved results with diabetic below-knee amputees, *Arch Surg* 120:777–780, 1985.

20. Gonzalez EG, Corcoran PJ, Reyes RL: Energy expenditure in below-knee amputees: correlation with stump length, *Arch Phys Med Rehabil* 55:111–119, 1974.

21. Harris JP, Page S, Englund R, et al: Is the outlook for the vascular amputee improved by striving to preserve the knee? *J Cardiovasc Surg* 29:741–745, 1988.

22. Harris PD, Schwartz SI, DeWeese JA: Midcalf amputation for peripheral vascular disease, *Arch Surg* 82:381–383, 1961.

23. Harris RI: Syme's amputation: the technical details essential for success, *J Bone Joint Surg (Br)* 38B:614–632, 1956.

24. Hoar CS, Torres J: Evaluation of below-the-knee amputation in the treatment of diabetic gangrene, *N Engl J Med* 266:440–443, 1962.

25. Kacy SS, Wolma FJ, Flye MW: Factors affecting the results of below-knee amputation in patients with and without diabetes, *Surg Gynecol Obstet* 155:513–518, 1982.

26. Keagy BA, Schwartz JA, Kotb M, et al: Lower extremity amputations: the control series, *J Vasc Surg* 4:321–326, 1986.

27. Kendrick RR: Below-knee amputation in arteriosclerotic gangrene, *Br J Surg* 44:13–17, 1956.

28. Kritter AE: A technique for salvage of the infected diabetic foot, *Orthop Clin North Am* 4:21–30, 1973.

29. Lim RC, Blaisdell FW, Hall AD, et al: Below-knee amputation for ischemic gangrene, *Surg Gynecol Obstet* 125:493–501, 1967.

30. Lind J, Kramhoff M, Bodtker S: The influence of smoking on complications after primary amputations of the lower extremity, *Clin Orthop Related Res* 267:211–217, 1991.

31. Moore WS, Hall AD, Lim RC: Below-the-knee amputation for ischemic gangrene: comparative results of conventional operation and immediate postoperative fitting technique, *Am J Surg* 124:127–134, 1972.

32. Murdoch G: Amputation surgery in the lower extremity, *Prosthet Orthot Int* 1:72–83, 1977.

33. Murray DG: Below-knee amputations in the aged: evaluation and prognosis, *Geriatrics* 20:1033–1038, 1965.

34. Paloschi GB, Lynn RB: Major amputations for obliterative peripheral vascular disease with particular reference to the role of below-knee amputation, *Can J Surg* 10:168–171, 1967.

35. Pedersen HE, LaMont RL, Ramsey RH: Below-knee amputation for gangrene, *South Med J* 57:820–825, 1964.

36. Perry T: Below-knee amputations, *Arch Surg* 86:199–202, 1963.

37. Pinzur MS: Knee disarticulation: surgical procedures, in Bowker JH, Michael JW, editors: *Atlas of limb prosthetics: surgical, prosthetic and rehabilitation principles,* ed 2, St Louis, 1992. Mosby-Year Book, Chapter 19A.

38. Pohjolainen T, Alaranta H: Lower limb amputations in Southern Finland, *Prosthet Orthot Int* 12:9–18, 1988.

39. Rizzo RL, Matsumoto T: Above vs. below-knee amputations: a retrospective analysis, *Int Surg* 65:265–267, 1980.

40. Robinson K: Long-posterior-flap myoplastic below-knee amputation in ischaemic disease: review of experience in 1967–1971, *Lancet* 1:193–195, 1972.

41. Robinson K: Skew flap myoplastic below-knee amputation: a preliminary report, *Br J Surg* 69:554–557, 1982.

42. Roon AJ, Moore WS, Goldstone J: Below-knee amputation: a modern approach, *Am J Surg* 134:153–158, 1977.

43. Smith BC: A twenty year follow-up in fifty below-knee amputations for gangrene in diabetics, *Surg Gynecol Obstet* 103:625–630, 1956.

44. Termansen NB: Below-knee amputation for ischaemic gangrene, *Acta Orthop Scand* 48:311–316, 1977.

45. Wagner FW Jr: Orthopaedic rehabilitation of the dysvascular limb, *Orthop Clin North Am* 9:325–350, 1978.

46. Wagner FW Jr: Partial foot amputations: surgical procedures, in Bowker JH, Michael JW, editors: *Atlas of limb prosthetics: surgical, prosthetic and rehabilitation principles,* ed 2, St Louis, 1992, Mosby-Year Book, Chapter 16A.

47. Waters RL, Perry J, Antonelli D, et al: Energy cost of walking amputees: the influence of level of amputation, *J Bone Joint Surg (Am)* 58A:42–46, 1976.

# CHAPTER 21

# Surgical Pathology of the Foot and Clinicopathologic Correlations

**Lawrence W. O'Neal, M.D.**

A knowledge of the anatomy of the foot is essential so that progression of pathologic changes in the diabetic foot can be understood and proper surgical treatment applied. Effective clinical evaluation and surgery are based on an understanding of gross anatomy and of alterations produced by disease. In treatment of diabetic foot problems, success is often uncertain, limited, and temporary even under the care of the most knowledgeable and diligent physician. Close attention to detail is necessary to obtain optimum results.

## ANATOMY

Some of the externally visible landmarks of the foot are shown in Figure 21–1.

### Skin

The skin of the dorsum of the foot is flexible and unspecialized. It contains hair follicles, sweat glands, and scanty sebaceous glands. Over the dorsum of the foot the skin is about 2 mm thick. In the dorsum few fibrous septa penetrate to deeper fascial structures except in the areas of wrinkle in the dorsal skin, overlying the metatarsophalangeal joints and the interphalangeal joints, where fibrous septa attach the dermis to the deep fascia. The skin in these sites is rela-tively more fixed than at other dorsal sites.

The plantar skin is 4 or 5 mm thick, with the thickest areas covering the heel and the distal metatarsals. The skin of the plantar surface is richly innervated; it has no hair follicles or sebaceous glands but has numerous sweat glands. Throughout the plantar skin the collagenous fibers of the dermis are connected to the deep fascia by heavy fibrous septa, which separate the subcutaneous fat into firm, partly discontinuous lobules. These septa are particularly heavy at the creases. Because of this dermal fixation to deep fascia, the skin of the sole is relatively fixed. Dorsal skin will glide 2 or 3 cm, but plantar skin will glide over deeper structures only 1 cm or less.

### Nails

The nails are specialized skin appendages. The nail itself is composed of keratinous flattened epithelial cells derived from the generative areas of the nail fold and nail bed (Fig 21–2). The adult nail is composed of three ill-defined layers: the dorsal nail, the intermediate nail, and the ventral nail.[26]

The dorsal nail arises from the proximal half of the roof of the nail fold and from the most proximal part of the floor of the nail fold. The intermediate nail arises from the distal part of the nail fold and the proximal nail bed up to the distal margin of the

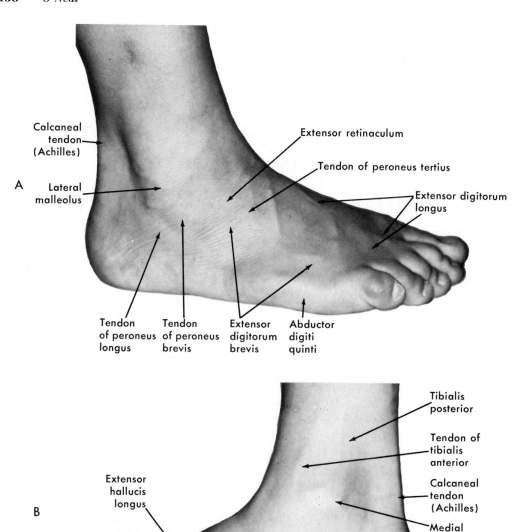

**FIG 21–1.**
Surface anatomy of lateral **(A)** and medial **(B)** aspects of foot.

lunula. The ventral nail arises from the distal half to two thirds of the nail bed up to the hyponychium (Fig 21–3).

The nail is bedded firmly on the epithelium of the nail bed, which apparently advances with nail growth, as is seen with the forward migration of small subungual hematomas.

The margins of the nail are overhung with skin folds called the nail wall.

## Nerves

Elements of the sciatic nerve furnish the motor and sensory innervation of the foot (Fig 21–4). The fourth and fifth lumbar segments and the first and second sacral segments contribute. The *saphenous nerve* reaches the skin over the anteromedial side of the lower tibia and as far distally as the medial side of the first metatarsophalangeal

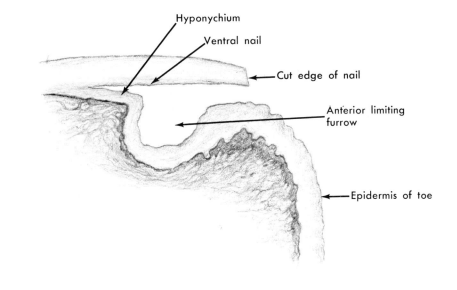

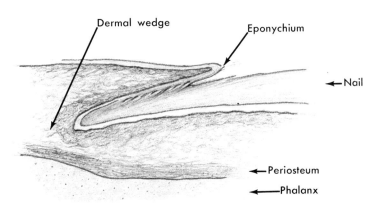

**FIG 21–2.**
Anatomy of nails with longitudinal sections of digits. *(Modified from Lewis BL:* Arch Dermatol Syphilis *70:732, 1954.)*

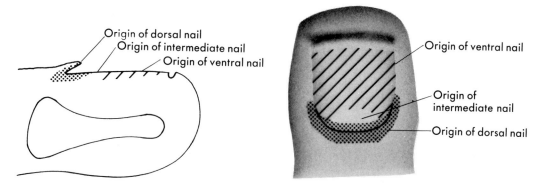

**FIG 21–3.**
Generative areas of nail lamellae. Most of nail bed and nail folds contribute some elements to ill-defined nail layers. *(Modified from Lewis BL:* Arch Dermatol Syphilis *70:732, 1954.)*

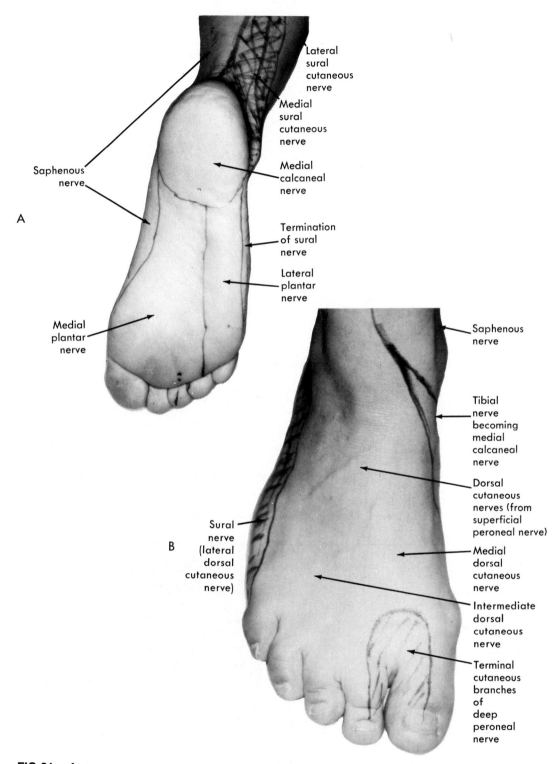

**FIG 21—4.**
Cutaneous nerve distribution of sole **(A)** and dorsum **(B)** of foot.

joint. The *common peroneal* branch of the sciatic nerve reaches the leg at the fibular head. It crosses anterior to the fibular neck deep to the origin of the peroneus longus muscle. The musculocutaneous *(superficial peroneal)* branch stays at first in the peroneal compartment and supplies the motor nerves of the peroneus longus and brevis muscles. The superficial peroneal nerve then pierces the fascia in the lower one third of the leg. A medial dorsal cutaneous branch descends in front of the ankle joint to the medial side of the hallux and to the adjoining portions of the second and third toes. The intermediate dorsal cutaneous branch of the superficial peroneal nerve lies anterior to the lateral malleolus and innervates the skin of the third and fourth interdigital spaces and corresponding digital segments.

The deep branch of the common peroneal nerve enters the extensor compartment of the leg and is distributed to the extensor muscles of the ankle and toes. Its termination is a dorsal digital nerve to the first interdigital web and adjoining segments of toes (lateral half of the hallux and medial half of the second toe).

The lateral margin of the foot derives its nerve supply from the *sural nerve*, which is known in the foot as the lateral dorsal cutaneous nerve. The medial calf and medial side of the ankle are supplied by the *saphenous nerve*.

The sensory innervation of the heel is from a medial calcaneal branch of the *tibial nerve*. The tibial nerve divides deep to the plantar fascia into the medial and lateral plantar branches. The cutaneous distribution of the *medial plantar nerve* includes the medial three and one-half digits and the distal two thirds of the medial sole. Small interdigital twigs from the medial plantar nerve innervate the nail beds of the medial three toes. The *lateral plantar nerve* supplies the lateral portion of the sole of the foot and the lateral one and one-half toes.

## Vessels

All of the arterial supply of the foot is derived from the popliteal artery, which lies on the knee joint and on the popliteal muscle. At the lower border of the popliteal muscle the popliteal artery divides into anterior and posterior tibial arteries.

The *anterior tibial artery* penetrates the upper part of the interosseous membrane and enters the extensor compartment of the leg. Distally it lies between the tibialis anterior and extensor muscles. At the ankle it lies more medially and crosses the ankle joint anteriorly, becoming in the foot the *dorsalis pedis artery*. The dorsalis pedis artery usually lies lateral to the extensor hallucis longus muscle. In the space between the first and second metatarsal, the posterior tibial artery generally divides into a deep plantar and a dorsal metatarsal branch.

The *posterior tibial artery* accompanies the tibial nerve. The artery lies between the tibialis posterior and flexor digitorum longus muscles and the soleus muscle and tendon of the calcaneus. Near the medial malleolus it sends a branch to the heel pad along the medial calcaneal nerve.

In the plantar space the posterior tibial artery divides into medial and lateral plantar arteries. These arteries course with the medial and lateral plantar nerves. The plantar arch is formed by anastomosis between the medial and lateral plantar arteries, with a contribution from the dorsalis pedis artery at the first intermetatarsal space. Small dorsal digital arteries arise from a variable dorsal arcuate branch of the dorsalis pedis artery.

The plantar digital vessels arise from the plantar arch. The plantar arch is variable in detail but in the healthy individual provides abundant opportunity for collateral circulation in the distal foot. The arterioles to the skin form an *internal vascular belt* at the junction between the subcutaneous tissue and the dermis. Arising from this internal vascular belt are dermal plexuses that are intimately interconnected, forming a reticular network of vessels of different sizes. From this network arboreal terminal branches form a subpapillary plexus with capillary loops into the dermal papillae, integrating a number of papillae into *vascular districts*, which are also interconnected.

## Muscles, Tendons, and Fascia

The muscles in the extensor group are located anteriorly in the leg. They include the tibialis anterior, the extensor hallucis longus, and the extensor digitorum longus. Laterally are the peroneal muscles. Both the anterior and the lateral muscle groups are innervated by the common peroneal nerve.

The flexors of the foot and toes are innervated by the tibial nerve. The flexors are in the posterior compartment of the leg behind the interosseous membrane.

The deep muscular fascia encloses the muscles in the leg and adheres to the periosteum of the superficial portion of the tibia and of the lateral malleolus. At the anterior ankle thickened areas of this fascia form the extensor retinacula (the transverse crural ligament and the cruciate crural ligament), under which the extensor tendons course. The fascia is then continuous with the thinner fascia of the dorsum of the foot and toes.

The gastrocnemius muscle arises from medial and lateral attachments on the distal posterior femur. These heads of the gastrocnemius form the distal margin of the popliteal fossa. The soleus muscle arises from the proximal tibia and fibula. Its tendon joins the tendon of the gastrocnemius and is attached to the calcaneus as the calcaneal tendon (Achilles tendon). The small plantaris muscle arises from the lateral femoral condyle. The plantaris tendon crosses between the soleus and the gastrocnemius and forms the medial portion of the calcaneal tendon. The gastrocnemius, soleus, and plantaris are innervated by branches of the tibial nerve.

Across the ankle the long tendons maintain their relative position to each other and are held in place by fascial condensations.

In the sole of the foot the plantar aponeurosis is the most superficial fascia (Fig 21–5).[20] Its central portion is the thickest and is attached to the medial tubercle of the calcaneus. The plantar fascia spreads fan-like distally. Near the metatarsal heads the fascial fibers divide into five processes, which form bundles surrounding the metatarsal heads. Distally the plantar aponeurosis joins with transverse fibers (the superfi-

cial transverse metatarsal ligament) and anchors the dermis at the distal plantar crease. Some deeper fibers extend to the flexor sheaths near the metatarsophalangeal joints.

The dermis of the sole is attached to plantar fascia by fibrous septa that enclose the fat lobules. In the central plantar space the flexor digitorum brevis muscle arises from the proximal portion of the plantar fascia. The lateral and medial portions of the plantar fascia are thinner than the central portion. Medially the fascia covers the abductor hallucis and laterally the abductor digiti quinti muscles. The strong plantar aponeurosis forms the principal stay of the longitudinal arch.

Beneath the plantar fascia the muscles in the sole of the foot are categorized into four layers. The most superficial *first layer* (Fig 21–6)[20] consists of the flexor digitorum brevis, the abductor hallucis, and the abductor digiti quinti muscles. The flexor digitorum brevis originates from the medial tubercle of the calcaneus and from the deep surface of the plantar aponeurosis. Its four tendons insert into the middle phalanges of the four lateral toes. The abductor hallucis arises from the medial tubercle of the calcaneus and inserts on the medial side of the base of the proximal phalanx of the hallux. The abductor digiti quinti arises from the medial and lateral tubercle of the calcaneus and inserts into the base of the proximal phalanx of the little toe.

The *second layer* is composed of the tendons of the flexor hallucis longus and the flexor digitorum longus muscles. These tendons insert in the proximal portion of the distal phalanges on their plantar aspect. The quadratus plantae, or accessory flexor, arises from the calcaneus and inserts on the flexor digitorum longus tendons. The four lumbrical muscles arise from the medial side of the tendons of the flexor digitorum longus group, pass to the hallux side of the toes, and insert on the capsule of the metatarsophalangeal joint and on the dorsal expansion of the extensor tendon of the lateral four toes. The tendons of the lumbricals lie superficial to the deep transverse metatarsal ligament. The lumbrical muscle, as in the

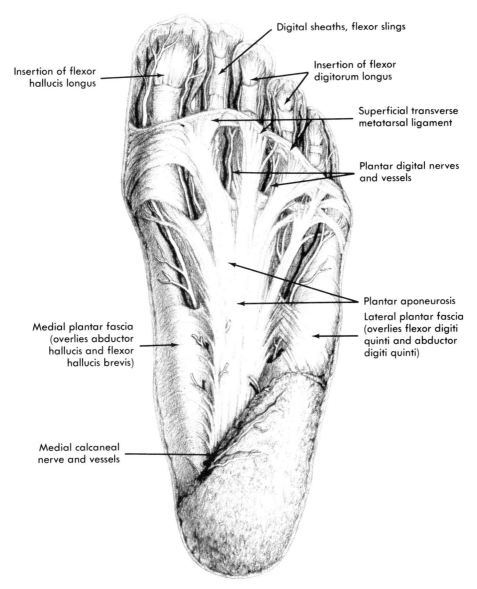

**FIG 21–5.**
Plantar fascia. Note separating bundles near metatarsal heads. *(Redrawn from Grant JCB: An atlas of anatomy, ed 6. Baltimore, 1972, Williams & Wilkins.)*

hand, extends the proximal interphalangeal joint and assists in flexion of the metatarsophalangeal joint.

In the *third layer* (Fig 21–7)[20] lie the flexor hallucis brevis, the flexor digiti quinti, and the two adductor hallucis muscles—the oblique and the transverse. The flexor hallucis brevis originates from the dense fibrous plantar tarsometatarsal ligaments and from the cuboid. It splits into a medial and lateral tendon, each of which encases a sesamoid bone under the metatarsal head. At their in-

sertion on the proximal phalanx of the hallux they are joined by the tendon of the abductor hallucis medially and the tendons of the oblique and transverse heads of the adductor hallucis to form a composite flexor tendon. The oblique head arises from the bases of the second, third, and fourth metatarsal heads and from the fascial sheath of the peroneus longus. The transverse head of the adductor hallucis arises from the plantar aspect of the four lateral metatarsophalangeal joints and the deep transverse meta-

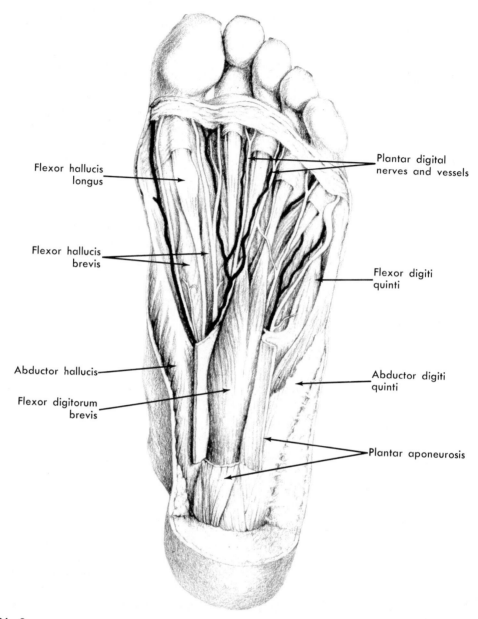

Flexor hallucis
longus

Flexor hallucis
brevis

Abductor hallucis

Flexor digitorum
brevis

Plantar digital
nerves and vessels

Flexor digiti
quinti

Abductor digiti
quinti

Plantar aponeurosis

**FIG 21–6.**
First layer of plantar muscles. *(Redrawn from Grant JCB: An atlas of anatomy, ed 6. Baltimore, 1972, Williams & Wilkins.)*

tarsal ligament. The small flexor of the little toe arises from the base of the fifth metatarsal and inserts in the base of the proximal phalanx of the little toe.

The plantar interossei, the dorsal interossei, and the tendons of the tibialis posterior and peroneus longus muscles lie in the *fourth layer* (Fig 21–8).[20] The three plantar interossei arise from metatarsal shafts of the third, fourth, and fifth metatarsals and insert in the medial side of the bases of the corresponding proximal phalanges. They are adductors to these toes. The four dorsal interossei muscles each arise from adjoining metatarsal surfaces in the first, second, third, and fourth intermetacarpal spaces and attach at the bases of the proximal phalanges of the second, third, and fourth toes. The dorsal interossei abduct from the axis of the second toe. The tendon of the peroneus

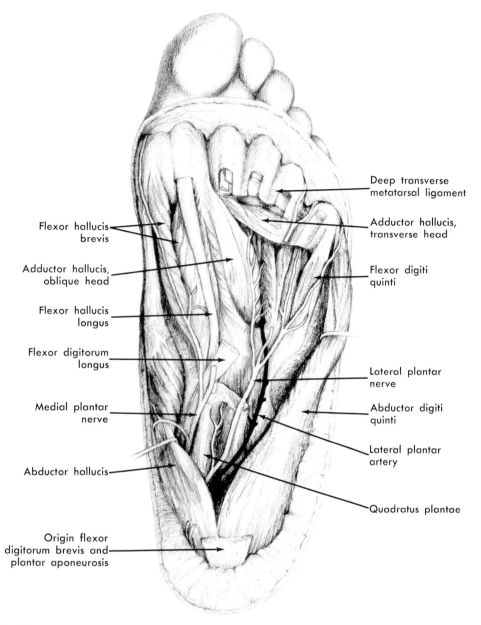

**FIG 21–7.**
Third layer of plantar muscles. *(Redrawn from Grant JCB:* An atlas of anatomy, *ed 6. Baltimore, 1972, Williams & Wilkins.)*

Labels on figure:
- Deep transverse metatarsal ligament
- Flexor hallucis brevis
- Adductor hallucis, transverse head
- Adductor hallucis, oblique head
- Flexor digiti quinti
- Flexor hallucis longus
- Flexor digitorum longus
- Lateral plantar nerve
- Medial plantar nerve
- Abductor digiti quinti
- Lateral plantar artery
- Abductor hallucis
- Quadratus plantae
- Origin flexor digitorum brevis and plantar aponeurosis

longus lies in a groove in the cuboid, passes deep to the flexor hallucis brevis, and inserts in the base of the first metatarsal and the first (medial) cuneiform. The tibialis posterior inserts chiefly on the medial aspect of the navicular tubercle but sends fibrous attachments to the complex ligaments of the hole plantar tarsus and tarsometatarsal ligaments.

The collagenous structures of the distal foot intermingle to a degree not made clear by the preceding descriptions. In the 2 cm between the heads of the metatarsals and the plantar metatarsophalangeal crease, the dermal collagen, plantar fascia, flexor sheaths, joint capsule, and periosteum of sesamoid, metatarsal, and proximal phalanges are closely approximated to one another and attached more or less by commonly used fibrous sheaths and septa. The superficial

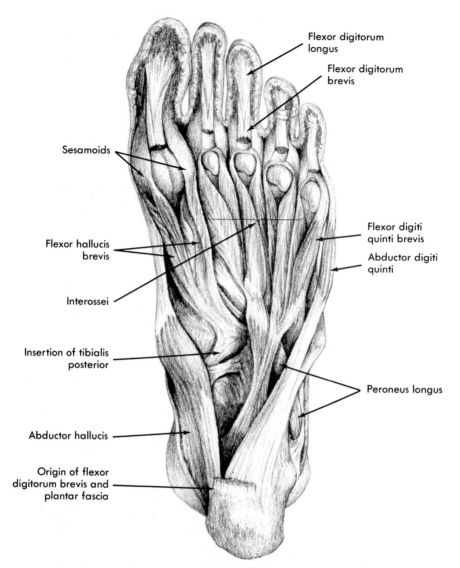

**FIG 21–8.**
Fourth layer of plantar muscles. *(Redrawn from Grant JCB:* An atlas of anatomy, *ed 6. Baltimore, 1972, Williams & Wilkins.)*

transverse metatarsal ligament is a local condensation of this fibrous tissue. Adjacent to joint capsule and commingling with joint capsule fibers is the deep transverse metatarsal ligament.

The *bones* of the foot and some of the major tendon insertions are shown in Fig 21–9.

## FASCIAL COMPARTMENTS [31]
(FIG 21–10)

The *medial compartment* is bounded by the inferior surface of the first metatarsal dorsally, an extension of the plantar aponeurosis medially and intermuscular septum laterally. The medial compartment contains the abductor hallucis and the flexor hallucis brevis muscles and the flexor hallucis longus, peroneus longus, and posterior tibial tendons.

The *central compartment* is bounded by the plantar aponeurosis inferiorly, intermuscular septa medially and laterally, and the tarsometatarsal structures dorsally. The central compartment contains the flexon digitorum brevis muscle, the flexor digitorum longus tendons, the lumbricales, quadratus

**A**

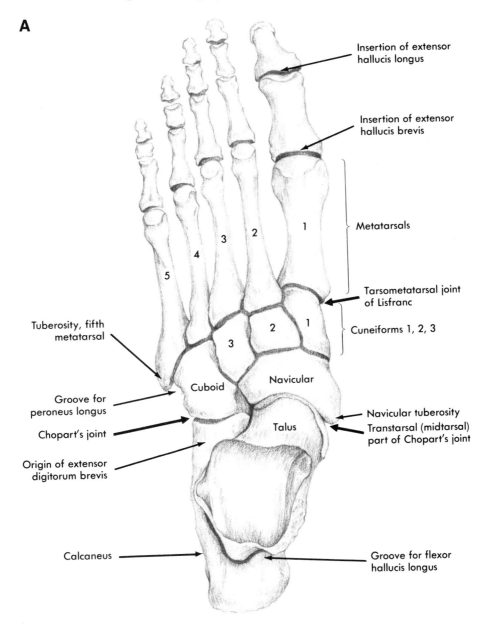

Insertion of extensor
hallucis longus

Insertion of extensor
hallucis brevis

Metatarsals

Tarsometatarsal joint
of Lisfranc

Cuneiforms 1, 2, 3

Tuberosity, fifth
metatarsal

Groove for
peroneus longus

Chopart's joint

Origin of extensor
digitorum brevis

Cuboid

Navicular

Navicular tuberosity

Transtarsal (midtarsal)
part of Chopart's joint

Talus

Calcaneus

Groove for flexor
hallucis longus

**FIG 21–9.**
**A,** bones of foot from dorsal aspect. **B,** bones of foot from plantar aspect.          *(Continued.)*

plantae, adductor hallucis muscle, and the peroneal and posterior tibial tendons.

The *lateral compartment* is bounded by the fifth metatarsal dorsally, an intermuscular septum medially, and the edge of the plantar aponeurosis laterally. The lateral compartment contains the abductor digiti quinti, the flexor digiti quinti, and the opponens muscles of the fifth toe.

The *interosseous component* is bounded by the interosseous fascia of the metatarsals and contains the seven interossei.

## CANDIDATE FOR FOOT PROBLEMS

Anyone who has diabetes for 15 years or more is a potential candidate for foot problems, because neuropathy progresses enough in that time to cause clinical problems. However, in some patients the diagnosis of diabetes is made when the patient is examined for foot ulcers or infections. A tendency of many authors is to classify diabetic foot lesions as "ischemic" or "neuropathic." Although an ischemic or neuropathic pattern

**B**

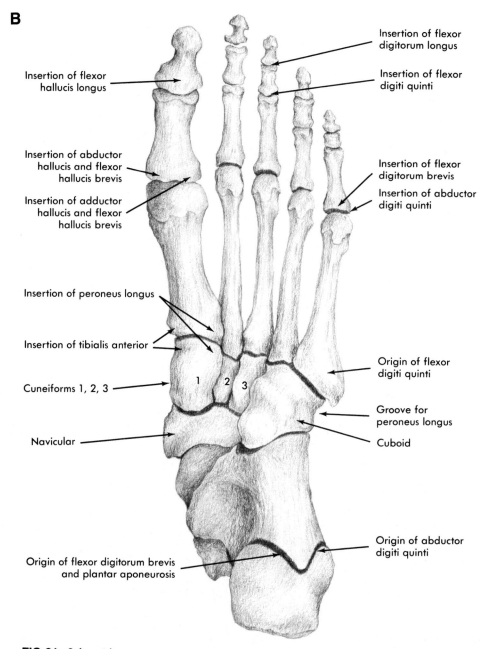

Insertion of flexor
hallucis longus

Insertion of flexor
digitorum longus

Insertion of flexor
digiti quinti

Insertion of abductor
hallucis and flexor
hallucis brevis

Insertion of adductor
hallucis and flexor
hallucis brevis

Insertion of flexor
digitorum brevis

Insertion of abductor
digiti quinti

Insertion of peroneus longus

Insertion of tibialis anterior

Cuneiforms 1, 2, 3

Origin of flexor
digiti quinti

Groove for
peroneus longus

Navicular

Cuboid

Origin of abductor
digiti quinti

Origin of flexor digitorum brevis
and plantar aponeurosis

**FIG 21–9 (cont.).**

may predominate, most ulcers have an element of each. Deterioration of the pedal vessels and nerves is accompanied by other problems of diabetes, such as retinopathy and nephropathy (see Chapter 2). Changes in the foot develop so gradually that many patients are unaware of the degree of deterioration and become distressed when minor injury precipitates major disability. Although most diabetics are aware of the risk

for foot infections and amputations, few understand the causes and mechanisms of the process or the measures needed to maintain an intact foot.

## Vulnerable Foot

Many deformities develop in the feet of older persons. In diabetes of long duration, foot deformities are nearly universal. In a

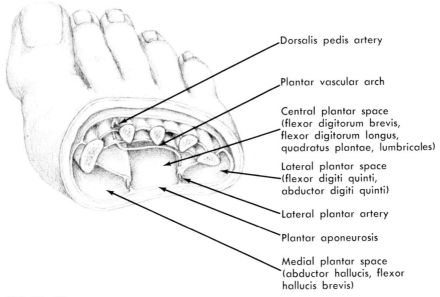

Dorsalis pedis artery

Plantar vascular arch

Central plantar space
(flexor digitorum brevis,
flexor digitorum longus,
quadratus plantae, lumbricales)

Lateral plantar space
(flexor digiti quinti,
abductor digiti quinti)

Lateral plantar artery

Plantar aponeurosis

Medial plantar space
(abductor hallucis, flexor
hallucis brevis)

**FIG 21–10.**
Plantar spaces in distal foot.

survey of diabetic patients at a Veteran's Affairs Hospital clinic, 50% had vascular insufficiency, neuropathy, and a coexisting foot deformity, indicating a high risk for morbidity.[39] The common abnormalities were angular, usually hallux valgus and hammer digit. Less common, but significant, abnormalities were submetatarsal head calluses, interdigital soft corns, and Charcot's foot. Several of the deformities of the foot in this study were ulcerated; one patient had osteomyelitis and one had gangrene of the hallux. Two patients previously had distal amputations.

A survey[38] of foot problems in 742 diabetics in a Stockholm hospital showed that only one third of the patients were free of foot-related symptoms. A significant number of those with foot problems, even with infection, gangrene, and neuropathic ulcer, were not receiving any medical care. The foot deformities seen so often in the elderly[35] are more frequent in the diabetic and require more close monitoring and maintenance care.[43]

Foot deformities in the diabetic patient have several causes. Of course some are old, long-tolerated abnormalities that become problems only when circulation and sensation diminish.

Neuropathy of the motor nerves contrib-

utes to angular deformities of the toes and distal foot. At first the most distal muscles, the intrinsic muscles of the foot, seem to be affected. The loss of balancing lumbrical function results in extension of the metatarsophalangeal joint of the toes and flexion of the proximal interphalangeal joints (the "intrinsic minus foot").[9] The result of this imbalance is hammertoes. In addition, loss of abduction function of the dorsal interossei causes the toes to become crowded on the axis of the second digit, accentuating the angular prominences at the first and fifth metatarsophalangeal joints (bunion and bunionette). The neuropathic arthropathy of diabetes, or Charcot's foot, eventually results in a collapse of the midfoot.[17, 37] The subsequent rocker-bottom foot, medial tarsal subluxation, digital subluxation, and bone fragments offer additional opportunity for ulceration, including the unique midplantar ulcer. Autonomic neuropathy often portends development of foot ulcers,[8] although the loss of pain sensation is also a prerequisite. In addition to the osseous abnormalities, a loss of soft tissue mass in the sole of the foot (particularly in diabetics with plantar ulcerations) causes less padding and dispersion of mechanical forces than in the normal foot.[19] Although the contribution of vascular deficiency to the development of first ulceration has been challenged by LoGerfo and Coffman,[27] most functional and histologic studies indicate disease of arteries, arterioles, and capillaries distinctive to diabetics. That these vascular lesions may be present and distinctive in diabetes does not undermine LoGerfo and Coffman's thesis that many of the ulcerated and gangrenous feet of diabetics can be salvaged by arterial surgery (see Chapter 18).

LoGerfo et al.[28] have recently reported dramatic improvement in rates of foot salvage with distal bypass grafting, often to a patent dorsalis pedis artery. Figures 21–11 and 21–12 show a summary of their total operations for diabetic foot problems in their series. A dramatic fall in the rates of below-knee and above-knee operations was

clearly associated with the increased use of pedal vascular bypass.[28]

With careful supervision, the intact foot of an educated patient can be maintained despite low blood flow. Injury, including surgery or infection, requires an increased blood flow to contain and heal the damage. The arteries and arterioles of the diabetic often cannot deliver the required relative hyperemia. The capillaries and arterioles seem to be particularly vulnerable to occlusion from the angiotoxic enzymes of invading bacteria. *Staphylococcus* is a common bacterial pathogen.[33]

## The Vulnerable Patient

Walsh et al.[41] described a group of patients with newly diagnosed diabetes who

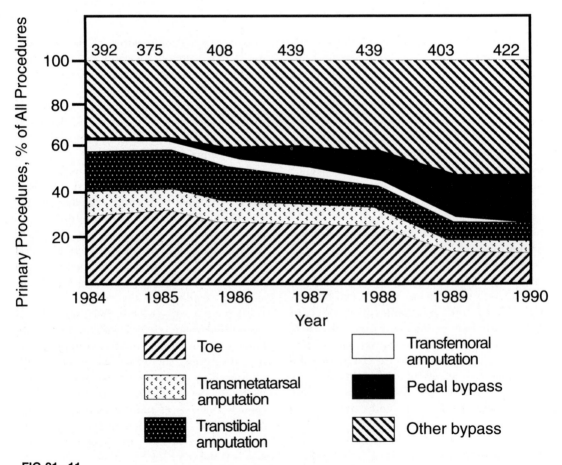

**FIG 21–11.**
The changing pattern of surgery for diabetic foot problems of New England Deaconess Hospital, Boston. The reduction in the rate of all lower limb amputations associated with the increased use of pedal arterial reconstruction is seen. *(From LoGerfo FW, Gibbons GW, Pomposelli FB Jr, et al: Arch Surg 127:617, 1992. Used by permission.)*

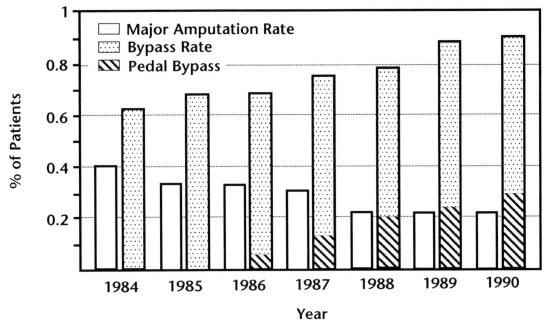

**FIG 21–12.**
Reduction in major amputation rates in New England Deaconess Hospital, Boston, is correlated with increased use of femoropopliteal and distal bypass operations. *(From LoGerfo FW, Gibbons GW, Pomposelli FB Jr, et al: Arch Surg 127:617, 1992. Used by permission.)*

had retinopathy and foot lesions at the time of diagnosis. The patients were remarkably unconcerned about their condition. Their self-neglect and lack of insight contributed to a poor prognosis.

It is well known that preventive care and education are extremely important in maintaining the intact foot. These factors are, however, difficult to implement and evaluate. In the Nottingham study,[43] 93% of those interviewed (all patients previously hospitalized for diabetic foot ulceration, infection, or gangrene) later claimed that they had not been told or offered anything to read about preventing foot problems. Many of these patients were, when interviewed, using the services of the diabetic clinic or the district nurse. Few had used these services before hospitalization. Only 66% of the Stockholm diabetic patients with severe foot disease used hospitals for their diabetic care.[37] The remainder received insufficient care or no care.

Any physician who treats diabetics with foot problems recognizes patients who are doomed to serious foot infections and amputations. The bravado of the late-stage juvenile diabetic who wants to match the activities of peers is ominous. The type II diabetic who "has to" walk, work, or even dance and hike with an ulcerated foot presents an educational challenge. Physicians often call these patients "noncompliant." The closer the physician can bring the patient to understanding the problems of collaborative health maintenance, the more likely the patient is to keep an intact foot.

The aim of education in this field is to prevent the development of a foot ulcer, or if the patient gets one, to never get another.[3] Unfortunately, this goal is not achieved often enough. Amputation of one leg is too often followed by the need for amputation of the other leg (see Chapter 2). The contralateral leg usually has all of the signs of severe vascular insufficiency (Fig 21–13).

## INITIAL LESIONS

Although the end of the process may be loss of limb or life or both, the initial event is a break in the skin somewhere in the foot, followed by penetration of bacteria and local

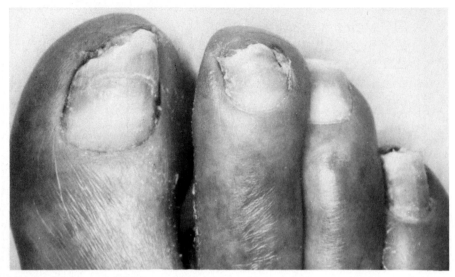

**FIG 21–13.**
Foot in patient with advanced diabetes shows shiny, thin, dry, hairless skin; dermal hemosiderin deposits; and irregular growth of nails, with evidence of poor care. This man, in his fifties, had had his left leg amputated and was nearly blind from retinopathy.

infection. Ordinarily most of the initial incidents leading to severe infections, gangrene, amputation, and disability in the diabetic seem trivial and indeed would be trivial or negligible to younger nondiabetics. The initial lesion may be *acute mechanical trauma* in which skin is torn or punctured. Frequently the poor eyesight of the diabetic patient contributes to stubbing the toes, stepping on sharp objects, or gouging the skin in trimming nails. *Thermal trauma* from foot baths and heating pads may destroy skin in the neuropathic foot (see Chapter 2). *Incessant friction* over angular prominences is often associated with improperly fitting shoes. One brief episode of walking on an insensitive foot may result in blistering and erosion. If the circulation is adequate, healing usually occurs with rest. If circulation is inadequate to deliver the hyperemic response needed for healing, a patch of gangrene may result.

Several of the deformities of the foot result in concentrated weight bearing, predisposing to callus formation and ulceration. The toes play an important part in increasing the weight-bearing area during walking.[23] In the intrinsic minus foot, with the toes in dorsiflexion, more concentrated weight bearing is placed on the metatarsal heads. Areas of callus and ulceration correlate well with areas of maximal vertical and sheer forces (see Chapter 9 and 10).

In bedridden disabled patients the heel is vulnerable to ulceration. The simple weight of the immobile foot on the mattress will obliterate blood perfusion in the posterolateral side of the heel. The consequence of these initial events, which seem minor and are often ignored or minimized, may be midthigh amputation when ulcers occur in a foot debilitated by diabetes. The degree of vulnerability of the debilitated foot is often not appreciated by the patient, who may have difficulty in understanding why "such a little thing" can result in tissue loss and progessive disability. The diabetic with severe neuropathy frequently does not know how the lesions happened.

## Local Progression

The initial problem is minor trauma, followed by minor infection. The progression to major infection with necrosis of tissue results from (1) a circulation inadequate to confine the infection and (2) a neuropathy so profound that the part is not voluntarily put at rest as a foot with normal sensation would be, resulting in milking of the infection through the natural fascial pathways. Although the "ischemic" foot may have a somewhat different pattern than the "neuropathic" foot and one pattern or the other may predominate, both vascular lesions and nerve lesions contribute to the problem. Treatment for the predominantly ischemic foot differs substantially from that of the predominantly neuropathic foot.

## Septic Arteritis and Tissue Necrosis

In tissues adjoining infection, small vessels commonly develop thrombotic occlusion. This process is seen in arterioles of the skin adjoining stasis ulcers, in small vessels in the base and margins of duodenal ulcers, and in small pulmonary arterioles in the wall of tubercular cavities. Thrombosis of small vessels is partly responsible for the necrosis of tissue in these lesions and for the frequent chronicity of these and other types of infections. Usually in tissues with otherwise normal small vessels, this process occurs only at the margin of the infection. After sloughing, draining, or other control of the infection, normal arterioles recanalize and form abundant granulation tissue, which is the first stage in wound healing.

Numerous bacteria elaborate angiotoxic (necrotizing) substances. For example, particularly injurious is the α-toxin of staphylococci, which, when injected into the skin, results in the local development of an impressive necrotic lesion. Streptokinase and streptococcal hyaluronidase have been implicated in the rapid extension of cellulitis by digestion of fibrin barriers and intracellular ground substance. In the mixed infections so common in the diabetic foot, the necrotizing toxins following the spreading factors can produce a devastating lesion.

In the already diseased small vessels in the diabetic patient, the occlusive process is exaggerated, and one sees paronychia, ingrown nails, and minor injuries proceeding to ever-enlarging areas of necrosis rather than staying limited. More arterioles are obliterated, larger arterioles are obliterated, and the original lesions become converted from trivial infections to areas of gangrene. Creeping advancement of this process of infective obliterative microangiopathy (Fig 21–14) can occur until a plane or space is reached, such as a tendon sheath, into which the bacteria will spill and spread. As more of the arterioles and small arteries become involved, the infection and necrosis progress (Fig 21–15).

Regardless of any debate about the significance of microangiopathy in diabetes,[27] the

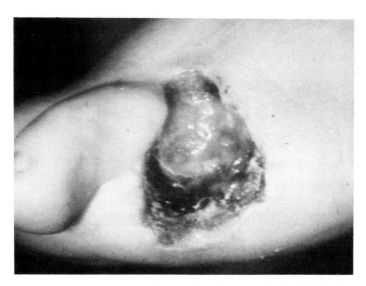

**FIG 21–14.**
Creeping gangrene after amputation of fifth toe. Small skin vessel thrombosis has led to patch of gangrenous skin inferior to base of toe.

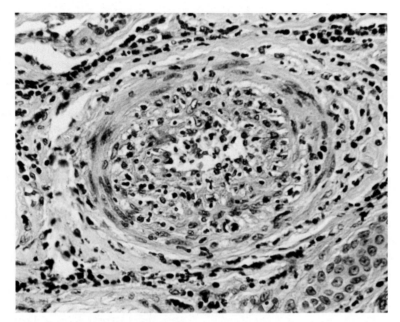

**FIG 21–15.**
Obliteration of lumen of small dermal arteriole by intimal hyperplasia and septic thrombus. Note cellular evidence of inflammation in areolar tissues near arteriole.This arteriole was about 1 mm from margin of area of dry gangrene.

potential virulence of infection arising in local lesions is greater in the diabetic than in other neuropathic conditions (paraplegia, syringomyelia, tabes, Hansen's disease). The greater risk to the diabetic foot may indicate that the capillaries and arterioles of diabetics are more likely to occlude when exposed to bacterial toxins.

Many authors have taken a static view toward the role of microangiopathy in the progression of foot infections. It seems apparent now that the maximum vasodilator capacity of the resistance vessels and the autoregulation of blood flow are reduced in long-term diabetics.[24] Consequently, when increased blood flow is required to contain infection in the foot, it is not readily available.

Although the plantar fascia, tendon sheaths, and other structures in and near the superficial transverse metatarsal ligament form barriers to infection when the arterial circulation is good, creeping infective microangiopathy can destroy fibrous barriers, as well as skin, and allow spread through and along structures in the distal foot that would ordinarily retard the spread of infection.

## "End-Artery" Disease in the Diabetic Foot, Angiopathy, and Microangiopathy

The normally rich collateral circulation in the foot, with extensive complex communications in the plantar arches and the dorsal arch and between the two arches, as well as smaller unnamed communications everywhere in the normal foot, allows major trauma, major operations, and major infections to be tolerated in the normal foot with little attention being required for the arteries distal to the ankle.

In the diabetic, however, multiple complete and partial arteriosclerotic blockades of large, medium-sized, and small arteries result in a situation comparable with end-arteries as in the heart or kidney, where opportunity for collateral circulation is barred. If the end-artery becomes blocked, there is no replacement for its function, and the tissue supplied by the artery dies (Fig 21–16). Foot angiography in diabetics with foot infections tends to support this concept.[22]

Examples are seen in plantar space abscesses. After penetrating wounds of the sole of the foot (e.g., from a tack, pin, glass, or

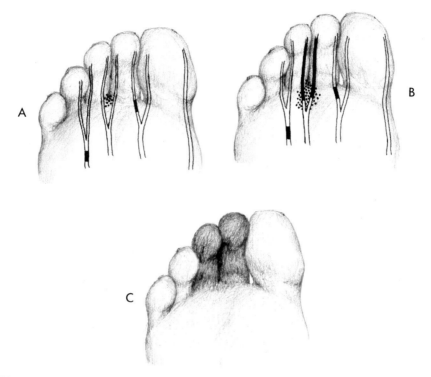

**FIG 21–16.**
Schematics of mechanisms whereby advancing infection causes obliteration of small arteries that have been converted into end-arteries by arteriosclerotic disease process, with resultant gangrene. **A,** early web space infection in foot with patchy segmental arteriosclerotic occlusion of digital and metatarsal vessels. **B,** thrombosis of arteries adjacent to web space infection. **C,** gangrene of second and third toes.

nail in shoe), the plantar space may be directly entered and an abscess formed, or the infection may at first be subcutaneous and follow the dermal fibrous septa to and through the plantar fascia.

In the inexpansile central plantar space, infection can quickly obliterate the plantar arterial arch and its branches, to be followed by necrosis not only of tissue in the central plantar space but also of the second, third, and fourth toes, which receive most of their blood supply from the plantar arch (Fig 21–17). The fifth toe and the hallux receive some of their circulation through the lateral and medial plantar spaces, respectively, and may survive central plantar space abscesses.

Frequently digital and web infections will produce localized gangrene that spreads by means of septic obliterative angiopathy until the digital arteries are reached. Occlusion of these may lead to gangrene of the adjoining digits if the neighboring small vessels are obstructed and an end-artery

situation exists (Fig 21–18). Older anatomic studies[16] showed no clear-cut histologic differences between the lower limb arteriosclerosis of diabetics and nondiabetics. The major difference was that in the diabetic limb the obstructive disease tended to spread more distally and in particular to involve the metatarsal arteries. These findings have been amply confirmed and are often seen in lower limb angiograms (see Chapter 16).

The distal arteriosclerosis occurs at an earlier age in diabetics than in nondiabetics. In type II diabetes, progression of lower limb arterial occlusive disease was seen in 87% of patients followed for more than 2 years.[2]

Serial sections of material from amputated specimens by Pederson and Olsen[36] confirmed the segmental nature of the obstruction in small arteries of the foot and toe. Arterial calcification, however, bears no relationship to the presence or location of arterial occlusion.[13] Better methods of eval-

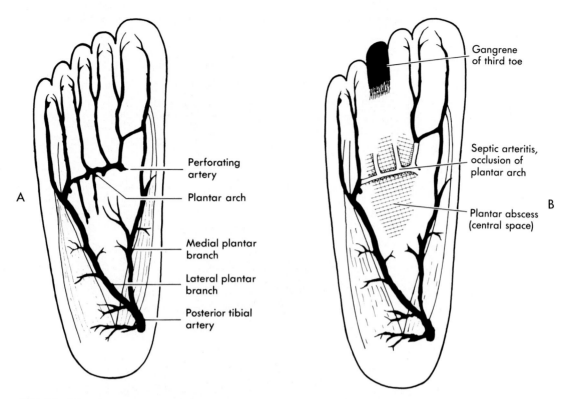

**FIG 21–17.**
**A,** normal plantar arch receives contributions from medial and lateral plantar branches of posterior tibial artery and from dorsalis pedis via a perforating artery or arteries. **B,** if central plantar space abscess causes occlusion of plantar arch, gangrene of middle toe will result.

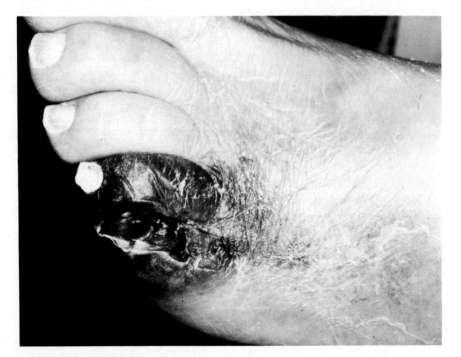

**FIG 21–18.**
Tissue necrosis by both microangiopathy (fifth toe) and end artery disease (fourth toe) in same foot. After fifth toe was stubbed, gangrene began in injured tissue near avulsed nail. When infection reached foot, fourth toe became gangrenous as lateral digital artery of fourth toe became obliterated. Inflammatory changes in dorsum of foot are called dorsal foot phlegmon. When photograph was taken, dorsalis pedis pulse could be felt.

uating the smaller distal arteries of diabetic patients are needed.[16]

The distinctive distal patchy atherosclerosis in the diabetic with multiple blockades in capillaries, arterioles, small arteries, and named larger arteries converts tissue that in health is perfused by interlocking and alternate channels of blood flow to tissue supplied by only one artery, sometimes tenuously. The amount of tissue thus dependent on its single artery may vary from a few square millimeters of skin in a *vascular district* to the entire area of the foot or leg (Fig 21–19).

## The Nails (Table 21–1)

The initial break in the skin often originates near the nails. Nail deformities after trauma, fungus infection, systemic disease, and poor care are common in the general population. In the ischemic neuropathic foot of diabetics, some nail abnormality appears to be universal. Nails lead to difficulty in several ways. The reduced vision and frequent obesity of many diabetic patients make it difficult for them to reach the nails, and they may cut the adjacent skin. With neglect the nails grow too long, and a nail may gouge the skin of the neighboring toe (Fig 21–20). Frequently in the elderly, as the nail grows long, it incurves and partly encircles the distal nail bed. Then stubbing the toe or wearing new shoes can break the skin. In some of the nail abnormalities, excess keratin and debris accumulate under the nail and in the nail folds, where bacteria might grow.

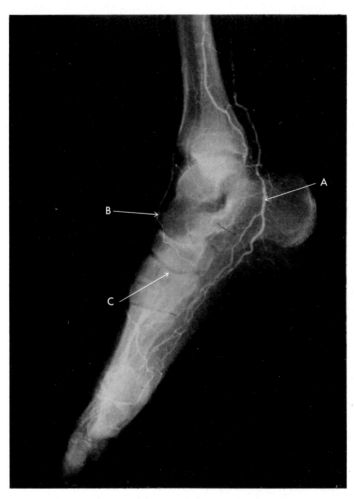

**FIG 21–19.**
Posterior tibial artery **(A)** as end-artery in foot. Dorsalis pedis **(B)** is reconstituted by collateral artery **(C)**.

**TABLE 21–1.**

Glossary of Nails*

**Onych-, onycho-** Gr. onyx, meaning nail
**Onychatrophy** Atrophy of the nails
**Onychauxis** Marked overgrowth of the nails
**Onychectomy** Ablation of a nail
**Onychia** Inflammation of the matrix of the nail;
  onychitis
  **O. lateralis** Paronychia
  **O. maligna** Acute onychia in debilitated patients
  **O. parasitica** Onychomycosis
  **O. periungualis** Paronychia
  **O. sicca** Brittle nails
**Onychitis** Onychia
**Onychodystrophy** Dystrophy in the nails occurring
  as a congenital defect or due to any illness or
  injury that may cause a malformed nail
**Onychogryposis** Enlargement with increased
  curvature of the nails (Fig 21–21)
**Onycholysis** Loosening of the nails, beginning at the
  free border and usually incomplete
**Onychomadesis** Complete shedding of the nails,
  usually with systemic disease
**Onychomalacia** Abnormal softness of the nails
**Onychomycosis** Fungus infection of the nails
  **O. favus** Favus of the nails
  **O. trichophytina** Tinea unguium
**Onychonosus** Any disease of the nails;
  onychopathy; onychosis
**Onychophosis** Growth of horny epithelium in the
  nail bed
**Onychophyma** Swelling or hypertrophy of the nails
**Onychoptosis** Falling off of the nails
**Onychorrhexis** Abnormal brittleness of the nails with
  splitting of free edge
**Onychoschizia** Loosening of the nail from the nail
  bed
**Unguis incarnatus** Ingrowing nail; onychocryptosis
  (Figs 12–22 and 12–23)

*Adapted from Sutton RL Jr: Diseases of the skin, ed 11, St
Louis, 1956, Mosby-Year Book.

Infections beginning in the nail bed, paronychium, or nail wall spread on the dorsal and lateral aspects of the toes. The infections are often prohibited from reaching the pad by fibrous septa that extend from the dermis to the periosteum. Characteristically the infections spread on the dorsum of the digit to reach the dorsum of the foot by way of the lymphatics.[30] However, if the distal digit becomes necrotic, the flexor tendon sheath may be entered.

After the initial break in the skin, the rate of spread of the infection depends on the virulence of the pathogenic bacteria and the degree of ischemia. Indolent small infections may be confined to the tissues adjacent to the nail for a long time. Relief of infections near the nails usually requires removal of a portion of the nail, which must be done cautiously, or further tissue damage may be caused.

## Toes and Webs

Toe deformities seem more common in diabetics than in the general population (Fig 21–24) in part because of neuropathy involving the nerve supply to the small intrinsic muscles of the foot. Neuropathy of motor nerves supplying the lumbrical muscles and the interossei results in claw toes, hammertoes, crowding of toes, and exaggeration of bunions and bunionettes. Less weight is borne on the toes, and more is borne on the metatarsal heads. The angular prominences are susceptible to skin-on-shoe friction and the crowded toes to skin-on-skin friction. Friction is ignored in the insensitive foot, and blisters, ulcers, and ulcerated calluses appear (Fig 21–25).

### Cock-Up Deformity

Cock-up deformity is seen in the great toe. The interphalangeal joint is flexed, and the metatarsophalangeal joint is extended. The deformity appears to be caused by an imbalance between the flexor and extensor muscles of the great toe. In the diabetic patient ulceration of the callus on the dorsum of the interphalangeal joint may quickly permit the joint to become infected.

### Hammertoe

In hammertoe the metatarsophalangeal joint of the digit is extended, and the proximal interphalangeal joint is flexed. A painful corn (clavus) overlies the bony prominence of the proximal interphalangeal joint (Fig 21–26). When the clavus ulcerates, septic arthritis of the proximal interphalangeal joint may result. Occasionally calluses and penetrating ulcers may develop on the tips of the toe, which in the hammertoe is subject to friction on the insole of the shoe.

### Varus Deformity of Toes

Varus deformity, in which the third, fourth, and fifth toes drift medially, may cause nails to gouge adjacent toes, produc-

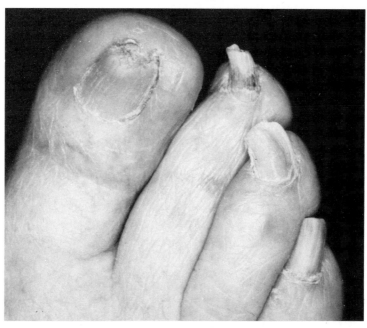

**FIG 21–20.**
Toes of obese diabetic patient with onychomycosis of nail of hallux and incurving distal growth of all nails. Nails have grown long because of neglect. Note that nail of third toe gouges skin of second toe.

ing small ulcers. Crowding, sometimes with overlap, causes skin friction of toe on toe.

### Web Infections

Web infections are particularly hazardous, because they may occur without pre-existing anatomic deformity. They may simply occur because of poor foot hygiene and accumulation of moist detritus in the webs, fissuring of skin, and entrance of infection. Infections beginning in the interdigital webs are especially dangerous because of the proximity of the digital arteries and because of ready access to the deeper structures of the foot by way of the lumbrical tendons.

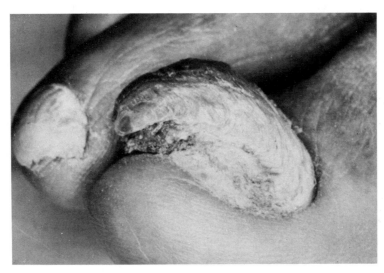

**FIG 21–21.**
Onychogryposis. In diabetic patient infection may begin in debris covering nail bed. This type of nail easily hooks bedding, socks, or furniture, causing avulsion of nail and trauma to proximal nail fold.

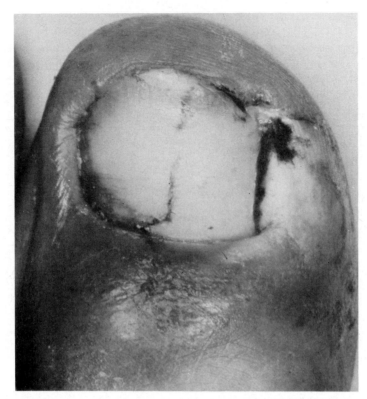

**FIG 21–22.**
Ingrowing nail with infection and granulation tissue of medial nail wall and cellulitis near base of nail.

### Heloma Molle

Heloma molle is a soft corn between the toes caused by a combination of osteoarthritis of the toe and crowding. The most common location is on the lateral side of the base of the fourth toe from pressure and friction of the adjacent head of the proximal phalanx of the fifth toe. Heloma molle can occur in other areas where a knobby joint of one toe crowds in on an adjoining toe (Fig 21–27). Heloma molle can lead to web space abscess.

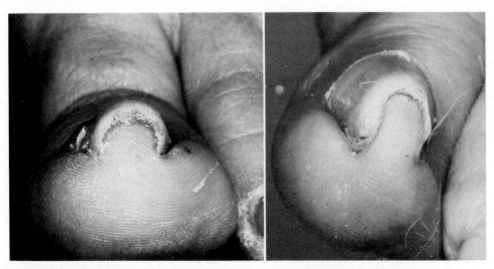

**FIG 21–23.**
Type of nail that is particularly hazardous in diabetic patient. It starts from wide base at nail root and incurves distally, pinching nail bed. These two nails form arcs of greater than 200 degrees at distal toe. If neglected, medial and lateral nail margins may meet beyond distal toe, forming full circle and brittle claw.

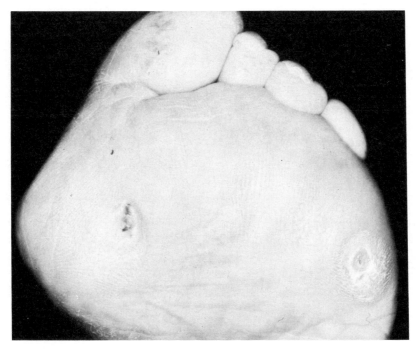

**FIG 21–24.**
Diabetic foot with crowding of toes, hammertoes (note position of nails), bunion, and distal plantar calluses.

## Distal Foot

### *Hallux Valgus*

Hallux valgus is a deformity of the great toe at the metatarsophalangeal joint. The hallux deviates laterally (adduction) in rela-

tion to the first metatarsal shaft and head. A bony prominence, exostosis, appears over the head of the metatarsal medially, and a swollen bursa forms. Erosion and ulceration of the skin over the bony prominence allow

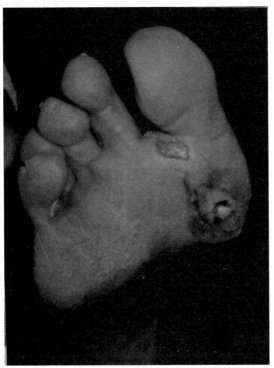

**FIG 21–25.**
Concentrated weight bearing in intrinsic minus foot with resultant ulcer over first metatarsal head.

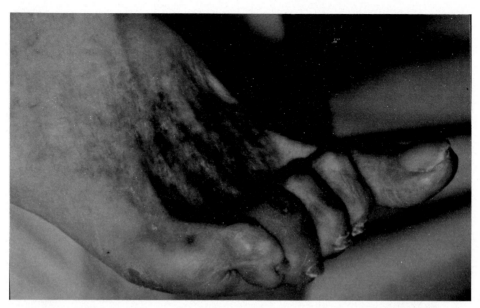

**FIG 21–26.**
Intrinsic minus foot with hammertoes and ulcer over proximal interphalangeal joint of fourth toe. Such ulcers can readily enter joint.

infection to enter the bursa. Subsequently the infection may spread along the abductor hallucis and flexor hallucis brevis muscles, causing medial plantar space infections. More indolent infections can erode the metatarsophalangeal joint and enter the joint with resultant septic arthritis and osteomyelitis.

### Tailor's Bunion

Tailor's bunion (bunionette of the fifth toe) is an exostosis of the lateral part of the fifth metatarsal head often associated with varus deformity of the fifth toe. As in hallux valgus, ulceration may occur in the diabetic with this deformity, and infection may

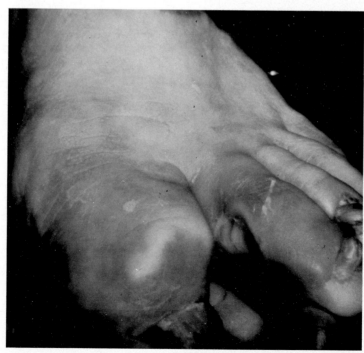

**FIG 21–27.**
Heloma molle of base of second toe from pressure of deformed adjacent interphalangeal joint of hallux.

spread into a joint or into the lateral plantar space (Fig 21–28).

### Distal Foot Calluses

Distal foot calluses are a frequent source of problems for the diabetic (Fig 21–29). Ulceration of the calluses causes mal perforans, which is discussed later in this chapter. The majority of foot ulcers occur under the metatarsal heads. The first, second, and fifth joints are involved in that order. All of the patients with ulcers exert maximum loads at the site of the ulcer. See also Chapters 9 and 10 for a discussion of detecting loads and pressure points.

## Middle Part of Foot

The middle part of the foot is not subject to calluses and deformities with ulcerations as are the toes but is frequently injured by penetrating objects. In the patient with advanced diabetes who cannot see well and cannot feel pain, infection spreads either directly to the central plantar space or along collagenous septa that connect the dermis to the plantar fascia. Inadequate circulation and failure to put the foot at rest contribute to worsening of the infection.

Central planter space abscesses can rupture in the sole of the middle part of the foot. When Charcot's foot collapses into a rocker sole, the weight on walking can be concentrated on the middle of the sole rather than on the metatarsal heads. Midsole ulcers may result.

## Heel

Because of the bony prominences of the calcaneus, the heel is sometimes the site of neurotrophic ulcers. When ulceration and gangrene occur in the heel, the foot is sel-

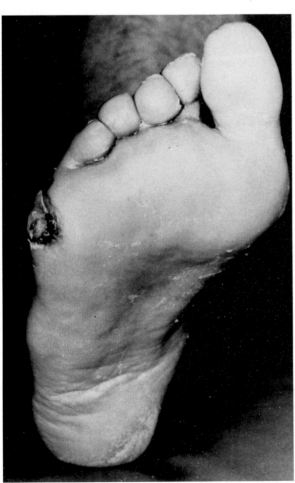

**FIG 21–28.**
Ulcerated callus at bunionette. Amputation of fifth ray was required because of penetration to joint. Ulcerated bunionette often is associated with shoes that are too snug.

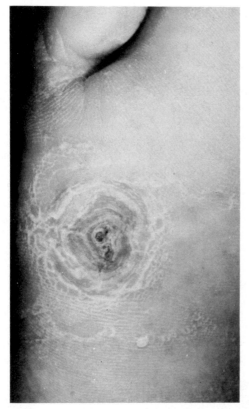

**FIG 21–29.**
Callus of distal part of lateral sole. Cracking and fissuring allow entry of bacteria.

arterial flow is adequate. Commonly these deformities are ignored at this time because they are being tolerated. Later, when they are being poorly tolerated, elective correction is hazardous and may itself precipitate disaster. Serious consideration should be given to correction of deformities early. Most of them can be palliated and the difficulty deferred by good podiatric treatment and follow-up (see Chapters 23 and 24). The physician should take into consideration the intelligence and educability of the patient, opportunity for observation, general condition and associated systemic diseases, age, occupation, activity, and evaluation of circulation, and neuropathy and should definitively treat many more of the nail, toe, and distal foot abnormalities while the opportunity exists. Treatment after entry of infection and beginning local spread is often unavailing.

The nail, toe, and distal foot abnormalities in the diabetic foot are numerically so overwhelming that not all of them can be attended to, but certainly lesions that have already given rise to minor infections should be corrected. With the passage of time in-

dom salvagable because debridement and amputations in this area often preclude functional weight bearing. Ulcers and patches of gangrene can develop on the posterolateral surface of the heel as the immobile foot of the supine patient lies abducted on the mattress (Fig 21–30). Lesions of the more posterior portion of the heel usually indicate excessive walking on the insensitive foot (Fig 21–31). Heel lesions present exceedingly difficult surgical problems. Leg or thigh amputations are often necessary.

## Question of Prophylactic Surgery

Many of the aforementioned abnormalities that can later lead to a break in the skin, infection, and progression to gangrene and major debridements and amputations are seen in younger diabetics, perhaps at a time when neuropathy is insignificant and

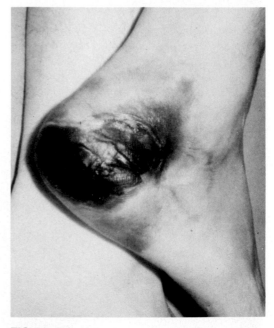

**FIG 21–30.**
Gangrene of heel in bedridden diabetic patient caused by weight of immobile neuropathic foot on mattress.

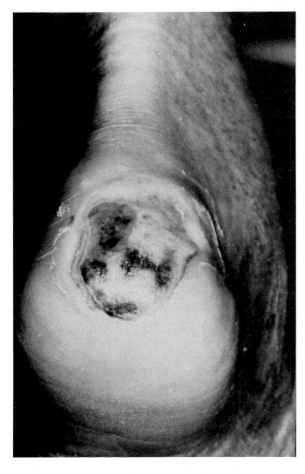

**FIG 21–31.**
Heel ulcer began as blister after one episode of excessive walking in patient with severe neuropathy.

grown nails, incurving nails, bunions, calluses, and hammertoes only become worse and do not improve.[19, 31] After a minor infection arising in a friction ulcer has been contained and the ulcer has healed, the scar is more vulnerable to later friction and is likely to ulcerate again. The scar epithelium is less durable than the originally intact skin. The capillaries and arterioles beneath this epithelium have been thrombosed, and on healing they only partly recanalize and reform.

The following are requirements for prophylactic operations for toe and foot deformities in diabetes. Amputation and debridements for infection and gangrene are discussed in Chapter 20.

1. The deformity should no longer be amenable to foot maintenance techniques such as nail clipping, protuberance padding, and callus trimming (see Chapter 23).

2. The deformity should be of such a character that ulceration can be expected or may have already occurred despite a good, supervised, foot maintenance program.

3. If the foot is ischemic, no procedure should be done unless revascularization has been successful (see Chapter 18).

4. The operation should be definitive and the deformity permanently corrected. For example, when a nail or portion of a nail needs to be removed, the corresponding generative area of the nail should also be removed.

5. Simple operations should be used. Osteoplastic operations and tendon transfers require more tissue handling than do the more simple amputations, osteotomies, ostectomies, and removal of exostoses.

6. Scar on weight-bearing sites should be avoided. In distal toe amputations the plantar flap should be longer than the dorsal flap. Incisions for removal of metatarsal heads should be made in the dorsum of the foot.

7. Muscle imbalances should be avoided. An amputation through the middle phalanx of a toe will often result in the toe being pulled into extension unless an extensor tenotomy is also done.

## MAJOR INFECTIONS

Mead and Mueller[30] recognize three basic anatomic types of major foot infection. These three types, which represent different problems and require different treatments, are (1) abscess occurring in the deep spaces of the foot, chiefly in the central plantar space; (2) nonsuppurative phlegmon of the dorsum of the foot; and (3) mal perforans ulcer of the plantar surface of the foot. In a prospective study of major foot infections in 300 diabetic patients, Bose[4] found that the distribution of these lesions was as follows: abscesses in the deep spaces of the foot in 240 patients (80%), cellulitis of the dorsum of the foot in 24 patients (8%), and perforating ulcer in 36 patients (12%).

The frequently unshod foot of the diabetic in the Third World is subject more often to central plantar space abscess from penetration.[1] Central plantar space abscess can be the most devastating infection in the foot.[6, 14] Infection may enter the deep plantar space in several ways. Direct penetration by foreign bodies in the insensitive foot may not be recognized until the abscess is well established and has produced swelling so pronounced that it can be seen or can prevent putting on shoes.

Web space infections may begin with superficial breaks in the skin caused by fungus infections or by maceration associated with poor hygiene. Infection in the web space extends to the bursa of the lumbrical tendons and then follows the lumbrical muscle into the central plantar space. Infections of the plantar surfaces of the toes may spread into the central plantar space by means of involvement of the flexor tendon sheath.

Of Bose's[4] 240 cases of plantar abscess, 70 began as initial lesions near the nail or nail bed, 140 began as web space infections, and 30 were caused by direct penetration of the soles.

Infection anywhere in the toe may reach the plantar space by local spreading of infection until the flexor tendon sheath is involved by suppurative tenosynovitis. Consequently, it is common for infection to originate from areas near the toenails.

Once the infection is established in the plantar space, the characteristic signs of plantar abscess appear. The longitudinal arch and the skin creases disappear, and the area of the longitudinal arch may bulge. The sole of the foot becomes edematous. Frequently in the diabetic patient, pain and tenderness are absent and ambulation may continue, adding dependency and the milking action of motion to factors influencing spread of the infection. In a few days edema of the dorsum of the foot appears. The usual systemic signs of severe infection such as fever and malaise occur. Loss of diabetic control and ketoacidosis are often present. The appearance of glucosuria is sometimes the first abnormality noted by the patient and even sometimes is the feature that precipitates a visit to the physician.

Further spread of central plantar abscess may occur in the proximal part of the central plantar space, particularly in bedridden patients because the pus may gravitate. At the proximal end of the central plantar space, the long flexor tendons of the toes are again surrounded by bursa sheaths. After exiting from the plantar space, the tendons lie posterior to the medial malleolus. Through this route infection may be carried to the leg.

Thrombotic obliteration of small- and medium-sized vessels may occur in established plantar abscess, resulting in progressive necrosis of the plantar fascia, tendon, and tendon sheath. If extensive, this necrosis may prohibit salvage of the foot. Creeping necrosis can occur in fasciae, as well as in skin. The plantar digital arteries of the second, third, and fourth toes arise from the plantar arch; with nearby infection, thrombotic occlusion of the plantar arch can appear and lead to necrosis of all or portions of those toes, particularly the middle toe.

The *lateral* and *medial plantar spaces* contain the abductor and short flexor muscles of the first and fifth toes. In addition to infection by direct penetrating trauma, infection may enter these spaces from infected bunions. Frequently these difficulties start with new shoes, which abrade the skin in the first and fifth metatarsophalangeal areas. Penetration through the subcutaneous tissue and erosion of the joint capsule with septic arthritis may follow (Fig 21–32). Medial and lateral plantar space abscesses seldom spread into the central plantar space.

## Dorsal Foot Phlegmon

The extensor tendons are not encased in sheaths but lie in loose areolar tissue on the dorsum of the foot. Deep to the extensor tendons, a dense fascia overlies the interossei and metatarsal muscles. The extensor tendons are covered by a thin superficial fascia, which is continuous with the extensor retinaculum of the anterior ankle. This fascia serves to contain the tendons and prevent bowstringing.

Heavy fibrous bands extend from the dermis to the periosteum and tendon sheath on the plantar surface of the digits, compacting the fat lobules on this weight-bearing surface. These fibrous septa do not exist on the dorsum of the digit. Consequently, infections of the dorsum of the toes arising in nails and calluses are partly restricted from going around the toe by these bands. Paronychias and ulcerated calluses on hammertoes seldom spread at first to the toe pad or the flexor tendon and may not reach the central plantar spaces.

Spread in the dorsum of the foot is by the lymphatics. First, the soft tissues of the dorsum become red and edematous. Again, as in the diabetic foot in general, pain and tenderness depend on the degree of neuropathy. Second, fever, malaise, and loss of diabetic control occur. The edema may be of impressive proportions in diabetics with neuropathy whose lack of pain permits dependency and motion. The dorsal phlegmon of the diabetic foot does not differ from cellulitis in nondiabetics except that the infection is perpetuated and spread by continuing use of the foot in diabetics with neuropathy, whereas persons with normal sensation elevate and rest the foot of their own volition. With infective occlusions of small vessels in the skin and lack of opportunity to develop collateral flow, the result may be necrosis of the skin overlying the

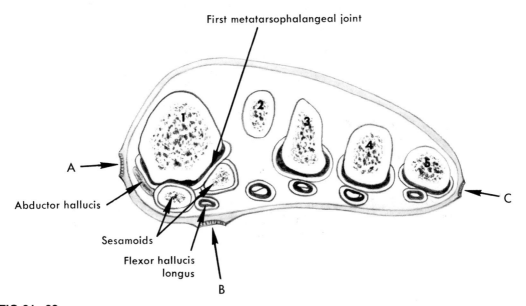

**FIG 21–32.**
Common modes of spread of infection in distal foot. **A,** infection from ulcerated bunion may enter lateral plantar space or first metatarsophalangeal joint fairly readily. Joint infection then can penetrate into central plantar space. **B,** mal perforans fixes flexor tendons. With progression of infection, plantar space or joint may be entered. **C,** ulcerated tailor's bunion finds meager tissue barrier to entry into fifth metatarsophalangeal joint.

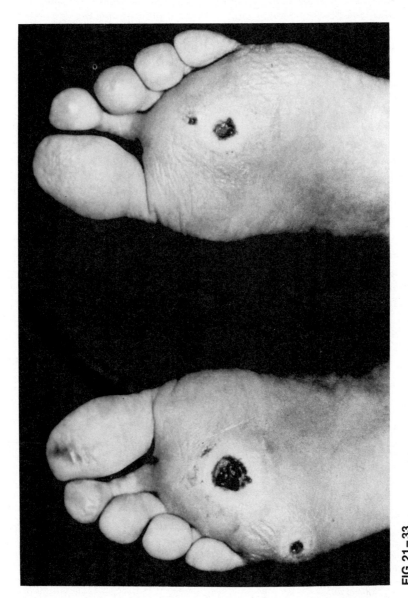

**FIG 21–33.**
Mal perforans ulcers of both feet over metatarsal heads.

phlegmonous area. Infections that may be controlled in nondiabetics lead in the diabetic, with microangiopathy, to death of tissue.

## Mal Perforans

Mal perforans is a chronic, indolent ulcer of the sole of the foot, usually over the head of the first, second, or fifth metatarsal (Fig 21–33). Ordinarily it is caused by ulceration of a preexisting callus. After the ulceration occurs, the hard, thickened area of hyperkeratinization continues to surround the crater. When seen, mal perforans is uniformly associated with neuropathy and probably is a direct consequence of it. Most of the patients with mal perforans do not have ischemia.[15] Characteristically the mal perforans implies severe neuropathy in the presence of good blood flow. The neuropathy is both autonomic and somatic.

The initial calluses are the result of concentrated weight bearing, chronic friction, and minor irritation in the insensitive foot. The high incidence of calluses in the diabetic foot is associated with a combination of sensory deficit and neurogenic small-muscle atrophy. The small-muscle atrophy produces abnormal foot alignment, which forces the body weight to be borne on surfaces poorly designed, anatomically, for that purpose. Fissuring and cracking in the calluses allow a variety of organisms to enter. The subsequent minor infection is ignored, and continued walking results in central excavation of the callus.

Penetration in the subcutaneous tissue in the sole of the foot is limited from lateral spread by the dense fibrous septa that partition the subcutaneous fat into lobules, giving resiliency to the walking surface. For a long time deep penetration may be limited to skin and subcutaneous tissue. The plantar fascia is partly deficient over the metatarsal heads, because the fibers of the plantar aponeurosis split and pass between the metatarsal heads. The flexor tendon may then form the base of the ulcer. Notwithstanding the presence of the flexor tendon in the ulcer, acute tenosynovitis and acute extension to the plantar spaces with acute abscess formation seldom occur. The slow progression of the ulcer, often in a foot with adequate circulation, allows the buildup of fibrous tissue in advance of the ulcer. The tendon sheaths and tissue spaces become obliterated. The flexor tendon becomes fixed to its sheath and to the underlying metatarsophalangeal joint capsule and periosteum. Ultimately the tendon is eroded and the joint entered, with subsequent septic arthritis and osteomyelitis. The

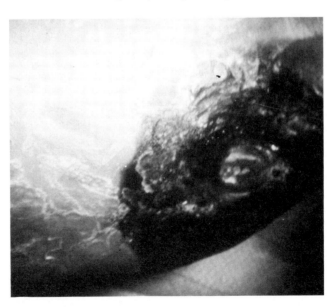

**FIG 21–34.**
Gangrene spreading radially from mal perforans after superficial femoral artery thrombosis.

depth of penetration of the plantar ulcer is often misjudged on clinical examination. More of them penetrate to deeper structures than is ordinarily suspected. Newman et al.,[33] by bone biopsy and bone culture, found underlying osteomyelitis in 68% of diabetic foot ulcers. Only 32% of those with osteomyelitis had been diagnosed clinically by the referring physician. The majority of those with osteomyelitis were ambulatory outpatients. Leukocyte scanning[33] and magnetic resonance imaging[13, 32, 34] may assist in the diagnosis of bone infections.

Episodes of quiescence alternate with flareups of infection, and periodically the foot becomes red and swollen. The arterial circulation is usually good; otherwise this infection would not be tolerated. Gangrene of the skin spreading radially from the mal perforans center often means that occlusion of a major vessel (superficial femoral, popliteal) higher in the leg has occurred and is an indication for angiography (Fig 21–34).

## REFERENCES

1. Akanji AO: The pattern of presentation of foot lesions in Nigerian diabetic patients, *West Afr J Med* 9:1, 1990.

2. Beach KW, Bedford GR, Bergelin RO, et al: Progression of lower-extremity arterial occlusive disease in type II diabetes mellitus, *Diabetes Care* 11(suppl):464, 1988.

3. Bild DE, Selby JV, Sinnock P, et al: Lower extremity amputation in people with diabetes: epidemiology and prevention, *Diabetes Care* 12:24, 1989.

4. Bose K: A surgical approach for the infected diabetic foot, *Int Orthop* 3:177, 1979.

5. Brodsky JW: Diabetic foot infections, *Orthop Clin North Am* 22:473, 1991.

6. Carson JD, Jacobs RL, Karmody AM, et al: The diabetic foot, *Curr Probl Surg* 23:722, 1986.

7. Ctercteko GC, Dhanendran M, Hutton WC, et al: Vertical forces acting on the feet of diabetic patients with neuropathic ulceration, *Br J Surg* 68:608, 1981.

8. Deanfield J.E., Daggett PR, Harrison MJG: The role of autonomic neuropathy in diabetic foot ulceration, *J Neurol Sci* 47:203, 1980.

9. Delbridge L, Ctercteko G, Gowler C, et al: The aetiology of diabetic neuropathic ulceration of the foot, *Br J Surg* 72:1, 1985.

10. Duckworth T, Boulton AJM, Betts RP, et al: Plantar pressure measurements and the prevention of ulceration in the diabetic foot, *J Bone Joint Surg* 67B:79, 1985.

11. Fagrell B, Hermansson I-L, Karlander S-G, et al: Vital capillary microscopy for assessment of skin viability of microangiopathy in patients with diabetes mellitus, *Acta Med Scand* 687(suppl):25, 1984.

12. Faris I, Duncan H: Vascular disease and vascular function in the lower limb in diabetes, *Diabetes Res* 1:171, 1984.

13. Ferkel RD, et al: Magnetic resonance imaging of the foot and ankle: correlation of normal anatomy with pathologic conditions, *Foot Ankle* 11:289, 1991.

14. Fernando DJ, et al: The diabetic foot, *Diabetic Med* 8:82, 1991.

15. Fernando DJ, et al: Risk factors for nonischemic foot ulceration in diabetic nephropathy, *Diabetic Med* 8:223, 1990.

16. Ferrier TM: Comparative study of arterial disease in amputated lower limbs from diabetics and nondiabetics (with special reference to foot arteries), *Med J Aust* 1:5, 1967.

17. Frykberg RG: Neuropathic arthropathy: the diabetic Charcot's foot, *Diabetes Educ* 9:17, 1984.

18. Giannestras NJ: *Foot disorders*, Philadelphia, 1967, Lea & Febiger.

19. Gooding GAW, Stess RM, Graf PM, et al: Sonography of the sole of the foot: evidence for loss of foot pad thickness in diabetes and its relationship to ulceration of the foot, *Invest Radiol* 21:45, 1986.

20. Grant JCB: *An atlas of anatomy*, ed 6, Baltimore, 1972, Williams & Wilkins.

21. Harris R, Linn MW: Health beliefs, compliance, and control of diabetes mellitus, *South Med J* 78:162, 1985.

22. Hietala S-O, Lithner F: Foot angiography in diabetic patients with gangrene, *Acta Med Scand* 687(suppl):61, 1984.

23. Hughes J, Clark P, Klenerman L: The importance of the toes in walking, *J Bone Joint Surg (B)* 72:245, 1990.

24. Kastrup J, Lassen NA, Parving H-H: Diabetic microangiography: a factor enhancing the functional significance of peripheral occlusive arteriosclerotic disease, *Clin Physiol* 4:367, 1984.

25. Leventhal H, Zimmerman R, Gutmann M: Compliance: a self-regulation perspective, in Gentry WD, editor: *Handbook of behavioral medicine*, New York, 1984, Guilford Press.

26. Lewis BL: Microscopic studies of fetal and mature nail and surrounding soft tissue, *Arch Dermatol Syph* 70:732, 1954.

27. LoGerfo FW, Coffman JD: Vascular and microvascular diseases of the foot in diabetes: implications for foot care, *N Engl J Med* 311:1615, 1984.

28. LoGerfo FW, Gibbons GW, Pomposelli FB Jr, et al: Trends in the care of the diabetic foot: expanded role of arterial reconstruction, *Arch Surg* 127:617, 1992.

29. Margo MK: Surgical treatment of conditions of the fore part of the foot, *J Bone Joint Surg* 49A:1665, 1967.

30. Meade JW, Mueller CB: Major infections of the foot, *Med Times* 96:154, 1968.

31. Meyerson MS: Management of compartment syndromes of the foot, *Clin Orthop* 271:239, 1991.

32. Moore TE: Abnormalities of the foot in patients with diabetes mellitus: findings on MR imaging, *AJR* 157:813, 1991.

33. Newman LG, Waller J, Palestro CJ, et al: Unsuspected osteomyelitis in diabetic foot ulcers, diagnosis and monitoring by leukocyte scanning with indium In 111 oxyquinoline, *JAMA* 266:1246, 1991.

34. O'Hanlan JM: Osteomyelitis of the foot in diabetic patients: evaluation with magnetic resonance imaging, *J Foot Surg* 34:397, 1991.

35. Osterman HM, Stuck RM: The aging foot, *Orthop Nurs* 9:43, 1990.

36. Pederson J, Olsen S: Small vessel diseases of the lower extremity in diabetes mellitus: on the pathogenesis of the foot lesions in diabetics, *Acta Med Scand* 171:551, 1962.

37. Raju UB, Fine G, Partamian JO: Neuropathic neuroarthropathy (Charcot's Joint), *Arch Pathol Lab Med* 106:349, 1982.

38. Rosenquist U: An epidemiologic survey of diabetic foot problems in Stockholm County 1982, *Acta Med Scand* 687(suppl)55, 1984.

39. Spencer F, Sage R, Graner J: The incidence of foot pathology in a diabetic population, *J Am Podiatr Assoc* 75:590, 1985.

40. Sutton RL Jr: *Diseases of the skin*, ed 11, St Louis, 1956, Mosby-Year Book.

41. Walsh CH, Soler NG, Fitzgerald MG et al: Association of foot lesions with retinopathy in patients with newly diagnosed diabetes, *Lancet* 1:878, 1975.

42. Wessler S, Schlesinger MJ: Studies in peripheral arterial occlusive disease: I. Methods and pathologic findings in amputated limbs, *Circulation* 7:641, 1953.

43. Worth CT, McEwen J: A follow-up study of diabetic patients with foot problems in Nottingham, 1971–1978, *Practitioner* 226:2085, 1982.

# CHAPTER 22

# Rehabilitation

**Phala A. Helm, M.D.**

**Karen J. Kowalske, M.D.**

Diabetes with serious complications secondary to the disease requires a well-organized, knowledgeable, comprehensive health care team to deliver optimal, staged care. In spite of the estimated 14 million diabetics in the United States, in most health care settings, treatment is fragmented and the center concept has been slow to develop.

Reiber[22] reported that foot pathologic conditions were the most common diabetic complication leading to hospitalization, and the actual cost of diabetic foot problems was unknown. In a cost of illness study assessing United States economic costs of non-insulin-dependent diabetes mellitus (NIDDM), it was estimated that chronic skin ulcers accounted for $150 million of the $11.6 billion spent in direct NIDDM costs. Reiber[22] also reported that a 1987 survey of United States hospitals (excluding military and Veterans Affairs hospitals) indicated 56,000 diabetics had at least one amputation.

This monumental problem mandates that rehabilitation of the diabetic patient begin before complications develop. Preventive programs to maintain cardiovascular fitness, mobility, strength, endurance, and care for one's feet should be emphasized by all team members. To design a comprehensive rehabilitation program for the diabetic, a thorough history, physical examination, and diagnostics are essential.

## EVALUATION

The evaluation should include assessment for mobility, ulcerations, edema, bony and soft tissue deformities of the feet, and inspection for skin changes. Sensation, strength, peripheral pulses, and a thorough cardiovascular examination should also be included in the total examination.

### Mobility: Proximal Limitations

When a patient is initially evaluated for diabetic foot problems, the clinician is remiss if assessment does not include deviations of the trunk, leg length discrepancies, and hip and knee deformities. Preexisting problems such as kyphoscoliosis, congenitally shortened limb, or proximal contractures may cause a difference in leg length that can result in abnormal pressure distribution on the feet. In some cases this can be easily corrected with inlays for the shoes or with external elevation of the heel and sole of the shoe.

By watching our patients walk while they are undressed, we can easily detect other abnormalities. In diabetic foot clinics, it is customary to remove shoes and socks; however, one can become so focused on the foot that looking at the total person unclothed is frequently neglected. Degenerative joint disease (DJD) of the hips and knees is not an uncommon finding in the overweight population and is often found in patients with diabetic foot problems. Degenerative joint disease of the hip can result in pain, as well as hip and knee contractures, producing abnormal foot pressures. For example, contracture of the hip in an externally rotated position causes increased pressure on the medial foot and great toe when the patient is ambulating.

Degenerative joint disease of the knees can cause genu valgum or varum with associated limitation of knee motion and an abnormal gait pattern. High-pressure areas may occur on the medial foot with valgus deformity and on the lateral foot with varus deformity of the knee.

Treatment of these conditions with range of motion and strengthening exercises may be beneficial if the disease has not progressed to an advanced state. With hip and knee deformity, secondary to DJD, modifications of footwear are not usually beneficial.

### Limited Joint Mobility: Foot and Ankle

Diabetics often have limitation in range of motion with feet that are rigid, firm, and dry. Several studies have shown that limitation of joint mobility of the foot and ankle causes abnormally high plantar foot pressures.[8, 16] There are multiple reasons why joint mobility can be compromised. With a motor neuropathy, muscle imbalance may occur and contractures develop. Intrinsic muscle weakness of the foot causes the toes to claw, resulting in contractures of the toes in hyperextension at the metatarsophalangeal joints and in flexion at the proximal interphalangeal joints. Claw toes increase loading on the metatarsal heads because they are contracted in an extended position; therefore, they do not sustain normal load at terminal stance in the gait cycle. High arches are also seen with an intrinsic minus foot; thus, secondary contracture of the plantar fascia can cause an even greater increase of pressure on the plantar forefoot. The extensor hallucis longus muscle can be weak, causing the great toe to become tight in plantar flexion.

When the peroneal nerve is compromised (as we often see in diabetics), weakness in toe extension, foot eversion, and ankle dorsiflexion occurs and the foot inverts and plantar flexes; thus, contractures of the triceps surae, posterior tibialis, and toe flexors occur, causing limited joint mobility and increased plantar pressures. Because of muscle weakness there is altered loading of the foot with longer duration of ground contact and an increase in forefoot pressure. Antigravity weakness of the anterior tibialis and the toe extensors causes the foot to slap when decelerating from dorsiflexion to plantar flexion, loading the forefoot with greater force and increasing the pressure on the metatarsal heads. A metabolic reason for limitation of joint mobility is impaired degradation of collagen, leading to its accumulation, causing periarticular stiffness. Soft tissue changes, such as very dry, cracked skin, can limit joint and skin mobility and result in open wounds that are more susceptible to infection.

Mueller et al.[17] found decreased sensation and limited joint mobility of dorsiflexion and subtalar joint motion in patients with diabetes mellitus and foot ulcerations. They believed that limited dorsiflexion and subtalar motion restricted the foot's ability to absorb shock and transverse rotation, therefore increasing the risk of plantar ulceration in the insensate foot. They[17] concluded that less than 5 degrees of dorsiflexion or 30 degrees of subtalar motion should be treated with mobility exercises and protective footwear.

Treatment of the rigid, contracted foot can be accomplished by massage with total foot mobilization, including the metatarsal bones (an up and down motion), stretching the toes in flexion and extension, the foot in inversion and eversion, the forefoot in adduction and abduction, and the ankle in dorsiflexion and plantar flexion (Figs 22–1 to 22–3). Massage and stretching may result in increased mobility (Figs 22–4 and 22–5).

### Ulcerations

Diabetics have various types of skin ulcerations and other types of dermatologic problems that must be differentiated because methods of treatment differ. Neuro-

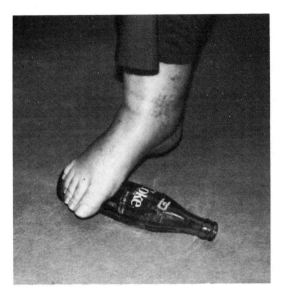

**FIG 22–1.**
Foot mobilization exercises.

pathic ulcers are located primarily on the plantar aspect of the feet and with claw toe deformities on the tips and dorsal aspect of the toes. Ischemic ulcers occur more on the dorsolateral foot and tips of the toes, whereas stasis ulcers are more likely to occur over the medial ankle above the malleolus. Ulcer size, location, appearance, odor, and surrounding skin changes all should be recorded and changes noted on follow-up visits (see Chapter 2). If erythema, warmth, or drainage is present, infection should be suspected and treatment with a broad-spectrum antibiotic considered (see Chapter 8). The issue of culturing foot ulcers remains controversial. Swab cultures may be misleading. Sterile saline irrigation, followed by

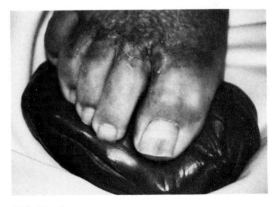

**FIG 22–2.**
Active and resistive exercises to increase mobility of toes.

curettage of the base of the ulcer, is the clinical practice recommendation of the American Diabetes Association.[9] Underlying osteomyelitis is often clinically silent and must be ruled out, especially in nonhealing, deep or draining wounds, or wounds with exposed bone.[19] If neuroarthropathy is present, the differentiation of osteomyelitis becomes more difficult. Bone scans may be of some use but are often positive in both conditions. Of the imaging tests, leukocyte scan has a high sensitivity but may not be readily available.[19] Magnetic resonance imaging (MRI) appears to be specific for osteomyelitis and is becoming more accessible in most areas. Bone biopsy to evaluate for osteomyelitis is invasive and should be reserved for equivocal cases.

## Edema

Lower limb edema is often seen in diabetics with foot ulcerations and may be caused by the inflammatory process or secondary disease complications such as renal or cardiac conditions. Apelqvist et al.[1] reported that ulcers in patients with pitting edema were less likely to heal. Edema, especially fluctuating edema, makes lower limb orthotic application for deformity and casting for foot ulcers much more difficult. Erythema with associated edema may indicate neuroarthropathy (Charcot joint), which requires a thorough evaluation and immediate treatment if the diagnosis is made. When acute Charcot joints or ulcerations are treated with immobilization by total contact casting, cardiac demands increase; thus, close monitoring, especially of the elderly, is advisable.

## Bony and Soft Tissue Deformity

An insensate foot that is deformed or malaligned because of bony or soft tissue abnormalities is a foot at risk. The examiner must recognize and record these changes before prescribing correct footwear and orthoses for preventive treatment. The list of problems is almost endless, but a few of the more common deformities in combination with a neuropathy that can cause serious complications are hallux valgus, hallux rigidus, claw toes, hammertoes, pronated

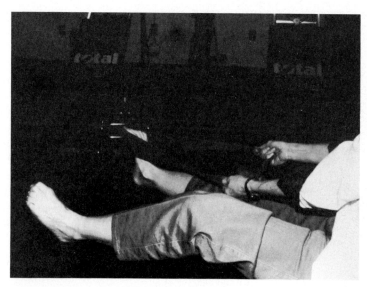

**FIG 22–3.**
Stretching combined with active exercise to increase foot mobility.

foot, supinated foot, Charcot joint, previous surgeries or amputation, healed ulcer scars, tight plantar fascia, rigid foot, and skin atrophy.

It has been shown that foot deformity results in increased plantar pressures but that deformity alone does not cause ulceration.[8] Fernando et al.[8] found the incidence of plantar ulceration in diabetics with limited joint mobility and neuropathy to be 65%. In patients with neuropathy without limited joint motion, ulcer incidence was 5%. In those patients with limited joint motion without neuropathy, the incidence was 0%.[8]

## Sensation

Peripheral neuropathy with loss of distal sensation is a common complication of diabetes[4] and may be related to metabolic ab-

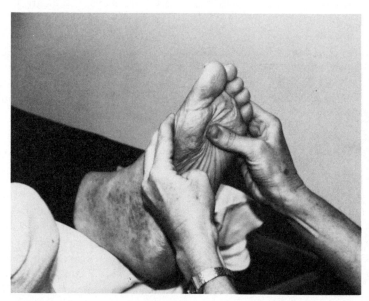

**FIG 22–4.**
Foot masssage and stretching yield good results in increased mobility.

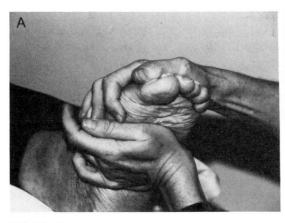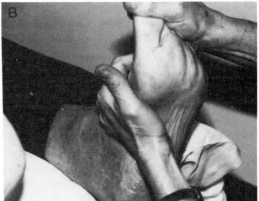

**FIG 22–5.**
Stretch toes in flexion, **(A)** and extension **(B)** to increase mobility.

normalities in neural tissues that are related to hyperglycemia.[2, 4] Although touch sensation can easily be evaluated using a cotton swab, it does not provide the quantifiable information essential for following disease progression or for research comparisons. The Semmes-Weinstein monofilament test is a commonly used quantitative tool for evaluation of touch sensation.[12, 17] Other authors have used vibratory testing to evaluate for a peripheral neuropathy.[3] It can be measured grossly with a tuning fork or more accurately by the bioesthesiometer.[3, 18]

## Motor Status

Motor examination includes both inspection for muscle wasting and formal muscle testing. Proximal muscle testing is essential to rule out some of the common conditions that cause muscle weakness that influence patient's gait and balance and cause unequal pressure distribution on the feet. Radiculopathies, mononeuropathies, and mild paresis secondary to a cerebrovascular accident are problems frequently overlooked when one is testing the diabetic. Proximal muscles of the upper limbs may also be weak for a variety of reasons, and this too can affect ambulation. Good strength is necessary in the shoulder depressors and abductors and elbow and wrist extensors to walk safely with crutches or a walker.

A severe peripheral neuropathy may result in balanced weakness of both the ankle and toe flexors and extensors, resulting in a steppage gait and no muscle power for terminal stance. The peroneal nerve is easily compromised in the diabetic patient, resulting in an unbalanced foot with weakness of only the dorsiflexors, evertors, and toe extensors. Functionally the foot assumes a plantar flexed, inverted position, again applying unequal forces on the plantar surface.

## Vascular Status

When the total rehabilitation program is considered, the patient's vascular status must be determined. Peripheral vascular disease (PVD) with associated claudication may limit ambulation distance and tolerance and thus may be an indication for a progressive walking program. Peripheral vascular disease is a major consideration when one is prescribing casting or prosthetic training because these activities increase the vascular demand on the uninvolved limb and may result in ischemia. Examination begins with inspection for skin atrophy, dependent erythema, hair loss, and nail changes, because all are suggestive of ischemia. Skin temperature, easily tested with the dorsal hand, can be compared side to side and proximal to distal.

## Cardiovascular Status

A thorough cardiac examination, including heart rate and blood pressure monitoring, lying, sitting and standing, and with activity, can be used to determine the therapeutic range for heart rate and evaluate cardiac response to activity. Certainly unstable angina would be a contraindication for exercise, but the majority of other cardiac diagnoses do not prevent ambulation, strengthening, functional retraining, or other therapeutic interventions. In fact, rehabilitation of patients after myocardial infarction has been shown to decrease mortality.[20] Cardiac patients can improve exercise tolerance by increasing the efficiency of the skeletal muscles. If functionally limiting cardiac disease is present, preconditioning before intervention may be necessary. This would include a generalized conditioning program before prosthetic fitting or casting for an ulcer.

Autonomic neuropathy is an uncommon but significant complication of diabetes and has an effect on cardiovascular reflexes. The reported incidence of autonomic neuropathy ranges from 17% to 74% in unselected patients.[8, 13] The most commonly measured parameters are variations in heart rate with a single breath, Valsalva's maneuver, or with six respirations/minute. Although these tests of heart rate variation are scientifically interesting, their relevance to clinical practice is controversial. The most significant factors affecting rehabilitation regulated by the autonomic nervous system are orthostatic hypotension, difficulty regulating heart rate, and anhidrosis. In the Neil et al.[18] population-based study of these cardiovascular reflexes, no difference in postural hypotension was seen between patients with normal and abnormal heart rate variation. This suggests that orthostatic hypotension is a multifactorial problem affected by fluid status and hormonal regulation and is only partially regulated by the autonomic nervous system.[18]

## Psychologic Evaluation

The psychologic aspects of the diabetic with foot problems have not been well studied. In a recent study of diabetics, Lloyd et al.[15] showed that quality of life was significantly lower and fewer type A behaviors were seen in patients with four or more disease-related complications. Because multiple complications may result in a lower quality of life and less type A behaviors, a prospective study is needed to determine if having a type A personality or a good quality of life provides a protective effect.[15]

## AMPUTATIONS: THE AMPUTEE

Preventing amputation in the diabetic patient requires a thorough understanding of the causes to intervene in a timely, effective manner. Pecoraro et al.[21] reported that most diabetic lower limb amputations result from a combination of causes rather than from a unitary cause. They found that there were seven potential causal pathways: (1) ischemia, (2) infection, (3) neuropathy, (4) faulty wound healing, (5) minor trauma, (6) cutaneous ulceration, and (7) gangrene. In their study of 80 lower limb amputations, the sequence of minor trauma, resulting in cutaneous ulceration and subsequent faulty wound healing, preceded 72% of the amputations. Lack of protective sensation was a component cause in 82% of those amputations. A single cause was found to be responsible for amputations in those patients who had ischemia from acute arterial occlusion.[21]

For patients with an amputation, ambulation with a prosthesis is not always possible. Steinberg et al.[25] studied 116 lower limb amputees 65 years and older. Of 59 unilateral transtibial amputees who were fitted with a prosthesis, 73% became functional wearers (using it full time to ambulate), and 25% became part-time wearers. Of 30 persons who had unilateral transfemoral amputations, 50% were functional wearers; 14% were part-time wearers. Of the bilateral amputees, only 33% became full-time users. In this study, functional outcome difference between diabetic and nondiabetic patients was not statistically significant.[25]

Volpicelli et al.[27] reported on the ambulation level of 103 bilateral lower limb amputees. Of 38 bilateral transfemoral amputees, 2 with traumatic amputation were prosthetically rehabilitated, whereas 35 with dysvascular amputation were not. Combination of transfemoral and transtibial amputations were reported in 21 patients. Of these, five were prosthetically rehabilitated, including four dysvascular amputees. Forty-four patients had bilateral transtibial amputations, with 35 prosthetically rehabilitated.[27] In general, with greater length of the amputated limb, function is better and energy cost is less. It is thus very important to save the knee joint.[30]

Clinicians must use common sense in deciding whether a patient should be fitted with a prosthesis. A lower limb prosthesis is extremely expensive, not including the cost of rehabilitation to prepare the patient to become a prosthetic user. The major indication for a prosthesis is the prospect of ambulation; however, there are patients who cannot ambulate but need a prosthesis to improve body mechanics and conserve energy to stand, pivot, and transfer. Kirby and Vinjamuri[14] tested nonambulatory sitting amputees with and without a prosthesis and concluded that a prosthesis improves the anterolateral reach of unilateral transtibial amputees and the straightforward and anterolateral reach of bilateral amputees. When a prosthesis was not being worn, a sitting surface that provided support of the residual limbs improved forward reach.[14]

There are patients who should not be fitted with a prosthesis for ambulation. Contraindications for prosthetic fitting may include a compromised residual limb (i.e., ulceration or dysvascularity), severe contracture of the hip or knee, a neurologic problem causing spasticity or weakness, mental deterioration, severe cardiac and respiratory disease, or failure to ambulate for a significant period before amputation. Chronologic age in itself is not a contraindication to fitting.

## ENERGY EXPENDITURE: FACTORS TO CONSIDER FOR AMBULATION

Energy expenditure is a major factor when decisions about ambulation are made. Reuter and Pierre[23] studied energy expenditure in normal and pathologic gait and found that there were greater than normal rates of energy expenditure and a decrease in walking velocity with progressive increases in knee flexion contracture. Loss of 15 degrees of knee extension caused a 7% rise in the rate of oxygen consumption and an 11% decrease in walking efficiency. A 30-degree loss caused a 15% rise in oxygen uptake and a 19% drop in efficiency. A 45-degree limitation resulted in a 21% increase in oxygen consumption and a 32% loss of walking efficiency. Energy cost increased progressively to 46% at the 45-degree knee flexion contracture level.[24] The energy cost may be more than older persons can tolerate, and they may stop walking. Because the body tries to compensate for this abnormality in increasing hip flexion and plantar flexion, there is an increase in forefoot contact with the floor during the stance phase. This must be kept in mind when one is evaluating patients with insensate limbs because it could cause an increase in forefoot pressure and skin breakdown; therefore, therapeutic intervention, including range of motion of the foot to alleviate the contracture, is indicated.

Waters et al.[29] also studied the effects of crutch walking. They found that a swing-through gait with weight bearing on one leg is "a high energy consumption experience." Compared with normal walking, the rate of oxygen consumption increased 70%, heart rate increased 48%, velocity decreased 23%, oxygen cost increased 233%, and gait efficiency dropped 57%.[29] Again, older persons may not be able to perform at this level.

For comparison in energy expenditure of the amputee, normal walking serves as the baseline. For men and women, the average rate of energy expenditure is 12.0 mL of oxygen/g per minute, at an average comfortable walking speed of 80 m/min. The average energy cost per unit of distance traveled is 0.15 mL of oxygen/g per minute. Regardless of age, the rate of energy expenditure for walking is the same for adults. Walking speed of the amputee is affected by the level of amputation and the physical condition resulting in amputation. Walking speed slows for higher levels and for amputations secondary to vascular disease. For dysvascular amputees, velocity for the transtibial level was 37% slower (45 m/min vs. 71 m/min) and at the transfemoral level 31% slower (36 vs. 52 m/min) compared with the traumatic amputee.[28]

In view of energy expenditure, the total rehabilitation program may need modification to accommodate the older patient who has a lower aerobic reserve and who therefore is less able to tolerate added physical stress. Our expectations of the ambulator must be based on physical evidence that the patient can perform at a level commensurate with his or her disability; otherwise, unrealistic demands are made on the patient (Table 22–1).

# PREOPERATIVE AND POSTOPERATIVE AMPUTEE REHABILITATION

A neglected part of total patient management is the preamputation stage. When amputation is anticipated or planned, rehabilitation clinicians have the opportunity to help prepare the patient physically and psychologically (Table 22–2). Questions can be answered and instructions given to alleviate anxieties of the unknown. Patients want to know what a prosthesis looks like, of what it is made, and how much it costs. The patient should be shown what type of exercise program is expected and how ambulation is performed with crutches or a walker on flat

**TABLE 22–1.**

Considerations for Amputation Levels

| Level | Considerations | Disadvantages |
|---|---|---|
| Transfemoral | Ideal length is at least 10 cm below the inguinal ligament[10] or 5–7 cm proximal to the knee joint[6]<br>Greater energy expenditure<br>Consider only if distal amputation is impossible | Very few become prosthetic users |
| Transtibial | Any length is better than transfemoral<br>Optimum length is three fourths the distance from knee joint to the musculotendinous junction of gastrocnemius and soleus<br>Very functional level | Knee flexion contractures<br>Short stumps, inadequate lever arm |
| Syme ankle Disarticulation | Disarticulation at talus<br>Longer lever arm<br>End bearing, more comfortable stump<br>Good for balance and stability | Less cosmetic design of prosthesis<br>End bearing sometimes a problem because of poor fit with insensate heel pad |
| Chopart Lisfranc | Chopart amputation at the midtarsal joints<br>Lisfanc amputation at the tarsometatarsal junction | Equinovarus deformity may occur if dorsiflexors and evertors are not reattached<br>Secondary skin breakdown<br>Prosthetic fitting is demanding |
| Transmetatarsal | Good primary healing<br>Preferred if more than two rays to be amputated<br>Longer lever arm for better push off<br>Stability in midstance | Short stump can piston up and down in shoe<br>Skin breakdown with improper footwear<br>High reamputation rate if preoperative level selection is not properly done |
| Ray | Toe phalanges and metatarsal shaft<br>Best is central ray<br>Requires only custom insoles and sometimes shoe modifications<br>Poor risk with localized gangrene | First ray resection can collapse medial arch causing increased pressure and ulceration<br>Fifth ray resection may cause foot supination and increased pressure over fourth metatarsal head |
| Hallux | Lateral shoe wear pattern<br>Functionally, little or no walking disability | Compromises stability of first ray<br>Slight callus formation beneath second and third metatarsal heads[5, 24] |

**TABLE 22–2.**

Comprehensive Treatment Program After Amputation

| Activity | Purpose | Treatment |
|---|---|---|
| Bed rest | Prevent pressure ulcers<br>Prevent contractures | Therapeutic mattress<br>Proper stump positioning<br>Splinting for knee extension<br>Prone positioning |
| Range of motion exercises | Prevent contractures, knee flexion, hip flexion, hip abduction, and external rotation | Passive and active range of motion to joints proximal to amputationabduction, and external rotation |
| Strengthening | Preparation for ambulation | Strengthen key crutch muscles<br>Stress hip and knee extensors<br>Strengthen both lower limbs |
| Transfer activities | Increase mobility | Mat activities and movement from bed to chair |
| Stump care | Reduce edema | Airsplint<br>Elastic shrinker<br>Semirigid dressing (Unna)<br>Rigid dressing (plaster of paris cast)<br>Ace wraps (less desirable) |
| Gait training | Maintain endurance<br>Preparatory for prosthesis | Balancing exercises<br>Instruct in use of crutches or walker |
| Prosthetic training | Prevent faulty gait pattern | Instruction by qualified clinician |

surfaces and stairs. Addressing these issues before amputation not only shortens recovery time but also gives the patient a psychologic edge.

Amputees at various levels have distinctive problems of anatomic and functional loss, fitting and alignment of the prosthesis, gait abnormalities, and medical issues that require continued care for the remainder of their lives. One major medical difficulty is skin problems secondary to wearing an artificial limb (Table 22–3). If the skin is sufficiently abused, the patient will no longer be able to wear a prosthesis until the condition is corrected.

## EXERCISE

General exercise programs are individualized to the patient's age, cardiovascular status, mentality, musculoskeletal limitations, and condition of the feet, particularly if the feet are insensate. Under sedentary conditions, energy expenditure with physical activity is about 30% of total daily caloric requirement (less for obese patients); this can increase to 40% or 50% with the addition of an exercise program. Exercise is excellent for weight reduction when combined with caloric restriction, and it also helps reduce the risk of vascular disease. There are also beneficial effects for those with hyperglycemia, hyperinsulinemia, or hyperlipidemia.[31]

For an exercise program to be beneficial, it must be done on a regular basis (three to four times each week), include both upper and lower limbs, and consist of low resistance but high repetitions. Waters and Yakura[31] reported that measurement of the rate of oxygen consumption after several minutes of exercise at a constant submaximal work load reflected the energy expended during the activity. The maximal aerobic capacity ($Vo_2max$) is the highest oxygen uptake one can attain during physical work and is the single best indicator of physical fitness. Usually an individual can reach the $Vo_2max$ in 2 to 3 minutes of exhausting work. The $Vo_2max$ is influenced by age, and after age 20 years, maximum oxygen uptake declines because of a decrease in maximum heart rate and stroke volume and a more sedentary life-style. The $Vo_2max$ also depends on the type of exercise. Oxygen demand is directly related to muscle mass involved. The $Vo_2max$ is lower with upper limb exercise

**TABLE 22–3.**

Commonly Occurring Skin Problems in Amputee Stump

| Problem | Cause | Treatment |
| --- | --- | --- |
| Maceration | Moist skin | Cornstarch in socket and on stump |
| | | Absorbent stump socks |
| | | More frequent sock changes |
| Folliculitis, cysts, boils | Hair follicle and sweat gland occlusion | Eliminate high pressure points in socket |
| Open wound/ulcer | Multiple causes, e.g., high-pressure area is common cause (Fig 22–6) | Remove prosthesis until healed |
| | | Local wound care |
| Friction and skin stretch | Secondary to socket design | Elasto-Gel (SW Technologies, Inc., Kansas City, Mo.) |
| | | Thin nylon stump sock |
| Excessive sweating | Lack of evaporation | Antiperspirants |
| Hypersensitivity | Failure to desensitize | Massage and handling |
| Skin adherence | Scar tissue | Massage |
| | | Socket modifications; plastic surgical revision |
| Poor hygiene | Bacterial and fungal infections, dermatitis, odor | Wash stump and socket and stump socks with sudsing detergent at night |
| Contact dermatitis | Secondary to prosthetic parts and finishes | Patch test; remove contact |
| | | Cool compress |
| | | Topical corticosteroids |
| Epidermoid cysts | Follicular keratin plugs very sensitive; usually found along upper margins of prosthesis | Surgical incision and drainage or excision |
| Fungal infections inside socket | Secondary to moisture | Fungistatic creams |
| Painful neuromas | | Desensitize by tapping |
| | | Local injection |
| | | Surgical removal |

than lower limb exercise; however, heart rate and blood pressure are higher in upper limb than lower limb exercise.[31]

A conditioning program can increase aerobic capacity by improving cardiac output, increasing capacity of cells to extract oxygen from the blood, increasing hemoglobin level, and increasing muscular mass; this leads to increased fat utilization as a source of energy, resulting in decreased lactate production during exercise and increasing endurance. Other healthy side effects include decrease in heart rate and blood pressure and increase in stroke volume and cardiac output.[31]

Recent studies have described both the advantages and disadvantages of exercise programs, depending on whether a person has type I or II diabetes. Horton[11] did an extensive review of the literature and reported that in insulin-deficient diabetics with poor metabolic control, exercise may cause a rise in blood glucose levels and cause the acute onset of ketosis. Even in patients with well-controlled diabetes, exercise of high intensity may produce sustained hyperglycemia. It has also been demonstrated that exercise potentiates the hypoglycemic effect of injected insulin and that the combination of insulin and exercise can lead to symptomatic hypoglycemia and decreased insulin requirements.[11] It is reported that exercise can cause soft tissue and joint injuries in patients with peripheral neuropathy and that vigorous exercise increases proteinuria. Patients with proliferative retinopathy are reported to be at risk for retinal and vitreous hemorrhages during vigorous exercises. Autonomic neuropathy may cause a significant decrease in physical working capacity. This in turn is associated with an increased resting pulse, decreased cardiovascular response to exercise, lower $Vo_2max$, and poor response to dehydration. Patients with type

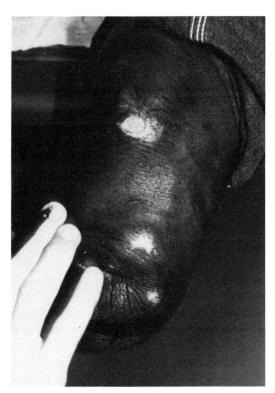

**FIG 22–6.**
Open wound associated with high pressure area in prosthesis

I diabetes who want to be involved in an exercise program and who do not have any major contraindicators should be encouraged to do so; however, a well-planned individualized program should be outlined so that the individual can exercise safely.[11]

Patients with type II diabetes, with insulin-resistant and impaired insulin secretion, commonly are obese with hyperlipidemia and hypertension. Treatment of these conditions generally involves dieting and regular physical exercise to improve insulin sensitivity. It has been shown that after physical training there is a 30% to 35% increase in insulin-stimulated glucose disposal. Type II diabetics who are involved in high-intensity exercise programs need adequate amounts of carbohydrates to maintain normal muscle glycogen.[11]

A major consideration for all diabetics when an exercise program is planned is the condition of the feet and proper footwear. If a patient has insensate limbs, certain physical activities or exercise programs must be avoided to prevent tissue destruction. Sustained brisk walking, running, and high-impact aerobic programs are contraindicated, whereas swimming, biking, and upper limb, high repetition–low resistance programs are well tolerated. Footwear should be protective and appropriate for the activity. For example, walking in a swimming pool can frequently damage insensate feet because of the rough surface; therefore, protective pool shoes are advisable. Good-fitting walking shoes with custom-molded insoles help distribute pressure equally over the foot and allow walking for longer distances without tissue damage. Diabetics with rigid or deformed feet do not have the flexibility to perform strenuous activities requiring quick agile movements; therefore, they must adjust their physical activities to primarily non–weight bearing exercise programs. Before an exercise prescription is written, precautions must be taken into account and activity programs individualized to provide a safe, healthy experience.

## RESULTS OF AN ORGANIZED APPROACH TO FOOT CARE

Foot problems in the diabetic population are multiple and require treatment by many disciplines. This treatment is generally fragmented or many times nonexistent. There are, however, a few foot centers where specialists in foot care are available to evaluate and treat the total patient. The organized approach to foot care in the diabetic population has been shown to be very effective in preventing complications. Edmonds et al.[6] reported 9,000 results from treatment in a specialized foot clinic where multiple disciplines were available. After 3 years this approach had achieved a high rate of ulcer healing and a reduction in major amputations. They reported healing in 86% of neuropathic ulcers and ischemic ulcers. The ulcer relapse rate in special shoes was 26% compared with 83% in those who reverted to their usual footwear. The number of major amputations for 2 years before the foot clinic were 11 and 12 amputations per year, respectively. This dropped to seven, seven, and five major amputations, respectively, over the next 3 years.[26] Thompson et al.[26] reported in a similar study the results of a multidisciplinary foot clinic in the United Kingdom. Over a 3-year period the annual number of amputations in diabetic patients was reduced overall 42%. Clearly, organized interdiscipline foot clinics, centers, and programs can save feet, and probably lives.

# REFERENCES

1. Apelqvist J, Larsson J, Agardh CD: The importance of peripheral pulses, peripheral edema and local pain for the outcome of diabetic foot ulcers, *Diabetic Med* 7:590–594, 1990.

2. Boulton AJM: The diabetic foot: neuropathic in aetiology, *Diabetes Med* 7:852–858, 1990.

3. Boulton AJM, Hardisty CA: Dynamic foot pressure and other studies as diagnostic and management aids in diabetic neuropathy, *Diabetes Care* 6:26–33, 1983.

4. Boulton AJM, Knight G: The prevalence of symptomatic diabetic neuropathy in an insulin treated population, *Diabetes Care* 8:125–128, 1988.

5. Czerniecki JM: Lower extremity amputations, in *14th annual review course in physical medicine and rehabilitation*, Bellevue, Wash, vol II, 1991, section 73, pp 1–8.

6. Edmonds ME, Blundell MP, Morris ME, et al: Improved survival of the diabetic foot: the role of a specialized foot clinic, *Q J Med* 232:763–771, 1986.

7. Ewing DJ, Martyn CN, Young RJ, et al: The value of cardiovascular autonomic function tests, ten years experience in diabetes, *Diabetes Care* 8:491–498, 1985.

8. Fernando DJS, Masson EA, Veves A, et al: Limited joint mobility: relationship to abnormal foot pressures and foot ulceration, *Diabetologia* 33:A170 (suppl), 1990.

9. Foot care in patients with diabetes mellitus, *Diabetes Care*, 14(suppl 1):18–19, 1991.

10. Friedmann LW: Rehabilitation of the amputee, in Goodgold J, editor: *Rehabilitation medicine*, St Louis, 1988, Mosby-Year Book, p 602.

11. Horton E: Exercise and diabetes mellitus, *Med Clin North Am* 72:1301–1321, 1988.

12. Holewski JJ, Moss KM, Stess RM, et al: Prevalence of foot pathology and lower extremity complications in a diabetic outpatient clinic, *J Rehabil Res Dev* 26:35–44, 1989.

13. Kennedy WR, Navarro X, Sakuta M, et al: Physiological and clinical correlates of cardiorespiratory reflexes in diabetes mellitus, *Diabetes Care* 12:399–408, 1989.

14. Kirby RL, Vinjamuri RC: Prostheses and the forward reach of sitting lower-limb amputees, *Arch Phys Med Rehabil* 71:125–127, 1990.

15. Lloyd CE, Mathews KA, Wing RR, et al: Psychosocial factors and complications of IDDM, *Diabetes Care* 15:166–172, 1992.

16. Masson EA, Veves A, Boulton AJM: Relationship of limited joint mobility to abnormal foot pressures and diabetic foot ulceration, *Diabetes Care* 14:8–11, 1991.

17. Mueller MJ, Diamond JE, Delitto A, et al: Insensitivity, limited joint mobility, and plantar ulcers in patients with diabetes mellitus, *Phys Ther* 69:453–462, 1989.

18. Neil HAW, Thompson AV, John S, et al: Diabetic autonomic neuropathy: the prevalence of impaired heart rate variability in a geographically defined population, *Diabetic Med* 6:20–24, 1989.

19. Newman LG, Waller J, Palestro CJ, et al: Unsuspected osteomyelitis in diabetic foot ulcers: diagnosis and monitoring by leukocyte scanning with In-dium In[111] oxyquinoline, *JAMA* 266:1246–1251, 1991.

20. Oldridge NB, Guyatt GH, Fisher ME, et al: Cardiac rehabilitation after myocardial infarction: combined experience of randomized clinical trials, *JAMA* 260:945–950, 1988.

21. Pecoraro RE, Reiber GE, Burgess EM: Pathways to diabetic limb amputation: basis for prevention, *Diabetes Care* 13:513–521, 1990.

22. Reiber GE: Diabetic foot care: financial implications and practice guidelines, *Diabetes Care* 15:29–31, 1992.

23. Reuter KV, Pierre MA: Energy cost and gait characteristics of flexed knee ambulation, Master's thesis, Pathokinesiology laboratory, Rancho Los Amigos Medical Center, Downey, Calif, 1980.

24. Schoenhaus HD, Wernick E, Cohen RS: Biomechanics of the diabetic foot, in Frykberg RG, editor: *The high risk foot in diabetes mellitus*, New York, 1991, Churchill Livingstone, pp 125–137.

25. Steinberg FU, Sunwoo I, Roettger RF: Prosthetic rehabilitation of geriatric amputee patients: a follow-up study, *Arch Phys Med Rehabil* 66:742–745, 1985.

26. Thompson FJ, Veves A, Ashe H, et al: A team approach to diabetic foot care—the Manchester experience, *Foot* 2:75–82, 1991.

27. Volpicelli LJ, Chambers LB, Wagner FW: Amputation levels of bilateral lower-extremity amputees, *J Bone Joint Surg (Am)* 65A:599–604, 1983.

28. Waters RL, Perry J, Chambers R: Energy expenditure of amputee gait, in Moore WS, Malone JM, editors: *Lower extremity amputation*, Philadelphia, 1989, WB Saunders, pp 250–260.

29. Waters RL, Campbell J, Hugos L, et al: Energy costs of walking in lower-extremity plaster casts, *J Bone Joint Surg (Am)* 1982; 64:896–899.

30. Waters RL, Perry J, Antonelli D, et al: Energy cost of walking of amputees: the influence of level of amputation, *J Bone Joint Surg (Am)* 1976; 58:42–46.

31. Waters RL, Yahura JS: The energy expenditure of normal and pathologic gait, *Crit Rev Phys Rehabil Med* 1:183–209, 1989.

# CHAPTER 23

# Role of the Podiatrist

**Lawrence B. Harkless, D.P.M.**
**Kenrick J. Dennis, D.P.M.**

Because the accelerated vascular and neurologic complications of diabetes lead to distinct clinical manifestations in the foot, it is inevitable that many diabetic patients at some point will develop foot complications that ultimately may lead to amputation.[58, 78] Professional foot care is of paramount importance in preventing the sequelae of diabetes.[40] Diabetic patients may not specifically seek help for a foot problem for many reasons, including ignorance of the need for foot care, embarrassment, and fear of losing a leg. This fact was supported by Rosenqvist,[69] who found that only 54% of diabetics with severe foot disease sought professional help. The vital role of the podiatrist who routinely gives foot care to the diabetic patient was further supported by Bailey et al.,[5] who found that a foot examination was included in only 12.3% of all office visits for follow-up care of diabetes.

The foot is unique in structure and function. It is a means of locomotion and also accepts all the stresses of body weight during ambulation. These stresses can cause the microtrauma that leads to foot lesions.

The team approach to the management of diabetes is critical in the prevention of, or at least retarding the rate of, diabetic complications.[30, 43, 80] It is well documented that proper routine care and patient education decrease diabetic foot complications.[25] Lippman[44] reported on a 15-year follow-up of persons who had lower limb amputations and were living in a nursing home with 535 residents. Before a foot care program was instituted, an average of 8 to 15 amputations were performed each year. In the 15 years of the program, no amputations were necessary among residents who used the foot care service. Similar results were obtained in our training program from 1977 to 1982 in which the rate of below-knee amputations was decreased by approximately one half. This decrease was primarily attributed to the fact that podiatry residents were working in the diabetes clinic, actively educating each patient on the etiology and pathogenesis of diabetic foot lesions. Although other factors also have played a role in the diminution of the amputation rate, we agree that patient education and responsibility play a most significant role.[5, 44, 53, 65, 69]

Because diabetic vascular and neurologic diseases are frequently manifested in the foot, the podiatrist is often the first professional to suspect undiagnosed diabetes. It therefore is extremely important for the physician to understand the intimate interaction between vascular and neurologic disease.* A thorough review of systems may give an early clue to impending pathologic changes. For example, in our experience the feet mirror the eyes with regard to vascular disease, that is, if diabetic vascular changes are present in the eyes, vascular changes are

*References 14, 27, 32, 38, 48, 49, 61–63, 85.

usually present in the feet, even though the patient may be asymptomatic.

The history is important in evaluating the diabetic patient. The following questions should be asked:

- Are you diabetic?
- How long have you had diabetes?
- Has anyone in your family had diabetes?
- If so, did they have any problems from diabetes, such as foot or leg amputations or kidney problems?
- Did they ever receive dialysis or have cataracts or blindness?
- Do you have pain or cramping in your legs when you walk?[38]
- Do you smoke cigarettes?[46, 82]
- Do you have a history of numbness or burning in the feet?
- Are you taking insulin?
- How long have you been taking insulin?
- Do you have diabetes type I or II?
- Are you overweight?
- Is your diabetes under control?[74]
- What type of home monitoring do you use?

The answers to these questions will play a role in the overall evaluation of the diabetic.[54, 55, 84] When these are used in conjunction with the clinical examination, the patient can be categorized as high or low risk.

It is also important to ask diabetic patients if they know how diabetes affects their feet. Many patients who have had diabetes for several years do not know exactly how diabetes affects the foot. The patient may know that a foot or leg could be amputated because of diabetes but does not know why this happens. Therefore, patient education remains a key to any successful diabetic treatment program, along with routine diabetic foot care.[5, 8, 22, 69]

The podiatrist is a key member of the medical team in educating the diabetic patient about the cause and pathogenesis of diabetic foot lesions. During most office visits the podiatrist is performing a procedure, such as trimming the nails or debriding calluses. Office visits provide an excellent opportunity for the podiatrist to em-

phasize the importance of foot care.[8] Each time patients come to the office, we ask them: "Do you know how diabetes affects the feet?" If they say they do, we ask them to explain what happens or what is the worst thing that can happen to their feet from diabetes and why. We ask this question again and again, until their answers reflect understanding.

Physical examination of the diabetic foot and leg should include a systematic examination of the vascular, neurologic, dermatologic, and musculoskeletal systems. Initially one should observe the feet, noting differences in texture, turgor, color, hair growth, skin lesions (Fig 23–1), and any obvious osseous deformity, noting specifically if the feet are symmetric.

The vascular examination should include palpation of the dorsalis pedis and posterior tibial pulses and capillary filling time. Capillary filling time is probably a more accurate functional indicator of distal perfusion.[47, 64] Sizer and Wheelock[75] found that distal amputations would heal even in the pulseless foot as long as the capillary filling time was less than 20 seconds. Dependent rubor and pallor on elevation also are excellent indicators of distal perfusion.[37] Noninvasive vascular analysis today has reached a level of sophistication such that it provides an excellent adjunct to the clinical examinations (see Chapter 15).[3, 9, 17, 32, 60]

Atrophy of the subcutaneous tissue, what one resident called "baked potato toe," is another clinical sign that the patient has advanced vascular disease. A toe is called "baked potato toe" if on palpation of the distal end of the hallux the soft resiliency of the tissues underneath is absent and the toe looks and feels like a baked potato.

The neurologic examination should include evaluation of the deep tendon reflexes, both patellar and Achilles, as well as sharp and dull, vibratory, temperature, and proprioceptive sensations (Fig 23–2).[1, 2, 24, 36, 51] The vibratory sensation test is used to evaluate the onset of neuropathy, because vibration is one of the first sensations to be affected.[4, 24, 50, 79] Usually when neuropathy is present, the vibratory sensation is markedly decreased from the metatarsopha-

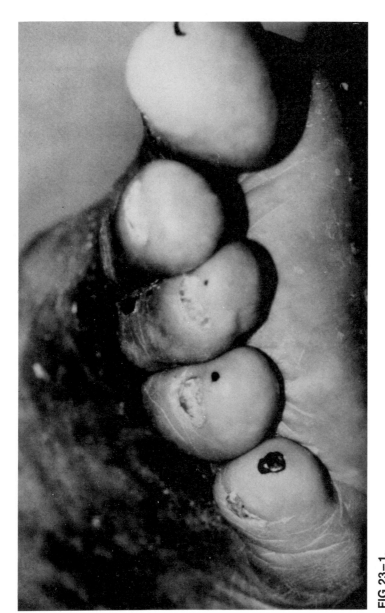

**FIG 23–1.**
Multiple distal areas of focal gangrene secondary to "microembolic shower."

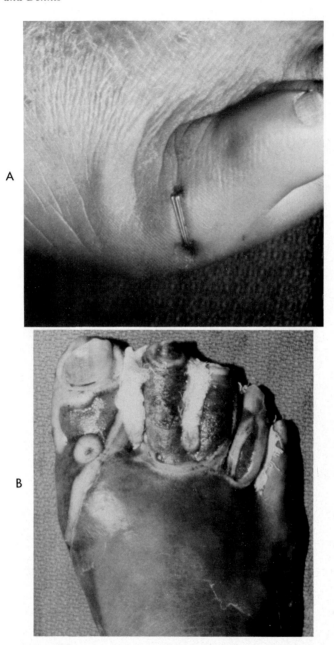

**FIG 23-2.**
**A,** staples in lateral aspect of fifth toe were incidental finding on routine visit, depicting significance of neuropathy. **B,** this patient checked bath water with toes instead of hand, resulting in full-thickness burn; injury indicates importance of recognizing extent of neuropathy and proper patient education.

langeal joints distally.* Sometimes it can be 20% decreased at the malleoli but 50% decreased at the metatarsophalangeal joints, which is why the lesions tend to develop at the metatarsophalangeal joints and distally.

Thickened mycotic nails, tinea pedis,

*References 4, 6, 10, 15, 42, 76, 77.

macerated interspaces, xerosis with scaling, corns, calluses, and ulcers are among the most common diabetic skin lesions. One of the primary reasons why a patient visits a podiatrist is for nail care. Fungal infections of the nails are a common finding in the diabetic. In the nondiabetic population, fungal infections are normally found in the hyper-

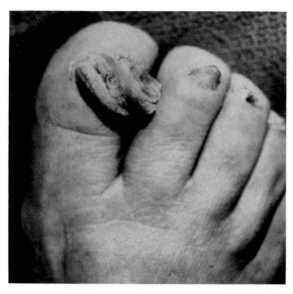

**FIG 23–3.**
Thickened mycotic nails in neurotrophic foot may
lead to subungual hemorrhage and ulceration.

hydrotic foot or after nail trauma. A subungual hematoma that is simply drained and not avulsed serves as an excellent culture medium for fungus and often results in a mycotic nail. The etiology of diabetic fungal infections is much less clear. Diabetic neuropathy may lead to nail trauma, with subsequent subungual hemorrhage increasing the chance of fungal infections. Diabetic vascular disease works in conjunction with the neuropathy by decreasing the patient's intrinsic ability to combat the infection.

The fungus actually invades the nail bed, infecting the nail as it grows distally. The nail may become multilayered and disorganized as it grows out and will actually separate from the nail bed distally (Fig 23–3). The hallux is the toe most commonly affected, but any nail may be involved. As the nail thickens, the pressure from shoe gear will increase, and in the neurotrophic foot may lead to subungual hematoma and even ulceration.

Nail problems in the diabetic must be treated aggressively. A detailed clinical and laboratory evaluation is of primary importance in assessing the local vascular supply and hence the prognosis with either palliative or surgical treatment. Subungual hematomas are among the earliest signs of diabetic peripheral neuropathy and are secondary to poorly fitting shoe gear (Fig 23–4). If the manifestation is acute, the nail should be removed. Onycholysis, onychomadesis, and subungual ulcerations should be treated with

simple nail avulsions to avoid the catastrophic complications of infection and ischemia. Onychomycosis and onychocryptosis should be treated by permanent matricectomy to avoid subungual ulcerations and infections (Fig 23–5).

Permanent correction of nails that have had fungal infections is extremely difficult. The patient with mycotic nails has three choices for treatment. First, the nails can simply be trimmed on a regular basis. Patients who have sensation can be given instructions in using a fingernail file periodically to keep the nail thin.

The second treatment choice involves avulsing the nail, followed by aggressive local and systemic treatment of the fungus. The nail needs to be avulsed because the fungus actually invades the nail bed. Any conservative treatment plan is doomed if the infected tissue is not removed. As the nail bed heals, the patient is instructed to clean the nail bed thoroughly each day and add 1 drop of antifungal solution. This local treatment is used in conjunction with oral griseofulvin in patients who have no evidence of liver disease. Griseofulvin treatment normally is continued for 6 to 12 months. A complete blood cell (CBC) count and liver and renal function tests should be taken before treatment and then at 2-month intervals.

The third choice for treatment and our procedure of choice if the circulation is ade-

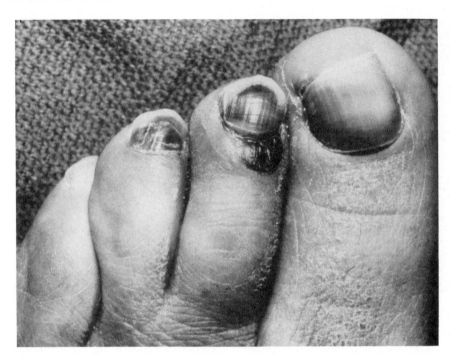

**FIG 23–4.**
Asymptomatic subungual hematomas are not uncommon in early neuropathy. Patient was unaware of poor shoe fit.

quate is a definitive nail eradication procedure.[59] In our institution the phenol alcohol technique is used for permanent eradication of nails, although the healing time may be slightly prolonged. In the past 9 years I have not had any significant complications (Fig 23–6).

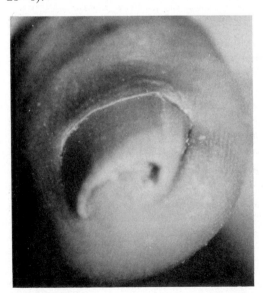

**FIG 23–5.**
Ingrown nails become significant source of infection in neurotrophic foot.

The diabetic with a specific nail problem should see a podiatrist on a routine basis for debridement. Debridement of fungally infected nails should be performed aggressively. When onycholysis is present, it is possible to debride almost the entire nail plate without risk to the patient. Routine professional care is extremely important, especially for the neurotrophic patient or the patient with decreased visual acuity (Figs 23–7 and 23–8).

Plantar xerosis (dry skin) is another common finding in the diabetic (Fig 23–9) and is often difficult to differentiate from a chronic tinea infection. Xerosis is a result of anhydrosis, which is caused by a loss of sympathetic nervous function secondary to diabetic autonomic neuropathy.[29] The medial and lateral margins of the heel, as well as the toe sulci, are the most common areas affected. When xerosis is present for a prolonged period, fissures may occur, leading to ulceration. If fissures occur, the initial treatment should consist of silver nitrate applied to the base, which cauterizes the raw edges. This should be followed by a mixture of a 20% urea cream, as a keratolytic, and hydrocortisone applied under the occlusion at night.

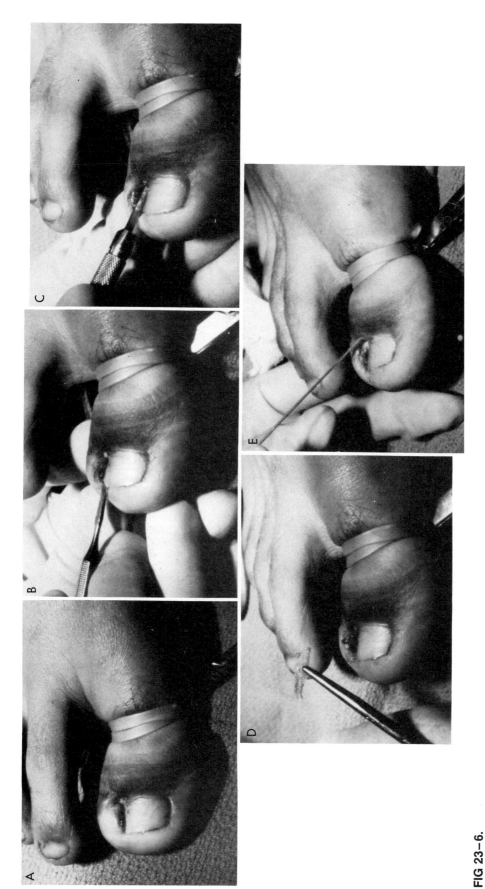

**FIG 23–6.**

**A,** acute manifestation of cryptotic nail with inflamed lateral border. Surgery and use of tourniquets should be done after evaluation of circulation. **B,** spatula is used to free offending area of nail from nail bed and eponychium. **C,** nail edge is split by placing chisel blade to most proximal edge of nail. **D,** nail border is removed with hemostat and closely inspected to make sure no spicules were left behind. **E,** phenol must be applied to nail matrix carefully to avoid spilling over digit. Phenol is applied only proximal to lunula. Three 30-second applications are used.

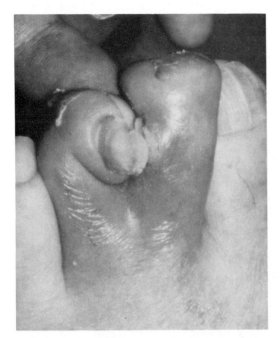

**FIG 23–7.**
After the patient missed one office visit for nail care, patient's nail became grade 2 ulceration by simply growing into adjacent toe.

Once the acute fissuring is controlled, prophylactic treatment consists of using any good emollient cream after bathing. Emollients trap the moisture in the skin and help counteract the transepidermal loss of water that originally caused the xerosis. Any good over-the-counter emollient cream will work

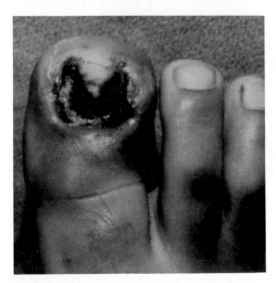

**FIG 23–8.**
This patient used "outgro" on nail for approximately 1 week before seeking professional advice.

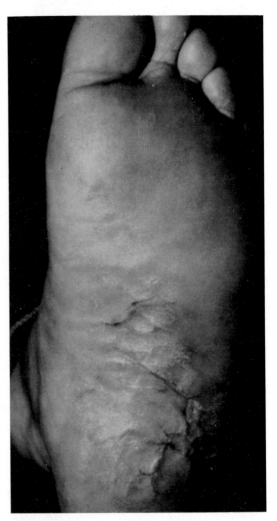

**FIG 23–9.**
Diabetic autonomic neuropathy leads to plantar xeroxis which may fissure and become secondarily infected.

for this routine care. The patient should apply six to ten "spots" of cream evenly over the entire foot. The spots should then be massaged in, taking care not to apply cream between the toes. Encourage the patient to apply the cream twice daily; in addition to moisturizing the skin, this routine also forces patients to inspect their feet.

Hard corns (heloma dura) are discrete areas of hyperkeratotic tissue over the proximal or distal interphalangeal joints or the distal end of the toe. They are the cutaneous manifestations of rigid flexion contractures of the toe (hammertoe, claw toe, or mallet toe). Rigid flexion contractures of the digits are commonly the result of diabetic motor

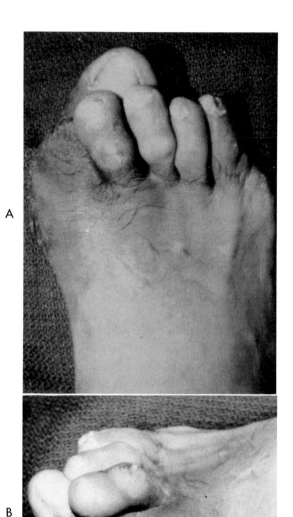

**FIG 23–10.**
**A,** diabetic motor neuropathy leads to loss of intrinsic musculature and contractures of lesser digits and hallux deformities. **B,** same foot with neurotrophic ulcer on plantar medial aspect of bunion.

neuropathy.[13, 44] The function of the intrinsic muscles is lost with motor neuropathy, and without the stabilizing effect of the intrinsic muscles, the digit buckles as the long flexor and extensor muscles become imbalanced. The plantar fat pad displaces anteriorly as the intrinsic muscles atrophy. The metatarsal heads become more prominent plantarly because of the fat pad loss but also because of the retrograde force of the contracted digits driving the metatarsal heads down. Lippman[44] described this as the "intrinsic minus" foot, stating that loss of intrinsic musculature leads to the classic claw foot of long-standing diabetes (Fig 23–10).

Limited joint mobility has been, until recently, a relatively unrecognized contributing factor to the intrinsic minus foot.[16, 19, 20, 31, 41] It has been reported that between 18% and 30% of patients with diagnosed diabetes for more than 2 years have significant soft tissue changes.[18, 68] This decrease in soft tissue elasticity results in skin, pulmonary, cardiovascular, and musculoskeletal pathologic conditions.

The motor neuropathy described by Lippman[44] leads to the structural deformity of the intrinsic minus foot. Limited joint mobility also may participate in callus and ulcer formation. The joint is no longer able to move through a full range of motion to accommodate the abnormal shape of a rigid shoe or able to move a prominent metatarsal head from its plantarflexed position.

The unique and deadly combination in diabetes mellitus is the combination of motor neuropathy, limited joint mobility, and the ultimate insult of sensory neuropathy. Sensory neuropathy will eliminate the protective mechanism inherent to us all, allowing the cascade of events to occur.[52, 73] Pressure over these bony prominences causes skin irritation and the resultant hyperkertosis and ulceration (Fig 23–11).

Soft corns (heloma molle) have a similar etiology as hard corns, but their location is different. They are found in the interspaces of the toes and are soft and white because of chronic maceration. Repetitive mechanical shearing between adjacent bony prominences may lead to hyperkeratotic buildup and ultimately tissue breakdown (Fig 23–12). Soft corns are white, not yellow like hard corns, and are therefore often misdiagnosed as either tinea or *Candida* infections. When they are coupled with maceration of the web space, there is a high propensity for tissue breakdown and secondary infection (Fig 23–13). Because of the proximity of the long flexor tendons and the deep plantar

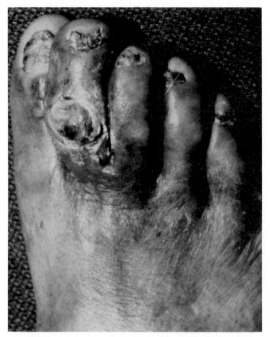

**FIG 23–11.**
Neurotrophic ulcer on dorsal aspect of second proximal interphalangeal joint secondary to shoe irritation over rigid hammertoe.

spaces, interdigital lesions should be carefully monitored.

Hard and soft corns need routine follow-up care (at least monthly). Palliative care involves debridement of the hyperkera-

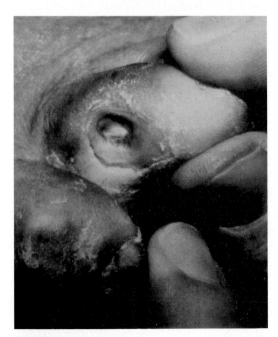

**FIG 23–12.**
Ulceration of interdigital soft corn.

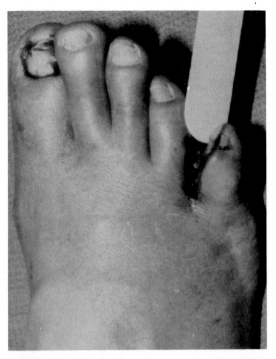

**FIG 23–13.**
Macerated interspaces frequently are source of infection. With proximity of flexor tendons, deep plantar space spread may occur.

totic buildup and relief of the pressure over these prominences. Shoe gear should be inspected to assure adequate depth of the toe box. Removable pads may be useful and are constructed of either foam, felt, or occasionally latex. If pads are dispensed, detailed instructions must be given about their use, so that the patient avoids wearing the pads while bathing or sleeping. If the vascular status is adequate, surgical correction of corns to prevent complications may actually be the true conservative treatment.

The most commonly encountered plantar calluses include the plantar medial aspect of the great toe (pinch callus), directly plantar to the metatarsal head and around the heel margin. Callus formation is a protective reaction resulting from the shearing forces of a prominent bone against unyielding shoe gear. The location of the callus is the result of either foot type or bone pathologic condition.[57] The overlying soft tissue reacts by increasing keratin production. The underlying bony pathologic condition has a myriad of etiologies, including an elongated or plantar-flexed metatarsal, retrograde plantar flexory force from digital deformities, soft tissue at-

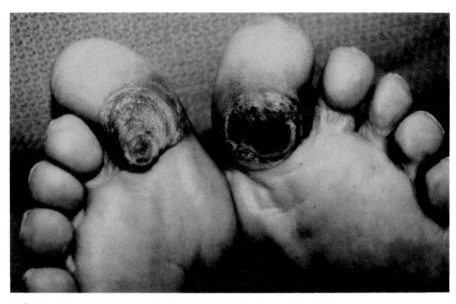

**FIG 23–14.**
Plantar interphalangeal preulcerative calluses secondary to hallux extensus.

rophy or displacement, prominent sesa-moids,[33] or hallux deformities (hallux extensus, valgus, interphalangeus abductus, or hallux hammertoe) (Fig 23–14).

Treatment of these calluses must include routine professional attention. Shoe accommodations are discussed in detail in Chapter 25. The patient without any sensory deficit may be instructed in the use of a pumice stone two or three times per week after bathing to help decrease hyperkeratotic buildup. We do not recommend the commercially available "corn removers" in any situation. We prefer periodic office visits for debridement at intervals specific for each patient.

When left unattended, especially in the neurotrophic foot, calluses will increase in thickness. As they continue to thicken, they also become rigid and unyielding, creating a new shear force with the bony prominence. This repetitive shear leads to inflammation, hemorrhage, and finally breakdown of the interposed soft tissue.[39] If this mechanical tissue destruction is allowed to continue unchecked, it is not uncommon to have a foul odor, swelling, or cellulitis as the first sign of a problem. Because there is a sevenfold increase in abnormally high pressure below the metatarsal heads in the neuropathic foot, we strongly believe that accommodative shoe gear is a mandatory part of the treat-

ment plan in any patient with clinical signs of neurovascular disease.[11, 12, 22, 28]

When the physician is confronted with a swollen and inflamed foot, Charcot's arthropathy must be ruled out (see Chapter 7). Charcot's arthropathy is a commonly misdiagnosed and improperly treated finding in the diabetic foot. [81] An edematous erythematous foot with increased skin temperature is often mistaken for an acute infection (Fig 23–15,A). The use of appropriate laboratory data, including the CBC count, sedimentation rate, x-ray films, and nuclear medicine studies, will help establish a differential diagnosis. The lateral x-ray film is particularly useful in this diagnosis, showing multiple areas of dorsal lipping with joint narrowing and finally subluxation and dislocation (Fig 23–15,B). During the active stage of Charcot's arthropathy, the foot must be protected. This protection initially should take the form of a short-leg walking cast changed weekly to make sure no irritation has occurred. Once stabilized, the patient must wear a steel-shanked shoe with a rocker bottom to decrease stress across the midfoot.

## DIABETIC ULCERS

Diabetic ulcers are classified as ischemic or neurotrophic, depending on which cause

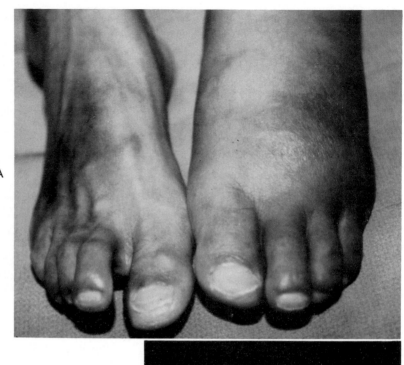

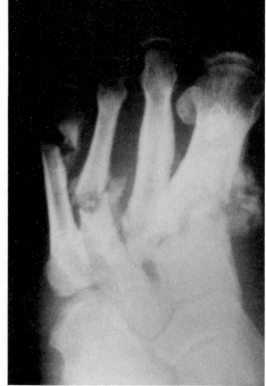

**FIG 23–15.**
**A,** patient in active stage of Charcot's anthropathy. Note marked edema of left forefoot. Charcot's arthopathy is commonly misdiagnosed as cellulitis. **B,** radiograph shows extraordinary destruction of midfoot.

predominates. Frequently diabetic ulcers have elements of both.

The hallmark of an ischemic ulcer is pain, pain that is out of proportion to the clinical appearance. This ulceration is char-

acterized by a yellow, punched-out, necrotic center with sharp margins that appear to be well vascularized (Fig 23–16). The ulcer tends to be extremely painful to any type of palpation or pressure.[34] The pain is often

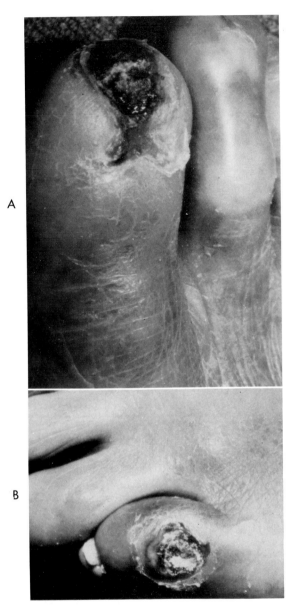

**FIG 23–16.**
**A,** classic ischemic ulceration with discolored "stuck-on" appearance to base. **B,** etiology of this ulcer was neuropathy, but central blackened necrotic area shows significant ischemic component.

exacerbated at night, and relief is obtained by sitting up in a chair or dangling the feet over the edge of the bed in a dependent position. On debridement of ischemic ulcers there is generally no bleeding from the deep central aspect. The wound bleeds only from the periphery. It is almost impossible to debride an ischemic ulcer without giving the patient a local anesthetic block.

The differential diagnosis includes all vascular ulcers such as Raynaud's disease and vasculitis. The cause of an ischemic ulcer may be neurotrophic, a pressure ischemia, but the ulcer is classified as ischemic because it has poor circulation, limiting the ulcer's ability to heal.[34, 35, 66] Although the prognosis for healing is poor, patients with ischemic ulcers do not necessarily have to lose the limb. We have treated several patients who have postponed the inevitable amputation for 1 to 3 years (leading a relatively normal life-style) by practicing meticulous foot care at home. The goal is to optimize the clinical situation by evaluating patients for possible vascular surgery and by encouraging patients to eliminate smoking, control their diabetes, control their weight, and eliminate shoe pressure. These goals require a great deal of education and motivation. However, life-style changes may tip scales in favor of healing. As long as the pain is tolerable and there are no clinical signs of infection, surgical intervention is not required.

The other type of diabetic ulcer is the neurotrophic ulcer, which is caused primarily by pressure. Boulton et al.[13] showed that in neuropathic feet an abnormally high pressure was transmitted through the metatarsal heads in 51% of feet compared with 7% in nondiabetic patients. In patients with a previous history of plantar ulceration an abnormally high pressure was found in 100% of the cases. This abnormally high pressure in conjunction with the repetitive moderate mechanical stress of walking will lead to tissue breakdown.

A neurotrophic ulcer is usually located in a weight-bearing area.[21] Musculoskeletal deformity tends to occur with callus formation, and the patient will have all the signs and symptoms of diabetic peripheral neuropathy in the foot. One of the earliest warning signs of impending breakdown is hemorrhage into a callus.[67] These "preulcerative" lesions are evident in approximately 10% of diabetic office visits (Fig 23–17). This is a time when aggressive intervention can successfully decrease the chance of ulcer formation.

The classic neurotrophic ulcer has a pink granulation base with a white fibrotic rim surrounded by hyperkeratotic tissue (Fig

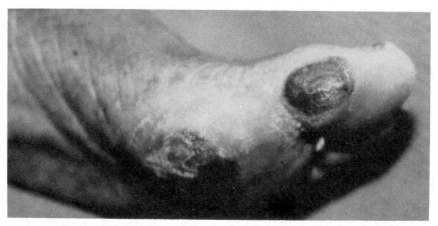

**FIG 23–17.**
High-risk areas for ulceration include plantar aspect of first metatarsophalangeal and interphalangeal joints.

23–18). The thickened white fibrotic and hyperkeratotic tissue is a response to the continuing pressure from weight bearing on an area that has already been traumatized.

Because a neurotrophic ulcer is simply the next step in the continuum of bony deformities and corn and callus formation, it would follow that the common ulcer locations are the same as the common sites of these skin lesions. A good vascular supply may be associated with neurotrophic ulcers; therefore, the foot is often warm, with an inflammatory reaction around the ulcer.[26]

Does this localized inflammation indicate that all ulcers are infected? It is true that a culture of ulcerations will grow some organism. But is this a true pathogen or simply an opportunistic contaminant? It is still common practice to give antibiotics to all diabetics with ulcerations. In our experience debridement of necrotic tissue and meticulous local wound care is the treatment of choice for an ulceration that has no clinical signs of proximal infection. It is important to make this clinical judgment after debridement of the necrotic hyperkeratotic cover. Each patient must be evaluated and treated on an individual basis. If, after a thorough clinical evaluation, any question remains concerning infection, the practitioner is obligated to follow through with Gram's stain and a culture, including anaerobic culture, and sensitivity. It is not uncommon to debride a foul-smelling lesion only to find a beefy red granulation bed without any sinus tracts,

proximal erythema, proximal tenderness, or purulent drainage. Although the lesion smells infected, if there are no clinical signs of infection, we will give the wound meticulous wound care and close follow-up.

When the clinical signs of infection are present, immediate, decisive action must be taken.[45, 71] If the patient continues to walk on an infected foot, there may be proximal migration along the fascial planes, extending proximally into the leg. If proximal tenderness and erythema are present, immediate hospitalization with appropriate consultations, incision and drainage, and intravenous antibiotics are indicated. Just as in the clinical examination, a systematic treatment plan is necessary to treat a neurotrophic ulcer effectively.

What factors are necessary for an ulcer to heal? Three factors, if adequately addressed, will promote healing of an ulcer. First and foremost is an adequate blood supply. If the ulcer either does not bleed on debridement or bleeds for only a few seconds to 1 minute, it is a poor prognostic sign. In this case the patient should immediately be sent to the vascular surgeon for evaluation and possible revascularization.

The second factor is pressure distribution.[21] If the repetitive moderate stress that initially caused the ulcer can be dispersed over the entire plantar aspect of the foot, the focal area of increased pressure may be relieved. Putting the patient at rest either by complete bed rest or use of a total-contact

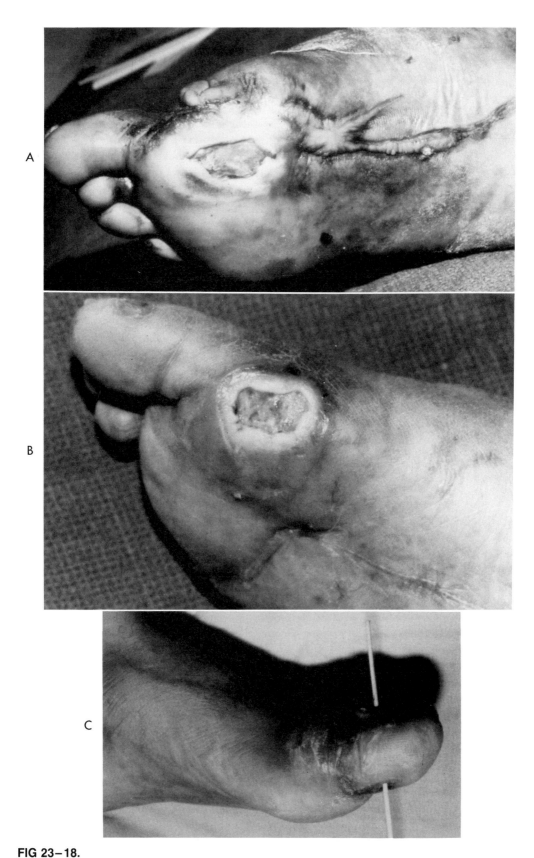

**FIG 23–18.**
**A,** classic neurotrophic ulceration below second metatarsal head. Lesion began as transfer lesion after previous hallux amputation. **B,** neurotrophic ulceration initiated by rat bites while patient was sleeping. Healing was prolonged because of weight-bearing location of lesion. **C,** grade 3 ulceration after home treatment of plantar first interphalangeal callus.

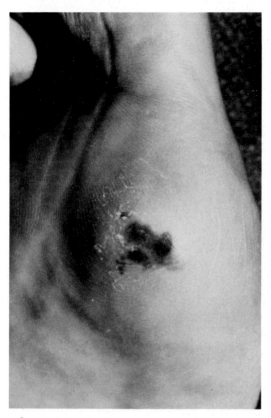

**FIG 23–19.**
Critical point is period when ulceration has just closed in.

cast or Plastazote insoles will decrease these areas of pressure.[7, 11, 56, 72, 83] For more information on the use of various footwear and molded insoles, see Chapter 25.

The final factor necessary for an ulcer to heal is debridement of all necrotic and infected tissue. Necrotic tissue serves as an excellent culture medium, as well as a barrier to new granulation tissue.[66]

Once the ulcer has closed over, it is at a critical point in the healing process. The critical point occurs when the lesion is in fragile balance between opened and healed (Fig 23–19). The most important period in ulcer healing is the first month after clinical resolution of the lesion. If the patient is given a return appointment for 2 months, on examination the ulcer will commonly be present again, appearing hyperkeratotic, with hemorrhage into the callus. There is no gross ulceration, but the lesion is preulcerative, with impending tissue breakdown.

What improves the long-term prognosis of ulcers? Probably the single most important aspect of intervention after patient education is the effective use of shoes and shoe modification.[12, 22, 26] Even while the patient is still wearing the total contact cast, shoes should be ordered. On the day the total-contact cast is removed, the patient should be able to step directly into a pair of customized shoes. An inlay type of shoe with a Plastazote insole is appropriate. The addition of a rocker bottom to the sole decreases motion at the metatarsophalangeal joints, thereby decreasing the friction and chances of breakdown.

## WHEN IS SURGERY INDICATED?

Surgery is indicated in the diabetic patient who has uncontrolled infection, recalcitrant ulcers, or osseous deformities. When infection is uncontrolled, the affected necrotic tissue must be excised. Once necrosis is present, no antibiotic in any dose will cure the problem. Gram-negative and anaerobic organisms are commonly found in diabetic infections.[70] At the time of surgery it is not common to find gross purulence in a gram-negative infection. What will be evident are multiple black dots; the soft tissue appears dusky, with a brownish discolored serous exudate. It has been said that both good antibiotics and good surgery are needed to control a diabetic infection.

The second indication for surgery is the recalcitrant ulcer. This is the ulcer that has been resistant to all conservative therapy for longer than 3 months. If it is believed that the factor keeping the ulcer from healing is pressure, a thorough evaluation of structural deformities and surgical correction is pursued.[23]

Finally, aggressive prophylactic treatment is needed for the diabetic patient who has not developed the vascular sequelae of the disease but who has gross osseous deformity. The prognosis for the diabetic patient is poor in the best of situations; if a musculoskeletal deformity is added to the problem, the development of later foot complications is almost inevitable.

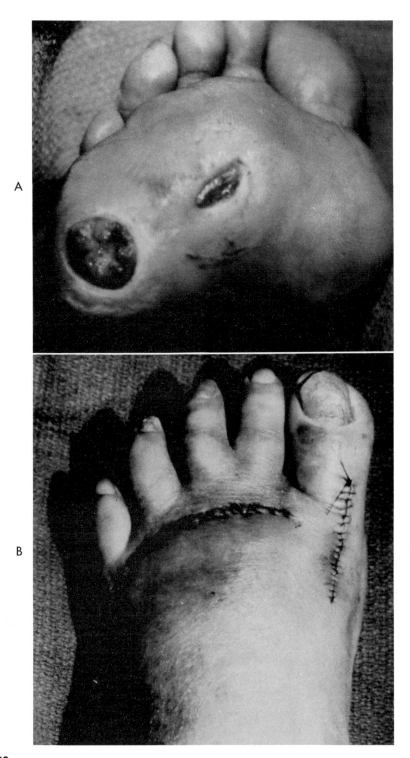

**FIG 23–20.**
**A,** plantar view of left foot shows recalcitrant neurotrophic ulcers. **B,** transverse incision for complete metatarsal head resection.

## Case Histories

### Case 1

This 55-year-old man with a 15-year history of insulin-dependent diabetes worked as a salvage yard dealer and was constantly on his feet. He was being followed up in the podiatry clinic for a recalcitrant ulceration beneath the metatarsal heads of his left foot. He had received treatment for approximately 2½ years with various conservative modalities, including pads, rigid postoperative shoes with Plastazote covering, and debridement of hyperkeratotic tissue. The initial ulcer developed because of a thermal injury to his insensitive foot.

Physical examination revealed dorsalis pedis and posterior tibial pulses 2/4 bilaterally; capillary return was 3 seconds. The neurologic examination showed an absence of sharp and dull and vibratory sensations from the ankle joint distally. The patellar reflex was 3/5, and the Achilles reflex was absent bilaterally.

The patient exhibited xerotic skin and dystrophic mycotic nails. Inspection of the plantar aspect of the metatarsal heads revealed a well-demarcated full-thickness ulceration about 4 cm in diameter with a red granulation base and hyperkeratotic rim (Fig 23–20,A). The lesion had not extended down to bone, and no sinus tracts or exudate was present. Musculoskeletal examination showed a pes cavus deformity with an anteriorly displaced fat pad and prominent lesser metatarsal heads. Radiographs revealed forefoot equinus at the level of the metatarsal cuneiform joint.

Because of the recalcitrant nature of the ulcer and lack of response to conservative care, surgical intervention was elected. The patient had a panmetatarsal head resection performed under local anesthesia. The first metatarsal head was approached through a dorsal longitudinal incision. The lesser metatarsal heads were approached through a transverse dorsal incision (Fig 23–20,B). A Penrose drain was used to prevent postoperative hematoma.

The patient healed uneventfully and was given an extradepth shoe with a rocker sole and a molded Plastazote insole. At 4 years postoperatively the patient had no clinical signs of ulceration.

### Case 2

A 27-year-old man with a 13-year history of insulin-dependent diabetes came to the clinic with nonpainful lesions on the distal hallux and over the second proximal interphalangeal joint. He said he first noticed the lesions after wearing a new pair of shoes and that they had been present for 2 to 3 weeks. A review of the patient's chart showed a long history of poor compliance, with three hospitalizations in the previous 18 months for diabetic ketoacidosis.

The podiatric physical examination revealed no palpable pedal pulses and a capillary filling time of approximately 10 seconds bilaterally. The neurologic examination showed that the sharp and dull sensation was absent distal to the malleoli. On the distal aspect of the right hallux was a 1-cm diameter ulceration with a yellowish "stuck-on" appearance centrally. A similar lesion was present on the dorsal aspect of the right second proximal interphalangeal joint. There were no clinical signs of infection (Fig 23–21,A).

The initial impression was that of an ischemic ulceration secondary to pressure-induced ischemia from poorly fitting shoes. Orthopedic and vascular consultations were obtained with similar recommendations. It was agreed to protect the area, practice local wound care, and provide follow-up care two or three times each week to watch for infection. The patient was given a postoperative wooden shoe and instructed to clean the lesions twice daily with peroxide and cover them with sterile gauze.

The patient adequately cared for the wound during the first month; therefore visits were decreased to once per week after the first month. Complete resolution of the lesions required almost 6 months (Fig 23–21,B). The patient was given an accommodative shoe and has not had any recurrence of the lesion.

### Case 3

This 42-year-old man with a 12-year history of insulin-dependent diabetes worked as an auto mechanic and as such was constantly squatting and on his feet. He was being followed up at the podiatry clinic for a recalcitrant ulceration on the plantar aspect

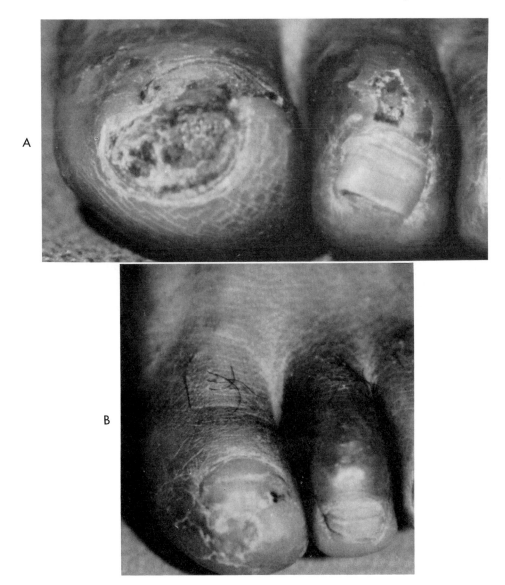

**FIG 23–21.**
**A,** ischemic ulceration on distal hallux and dorsum of second toes from poor shoe gear. **B,** with daily wound care and changing shoe gear, this lesion healed.

of the hallux interphalangeal joint. He had been treated for approximately 2 months with various pads in the shoes, rigid postoperative shoes, and debridement of hyper-keratotic tissue.

Physical examination showed dorsalis pedis pulses of 2/4 bilaterally and posterior tibial pulses of 1/4 bilaterally. The neurologic examination showed an absence of sharp and dull sensation distal to the midtarsal joint. Inspection of the plantar aspect of the left hallux showed a well-demarcated full-thickness ulceration of 1 cm diameter with a red granulation base and hyperkera-

totic rim (Fig 23–22,A). The lesion had not extended to bone, and no sinus tracts or exudate were present. Radiographs taken with a marker showed the lesion was directly below a hallux interphalangeal sesamoid bone.

Because of the recalcitrant nature of the lesion and the lack of response to conservative care, surgical excision of the interphalangeal sesamoid bone was elected.[33] The sesamoid was approached by extending the ulceration longitudinally and excising all necrotic tissue in the ulcer (Fig 23–22,B). The wound was lightly packed open, and this

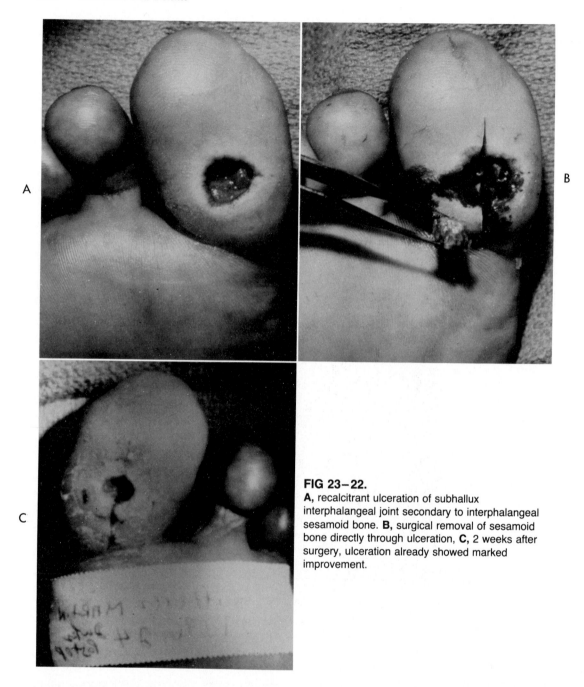

**FIG 23–22.**
**A,** recalcitrant ulceration of subhallux interphalangeal joint secondary to interphalangeal sesamoid bone. **B,** surgical removal of sesamoid bone directly through ulceration, **C,** 2 weeks after surgery, ulceration already showed marked improvement.

packing was changed daily. Within 2 weeks the lesion had responded significantly and had completely closed by 5 weeks postoperatively (Fig 23–22,C).

The patient was unable to afford an accommodative shoe and remained in a running shoe at work. Four years postoperatively, the patient was seen with a new lesion on the dorsomedial aspect of the hallux secondary to a new pair of shoes. The surgical site remained without any clinical signs of ulceration. This second ulceration became infected and did require a terminal Syme amputation of the hallux to heal.

## Case 4

The patient was a 58-year-old woman with a 20-year history of non-insulin-dependent diabetes mellitus. She was a long-standing patient of the podiatry clinic who had developed a plantar ulceration below her first metatarsal head. She also had an ulceration over the first metatarso-cuneiform joint dorsally, with a preulcerative area over the first interphalangeal joint. She had been treated unsuccessfully with debridement, immobilization, and shoe modifications.

The patient had a previous recalcitrant ulcer under the right forefoot. Three years before she had successfully undergone a

panmetatarsal head resection on the right foot, which had healed uneventfully. At the time of surgery, however, it was noted that she had significant arteriovenous shunting.

The podiatric physical examination revealed ¼ dorsalis pedis and posterior tibial pulses. Sharp and dull sensation was absent distal to the midfoot, and vibratory sensation was absent as well.

Grade 1 neurotrophic ulcerations were present plantar to the first metatarsal head, as well as over the dorsum of the first meta-

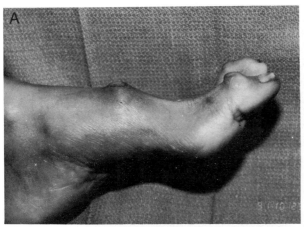
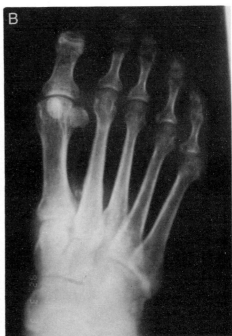
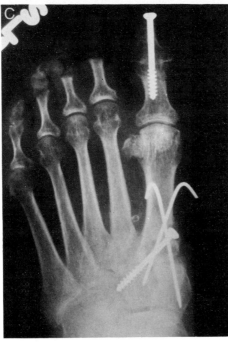

**FIG 23–23.**
**A,** lateral view of the left foot showing the contracture of the hallux interphalangeal joint and the first metatarso-cuneiform exostosis. **B,** preoperative radiograph showing contracture of all digits. **C,** postoperative radiograph showing fixation in the first ray and resection arthroplasties of digits 2 and 3.

tarso-cuneiform joints. She had a cavus foot type with a rigid plantar-flexed first metatarsal, hallux hammertoe, and first metatarso-cuneiform exostosis (Fig 23–23, A and B). Superficial ulcerations were present over the distal aspect of the second and third digits secondary to the rigid flexion contractures.

Surgical correction, consisting of a hallux interphalangeal fusion with a first metatarso-cuneiform fusion with a dorsiflexory wedge removed was performed. Resectional proximal interphalangeal arthroplasties were performed to reduce the rigid flexion contractures of the second and third digits (Fig 23–23,C).

The patient was kept non–weight bearing postoperatively. Nine weeks postoperatively, the patient was allowed to walk without any protection and began to have radiographic and clinical signs of the osteotomy site opening. The osteotomy was stabilized with a percutaneous K wire. After radiographic signs of union were evident, the patient was followed in an accommodative shoe with an ankle foot orthosis for 6 months.

# REFERENCES

1. Asbury AK: Report and recommendations of the San Antonio conference on diabetic neuropathy, *Diabetes Care* 11:592–598, 1988.

2. Asbury AK: Report and recommendations of the San Antonio conference on diabetic neuropathy, *Neurology* 38:1161–1165, 1988.

3. Apelqvist J, et al: Prognostic value of systolic ankle and toe blood pressure levels in outcome of diabetic foot ulcer, *Diabetes Care* 12:373–378, 1989.

4. Armstrong FM, et al: A study of peripheral diabetic neuropathy, The application of age-related reference values, *Diabetic Med* 8(suppl):94–99, 1991.

5. Bailey TS, et al: Patterns of foot examination in a diabetes clinic, *Am J Med* 78:371–374, 1985.

6. Birke JA, Sims DS: Plantar sensory threshold in the ulcerative foot, *Lepr Rev* 57:261–267, 1986.

7. Black JR: Management of diabetic plantar ulcers with a walking brace, *J Am Podiatr Med Assoc* 80:156–157, 1990.

8. Bloomgarden ZT: Randomized, controlled trial of diabetic patient education: improved knowledge without improved metabolic status, *Diabetes Care* 10:263–272, 1987.

9. Bongard O, Krahenbuhl B: Predicting amputation in severe ischaemia: the value of transcutaneous $PO_2$ measurement, *J Bone Joint Surg (Br)* 70B:465–467, 1988.

10. Boulton AJM: Clinical presentation and management of diabetic neuropathy and foot ulceration, *Diabetic Med* 8(suppl):52–57, 1991.

11. Boulton AJM, Bowker JH, Gadia M, et al: Use of plaster casts in the management of diabetic neurotrophic foot ulcers, *Diabetes Care* 9:149, 1986.

12. Boulton AJM, Franks CL, Betts RL: Reduction of abnormal foot pressures in diabetic neuropathy using a new polymer insole material, *Diabetes Care* 7:42, 1984.

13. Boulton AJM, Hardisty C, Betts RL, et al: Dynamic foot pressures and studies as diagnostic and management aids in diabetic neuropathy, *Diabetes Care* 6:26, 1983.

14. Boulton AJM, et al: Venous oxygenation in the diabetic neuropathic foot: evidence of arteriovenous shunting? *Diabetologia* 22:6–8, 1982.

15. Boulton AJM, et al: Impaired vibratory perception and diabetic foot ulceration, *Diabetic Med* 3:335–337, 1986.

16. Brink SJ: Limited joint mobility as a risk factor for diabetes complications, *Clin Diabetes* 5:122–127, 1987.

17. Buchbinder D, Flanigan DP: Arterial disease of the lower extremities *Diagnosis* 8:79–80, 1985.

18. Buckingham BA, et al: Scleroderma-like changes in insulin-dependent diabetes mellitus: clinical and biochemical studies, *Diabetes Care* 7:163–169, 1984.

19. Campbell RR, et al: Limited joint mobility in diabetes mellitus, *Ann Rheum Dis* 44:93–97, 1985.

20. Crisp AJ, Heathcote JG: Connective tissue abnormalities in diabetes mellitus, *J Royal Coll Physicians Lond* 18:132–141, 1984.

21. Ctercteko G, Dhanendran M, Hutton W, et al: Vertical forces acting on the feet of diabetic patients with neuropathic ulcerations, *Br J Surg* 68:608, 1981.

22. Delbridge L, Ctercteko G, Fowler C, et al: The aetiology of diabetic neuropathic ulceration of the foot, *Br J Surg* 72:1–6, 1985.

23. Downs DM, Jacobs RL: Treatment of resistant ulcers on the plantar surface of the great toe in diabetics, *J Bone Joint Surg (Am)* 64A:930, 1982.

24. Dyck PJ: Evaluation procedures to detect, characterize, and assess the severity of diabetic neuropathy, *Diabetic Med* 00:S48–S51, 1991.

25. Ebskov LB: Epidemiology of lower limb amputations in diabetics in Denmark (1980 to 1989), *Int Orthop* 15:285–288, 1991.

26. Edmonds ME, et al: Blood flow in the diabetic neuropathic foot, *Diabetologia* 22:9–15, 1982.

27. Edmonds ME, et al: Medial arterial calcification and diabetic neuropathy, *Br Med J* 284:928–930, 1982.

28. Edmonds ME, Nicolaides K, Watkins P: Autonomic neuropathy and diabetic foot ulceration, *Diabetic Med* 3:56, 1986.

29. Fagius J: Aspects of autonomic neurophysiology in diabetic polyneuropathy: a brief review, *Diabetic Med* 8(suppl):58–62, 1991.

30. Fernando DJS, et al: The diabetic foot 1990, *Diabetic Med* 8:82–85, 1991.

31. Fernando DJS, et al: Relationship of limited joint mobility to abnormal foot pressures and diabetic foot ulcerations, *Diabetes Care* 14:8–11, 1991.

32. Gilbey SG, et al: Vascular calcification, autonomic neuropathy, and peripheral blood flow in patients with diabetic nephropathy, *Diabetic Med* 6:37–42, 1989.

33. Giurini JM, Chrzan JS, Gibbons GW, et al: Sesamoidectomy for the treatment of chronic neurotrophic ulcerations, *J Am Podiatr Med Assoc* 81:167, 1991.

34. Harkless LB, et al: Diabetic ulceration: classification and management, in *Proceedings of the first international symposium on the diabetic foot*, Amsterdam, 1991, Excerpta Medica.

35. Hietala S, Lithner F: Foot angiography in diabetic patients with gangrene, *Acta Med Scand* 687(Suppl):61–67, 1984.

36. Ijff GA, et al: Cold and warm cutaneous sensation in diabetic patients, *Diabetic Med* 8(suppl):71–73, 1991.

37. Kozol RA, et al: Dependent rubor as a predictor of limb risk in patients with claudication, *Arch Surg* 119:932–935, 1984.

38. Kreines K, et al: The course of peripheral vascular disease in non-insulin-dependent diabetes, *Diabetes Care* 8:235–243, 1985.

39. Kucan JO, Robson MC: Diabetic foot infections: fate of the contralateral foot, *Plast Reconstr Surg* 77:439, 1986.

40. Kwasnik EM: Limb salvage in diabetics: challenges and solutions, *Surg Clin North Am* 66:305, 1986.

41. Larkin JG, Frier BM: Limited joint mobility and dupuytren's contracture in diabetic, hypertensive, and normal populations, *Br Med J* 292:1494, 1986.

42. Lehtinen JM: Prevalence of neuropathy in newly diagnosed NIDDM and nondiabetic control subjects, *Diabetes* 38:1307–1313, 1989.

43. Levin ME: The diabetic foot: preventing its morbidity and mortality, *Med Times* 116:23–31, 1988.

44. Lippman HI: Must loss of limb be a consequence of diabetes mellitus? *Diabetes Care* 2:432, 1979.

45. Lipsky BA, et al: Outpatient management of uncomplicated lower-extremity infections in diabetic patients, *Arch Intern Med* 150:790–797, 1990.

46. Lithner F: Is tobacco of importance for the development and progression of diabetic vascular complications? *Acta Med Scand* 687(suppl):33–36, 1984.

47. Lithner F, Tornblom N: Gangrene localized to the feet in diabetic patients, *Acta Med Scand* 215:75–79, 1984.

48. Lithner F, et al: Skeletal lesions and arterial calcifications of the feet in diabetics, *Acta Med Scand* 687(suppl):47–54, 1984.

49. LoGerfo FW, Coffman JD: Vascular and microvascular disease of the foot in diabetes, *N Engl Med J* 311:1615–1618, 1984.

50. Maser RE: Measuring diabetic neuropathy, *Diabetes Care* 12:270–275, 1989.

51. Masson EA, Boulton AJM: The neurometer: validation and comparison with conventional tests for diabetic neuropathy, *Diabetic Med* 8(suppl):63–66, 1991.

52. Masson EA, et al: Abnormal foot pressures alone may not cause ulceration, *Diabetic Med* 6:426–428, 1989.

53. Mazzuca SA, et al: The diabetes education study: a controlled trial of the effects of diabetes patient education, *Diabetes Care* 9:1–10, 1986.

54. Morgensen CE: Microalbuminuria predicts clinical proteinuria and early mortality in maturity-onset diabetes, *N Engl J Med* 310:356, 1984.

55. Moss JM, Delawater DE: Self-monitoring of blood glucose, *Am Fam Phys* 33:225, 1986.

56. Mueller MJ, et al: Total contact casting in treatment of diabetic plantar ulcers, *Diabetes Care* 12:384–388, 1989.

57. Mueller MJ, et al: Relationship of foot deformity to ulcer location in patients with diabetes mellitus, *Phys Ther* 70:356–362, 1990.

58. Nelson RG, et al: Lower-extremity amputations in NIDDM: 12-yr follow-up study in Pima Indians, *Diabetes Care* 11:8–16, 1988.

59. Nicklas BJ: Prophylactic surgery in the diabetic foot, in Frykberg R, editor: *The high risk foot in diabetes mellitus*, New York, 1990, Churchill Livingstone, pp 513–516.

60. Oishi CS, et al: The role of non-invasive vascular studies in determining levels of amputation, *J Bone Joint Surg (Am)* 70A:1520–1530, 1988.

61. Osmundson PJ, et al: Course of peripheral occlusive arterial disease in diabetes, *Diabetes Care* 13:143–152, 1990.

62. Pecoraro RE, et al: Pathways to diabetic limb amputation, *Diabetes Care* 13:513–521, 1990.

63. Rayman G, et al: Blood flow in the skin of the foot related to posture in diabetes mellitus, *Br Med J*, 292:87–90, 1986.

64. Rayman G, et al: Impaired microvascular hyperaemic response to minor skin trauma in type I diabetes, *Br Med J* 292:1295–1298, 1986.

65. Rettig BA: A randomized study of the effects of a home diabetes education program, *Diabetes Care* 9:173–178, 1986.

66. Robson MC, Edstrom LE: Conservative management of the ulcerated diabetic foot, *Plast Reconstr Surg* 51:551, 1977.

67. Rosen RC, Davids MS, Bohanske LM, et al: Hemorrhage into plantar callus and diabetes mellitus, *Cutis* 35:339, 1985.

68. Rosenbloom AL, et al: Limited joint mobility in childhood diabetes mellitus indicate increased risk for microvascular disease, *N Engl J Med* 305:191–194, 1981.

69. Rosenqvist U: An epidemiological survey of diabetic foot problems in the Stockholm county 1982, *Acta Med Scand* 687(suppl):55–60, 1984.

70. Sapico FL, Witte JL, Canawate HN, et al: The infected foot of the diabetic patient: quantitative microbiology and analysis of clinic features, *Rev Infect Dis* 6:171, 1984.

71. Sartoris DJ, et al: Plantar compartmental infection in the diabetic foot: the role of computed tomography, *Invest Radiol* 20:772–784, 1985.

72. Schaff PS, Cavanagh PR: Shoes for the insensitive foot: the effect of a "rocker bottom" shoe modification on plantar pressure distribution, *Foot Ankle* 11:133–140, 1990.

73. Sims DS, et al: Risk factors in the diabetic foot, *Phys Ther* 68:1887–1902, 1988.

74. Sindrup SH, et al: Peripheral nerve function during hyperglycemic clamping in insulin-dependent diabetic patients, *Acta Neurol Scand* 79:412–418, 1989.

75. Sizer J, Wheelock F: Digital amputations in diabetic patients, *Surgery* 72:980, 1972.

76. Sosenko JM: Body stature as a risk factor diabetic sensory neuropathy, *Am J Med* 80:1031–1034, 1986.

77. Sosenko JM, et al: Neurofunctional testing for the detection of diabetic peripheral neuropathy, *Arch Intern Med* 147:1741–1744, 1987.

78. Spencer F, et al: The incidence of foot pathology in a diabetic population, *J Am Podiatr Med Assoc* 75:590–592, 1985.

79. Thivolet C, et al: Measuring vibration sensation with graduated tuning fork, *Diabetes Care* 13:1077–1080, 1990.

80. Thomson FJ, et al: A team approach to diabetic foot care—the Manchester experience, *Foot* 2:75–82, 1991.

81. Tuccio AT, Wertheimer SJ: Non-infectious osseous alterations in the diabetic foot, *J Foot Surg* 24:154, 1985.

82. Vaccaro O, et al: Peripheral arterial circulation in individuals with impaired glucose tolerance, *Diabetes Care* 8:594–597, 1985.

83. Veves A, et al: Use of experimental padded hosiery to reduce abnormal foot pressures in diabetic neuropathy, *Diabetes Care* 12:653–655, 1989.

84. Wagner MM: Pathophysiology related to peripheral vascular disease, *Nurs Clin North Am* 21:195–205, 1986.

85. Ward JD, et al: Venous distension in the diabetic neuropathic foot (physical sign of arteriovenous shunting), *J R Soc Med* 76:1011–1014, 1983.

86. Wetter L, et al: Is hemoglobin concentration a predictor for the outcome of distal gangrenous lesions in diabetics? *Acta Med Scand* 687(suppl):29–32, 1984.

87. Wyss CR, et al: Transcutaneous oxygen tension as predictor of success after an amputation, *J Bone Joint Surg (Am)* 70A:203–207, 1988.

88. Yuh WTC, et al: Osteomyelitis of the foot in diabetic patients: evaluation with plain film, 99m Tc-MDP bone scintigraphy, and MR imaging, *Diabetes Spectrum* 4:80–86, 1989.

# CHAPTER 24

# Footwear in a Management Program for Injury Prevention

## William C. Coleman, D.P.M.

In many medical centers, foot care for the diabetic patient begins with treatment of the first injury. In an ideal situation, however, the possibility of the first foot injury should have been anticipated. Proper care for diabetic foot problems should always include an aggressive program of injury prevention. Every medical practitioner treating diabetic patients needs to inspect the feet of these patients regularly. All diabetic patients need education on footwear selection and foot inspection. As soon as changes caused by diabetes are noted on the feet, persons who sell, modify, or construct medically indicated shoes need to be included as contributing consultants.

With the proper use of appropriate footwear and instruction related to foot care, most diabetic patients can expect to avoid skin wounds on their feet. Providing appropriate footwear for the diabetic patient who has never had a foot injury, however, continues to be a difficult problem. Few medical practitioners have sufficient education or training regarding the applications and prescription of protective footwear. Most shoe modifications are recommended as the result of trial-and-error experience and training, which is based on the empirical findings of shoemakers of previous generations. There are few objective, experimentally derived data to support most shoe therapy.[28]

Unlike many European countries, the United States does not have a formal training program for shoemakers or shoe-fitters. In many countries, representatives of large-

scale, regional companies that manufacture prescription footwear are present at clinics to contribute to the decision-making process and become familiar with the clinical goals of each patient's prescribed shoes.

One of the most frequently asked questions at seminars concerned with foot care for diabetics is, "What sort of shoe should a diabetic patient wear during the period of treatment for an ulceration on the bottom of their foot?" The response to such a question should be obvious. A person with an insensitive foot should never walk with an open wound on the bottom of their foot. Of course, this is not always possible or practical. Nonetheless, shoes are not reliable as part of the treatment and usually will prolong the time needed to heal the wound.[6] If the patient with neuropathy must walk, casts or splints are a more effective means of protection.[9]

Even if a shoe is perfectly fitted to the foot and relieves stress to an open ulcer, the shoe will be removed by the patient at home. Many diabetics need to urinate in the middle of the night. When they walk to and from the bathroom, they seldom wear their protective shoes. One unguarded step on an insensitive foot with an ulceration, fracture, or infection can be devastating to the prognosis of that foot.[6] Shoes have their best utility as a means of injury prevention and not as a means of treating active injuries.

Frequently, diabetic patients cannot afford the proper, medically indicated footwear. Many third-party reimbursement systems do not cover shoes intended for the prevention of injury to the feet of a diabetic. After the problem has worsened and hospitalization or amputation has become the only form of treatment that is appropriate, payment from these organizations can be readily obtained.

This chapter is formatted according to a prevention program now being implemented at the Gillis W. Long Hansen's Disease Center. The basic concept for the program was presented by Joseph Reed, R.P.T., in 1982. He believed it was easier to anticipate possible injuries if patients could be classified according to their potential risk of injury. Patients with the highest risk would need the most protective footwear and would return for evaluation more often than patients who have less chance of damaging their feet as a result of diabetes.

## RISK DETERMINATION

This system of risk determination is based on the ability of a clinician to determine the presence or absence of protective levels of sensation, peripheral vascular disease, or both. Protective levels of sensation, for the purpose of this chapter, are present when a person can perceive and react to a threatening stimulus in a manner to minimize or prevent injury.

### Sensory Examination

Clinicians have observed that occasionally a diabetic patient with an open ulceration on the bottom of the foot may walk without limping despite a "normal" sensory examination. This indicates that commonly used sensory evaluation techniques may not be adequate to reveal the presence or absence of protective sensation.[16] A more precise, quantifiable system of sensory testing was needed for diabetic patients. After extensive reliability testing and clinical trials, Semmes-Weinstein monofilaments seem to provide reproducible quantification to differentiate patients who have protective sensation from those who cannot feel that damage has occurred.[4, 12]

Semmes-Weinstein monofilaments (Fig 24–1) are a set of progressively thicker nylon filaments each attached at right angles to a small handle. They are a modification of a sensory testing system described by von Frey[32] in 1925. Pressure is applied to the skin with the filament until it bends. A series of filaments, graduated in diameter, is used, with larger diameter filaments requiring more force to bend them. Sensations of light touch and deep pressure can be determined by finding the threshold between filaments that can and cannot be felt by the patient.[2] When they are used on the feet, loss of protective sensation has been described at the level when the patient cannot feel the Semmes-Weinstein monofilament that bends at a linear force of 10 g.[4] Sets of filaments that bend with the forces of 1, 10, and 75 g are frequently used clinically. These filaments can easily be differentiated by a test subject with normal sensation. The 1-g filament can be felt by most persons with normal sensation. A person with protective sensory loss may have some sensation remaining, and the 75-g filament can help determine the presence of this sensation.

### Vascular Examination

Vascular evaluation is essential to develop a complete impression of a patient's degree of risk of developing a foot pathologic condition (see Chapter 15). Clinicians may be disproportionately focused, however, on the problems created by vascular disease and, as a result, are often unprepared to manage neuropathic complications. Although the knowledge of an individual's vascular status is very important, it needs to be kept in perspective. One still must help protect patients who are not vascular surgical candidates from injury. The fact remains that the majority of diabetic patients have limbs amputated as a result of injury secondary to sensory neuropathy.

Clinics that have incorporated new programs of foot examination and patient education managed by professionals trained regarding foot problems have dramatically reduced amputation rates and hospital days for foot-related problems. At Atlanta's Grady Memorial Hospital, the amputation rate was decreased by 50%.[15] The County

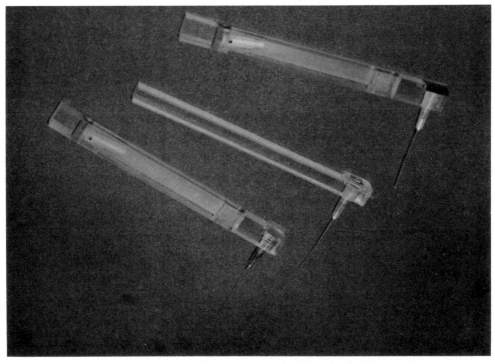

**FIG 24–1.**
Set of three Semmes-Weinstein monofilaments is used for sensory testing on feet. Here the monofilaments are attached to the end of lucite rods. Each of three filaments is a different thickness. The smaller filament bends with 1 g of force, the medium filament with a force of 10 g, and the largest at 75 g.

Health Department in Memphis reduced the number of days spent in the hospital by 68%.[27] The University Hospital in Geneva, Switzerland, was able to reduce the transtibial amputation rate by 85%.[1] All of these outcomes were achieved by innovative, multidisciplinary programs to manage the feet of persons with diabetes.

## RISK CATEGORIZATION

All of the risk categories presented here can be included within grade 0 (intact skin) of the foot lesion classification system described by Wagner.[33]

### Risk Category 0

Category 0 of risk (Table 24–1) includes all patients who have been diagnosed as having diabetes who retain protective levels of sensation and good tissue perfusion. Sensory systems within the foot and vascular supply to the foot, however, can be lost during any stage of the disease. Because this loss may be so gradual that it is not noticed by the patient, a periodic, objective evaluation of sensation should be done to help prevent tissue damage. A standardized record of foot risk factors should be maintained for the duration of the patient's life (Table 24–2).

### Risk Category 1

Patients in category 1 have not had ulcers of their feet but have lost protective levels of sensation. This places them at a higher risk of injury. The repetitive stress of walking alone can result in damage to their feet. For most patients an inability to feel the 5.07 Semmes-Weinstein monofilament that bends with a pressure of 10 g would place them in this category.

### Risk Category 2

Patients included in category 2 have lost sensation and also have a deformity in their feet but have not developed ulcers. Deformity results in the concentration of stress in a small area of the foot. The added stress

**TABLE 24–1.**

Risk and Management Categories

| Risk | Management |
|---|---|
| **Category 0** | |
| Protective sensation present | Foot clinic once/yr |
| No history of plantar ulcer | Patient education to include |
| May have foot deformity | proper shoe style selection |
| Has a disease that could lead to insensitivity | |
| **Category 1** | |
| Protective sensation absent | Foot clinic every 6 mo |
| No history of plantar ulceration | Review all footwear the patient |
| No foot deformity | wears |
| | Add soft insoles (Spenco,* nylon-covered PPT†) |
| **Category 2** | |
| Protective sensation absent | Foot clinic every 3–4 mo |
| No history of plantar ulcer | Custom-molded orthotic devices |
| Foot deformity present | are usually necessary |
| | Prescription footwear are often required |
| **Category 3** | |
| Protective sensation absent | Foot clinic every 1–2 mo |
| There is a history of foot ulceration and/or vascular laboratory findings indicate significant vascular disease | Custom orthotic devices are necessary |
| | Prescription shoes are often required |

*Spenco Medical Corporation, Waco, Tex.*
†*Professional Protective Technology, Deer Park, N.Y.*

usually occurs in a part of the foot that is not accustomed to additional pressure, resulting in injury. Surgical correction of deformity can result in moving a diabetic patient to a lower risk category.

## Risk Category 3

Persons in category 3 not only have lost sensation but also have a history of previous foot ulceration. Human skin and underlying soft tissues are more easily reinjured in areas where previous damage such as ulceration has occurred.

## PATIENT MANAGEMENT

As the risk of ulceration rises, so does the need for more frequent foot examination. With deformity or previous ulceration, these vulnerable areas need footwear modifications to limit stress even further. Also, as risk increases, the patient needs ever-increasing levels of education to ensure that

protective footwear is worn exclusively and that the patient identifies possible sites of injury early. In a survey of patients with diabetes at Kings College Hospital in London, the recurrence rate of ulceration was 26% among those with special footwear and 83% among those who returned to using their regular footwear.[13]

It is extremely difficult to indoctrinate most diabetic patients adequately in foot care and ulcer prevention before extensive damage has taken place. Many injuries can be prevented with a regular schedule of clinic visits and minimal guidelines for shoe modification. With this in mind, management categories have been established to complement the risk categories (see Table 24–1).

Education is essential at every visit for evaluation of the feet. It is also essential not to overwhelm the person with information. Each patient should be educated in accordance to his or her risk of developing a foot problem. As the risk increases, foot care education should also increase. To ensure that

## TABLE 24–2.

Insensitive Foot Examination*

| Examination | Justification |
| --- | --- |
| General | Inspect for possible ulceration, areas of inflammation, or other skin changes related to vascular disease |
| Sensory | Test vibratory sensation and perform a quantifiable sensory test to determine level of protective sensation |
| Temperature | With no sensation, a localized skin temperature increase >2°C in a localized area indicates an area of inflammation |
| Shoes | Identify the characteristics of the footwear that because of wear or style pose a threat to the feet |
| Muscle | Diseases that result in sensory loss can also lead to muscle paralysis; in the feet, intrinsic paralysis is the most frequent early involvement and results in clawed toe deformities |

*Patient education for self-examination should be provided to expand or reinforce the patient's active participation in his or her own care on every visit.

every patient obtains complete instructions, one can provide this form of education on video tape. The patient should view the tape, and then any questions would be answered by the clinical personnel. If a specific behavior is required of the patient, this behavior should be rehearsed by the patient under supervision of the clinical staff.

## Management Category 0

Patients in risk category 0 need to receive education on footwear selection. The feet of patients in this group could lose sensation before their next visit. If loss of sensation develops, they should begin to wear only shoes that pose no threat to their feet. A person with insensitive feet can no longer trust the feel of a shoe to determine proper fit, and therefore may buy a smaller shoe. Diabetics should always inform shoe-fitters of their disease. Because insensitivity or vascular disease can occur at any time, the peripheral sensory and circulatory status of

each diabetic should be reevaluated each year.

## Management Category 1

A patient in category 1 has exhibited loss of protective sensation. Because the only internal system providing protection has been lost, external behavioral changes have to be taught. Persons in this category need more complete information on common foot problems, such as callous formation, redness, and swelling. A recent study[34] in England has shown that callous tissue and the areas under the foot where callous forms are subjected to greater pressures than other tissues. Periodic reduction of callous reduces these pressures.

Patients with sensory loss in their feet should never walk barefoot. After stepping on a sharp object, the person with an insensitive foot will keep walking on the injured foot. This often results in added injury, delayed healing, or abscess formation. For these reasons, patients with insensitive feet need to maintain vigilance for possible dangerous circumstances at all times. Occasionally, injuries occur because of objects that have fallen into the shoe since it was last worn. Before a shoe is put on, the inside should be inspected for foreign objects, then turned upside down and shaken to be sure nothing is inside.

As a person walks, the bottom of the foot is subjected to repetitive stress. To minimize the effects of repetitive stress, persons in category 1 should have soft insoles made of materials such as microcellular rubber or polyurethane foam in all shoes they wear. These materials are available in precut insoles or in sheets of material that can be cut to the proper size. A nylon covering helps to minimize shear between the insole and the foot, and the soft cushion helps to reduce vertical (normal) stress.

Studies[7] in rats have shown that the likelihood of damage from repetitive stress increases as the number of steps increases. If walking is gradually increased over a long period, the tissues will adapt, thereby increasing the tissue ability to remain undamaged by repetitive stress. If the number of steps per day is significantly increased over a short period, however, tissue damage can develop. These studies should make the clinical staff aware that a patient leaving for vacation or expecting visitors is about to enter a high-risk situation. Either the number of steps taken needs to be minimized, or the tissues must be conditioned for greater stress over a long period. Added protection by footwear is also required.

Brand[3] describes the use of thermometry in determining the presence of inflammation on insensitive feet. This technique is particularly helpful in preventing injury to the feet when shoes are new and have not yet conformed to the shape of the foot.

Being at a higher risk of injury, people in this category need to visit their foot care physician more frequently than those in category 0. A visit every 6 months can help detect developing problems, such as claw-toe deformity. Clawed toes are a common finding, because as the denervation progresses, the toes contract as the result of paralysis of the intrinsic foot muscles.[33]

## Management Category 2

Deformity in the foot sometimes requires custom footwear to accommodate its shape (see Fig 24–5). Many custom shoes are manufactured from a plaster model of the foot that is sent to a manufacturer for last construction and shoe fabrication. This process creates a communication gap between foot care providers and shoe fabricators. This communication gap often results in less than ideal footwear. Most of the patients in category 2 do not require custom footwear. Depth footwear appropriately fit and modified by a prescription shoe-fitter will provide the necessary accommodations for most common deformities, such as clawed toes. Persons in this category need to visit a foot specialist at least every 4 months and probably more often until the problem is fully protected by shoes or the deformity is corrected by surgery.

## Management Category 3

Patients in category 3 have insensate feet that have been previously ulcerated. Ulcers occur most frequently under the insensate foot at the location of previous ulcers.[6] Scarring makes tissues less flexible and more likely to breakdown, particularly as the result of shear, a force applied parallel to the skin surface. Soft tissues withstand shear through the process of one layer of tissue gliding over adjacent tissues. Scar binds tissue layers together and prevents this gliding action. With this greater degree of susceptibility, these patients need a higher level of protection within their footwear.

Also in category 3 are patients with significant peripheral vascular disease. These patients have tissues that are more friable, which, once injured, have a much more difficult time healing. Often when peripheral vascular disease and neuropathy coexist, the injury occurs in a manner typical of neuropathic lesions but requires much more protection and time to heal because of poor tissue perfusion.

Category 3 patients require the most intense efforts of the medical community. With proper footwear and no current injury, these persons should routinely be seen by a foot specialist, with education reinforcement every 1 to 2 months.

## FOOTWEAR

When a shoe is too tight, ulcers usually develop medial to the first metatarsal head and lateral to the fifth metatarsal head (Fig 24–2). The ulceration is caused by pressure ischemia. This pressure is the result of tension within the leather of the upper portion of the shoe, which applies the greatest stress in areas of smallest circumference.[7] This breakdown is also related to the length of time a shoe is worn. For damage to occur, pressure from a shoe that is too tight must be maintained for hours with no relief. Diabetic patients should be taught to change their shoes at midday and perhaps again in the evening. By doing this, patients do not allow pressures to remain in one place on the foot for an excessive period of time.

The number given for a shoe size by a manufacturer can be used only as a general

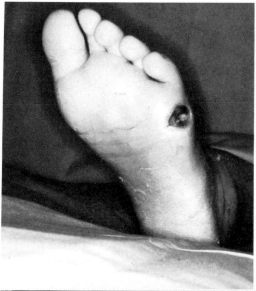

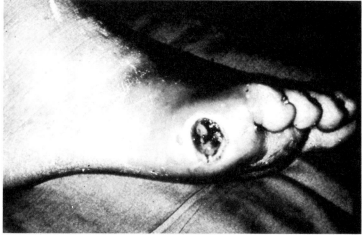

**FIG 24–2.**
Ulcerations on the feet of patients whose shoes were too tight. *(From Reed JK, Jr: Footwear for the diabetic, in Levin ME, O'Neal LW, editors: The diabetic foot, ed 3, St Louis, 1983, Mosby Year Book.)*

guideline for fitting a particular foot. Shoes of the same numbered size vary greatly in width and length because of differences in shoe lasts. Shoes for an insensitive patient should never be purchased just by asking for a specific numbered size.

The fit of a shoe should be determined by an experienced shoe fitter, such as a certified pedorthist, while the patient is standing in the shoe. The shoe should be ½ to ⅝ in. longer than the longest toe.[26] Length is only one of many factors that need to be evaluated to achieve good fit. Guess work can result in permanent damage to the foot (see Chapter 25).

Heels greater than 2 in. shift the body weight toward the forefoot, particularly onto the first and second metatarsal heads.[28, 29] This shift of body weight increases pressure under the metatarsal heads, increasing the risk of foot ulceration. Actual heel height is a vertical measurement from the top of the insole under the metatarsal heads to the top of the insole under the heel.

Pressure sensitive socks are available to help a shoe-fitter objectively evaluate fit (Fig 24–3).[5] These socks are coated with wax capsules containing dye that fracture when a certain pressure threshold is exceeded. The dye will stain the sock in areas of high pressure (Fig 24–4) in the shoe as the person walks.

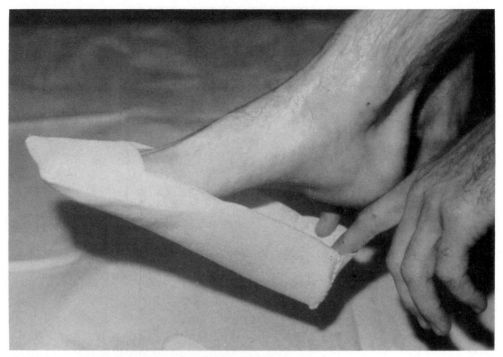

**FIG 24–3.**
Pressure-sensitive socks can be worn within the shoe to assist the clinician or shoe-fitter in determining proper fit for a diabetic patient with insensitive feet.

## SHOE INSERTS

Well-molded, custom inserts are usually required to adequately distribute forces around foot deformities. If a shoemaker, orthotist, or pedorthist wants to redistribute plantar forces with shoe inserts, the means of doing so fall into four general categories:

1. Pressure under one part of the foot can be relieved by increasing the pressure (elevating the insole) on an adjacent part. Metatarsal "cookies," buildups, or depressions in the insole are included into this group. These techniques are imprecise and can result in foot injury by greatly increasing local pressure on insensitive skin. Therefore, the following techniques are preferred.

2. Pressure under one part can also be reduced by exactly molding an insole to the plantar shape. Because pressure is equal to force (body weight) divided by the area (amount of foot in contact with the insole), exact molding reduces pressure under every part of the foot by increasing the area of contact.

3. The effects of pressure can be spread over time. Soft materials take time to compress. This compression slows the foot as it presses down into the insole. Thicker foam insoles are more effective than thinner insoles of the same material, but as the material used becomes thicker, the foot will begin developing blisters because of rubbing up and down against the side of the shoe.

4. In theory, dynamic, functional foot orthoses can reduce the pressure in one part of the foot by altering internal motions of the bones within the foot. If properly constructed, these inserts can successfully control the effects of mild to moderate pronatory deformities. Excessive pronation results in localized forces under one or two metatarsal heads and, in some cases, the first toe.[25] Effective control of pronation reduces these localized pressures by allowing all metatarsal heads to share the force of each step.

The toe region of an insole should not be molded under an insensitive foot. The foot elongates with pronation, and the toes must

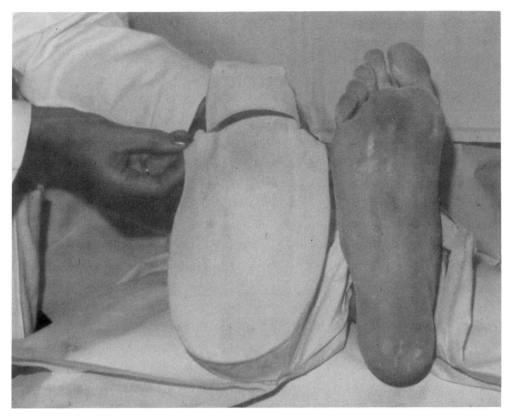

**FIG 24–4.**
Pressure-sensitive socks will localize areas of higher pressure within the shoe. Wax capsules within the sock fracture with high pressures and release a dye that stains the fabric.

be free to slide forward as this motion occurs. Ridges created by molding often result in distal toe ulceration.

There is a great variety of insole materials available from medical suppliers. Softer materials, such as polyethylene, polyurethane, or microcellular rubber foams, help to cushion the foot but cannot fully replace all characteristics of human soft tissues. These softer materials are molded and trimmed more easily than firmer ones. Unfortunately, this is often the only reason they are selected for insole construction. These materials are best used for a temporary or trial device.[14] Softer materials will not hold their molded shape for a long time because repetitive compression and decompression breaks down the cellular structure.

For long-term wear, the current preferences in insole design are a lamination of different materials or a single firm material. By combining materials in one insole, the manufacturer can take advantage of the good properties of one material while minimizing its weaknesses by using a second material with different mechanical characteristics (Figs 24–6 and 24–7). Rigid materials generally hold their shape for longer periods of time and are not as easily deformed as a person walks.

A laminated insole of Plastazote, cork, polyurethane foam, and leather was used in a study[8] in Germany. Patients who routinely wore the molded inserts greatly reduced their chance of developing foot ulceration compared with persons who returned to nonmolded footwear occasionally. This study reinforces the concept that a properly made insole must be worn all the time. A person cannot even occasionally wear shoes that are not especially designed to protect their feet.

Whenever possible, it is preferable to use the person's own soft tissue structures as a cushion. Human soft tissues have viscoelastic properties that provide more effective in-

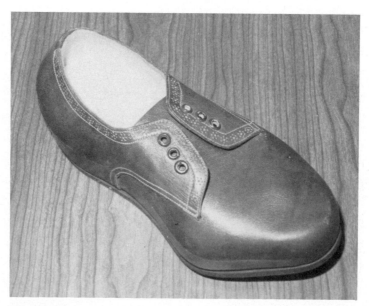

**FIG 24–5.**
Shoe custom made to accommodate a bunion deformity.

jury protection than any artificial materials. To hold soft tissues in place under bony prominences, frequently the site of localized pressure, firmer materials are usually needed.

Rigid materials are more effective in functional control of the foot. Because they retain a molded shape for longer periods, rigid materials are preferred when the intent is to hold a foot in a particular position or to

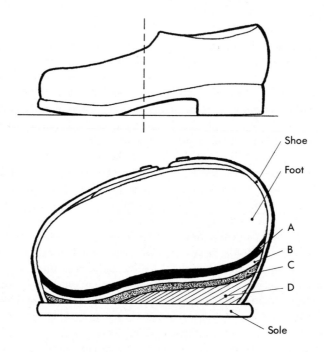

**24–6.**
Cross section of shoe shows layers of different materials in one type of laminated orthotic device. Layer **A** is nylon-covered PPT or Spenco; layer **B** is Subortholene (JMS Berkshire Resource, Inc., Clifton, N.J.); layer **D** is neoprene crepe. Nylon covering reduces shear stress, and underlying foam allows for cushioning. Pelite molds well to the shape of the positive model and is then reinforced by the rigid *Subortholene*. The neoprene crepe provides a firm support for the other materials.

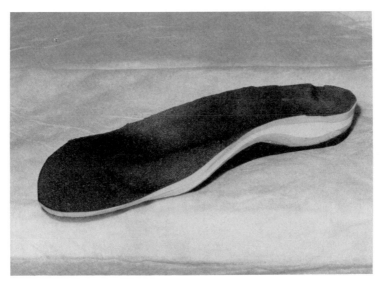

**FIG 24–7.**
Molded insert constructed of the materials illustrated in Figure 24–6.

resist motion in a given direction. If these rigid materials are used as the upper surface of insoles for insensitive feet, more precision and expertise are needed in their manufacture because rigid materials that are not properly formed can quickly result in severe injury to an insensitive foot.

Many insole devices require extra vertical room within the shoe because of the additional space needed for the insole. To accommodate these inserts, several shoe companies manufacture depth footwear. These shoes are ⅜ to ⅝ in. deeper than conventional oxford shoes (Fig 24–8).

## SHOE SOLE MODIFICATIONS

Common external shoe modifications such as metatarsal bars, Mayo crescent, anterior heels 20, and Hauser bars are not recommended for insensitive feet. These devices are intended to mold the inside of the shoe against the foot by applying pressure against the bottom of the sole (Fig 24–9). This type of molding is not precise and can result in injury to an insensitive foot.

The most frequent location of plantar ulceration on an insensitive foot is beneath the first metatarsal head, with the interphalangeal joint of the first toe and second metatarsal head almost as fr<sup></sup>

quent.[30] Recent studies have correlated the location of ulcers under the feet of diabetics with the region's higher vertical pressures.[11]

Studies have shown that a rigid shoe sole can reduce shear stress on the foot.[21] Rigid soles also limit the damage to toes that have limited motion at the metatarsophalangeal joint. An added sole rocker creates a fulcrum under the foot (Fig 24–10). As the shoe rotates over the fulcrum during walking, pressures on the metatarsal heads are reduced.

With a curved or roller sole (Fig 24–11), as the heel is lifted, the shoe will roll forward, keeping the heel of the shoe against the foot.[19] The rocker style is more effective than the roller at reducing forefoot pressures. As much as 50% of the pressure can be reduced by use of a rigid rocker sole.[10]

Shoes and insoles need periodic professional evaluation to maintain the proper shape as wear occurs. The temperature of the foot skin should also be tested during these visits. Elevation of the surface skin temperature is often the first clinical evidence of inflammation caused by an emerging injury on an insensitive foot.

Constant reinforcement concerning the essential use of appropriate footwear needs to be provided by all of the patient's health care providers.

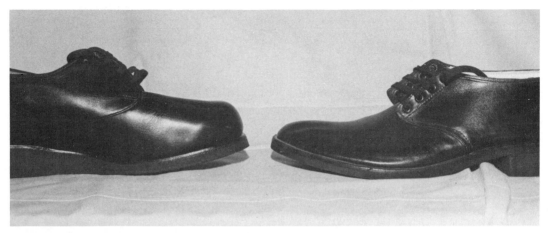

**FIG 24–8.**
Conventional oxford shoe *(right)* contrasted with shoe with extra vertical depth (left).

## SHORTENED FEET

Feet that have been shortened by destruction or amputation are a particularly difficult problem. A shortened foot has to compensate for the loss of length by performing more work. From a mechanical perspective, the shorter foot is a shorter lever. More force has to be applied to a shorter lever, compared with one of more length, to do the same amount of work. On a short foot this additional force is concentrated under what has become the front of the foot (Fig 24–12).

For cosmetic reasons, people want to wear shoes of equal length. To have shoes of equal length when one foot is much shorter, the shoe on the shorter foot will be excessively long. In this case, the short foot must do even more work by having a poor mechanical advantage to push down on the long shoe. The end of the foot will press against the middle of the shoe during walking rather than provide stability at the end of the shoe. The skin of the shortened foot will tend to ulcerate under the distal plantar surface. Because the foot is a shorter lever, additional work is needed for walking. Eventually the muscles in the back of the leg may accommodatively shorten, resulting in equinus. Both of these complications lead to greatly increased pressure under the front of the foot. Shoes for shortened feet should fit the foot in length. The sole of the shoe should be of a roller or rocker design to minimize the distal pressures under the forefoot.

To further redistribute the forces of body weight, a boot that fits snugly to the exact shape of the lower leg can be constructed. This boot, known as a fixed-ankle-brace walking boot (Fig 24–13), or FAB walker, has lacing in front of the leg. These laces allow for daily adjustment to compensate for variances in leg volume and to ensure snug fit at all times.

If the patient insists on a long shoe for a short foot, the sole should be rigid with a rocker fulcrum behind the distal end of the foot. The distal end of the shoe should not touch the ground as the person walks.

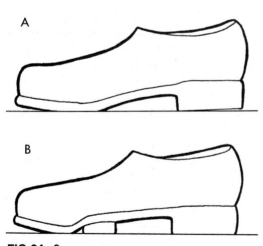

**FIG 24–9.**
**A,** conventional shoe. **B,** effffect of a properly constructed metatarsal bar, which molds the shoe sole behind the metatarsal heads to relieve stresses in this region.

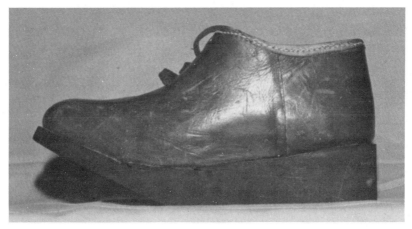

**FIG 24–10.**
Rocker-style sole is rigid, and as the wearer walks the shoe rotates over a ridge (fulcrum) in the sole located posterior to the metatarsal heads.

## TEMPORARY FOOTWEAR

The person with an insensate foot or significant peripheral vascular disease should never take an unprotected step. There are times, usually when shoes are being ordered, repaired, or modified, when the feet need some sort of interim protective shoes, which should be readily available. They should be custom molded to the individual's feet and made of materials that allow rapid construction. Because these shoes are not intended for definitive long-term use, they do not need to have long-term wear capability. When the definitive footwear is available, these shoes can continue to be useful as house shoes or shower sandals. Currently, ideal materials for these temporary shoes are thermoplastic polyethylenes such as Plastazote (Ali Med, Boston). Being water resistant, the closed-cell structure can be washed and will not absorb fluids. A commercially available total Plastazote shoe (Apex Foot Products Corporation, Englewood, N.J.) (Fig 24–14), in most cases, can be used for temporary use.[24] These shoes have soft uppers and enough space internally for the addition of a molded insole.

For severely deformed feet, during times when shoes are being repaired or before shoes have been provided, custom-molded Plastazote sandals can be constructed.[23] These sandals consist of an upper layer of

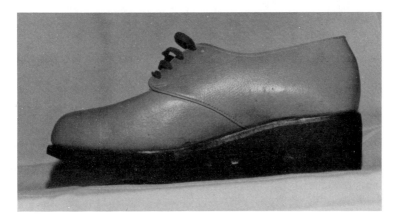

**FIG 24–11.**
Roller-style shoe also is rigid, but does not have a ridge like the rocker style. As the person walks and lifts the heel the shoe rolls forward on the curved sole. This prevents pressures from remaining in one location under the foot, because the point of contact with the ground is constantly moving forward as the heel is lifted.

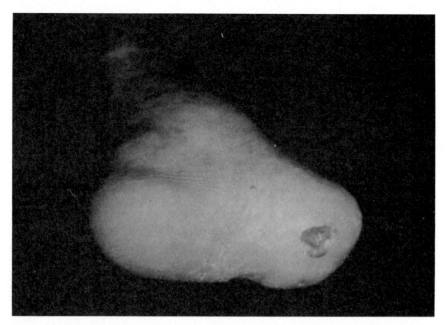

**FIG 24–12.**
Pressures under a shortened foot are much greater than under a foot of normal length. Extra protective measures must be taken to prevent plantar soft tissue destruction.

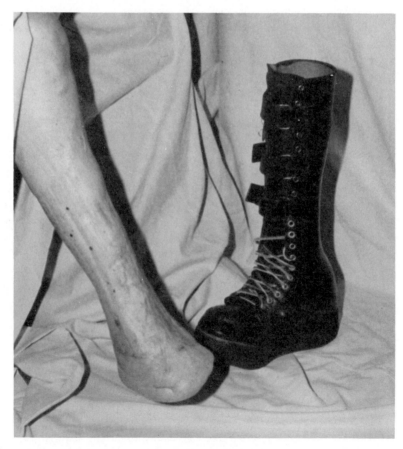

**FIG 24–13.**
Fixed-ankle-brace walking boot has been used by this patient with a shortened foot more than 20 years. The boot is made over a positive model of the patient's lower leg. The back of the boot is reinforced with ⅛-in polypropylene. Lacing allows for daily adjustment of fit over the foot and leg.

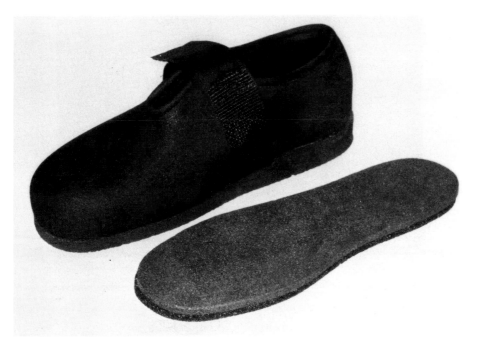

**FIG 24–14.**
Commercially available total Plastazote shoe with a polyethylene insert is available for temporary protection until definitive footwear is available. *(From Reed JK, Jr: Footwear for the diabetic, in Levin ME, and O'Neal LW, editors: The diabetic foot, ed 3, St Louis, 1983, Mosby Year Book.)*

medium-density Plastazote (which is actually the softest), reinforced beneath with a firmer Plastazote. A neoprene crepe sole and straps of either leather or cotton webbing complete the sandal (Figs 24–15 and 24–16).

## CONCLUSION

If clinical programs of injury prevention for insensitive feet are going to be successful, medical professionals will have to insist that people who fit and modify medically in-

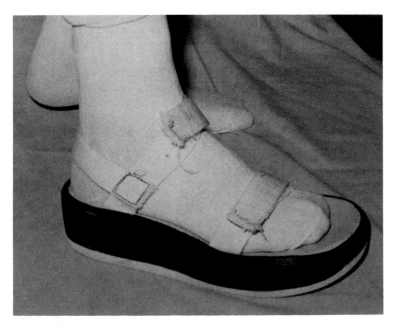

**FIG 24–15.**
Custom-made Plastazote sandal with cotton webbing for straps and Velcro closures.

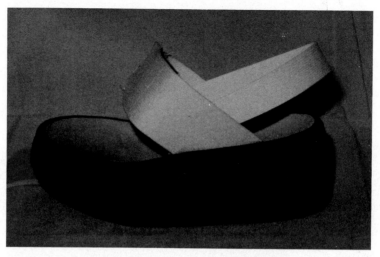

**FIG 24–16.**
For shorter feet a single strap can be used, but should be wider to prevent excessive pressures over the dorsal surface of the foot.

dicated footwear be knowledgeable, professional, and precise in their work. Shoes are the primary means of protecting insensitive feet. The responsibility to ensure proper shoe applications must rest with the physician.

Several publications have emphasized the need to develop multidisciplinary teams to adequately manage the foot problems of many diabetics.[1, 13, 15, 27] The best published data for developing programs to benefit patients with diabetic foot problems and reducing amputation rates have come from endocrinologists who have brought teams together (see Chapter 2). The primary day-to-day management of the majority of persons with diabetes must be under the supervision of medical professionals familiar with the pathologic conditions and biomechanics of the foot. Because foot problems can develop quickly and unexpectedly in the patient with diabetes, team members must be readily available. Medical and surgical expertise are needed on the team to make comprehensive diabetic foot care as seamless as possible. Physicians who accept the responsibility for the foot care of diabetic patients should be familiar with every aspect of shoe modification for therapeutic use. They should also accept the fact that the patient with an insensitive foot will always need life-long assistance to prevent tissue damage.

## REFERENCES

1. Assal JP, Muhlhauser I, Pernat A, et al: Patient education as the basis for diabetic foot care in clinical practice, *Diabetologia* 28:602, 1985.

2. Bell JA: Light touch-deep pressure testing using Semmes-Weinstein monofilaments. In:Hunter JM, Schneider LH, Mackin EJ, et al, editors: *Rehabilitation of the hand*, St Louis, 1984, Mosby–Year Book.

3. Bergtholdt HT: Thermography on insensitive limbs. In:Uematsu S, editor: *Medical thermography, theory and clinical applications*, Los Angeles, 1976, Brentwood Publishing.

4. Birke J, Sims D: Plantar sensory threshold in the ulcerative foot, *Leprosy Rev* 57:261, 1986.

5. Brand PW, Ebner JD: Pressure sensitive devices for denervated hands and feet, *J Bone Joint Surg [Am]* 51:109, 1969.

6. Brand PW: *Insensitive feet: a practical handbook on foot problems in leprosy*, London, 1981, Leprosy Mission.

7. Brand PW: The insensitive foot (including leprosy). In: Jahss MH, editor: *Disorders of the foot and ankle*, ed 2, Philadelphia, 1991, WB Saunders.

8. Chantelau E, Kushner T, Spraul M: How effective is cushioned therapeutic footwear in protecting diabetic feet? A clinical study. *Diabetic Med* 7:355, 1990.

9. Coleman WC, Brand PW, Birke JA: The total contact cast, *J Am Podiatr Med Assoc* 74:548, 1984.

10. Coleman WC: The relief of forefoot pressures using outer shoe sole modifications. In: Patil KM, Srinivasan H, editors: *Proceedings of the International Conference on Biomechanics and Clinical*

*Kinesiology of Hand and Foot*, Madras, India, 1985, Indian Institute of Technology.

11. Ctercteko GC, Dhanendran MK, Hutton WC, et al: Vertical forces acting on the feet of diabetic patients with neuropathic ulceration, *Br J Surg* 68:608, 1981.

12. Dellon AL: *Evaluation of sensibility and reeducation of sensation in the hand*, Baltimore, 1981, Williams & Wilkins.

13. Edmonds ME, Blundell MP, Morris ME, et al: Improved survival of the diabetic foot: the role of a specialised foot clinic. *Q J Med* 1986; 232:763.

14. Enna CD, Brand PW, Reed JP Jr, et al: The orthotic care of the denervated foot in Hansen's disease, *Orthot Pros* 30:33, 1976.

15. Hobgood E: Conservative therapy of foot abnormalities infections and vascular insufficiency. In: Davidson JK, editor: *Clinical diabetes mellitus*, New York, 1986, Thieme.

16. Lang-Stevenson AI, Sharrard WJW, Betts RP, et al: Neuropathic ulcers of the foot, *J Bone Joint Surg [Br]* 67:438, 1985.

17. Logerfo FW, Gibbons GW: Ischemia in the diabetic foot: modern concepts and management, *Clin Diabetes* 7:72, 1989.

19. Milgram JE: Office measures for relief of the painful foot, *J Bone Joint Surg [Am]* 46:1095, 1964.

20. Miller WE: The anterior heel for metatarsalgia in the adult foot, *Clin Orthop* 123:55, 1977.

21. Price EW: Studies on plantar ulceration in leprosy. VI: The management of plantar ulcers, *Leprosy Rev* 31:159, 1960.

22. Reed JK Jr: Plastazote insoles, sandals, and shoes for insensitive feet. In: McDowell F, Enna CD, editors: *Surgical rehabilitation in leprosy*, Baltimore, 1974, Williams & Wilkins.

23. Reed JK Jr: Footwear for the diabetic. In: Levin ME, O'Neal LW, editors: *The Diabetic Foot*, ed 3, St Louis, 1983, Mosby–Year Book.

24. Root ML, Orien WP, Weed JH: *Normal and abnormal function of the foot*, vol 2, Los Angeles, 1977, Clinical Biomechanics.

25. Rossi WA, Tennant R: *Professional shoe fitting*, New York, 1984, National Shoe Retailers Association.

26. Runyan JW: The Memphis chronic disease program. *JAMA* 231:264, 1975.

27. Schaff PS, Cavanagh PR: Shoes for the insensitive foot: the effect of a "rocker bottom" shoe modification of plantar pressure distribution. *Foot Ankle* 11:29, 1990.

28. Schwartz RP, Heath AL: A quantitative analysis of recorded variables in the walking pattern of "normal" adults, *J Bone Joint Surg [Am]* 46:324, 1964.

29. Snows RE, Williams KR, Holmes GB: The effects of wearing high heeled shoes on pedal pressure in women, *Foot Ankle* 13:85, 1992.

30. Stokes IAF, Faris IB, Hutton WC: The neuropathic ulcer and loads on the foot in diabetic patients, *Acta Orthop Scand* 46:839, 1975.

31. von Frey M: Gibt es tiefe Druckempfindungen, *Dtsch Med Wochenschr* 51:113, 1925.

32. Wagner FW Jr: A classification and treatment program for diabetic, neuropathic, and dysvascular foot problems, *AAOS Instructional Course Lecture*, vol 28, St Louis, 1979, Mosby–Year Book.

33. Young MJ, Cavanagh PR, Thomas SG, et al: The effect of callus removal on dynamic plantar foot pressure in diabetic patients, *Diabetic Med* 9:55, 1992.

# CHAPTER 25

# Pedorthic Care of the Diabetic Foot

**Dennis J. Janisse, C.Ped.**

## ROLE OF BOARD CERTIFIED PEDORTHIST

The pedorthist is a health professional who provides prescription footwear and related devices to patients referred by the medical profession.[23] To achieve the status of Board Certified Pedorthist (C.Ped.), a candidate must complete the certification process established by the Board for Certification in Pedorthics (BCP). The C.Ped. designation is intended to provide the prescribing physician and consumer with the assurance of competence in dispensing prescription footwear. The BCP works in cooperation with the Prescription Footwear Association (PFA) to establish standards and provide educational opportunities for individuals involved in the practice of pedorthics.[1]

To become certified, a candidate must pass a comprehensive written examination covering all aspects of the profession, submit an acceptable log of completed prescriptions and provide attestations of clinical competence from two physicians. In preparation for the examination, most have also completed a university short course in pedorthics and served a period of apprenticeship before attaining certification. To maintain certification, a pedorthist must participate in continuing education programs.[1]

As a member of the team involved in the long-term treatment of the patient with diabetes, the certified pedorthist plays an important role in the care of the insensate foot.[2, 8, 22] First, the pedorthist can provide the necessary prescription footwear by maintaining the required inventory to ensure that the patient receives the type of shoes prescribed and ensuring that they fit properly. He or she can also take foot impressions and provide any needed external shoe modifications and total contact inserts. When necessary, the pedorthist can also construct custom-made shoes.

The second part of the pedorthist's role is in the area of patient education. Levin[22] has stated, "Our best approach to saving the diabetic foot is patient education"; the importance of patient education has also been noted by Boulton[2] and others.[8, 10, 12, 15, 26] The pedorthist is a valuable resource for instructing patients in all aspects of footwear: the purpose and proper use of the prescribed footwear, criteria of a good fit, and appropriate shoe materials and styles for the diabetic foot. The pedorthist can reinforce information given by other team members, such as foot inspection and hygiene procedures and injury prevention. The need for follow-up is emphasized, including any necessary minor adjustments to the current footwear, as well as future changes in the prescription itself as the patient experiences changes in his or her feet.

Finally, the certified pedorthist plays an important role in monitoring patient progress. Ideally the pedorthist should meet in a clinic setting with both the physician and the patient to determine the patient's footwear needs and formulate an effective prescription. However, because pedorthists may work with a large number of referring physicians, seeing every patient in a clinic setting is often not practical, with the result that most patients come to the pedorthist with a written prescription from their physician. In these cases, the pedorthist must serve as the link between the physician and the patient. In return visits to the pedorthist the patient can report success or any problems experienced with the prescription footwear. The pedorthist should inspect both the footwear and the patient's feet, looking for signs of undue skin pressure. The overall effectiveness of the prescription footwear should be noted and reported to the prescribing physician with recommendations for additional modifications or adjustments. The pedorthist should see patients several times, until it is certain the prescription is filled correctly and functioning properly.

When patient progress is monitored, additional opportunities are created for patient education and reinforcement of important foot care concepts. The pedorthist will often be able to prevent a foot problem through early detection; for example, in a routine foot inspection the pedorthist might notice a red spot or a developing ulcer that the patient has overlooked, especially if he or she has any loss of sensation. (The importance of regular foot inspection has been noted by Levin[22] and others.[2, 8, 15]) In addition, detailed footwear records should be maintained for all patients, facilitating effective follow-up and long-term management of diabetic foot problems.

## OBJECTIVES IN THE PEDORTHIC CARE OF THE DIABETIC FOOT

Before the specific types of prescription footwear that a pedorthist can provide are discussed, it is first necessary to identify the objectives in the pedorthic care of the diabetic foot. These can be stated as follows[16]:

1. *Relief of areas of excessive plantar pressure.* Repetitive application of high pressures during the walking and standing activities of daily life can lead to ulceration on the plantar surface of the insensitive foot.[7] Specific high-pressure areas, such as the metatarsal heads, are particularly susceptible to neuropathic ulceration.* By relieving high-pressure areas and more evenly spreading forces over the plantar surface, one can attempt to reduce the incidence and recurrence of ulceration.†

2. *Reduction of shock.* Even moderate amounts of pressure, when repetitive, can lead to ulceration in the insensitive foot[2, 4, 34]; therefore, in addition to relieving specific high-pressure areas, a reduction in the overall amount of vertical pressure, or shock, on the plantar surface is desirable.[5, 27, 32, 35] This is especially important for a foot with undue bony prominences or with the abnormal bone structure associated with the Charcot foot.

3. *Reduction of shear.* The reduction of horizontal and vertical movement of the foot within the shoe, leading to skin shear, is also an important consideration in minimizing ulceration, callus buildup, and excessive heat because of friction.‡

4. *Accommodation of deformities.* Deformities resulting from conditions such as Charcot's involvement, loss of fatty tissue, and amputations must be accommodated.[10, 27, 35] It is also vital to minimize pressure from shoe uppers on hammertoes or claw toes.[2, 15, 35]

5. *Stabilization and support of deformities.* Many deformities need to be stabilized to relieve pain and avoid further destruction, whereas flexible deformities may need to be controlled or supported in a more normal or neutral position to decrease progression of the deformity.[8, 35]

6. *Limitation of joint motion.* Limiting

---

*References 2, 3, 10, 15, 22, 34.
†References 5, 7, 8, 15, 32, 35.
‡References 4, 5, 10, 14, 32, 34.

the motion of involved joints can often decrease inflammation, relieve pain, and result in a more stable and functional foot.[27, 35] For example, supporting the heel and arch to limit pronation can decrease pain and inflammation of the midfoot and subtalar joints.

It is important to note that pedorthic care for ulcers is intended strictly as a long-term management technique for maintaining healed ulcers and preventing further ulceration; it is not generally considered an appropriate treatment or healing measure for open ulcers.[8, 12, 22, 32] (For specific treatment methods for open ulcers, see Chapters 2, 11, 13, and 14.) Therefore, in this chapter, when I refer to ulcers, it is always with the understanding that pedorthic care for ulcers is limited to maintenance and prevention after healing.

## ACHIEVING PROPER SHOE FIT[17]

To meet the objectives in the pedorthic care of the diabetic foot, one must begin with a properly fitting shoe. The excessive pressure and friction from poorly fitting shoes can lead to blisters, calluses, and ulcers in the insensitive foot.* In this section, the two basic components of shoe fit, that is, shape and size, as well as guidelines for proper shoe fit, are discussed.

### Shoe Shape

Proper shoe fit is attained when shoe shape is matched to foot shape.[13, 18, 25] The shape of a shoe, including the shape of both the sole and the upper, is dependent on the *last*, the mold over which the shoe is made. The standard last is the single, basic shoe shape from which most mass-produced shoes are made. Prescription footwear, on the other hand, are made over a variety of last shapes: examples include the combination last, which has a narrower heel than the standard last; the inflare last, which provides more medial forefoot surface area[23]; and the in-depth last, which is shaped to allow extra volume for the foot inside the shoe and provides enough room for a generic insole or a custom insert.

Specific parts of the shoe upper also affect shoe fit. Terms useful in describing the shoe upper are (1) *counter*, the part of the

*References 2, 4, 8, 9, 11, 14, 22.

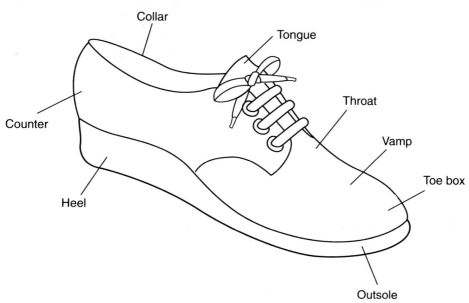

**FIG 25–1.**
Parts of a shoe.

shoe extending around the heel; (2) *toe box*, the part that covers the toe area; (3) *vamp*, the part that covers the instep; and (4) *throat*, the part at the bottom of the laces. These, along with other important parts of a shoe, are illustrated in Figure 25–1.

The counter controls the heel and determines heel fit. Strong counters are necessary to adequately control the foot inside the shoe.[8, 18] A shoe that has a high toe box and a rounded, or oblique, toe provides the best fit by allowing the toes to fit comfortably inside the shoe. A shoe with a tapered toe box or a pointed toe is therefore inappropriate for the diabetic foot, because it applies pressure to the toes and forces them into an unnatural shape, leading to calluses, ulcers, and eventual deformity.[8, 9] As with the toe box, the vamp should be high enough to prevent pressure on the instep. A shoe with laces is best for the diabetic foot because laces provide the adjustability needed for any edema or other deformities and allow the shoe to be fit properly without any danger of it slipping off. Pumps and slip-ons often have virtually no vamp, so that they must be fitted too snugly or they will fall off. Of the two types of throat openings, the blucher is preferred over the balmoral because it allows for greater adjustability, easier entry, and is more compliant to foot shape (Fig 25–2).[13, 25]

## Shoe Size

Once the properly shaped shoe has been found, the next step is to determine the proper size. There are three essential measurements in determining shoe size: overall foot length (heel to toe), arch length (heel to arch, or first metatarsal), and width. The proper shoe size is the one that accommodates the first metatarsophalangeal joint (i.e., the widest part of the foot) in the widest part of the shoe; it is for this reason that shoes must be fit by arch length rather than by overall foot length.[25] The feet in Figure 25–3 have the same overall foot length but require different size shoes because of the difference in arch length.

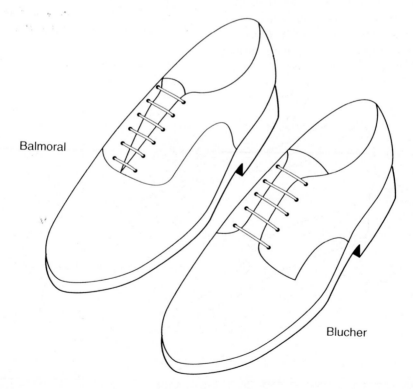

Balmoral

Blucher

**FIG 25–2.**
Two types of throat openings. *Left,* balmoral; *right,* blucher. *(Redrawn from Rossi WA, Tennant R: Professional shoe fitting, New York,1984, National Shoe Retailers Association. Used by permission.)*

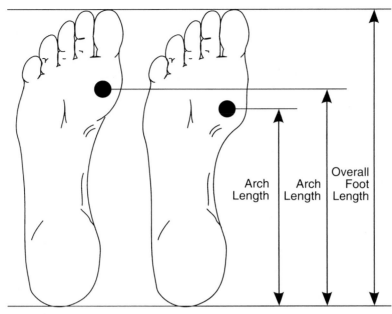

**FIG 25–3.**
Overall foot length vs. arch length. These feet have the same overall foot length, but the foot on the left would require a larger size shoe because it has a longer arch length *(Redrawn from Rossi WA, Tennant R: Professional shoe fitting, New York, 1984, National Shoe Retailers Association. Used by permission.)*

## Guidelines for Proper Shoe Fit

The following is a set of guidelines that can be used to achieve proper shoe fit[17, 25]:

1. Measure both feet with an appropriate measuring device; the Brannock measuring device is recommended.
2. Fit shoes on *both* feet while weight bearing.
3. Check for the proper position of the first metatarsophalangeal joint. It should be in the widest part of the shoe.
4. Check for the correct length. Allow ⅜ to ½ in. between the end of the shoe and the longest toe.
5. Check for the proper width, allowing adequate room across the ball of the foot.
6. Look for a snug fit around the heel.
7. Determine that proper fit over the instep has been achieved by an appropriately high vamp, preferably with laces to allow adjustability.

A properly fitting shoe is absolutely essential for the diabetic foot, especially if there has been any loss of sensation or previous instances of callusing, ulceration, or deformity, to prevent recurrence or further damage.[2, 8, 9] The patient with a loss of sensation will tend to purchase a shoe that is too tight; the size that feels right is often too small because of the loss of sensation.[2, 8, 22, 35] It is highly recommended that shoe fitting for these patients be done by a certified pedorthist or professionally trained shoe fitter.[2, 8, 17, 18]

## PRESCRIPTION FOOTWEAR FOR THE DIABETIC FOOT

For patients in the early stages of diabetes who have no history of foot problems and no signs of neuropathy, a properly fitted shoe made of soft materials with a shock-absorbing sole may be all that is necessary.[8, 35] However, for many patients the objectives listed previously can be achieved only with the use of prescription footwear. The following modalities are discussed in this section: (1) in-depth shoes, (2) external shoe modifications, (3) total contact inserts (TCIs), and (4) custom-made shoes.

## In-depth Shoes

The majority of diabetic footwear prescriptions begin with the in-depth shoe. It is generally a blucher-style oxford or athletic shoe with an additional ¼ to ⅜ in. of depth throughout the shoe. This provides the extra volume needed to accommodate both the foot and a TCI, a special insole custom made to fit the exact contours of the individual foot.[18] The additional depth is also useful in accommodating deformities associated with the diabetic foot, such as hammertoes and claw toes, as well as moderate medial and lateral bony prominences resulting from Charcot's deformities.[2, 11, 18]

Other features common to in-depth shoes that are especially useful in the care of the diabetic foot include their light weight, shock-absorbing soles, and strong counters. In-depth shoes are made with a variety of upper materials, including deerskin and cowhide; some have a heat-moldable lining material that allows the upper to be molded to the individual foot, especially useful for severe deformities. In-depth shoes also come in a wide range of shapes and sizes to accommodate almost any foot except those with severe skeletal distortion.

## External Shoe Modifications

The outside of the shoe can be modified in a variety of ways. The following external shoe modifications are covered in this section: rocker sole, stabilization, extended steel shank, cushion heel, wedge, and customized upper.

## Rocker Sole[19]

The rocker sole is one of the most commonly prescribed shoe modifications. As its name suggests, the basic function of a rocker sole is to literally rock the foot from heel-strike to toe-off without bending the shoe. However, the actual shape of rocker sole varies according to (1) the patient's specific foot problems and (2) the desired effect of the rocker sole. In general, the biomechanical effects of a rocker sole are (1) restoring lost motion in the foot, ankle, or both related to pain, deformity, or stiffness, resulting in an overall improvement in gait[18, 35]; and (2) relieving pressure on a specific area of the plantar surface.[4, 15, 18]

There are two terms relevant to a discussion of rocker soles: (1) the *midstance*, or the portion of the rocker sole that is in contact with the floor when in a standing position; and (2) the *apex*, or high point, of the rocker sole, located at the distal end of the midstance. These terms are illustrated in Figure 25–4. It is important to note that the apex must be placed behind any area for which pressure relief is desired. For example, a rocker sole designed to relieve pressure on the metatarsal heads must be made with the apex behind the metatarsal heads. This means that the apex must run in a slanted line across the sole so that it remains

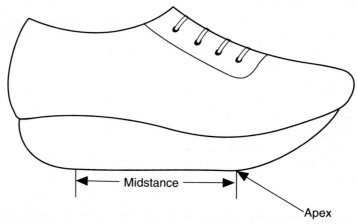

**FIG 25–4.**
Rocker sole, illustrating midstance and apex.

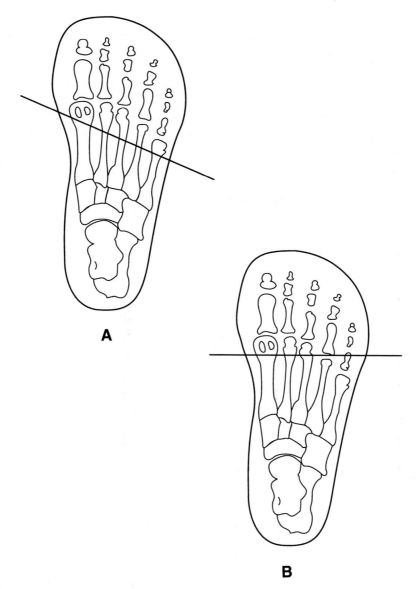

**FIG 25–5.**
Position of apex on rocker sole. **A,** apex must be placed behind the metatarsal heads to provide pressure relief. **B,** rocker sole with the apex in this position would relieve pressure on the first and second metatarsal heads but not on the third, fourth, or fifth. *(Modified from Rossi WA, Tennant R: Professional shoe fitting, New York, 1984, National Shoe Retailers Association.)*

behind all five metatarsal heads (Fig 25–5,A). If the rocker sole were instead made with the apex running straight across the sole (Fig 25–5,B), there would be pressure relief of the first and second metatarsal heads but not of the third, fourth, and fifth.[29]

In general, rocker soles are custom made for each patient; however, the following basic types of rocker soles can be identified.[19]

**Mild Rocker Sole.**—The most widely used and most basic of the rocker soles has a mild rocker angle at both the heel and the toe (Fig 25–6,A). This type of rocker sole can relieve metatarsal pressure and may assist gait by increasing propulsion and reducing the amount of energy expended in the effort of walking. It is appropriate for the foot that is not at risk and is typically found on athletic walking shoes. The other types of

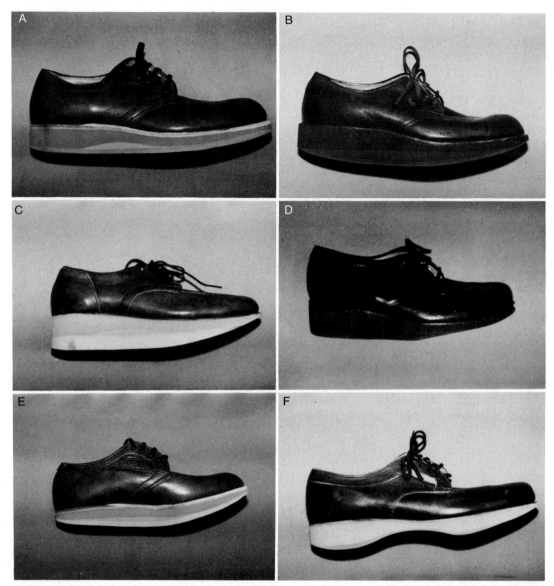

**FIG 25–6.**
Rocker soles. **A,** mild rocker sole. **B,** heel-to-toe rocker sole. **C,** toe-only rocker sole. **D,** severe angle rocker sole. **E,** negative heel rocker sole. **F,** double rocker sole.

rocker soles are essentially variations of this basic, mild rocker sole.

**Heel-to-Toe Rocker Sole.**— This type of rocker sole is shaped with a more severe angle at both the heel and the toe (Fig 25–6,B). It is intended to aid propulsion at toe-off, decrease heel-strike forces on the calcaneus, and reduce the need for ankle motion. The heel-to-toe rocker sole may be indicated for patients with a fixed claw toe or rigid hammertoe, midfoot amputation, or calcaneal ulcers.

**Toe-Only Rocker Sole.**— As the name suggests, the toe-only rocker sole has a rocker angle only at the toe, with the midstance extending to the back end of the sole (Fig 25–6,C). The purpose of this type of rocker sole is to increase weight-bearing proximal to the metatarsal heads, to provide a stable midstance, and to reduce the need for toe dorsiflexion on toe-off. Indications for the toe-only rocker sole include hallux rigidus, callus, or ulcer on the distal portion of a claw, hammer, or mallet toe, and metatarsal ulcers.

**Severe Angle Rocker Sole.**—This type of rocker sole also has a rocker angle only at the toe, but it is a much more severe angle than that found on the toe-only rocker sole (Fig 25–6,D). The purpose of the severe rocker angle at the toe is to eliminate the weight-bearing forces anterior to the metatarsal heads. It is indicated for extreme relief of ulcerated metatarsal heads.

**Negative Heel Rocker Sole.**—Shaped with a rocker angle at the toe and a negative heel, this type of rocker sole results in the patient's heel being at the same height or lower than the ball of the foot when in a standing position (Fig 25–6,E). The purpose of the negative heel rocker sole is to accommodate a foot that is fixed in dorsiflexion or to relieve forefoot pressure by shifting it to the hindfoot and midfoot. Its indications include an ankle that is fixed in dorsiflexion, prominent metatarsal heads with extreme ulcers or callusing, and distal toe ulcers. Also, because forefoot pressure relief is accomplished through the use of a negative heel, the depth or height of the sole itself can be minimized, thereby increasing overall stability of the shoe. It is therefore indicated for patients who feel unstable with the normal height of a rocker sole. The negative heel rocker sole is to be used with caution, however, because inability to attain the necessary ankle dorsiflexion will cause discomfort and may increase pressure on the problem area.

A variation of the negative heel rocker sole can be found on certain commercially made negative heel "healing" shoes. Made with a severe negative heel, these shoes can virtually eliminate weight bearing on the metatarsal and toe areas, allowing their use both as an ulcer healing method and a posthealing protection measure.[12]

**Double Rocker Sole.**—This type of rocker sole is a mild rocker sole with a section of the sole removed in the midfoot area, thereby giving the appearance of two rocker soles—one at the hindfoot and one at the forefoot—and two areas of midstance (Fig 25–6,F). Because the thinnest area of the double rocker sole is at the midfoot, it is used to relieve a specific midfoot problem area, such as a midfoot prominence associated with a rocker bottom foot or a Charcot foot deformity.

Clearly there are many types of rocker soles, and each must be individualized for a given patient's foot condition and the desired effect. A poorly or improperly designed rocker sole can actually worsen the problem it was supposed to help correct.[29] When a rocker sole is prescribed, it is essential that the physician clearly specify the desired effect or purpose of the rocker sole. A certified pedorthist is trained to know which type of rocker sole will best achieve that purpose. The pedorthist will also take measurements, obtain floor reaction imprints, and provide follow-up care to make sure that the rocker sole is performing properly for the individual patient.

### Stabilization

A second type of external shoe modification involves the addition of material to the medial or lateral portion of the shoe to stabilize some part of the foot.

**Flare.**—A flare is an extension to the heel, sole, or both of the shoe (Fig 25–7). Flares can be medial or lateral, and their purpose is to stabilize a hindfoot, midfoot, or forefoot instability. For example, a medial heel flare might be used to support a foot with a fixed valgus heel deformity.

**Stabilizer.**—A stabilizer is an extension added to the side of the shoe, including both the sole and upper (Fig 25–8). Made from rigid foam or crepe, a stabilizer provides more extensive stabilization than a flare and is used for more severe medial or lateral instability of the hindfoot or midfoot, for example, with a medially collapsed Charcot foot. Before a stabilizer is added, the patient must wear the shoe for a few weeks until it is "broken in" (i.e., has taken on the shape of the deformed foot). Adding a stabilizer to a new shoe can lead to serious skin breakdown in the diabetic foot.

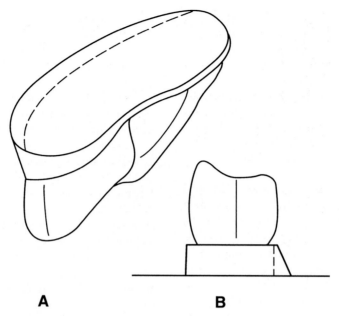

**A**                                **B**

**FIG 26-7.**
Lateral flare. **A,** plantar view; **B,** posterior view.

### Extended Steel Shank

An extended steel shank is a strip of spring steel inserted between the layers of the sole, extending from the heel to the toe of the shoe (Fig 25-9). It is most commonly used in combination with a rocker sole and, in fact, will often make the rocker sole more effective. An extended steel shank can also prevent the shoe from bending, limit toe and midfoot motion, aid propulsion on toe-off, and strengthen the entire shoe and sole. It is indicated for hallux limitus or rigidus, limited ankle motion, and more proximal partial foot amputations.

### Cushion Heel

A cushion heel consists of a wedge of shock-absorbing material added between the heel and sole of the shoe (Fig 25-10). Its purpose is to provide a maximum amount of

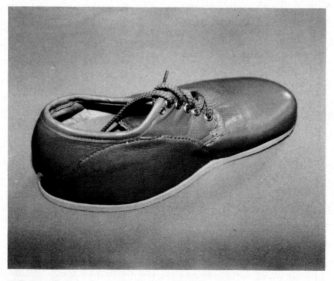

**FIG 25-8.**
Medial stabilizer.

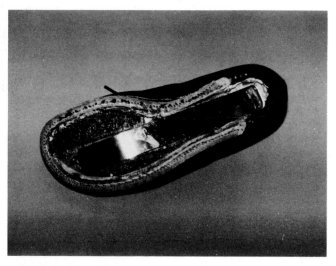

**FIG 25–9.**
Extended steel shank.

shock absorption under the heel (in addition to that provided by a total contact insert) while maintaining a stable stance. It is indicated for calcaneal ulcers or for a rigid ankle and hindfoot as a result of Charcot deformity.

### Wedge

A wedge of sole material is sometimes added medially or laterally to the heel of the shoe or to both the heel and sole (Fig 25–11). It can be inserted between the upper and the sole or added directly to the bottom of the shoe to redirect the weight-bearing position of the foot. A wedge is also useful in stabilizing a flexible deformity in a corrected position or in accommodating a fixed deformity (by essentially bringing the ground to the foot). A medial wedge is indicated in cases of extreme pronation, whereas a lateral wedge can be used for ankle instability or a varus heel deformity.

### Customized Upper

Occasionally, to accommodate a severe or unusual (but often localized) foot deformity, it becomes necessary to make a shoe modification that does not fit into any of the previous categories. By use of a customized shoe upper, the patient whose foot will otherwise fit into a stock in-depth shoe can avoid the expense and delay associated with a custom-

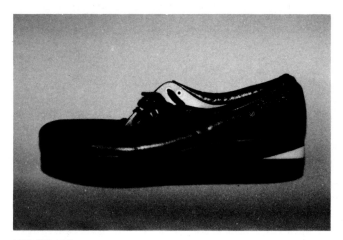

**FIG 25–10.**
Cushion heel.

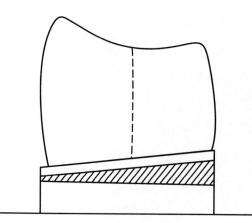

**FIG 25–11.**
Lateral wedge, inserted between the upper and the sole.

made shoe. A Charcot foot deformity is a good example of the type that might require a customized upper. For example, Figure 25–12 shows a shoe with a custom-molded lateral "pocket" designed to accommodate a severe Charcot deformity. Another type of customized upper, for patients who have difficulty tying their shoes, is the addition of a Velcro opening that maintains the appearance of shoelaces (Fig 25–13).

## Total Contact Insert[16]

The TCI is a special insole which is custom made over a model of the patient's foot, thereby achieving "total contact" with the plantar surface of the foot,[24] using the same total contact concept as the total contact

cast (see Chapter 13). The TCI is composed of a *shell*, the layer of material next to the foot and in total contact with the foot, and the *posting*, the material that fills in the space between the shell and the shoe (Fig 25–14). A properly designed TCI can achieve the objectives for pedorthic care of the diabetic foot in the following ways:

1. Relieve areas of excessive plantar pressure by evenly distributing pressure over the entire plantar surface.[3, 8, 10, 15, 34]
2. Reduce shock through the use of shock-absorbing materials in the TCI.[3, 10, 34]
3. Reduce shear, because the total contact minimizes horizontal and vertical foot movement.[4, 34]
4. Accommodate deformities with the use of soft, moldable materials in the TCI's shell.[34]
5. Stabilize and support deformities with the use of more rigid, supportive materials in the posting.[8, 31]
6. Limit the motion of joints, also through the use of supportive materials.[31]

The even distribution of plantar pressure made possible with a TCI is crucial in maintaining healed plantar ulcers and preventing their recurrence.[3, 10, 27, 35] It is important to note that even though premade insoles may provide some degree of shock absorption, they cannot fulfill the other objectives because of the absence of total contact.

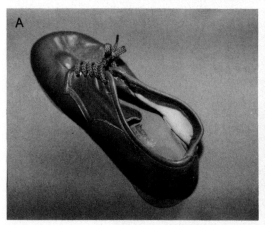
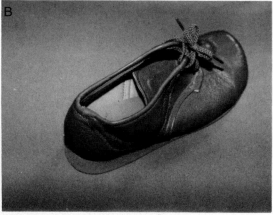

**FIG 25–12.**
Two views of custom-molded lateral "pocket" designed to accommodate a severe Charcot deformity. Notice that this shoe has also been stretched for a hammertoe deformity.

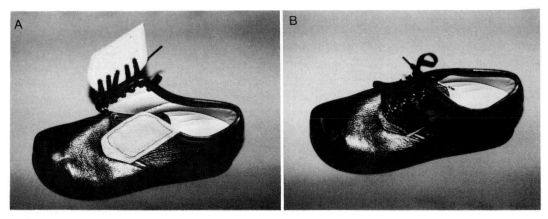

**FIG 25–13.**
**A,** customized Velcro opening addition. **B,** when closed, the shoe maintains the appearance of shoelaces.

### Design and Fabrication

For a TCI to accomplish the desired objectives, it should be designed and fabricated by an experienced professional who can:

1. Understand and evaluate the biomechanics of the lower limb.
2. Identify areas of excessive plantar pressure.
3. Utilize the appropriate impression techniques.
4. Select the appropriate TCI materials.

A certified pedorthist is an ideal choice, having been trained in all of these areas. In addition, a detailed diagnosis and explanation of the desired function of the TCI from the prescribing physician are essential.

**Evaluation of Lower Limb Biomechanics**[24, 26].—The position and relationship of the hindfoot, midfoot, and forefoot is simple, yet critical information to be obtained. For example, a patient with valgus heels may have compensatory deformities on weight bearing, such as varus forefeet; this must be taken into consideration when the TCI is designed.

The range of motion in the joints of the lower limb must also be evaluated. Ankle dorsiflexion and plantar flexion, as well as

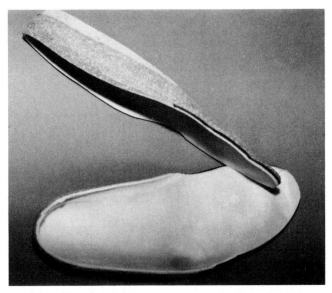

**FIG 25–14.**
Multiple-layer TCI. This TCI has a polyethylene foam shell, a middle layer of micropore rubber, and cork posting.

limited or fixed inversion or eversion, are important to observe. The midtarsal joints must be evaluated in terms of dorsiflexion and plantar flexion and pronation and supination. Range of motion in the metatarsophalangeal and phalangeal joints also needs to be noted, including clawed toes, hammertoes, mallet toes, and dropped metatarsal heads. Limited range of motion in any of these joints will have an impact on TCI design. For example, a fixed forefoot varus deformity that is not properly accommodated will result in excessive pressure being exerted on the lateral border of the foot with resultant strain in the midfoot area.

Finally, it is important that any examination of lower limb biomechanics be done in both static and dynamic states.[11, 26] Because the TCI must accommodate the foot while sitting, standing and walking, the changes that these activities produce in the foot must be determined.

**Identification of Areas of Excessive Plantar Pressure.**—Areas of excessive plantar pressure need to be defined so that they can be relieved by proper TCI design. This evaluation should begin with a physical examination of the plantar surface of the foot,[2, 11, 26] looking for calluses, blisters, ulcers, red spots, or any other indications of excessive pressure or shear. The examination should also identify bony prominences, such as depressed metatarsal heads, or bony deformity, such as a varus heel, associated with areas of soft tissue breakdown.

In addition to a physical examination of the foot, areas of excessive plantar pressure can be identified through more objective means, such as the Harris mat floor reaction system.[7, 31, 35] It consists of a rubber grid with ridges at three different heights. Ink is applied to the mat, and as the patient stands or walks over it, the ridges collapse under varying amounts of weight, thereby identifying areas of high pressure. Newer, more costly methods for evaluating plantar pressure use computerized force plate systems that provide detailed maps of the plantar surface, with quantitative measurements of plantar pressure (see Chapters 9 and 10). Either of these methods provides valuable information in determining the areas of high pressure that the TCI design must relieve.

**Foot Impression Techniques.**—As noted earlier, the TCI is made from a model of the patient's foot. There are four principal techniques used to take a foot impression, with the choice of technique determined by (1) the results of the biomechanical and pressure evaluations described earlier and (2) the desired function of the TCI. In terms of function, two basic types can be identified[31]: (1) *accommodative*, whose primary function is to accommodate a fixed deformity or one that places the foot particularly at risk; and (2) *functional*, which is designed to control a flexible deformity by providing support and stability. The function of the TCI depends on the specific foot condition. Many TCIs for the diabetic foot are both accommodative and functional to some degree.[24, 35] Foot impression techniques include the following:

1. *Plaster cast.* A traditional plaster cast is applied to the foot, similar to the process of total contact casting. This technique, when the foot is maintained in a neutral position, is useful when the purpose of the TCI is primarily functional.

2. *Wax.* A thin sheet of wax is heated in warm water and then molded to the foot. This procedure gives a good, clean impression and is a general purpose technique that can be used for both functional and accommodative TCIs.

3. *Sand and wax.* This technique is similar to the wax procedure, but as the sheet of wax is being molded to the foot, the patient stands in a tray of fine silica sand. As a consequence, the soft tissue is compressed, and the resulting TCI will be especially effective in relieving bony prominences.

4. *Foam box.* The patient's foot is pushed into a box of crushable rigid foam, or the impression can be taken with the patient weight-bearing. This technique is best used when the TCI is to be completely accommodative and results in a TCI with passive support and maximum accommodation.

**Selection of Appropriate TCI Materials.**—As with impression techniques, the selection of materials for the TCI is determined by its desired function. Total contact insert materials can be described in terms of their function and can be divided into three types[24, 31, 35]:

1. *Soft.* Cross-linked polyethylene foams are the most common soft materials currently in use. They are made by a large number of manufacturers and are rapidly being developed and improved. Generally they are moldable with application of heat (121° C–149° C) and come in a variety of densities. Their function is accommodative, and they are used close to the foot (i.e., in the shell). Studies show, however, that they decrease in thickness quickly, a phenomenon referred to as "bottoming out."[5, 10, 24, 35] Soft, nonmoldable materials such as closed-cell expanded rubber and polyurethane foam are accommodative but do not bottom out so quickly as moldable polyethylene. They often are used in conjunction with a moldable foam to provide an additional soft layer of shock absorption with minimal bottoming out.

2. *Semiflexible.* Leather and cork fall into this category. Many of the cork materials are being combined with plastic compounds to make them moldable when heated. Semiflexible materials are somewhat accommodative but provide more functional support than the soft type and do not bottom out as quickly.

3. *Rigid.* Acrylic plastics and thermoplastic polymers are considered rigid materials. They are moldable at very high temperatures and are primarily functional. They are the most durable and most supportive of the three types.

A study of five commonly used insole materials by Brodsky et al.[5] confirmed the characteristic properties just described. The study found that although the soft polyethylene foams had better pressure distribution characteristics when new, repeated exposure to the types of pressures insoles must withstand resulted in more rapid bottoming out than the more durable polymers. Other studies give similar results and show additionally that loss of thickness for the mold-

able polyethylene foam is inversely related to its density.[20, 21]

These studies would seem to suggest that to provide maximum moldability (essential for total contact) along with the necessary shock absorption and control, a TCI for the diabetic foot should be made from a combination of materials.[3, 5, 10, 31, 35] A triple-layer molded TCI can offer the needed combination of accommodative and functional properties. This type of TCI would consist of the following:

1. Top layer (shell): soft, moldable polyethylene foam.
2. Middle layer: closed cell neoprene rubber or a urethane polymer for long-lasting shock absorption.
3. Bottom layer (posting): cork, or possibly a denser polyethylene foam, for control.

The specific materials used for each layer can vary according to the needs of the individual patient.

## Custom-made Shoes

When extremely severe deformities are present, it may be that the foot cannot be fit with an in-depth shoe, even with extensive modifications. In these instances, a custom-made shoe, constructed from a cast or model of the patient's foot, is required. These cases are rare but can include severe Charcot's foot deformities and partial foot amputations.

## APPLICATIONS[19]

In this section, pedorthic care for the following problems associated with the diabetic foot are considered: uclers, amputations, and Charcot's joints and deformities. After the treatment objectives are identified, appropriate prescription footwear recommendations are made, including shoes, external shoe modifications, and TCIs. Most patients will not require all of the prescription footwear modalities described. Depending on the individual foot, the severity of the problems, and the degree of deformity, any or all of the footwear recommendations may be used. The use of in-depth shoes is recommended for all of the following unless otherwise indicated.

## Ulcers

As noted earlier in the chapter, pedorthic care for ulcers is intended strictly as a long-term management technique for maintaining healed areas and preventing further ulceration. Appropriate prescription footwear is considered an important factor in this effort, particularly in the insensate foot.*

### Plantar Ulcers

**Objectives.**—The objectives in the pedorthic management of plantar ulcers are (1) even distribution of plantar pressure by transfer from areas of high pressure, such as the metatarsal heads, to areas of lower pressure; (2) shock absorption; (3) reduction of friction and shear; (4) limiting of joint motion; and (5) accommodation of deformities.

**Shoes.**—Proper shoe fit is essential in maintaining healed plantar areas and preventing further ulceration. It is crucial that the shape of the shoe match the shape of the foot to limit overall pressure on the foot, to eliminate any particular high pressure areas, and to accommodate any deformities. A shoe with a heat moldable upper may be required for more severe deformities or in cases of mismated feet.

Other important characteristics for a shoe used in the pedorthic management of plantar ulcers include (1) a long medial counter to control the heel and medial arch and to decrease shear forces; (2) a blucher opening to allow easy entry into the shoe; (3) a shock-absorbing sole to reduce impact shock; and (4) a low heel to decrease pressure on the metatarsal heads and the toes.

**External Shoe Modifications.**—Addition of an appropriate rocker sole will aid in reducing overall pressure and impact shock; it will also limit motion of the joints and im-

*References 2, 6, 9, 12, 15, 22, 27, 35.

prove the weight-bearing transfer. Adding an extended steel shank will enhance the effects of the rocker sole. A negative heel rocker sole may be used for additional reduction of pressure and impact shock on the forefoot.

**TCIs.**—The use of a TCI can be quite effective in the distribution and transfer of plantar pressure and in reduction or elimination of weight bearing in problem areas. A TCI is also useful in stabilizing or restricting joint motion. To provide the maximum moldability essential for achieving total contact, along with the necessary shock absorption and control, a multiple-layer TCI is generally preferred.

### Dorsal Ulcers

**Objectives.**—Prescription footwear for dorsal ulcers should reduce friction and shear, accommodate any deformities, and, most important, reduce pressure from the shoe upper.

**Shoes.**—With dorsal ulcers, proper fit of the shoe upper is especially important. It should be made of a soft, pliable material such as deerskin; heat moldable uppers may be necessary for more severe deformities. The upper should also be free of unnecessary seams or designs in the toe area to minimize the possibility of skin irritation. A blucher opening allows easier entry, especially if a hammertoe deformity is present, and a low heel will prevent the foot from sliding forward in the shoe.

**External Shoe Modifications.**—The primary modification for dorsal ulcers is the stretching or molding of the shoe upper to accommodate deformities and reduce pressure in specific problem areas. For particularly severe deformities, a part of the shoe upper can be cut out and replaced with a moldable "pocket" (see Fig 25–12).

**TCIs.**—A TCI with a metatarsal pad can be especially helpful for dorsal ulcers on flexible hammertoes. The metatarsal pad aids in relaxing the hammertoe deformity, allowing the toes to extend slightly and reduce the possibility of pressure from the shoe upper.

## Partial Foot Amputations

Prescription footwear for several types of amputations are covered in this section: toe, ray, transmetatarsal, tarsometatarsal (Lisfranc) and midtarsal (Chopart). Although the pedorthic care for each type of amputation is different, several objectives are common to all amputations[30]:

1. *Provide shoe filler.* Unless the amputation is extensive and a custom-made or shortened shoe is used, some type of shoe filler is needed for the portion of the foot that has been amputated. In most cases, the filler can be incorporated into the TCI.[14]

2. *Equalize weight bearing.* Amputation of a portion of the foot will often result in uneven patterns of weight bearing on the remaining foot. Just as with the intact diabetic foot, any areas of excessive pressure must be eliminated and even distribution of weight bearing maintained.[8, 14, 27]

3. *Protect and accommodate remaining portion of the foot.* Because the occurrence of an amputation implies severe foot problems, special care must be taken to protect and accommodate the remaining portion of an at-risk foot.[14] The presence of skin grafts, scar tissue, or other postsurgical complications must also be taken into consideration when one is providing prescription footwear for a foot that has undergone partial amputation.

4. *Improve gait.* When part of the foot has been amputated, a natural gait pattern is no longer possible.[33] The addition of an appropriate type of rocker sole can often improve the gait pattern after an amputation.

The proper shoe for a partially amputated foot is determined by the extent of the amputation. If the metatarsal heads remain intact, shoe size does not change. Only when one or more metatarsal heads have been removed can the patient be fit with a shorter (i.e., smaller size) shoe.

## Toe and Ray Amputations

**Objectives.**— The first three of the objectives stated earlier are most relevant to toe and ray amputations; depending on the extent of the amputation, gait may not be significantly affected.[33] A shoe filler can help to minimize drifting of the remaining toes, which is particularly important after a great toe amputation. In the case of a ray amputation, especially the first ray, the removal of one or more metatarsal heads results in increased pressure on the remaining heads; it is therefore important to maintain even distribution of weight bearing to protect the remaining metatarsal heads.

**Shoes.**— As indicated earlier, shoe size after a toe amputation does not change because the metatarsal heads remain intact. Even after a ray amputation, where one or more metatarsals have been removed, a well-constructed shoe filler can usually allow the patient to wear a full shoe. Other important shoe features include a strong medial counter for stability, especially if the first ray has been removed, and a soft, moldable upper to protect and accommodate the remaining foot.

**External Shoe Modifications.**— Many shoes for toe and ray amputations do not require external modifications; however, possible modifications include a rocker sole with an extended steel shank (to improve gait and protect remaining metatarsal heads) and a flare (for additional stability, especially if more than one ray has been removed).

**TCIs.**— After removal of one or more toes, those remaining have a tendency to drift out of position. The use of a TCI with a filler will help to maintain the position of the remaining toes; it can also equalize weight bearing, thereby eliminating excessive pressure on the remaining toes and metatarsals.

## Transmetatarsal Amputation

**Objectives.**— The shoe filler provided for the amputated portion of the forefoot will help prevent creasing of the shoe at the point of the amputation, avoiding breakdown and eventual collapse of the shoe. A filler can also help control the remaining foot inside the shoe, decrease shear, and often eliminate the need for a costly, less cosmetically appealing custom-made shoe. Equalizing weight bearing is especially important after a transmetatarsal amputation.

**Shoes.**—A shoe with a blucher opening and a long medial counter can best control the remaining foot and help decrease shear. The upper should be made of a soft, moldable leather to accommodate and protect the remaining foot. A custom-made shoe is generally not necessary with a transmetatarsal amputation because enough of the foot remains to keep a shoe on with the aid of a filler; however, a smaller size shoe may be appropriate if the patient finds it cosmetically acceptable.

**External Shoe Modifications.**—An extended steel shank in conjunction with an appropriate rocker sole can reduce pressure and impact shock while aiding propulsion and reducing the amount of shoe distortion. The use of a cushion heel will further minimize impact shock. Medial and lateral flares may be added to stabilize and control the amputated foot and decrease shear.

**TCIs.**—A TCI with a filler will help to stabilize or restrict joint motion, accommodate bony prominences and deformities, decrease shear and shoe distortion, and equalize weight bearing. A custom-made sock may also be helpful in protecting and accommodating the remaining foot.

### Tarsometatarsal and Midtarsal Amputations

**Objectives.**—In addition to the objectives already listed, pedorthic care for a tarsometatarsal or midtarsal amputation should also be concerned with containing the remaining foot inside the shoe and preventing equinus contracture.[14, 33]

**Shoes.**—A high-top shoe is best after this type of amputation because it can most effectively contain the foot in the shoe and

provide the control necessary to prevent equinus contracture. A strong counter can also aid in providing control while improving medial and lateral stability. A wedge sole will provide a broader base of support, and a shorter shoe size will decrease the amount of shock on toe-off and aid in propulsion. For the smaller remaining foot, a custom-made shoe will best meet the treatment objectives by providing total accommodation of the foot.

**Shoe Modifications.**—An extended steel shank and appropriate rocker sole are needed to decrease shock impact, decrease shoe distortion, and aid in propulsion. A medial or lateral flare can improve stability and weight bearing. Because a smaller area must assume the weight that would normally be spread out over the entire foot, the use of a cushion heel will reduce shock at heel strike and further improve gait.

**TCIs.**—A TCI with any necessary filler will give maximum accommodation and protection of the remaining foot while stabilizing or restricting joint motion. A TCI will also decrease shear, decrease shoe distortion, and equalize weight bearing. Further protection of the remaining foot is made possible with the use of a custom-made sock.

As an alternative to incorporating the shoe filler into the TCI, a Chopart filler boot with a built-in shoe filler may be used. This orthotic device is made of leather, laces up the ankle, and resembles a high-top boot without a sole. Made to fit inside the patient's shoe, it offers additional control and helps maintain medial and lateral stability without the need for a high-top shoe.

### Charcot Joints and Deformities

**Objectives.**[11, 12, 22]—The objectives in pedorthic care of Charcot joints and deformities are (1) to accommodate fixed or flexible deformities, (2) to restrict or control unstable or painful joint motions, (3) to relieve or transfer pressure, and (4) to improve gait patterns.

**Shoes.**—The proper shoe for Charcot joints and deformities will be wide in the midfoot region to accommodate a collapsed midfoot. The extra midfoot width will also reduce or eliminate pressure on any bony prominences and provide a good base of support for the foot. A heat moldable upper may be necessary to accommodate deformities and relieve pressure. A blucher opening allows for easy entry of the foot into the shoe and will help control the foot, decrease shear, and accommodate edema. Further control and reduction of shear are accomplished with a long medial counter, and a shock-absorbing sole will reduce plantar pressure and shock. For severe deformities, such as a rocker bottom foot or extreme angulation or displacement of any part of the foot, a custom-made shoe will be necessary.

**External Shoe Modifications.**—A sole and heel flare (medial or lateral) can help to stabilize the Charcot deformity by providing a broader base of support, by reducing medial or lateral tilt, and by minimizing ligament strain. For the more severe deformity, such as a collapsed foot, a stabilizer can provide additional support and improve weight bearing. A properly designed rocker sole can assist in immobilizing unstable, damaged joints; it can also decrease midfoot pressure and strain, decrease impact shock, and improve gait.

Modifications to the counter of the shoe can accommodate some of the more severe deformities. A custom-molded addition to the medial or lateral counter, or counter "pocket" (see Fig 25–12), can be used for extreme medial and lateral deformities in the midfoot and hindfoot regions. For the rocker bottom foot, extending the height of the counter in the rear of the shoe may be necessary to help hold the foot inside the shoe.

**TCIs.**—A TCI with any necessary modifications to accommodate prominences and relieve pressure is an essential component of the pedorthic management of Charcot's joints and deformities.

# WRITING FOOTWEAR PRESCRIPTIONS

A complete written prescription from the physician is necessary to ensure that the certified pedorthist will be able to achieve the desired treatment results.[18, 31] It is often the only communication between the physician and the pedorthist. Even if a patient's footwear needs have been ideally determined in consultation with the physician in a clinic setting, a written prescription becomes a permanent part of the pedorthist's patient records, serving as a valuable resource for providing follow-up care, monitoring patient progress, and obtaining insurance reimbursement.

The written footwear prescription should include the following:

1. *Complete diagnosis.* It is important to provide the patient's complete diagnosis, including both primary and secondary diagnoses. The physician should never rely on the patient to communicate diagnoses to the pedorthist. It is also important that the diagnoses be as specific as possible; for example, a diagnosis of "foot sores" should more appropriately read, "diabetes, peripheral neuropathy, plantar ulcer under third metatarsal head."

2. *Desired effect.* The prescription should include a precise description of the desired effect or function of the footwear. For the previously mentioned diagnosis, this might say, "to relieve pressure on metatarsal heads."

3. *Specific footwear required to produce desired effect.* The physician should give the pedorthist some direction on how to accomplish the desired effect, such as in-depth shoes, external shoe modifications, and TCIs. Because the physician may not be familiar with the specific materials, shoes, construction techniques, or potential modifications, he or she may find it desirable to give the pedorthist some latitude in this area.

## Case Studies

The following case studies illustrate the broad range of pedorthic care for the diabetic foot.

568    *Janisse*

### Case 1: Plantar Ulcer

A 45-year-old man, 6 ft tall and 225 lb, with size 14 feet and a 20-year history of insulin-dependent diabetes had pes cavus feet with very little remaining fatty tissue, impaired sensation, and a history of numerous ulcers associated with severe callusing under the metatarsal heads (Fig 25–15,A). (The pes cavus foot does not absorb shock well; it puts extreme weight bearing on the metatarsal heads, which are already at risk because of the lack of fatty tissue and impaired sensation.)

His original prescription was for in-depth shoes and TCIs with a viscoelastic polymer added under the metatarsal heads to provide metatarsal pressure relief. Callus build-up improved somewhat but remained problematic on the first and fourth metatarsal heads. Addition of toe-only rocker soles provided further relief, but hemorrhaging under the first metatarsal calluses continued.

After consultation with the prescribing physician, it was decided that the TCI should be modified by adding posting material to transfer the excessive plantar pressure on the first and fourth metatarsal heads to the second and third. As seen in Figure 25–15,B, the new TCI has extreme posting proximal to the metatarsal heads, with plantar pressure transferred to the second and third metatarsal heads. The callus has virtually disappeared since the patient began wearing the new TCI.

### Case 2: Complex Plantar Ulcer

This 55-year-old, overweight man (5 ft, 6½ in., 225 lb), had a 15-year history of insulin-dependent diabetes. His vascular insufficiency had been improved with a vein bypass, but peripheral neuropathy had resulted in a completely insensate foot.

Visual examination revealed a severe calcaneal ulcer stretching from the plantar to the posterior part of the heel (Fig 25–16,A). Radiologic examination revealed soft tissue involvement only; no osteomyelitis was present (Fig 25–16,B). The ulcer was treated with total contact casting, which successfully closed the ulcer, except for a small area that was subsequently healed using a custom Plastazote sandal. Maintaining this healed area was especially challenging because the heel remained extremely susceptible to breakdown[22]; a very large deficit and a considerable amount of scar tissue were present.

The prescription called for a heat-moldable shoe to provide maximum accommodation of an at-risk foot. The shoe was modified with a heel-to-toe rocker sole and, very important, a cushion heel to absorb additional shock on heel strike (Fig 25–16,C). With the cushion heel and rocker sole, there was virtually no weight bearing on the post-ulcer heel area; significant weight bearing began at a position that was distal to the heel.

A triple-layer TCI served to further protect and accommodate the heel deficit, as

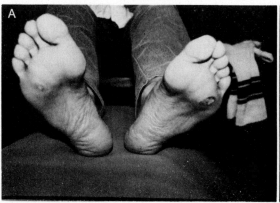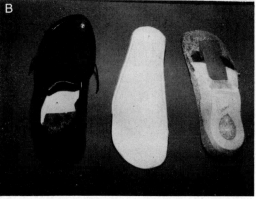

**FIG 25–15.**
Case 1. **A,** pes cavus feet with plantar ulcer under left fourth metatarsal head. **B,** in-depth shoe and TCI with posting to relieve pressure on first and fourth metatarsal heads.

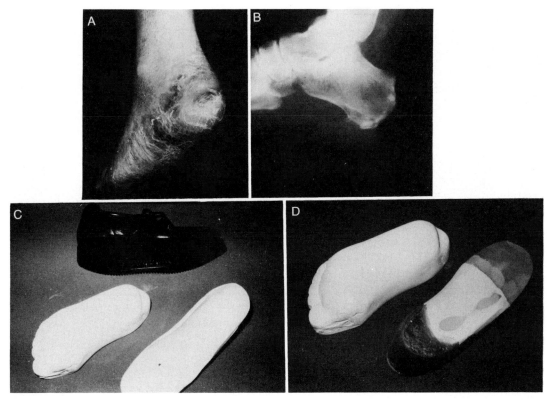

**FIG 25–16.**
Case 2. **A,** healed calcaneal ulcer. **B,** radiograph showing absence of osteomyelitis. **C,** heat-moldable shoe with rocker sole. (TCI and plaster foot model are also shown.) **D,** plantar view of TCI. Notice the heel deficit in the plaster model used to make the TCI.

well as other minor plantar prominences. The shell was made of soft Plastazote, and the deficit area of the heel was filled and supported with a soft density viscoelastic polymer (Fig 25–16,D). After 2 years, the patient has had no recurrence of ulceration or tissue breakdown.

### Case 3: Dorsal Ulcer

A 66-year-old woman with a 19-year history of insulin-dependent diabetes had a chronic dorsal ulcer on her second toe (Fig 25–17,A). Her insensate foot had collapsed medially, and she had a dynamic hammertoe deformity (i.e., the deformity worsened while walking).

Her first prescription was for a heat-moldable shoe and TCI. The shoe was stretched as much as possible over the second toe in an attempt to eliminate pressure from the shoe upper, but even after repeated attempts to further stretch the upper, reulceration of the toe occurred. The patient was treated in between shoe-stretching attempts with a custom Plastazote sandal with no pressure on the toes, and she would heal quickly.

The final solution was to remove all of the moldable lining material from the shoe in the area over the hammertoe. The remaining deerskin was extremely soft and even more stretchable without the lining material (Fig 25–17,B). For the past 4 years, there has been no recurrence of the ulcer.

This case illustrates the importance of evaluating the foot dynamically. In most cases the initial stretching of the shoe would probably have been successful, but this patient's toe position changed so dramatically while walking that normal stretching was ineffective in relieving dorsal pressure.

### Case 4: Ray Amputation

This 51-year-old man with a 32-year history of insulin-dependent diabetes had peripheral neuropathy resulting in completely

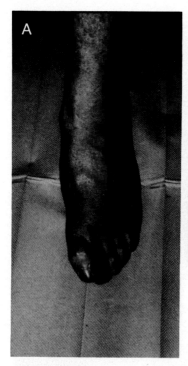
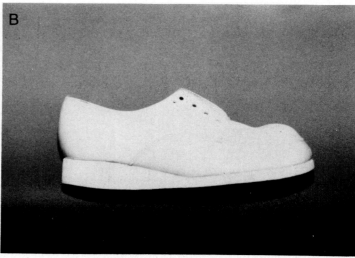

**FIG 25–17.**
Case 3. **A,** dorsal ulcer on second toe. **B,** shoe with stretched upper to reduce pressure on dynamic hammertoe.

insensate feet and a history of metatarsal ulcers.

He had a persistent plantar ulcer under the first metatarsal head of his left foot. His physician requested that we try to close the ulcer in-shoe so that the man could continue to work. This was done using in-depth steel-toed boots, rocker soles, and triple-layer TCI with extensive relief of the first metatarsal head. The ulcer had nearly closed when a sudden infection occurred. The bone infection was so severe that the first toe and a portion of the first metatarsal had to be amputated (Fig 25–18,A). The foot was closed with a skin graft, but the skin on the plantar surface remained intact and was therefore not especially difficult to maintain (Fig 25–18,B).

The new prescription made use of the patient's previous oblique-toed in-depth shoes (Fig 25–18,C). The rocker sole was modified to provide a small amount of heel rock but considerably more rock on the toe. An extended steel shank was also added. The new triple-layer TCI had a mild toe filler added to maintain the position of the lesser toes. Supportive material was added

under the remaining first metatarsal so that it would bear some weight and therefore balance overall weight bearing on the foot. This also served to eliminate excessive plantar pressure on the second through fifth metatarsal heads, thereby minimizing the chances of future callusing and ulceration (Fig 25–18,D).

## Case 5: Transmetatarsal Amputation

This 37-year-old man with a 15-year history of insulin-dependent diabetes was a heavy user of alcohol and was otherwise noncompliant. He had twice frozen his insensate feet, resulting in bilateral transmetatarsal amputations (Fig 25–19,A). His plantar skin was in good condition.

The choice of prescription footwear was made easy by the patient's desire to return to work. High-top work shoes with added rocker soles controlled his remaining feet well. (A smaller size was used because of the lack of metatarsal heads.) A TCI made with a combination of medium and firm density materials served to protect and balance the remaining foot and provide the necessary toe filler (Fig 25–19,B).

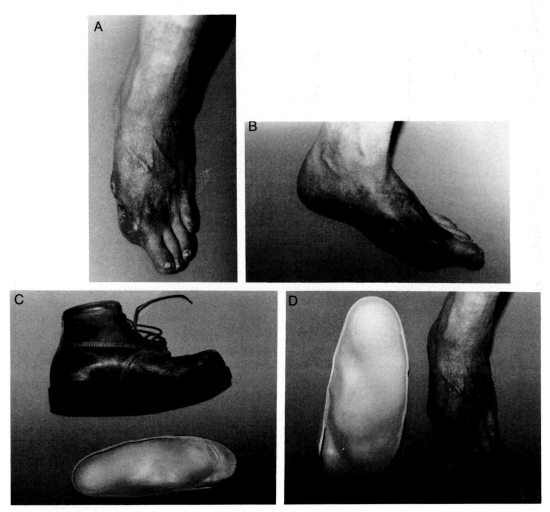

**FIG 25–18.**
Case 4. **A,** first ray amputation, dorsal view. **B,** medial view showing skin graft. **C,** oblique-toed in-depth boots with rocker sole; dorsal view of TCI. **D,** TCI with toe filler; dorsal view of foot.

### Case 6: Midtarsal Amputation

This 70-year-old man had a 25-year history of insulin-dependent diabetes. An infection occurred 2 years previously in his right foot, resulting in a midtarsal amputation (Fig 25–20,A). The original prescription after the amputation called for in-depth shoes (of the same size on both feet) and TCIs. The use of the same-size shoe on the amputated foot caused some gait problems and created the potential for breakdown in the distal portion of the stump.

The prescription was reevaluated, and the decision was made to use a custom-made shoe with a triple-layer TCI and a rocker sole (Fig 25–20,B). A custom-made sock was also fabricated for the amputated foot (Fig 25–20,C). Although the patient was initially concerned with the appearance of different-sized shoes, he was willing to give the shorter custom-made shoe a try. He found the comfort, protection, and ease of gait so much improved that acceptance came easily. He is now wearing his second pair.

### Case 7: Charcot Foot (Conventional Shoe)

A 66-year-old woman with a 20-year history of insulin-dependent diabetes had impaired sensation and a history of ulceration on the medial plantar aspects of her feet. She had bilateral medially collapsed Charcot foot deformities (Fig 25–21,A). The patient

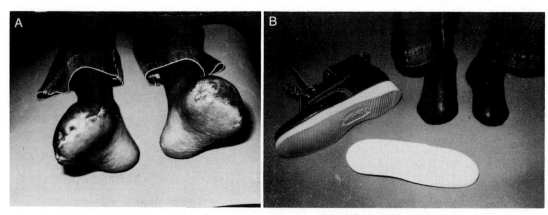

**FIG 25-19.**
Case 5. **A,** bilateral transmetatarsal amputations. **B,** high-top work shoe and TCI; dorsal view of amputated feet.

had been wearing standard cowhide in-depth shoes, which were hard to break in and caused callusing and discomfort until "deformed" enough to conform to the shape of her feet.

Her prescription included a triple-layer TCI (with a Plastazote shell) that molded well to the entire plantar surface of her foot; the TCI therefore had an increased midfoot width to accommodate her medially col-

lapsed midfoot. A viscoelastic polymer was added to the TCI under the bony promi-nences (Fig 25-21,B).

A thermal moldable shoe was used be-cause of its soft, accommodating upper, which was molded for some hammertoe de-formities also present. As shown in Figure 25-21,C, the sole of the shoe was cut length-wise (through both the outsole and insole) and split apart to accommodate her de-

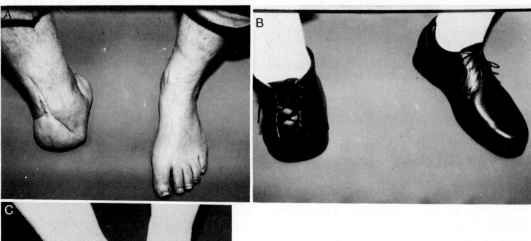

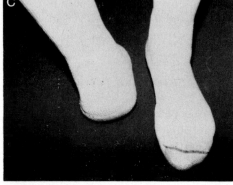

**FIG 25-20.**
Case 6. **A,** right midtarsal amputation. **B,** custom-made short shoe. **C,** custom-made short sock.

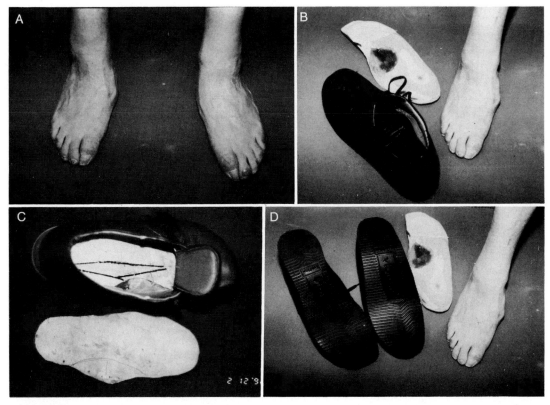

**FIG 25–21.**
Case 7. **A,** bilateral medially collapsed Charcot-foot deformities. **B,** plantar view of TCI showing addition of viscoelastic polymer. **C,** split-sole modification. **D,** plantar view of shoe before split sole modification *(left)* and after *(right).*

formed foot (i.e., making shoe shape match foot shape). Figure 25–21,D shows a plantar view of the patient's shoe both before and after the modification. A double rocker sole with an extended steel shank was also added.

This patient was extremely satisfied with the "split sole" modification, because her entire foot was contained within the shoe. Previously she had always felt that the medial aspect was either falling out of the shoe or off the side of the shoe.

### Case 8: Charcot Foot (Custom Shoe)

This 66-year-old man, 5 ft, 9 in. tall, weighing 280 lb, had had insulin-dependent diabetes for 18 years. He had a severely deformed left foot because of Charcot destruction. The foot was very large, with extremely prominent medial displacement and hallux varus (Fig 25–22,A and B).

In the past he had experienced plantar ulceration on the medial prominences. A plastic patella–tendon bearing (PTB) orthosis[28] had apparently contributed to the ulceration problem, because the foot was quite mobile and moved within the orthosis. The Charcot foot was stabilized with the use of total contact casting. The physician followed this with the use of a PTB orthosis attached to a shoe for 6 months. The brace was then removed, and the patient now needs only a custom-made shoe.

As the photographs illustrate, a conventional shoe would simply not be possible for this foot, even with extensive modifications. A custom-made shoe was therefore prescribed (Fig 25–22,C). It was able to accommodate the extensive deformities and was made with a padded collar because of the large size of the patient's legs. The TCI was extended quite high on the medial aspect of the foot for maximum protection. Velcro clo-

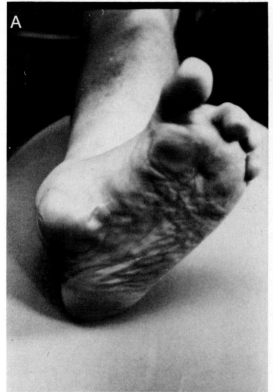

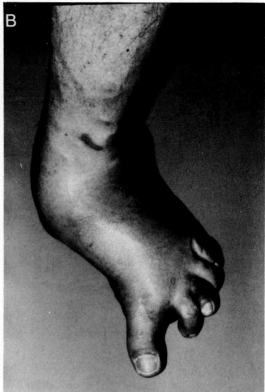

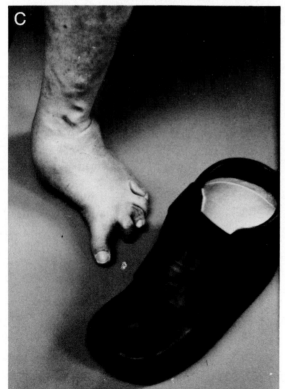

**FIG 25–22.**
Case 8. **A,** severe Charcot foot deformity with prominent medial displacement, plantar view. **B,** dorsal view showing hallux varus. **C,** high-top custom-made shoe with Velcro closures and padded collar. Notice medial extension of the TCI.

sures were added, because the patient cannot reach his feet to tie laces. The shoe was made as a high-top to offer added ankle support. This prescription has been highly successful for the past 3 years.

## SUMMARY

Current research in the care of the diabetic foot emphasizes (1) a team approach, (2) patient education, and (3) prevention. The certified pedorthist can make an important contribution in each of these areas. Whether on the staff of a diabetic foot clinic or in a private pedorthic practice, the pedorthist's specialized knowledge of prescription footwear for the diabetic foot and ability to provide properly fitting shoes, shoe modifications, and inserts make the pedorthist a valuable member of the treatment team. In addition, the pedorthist can educate patients not only in footwear but also in complete foot care. Foot and footwear inspections performed during follow-up visits and monitoring of prescription footwear effectiveness offer the opportunity for early detection and prevention of serious complications. Studies showing the importance of prescription footwear in preventing both ulcer recurrence and amputation point to its significance in the long-term management of the diabetic foot.[9, 10]

## Acknowledgment

I thank Susan Cronce for assistance in preparation of this chapter.

## REFERENCES

1. Board for Certification in Pedorthics: *Certification examination for pedorthics: candidate handbook*, Columbia, Md, 1990, Board for Certification in Pedorthics.
2. Boulton AJM: The diabetic foot, *Med Clin North Am* 72:1513–1530, 1988.
3. Boulton AJM, Franks CI, Betts RP, et al: Reduction of abnormal foot pressures in diabetic neuropathy using a new polymer insole material, *Diabetes Care* 7:42–46, 1984.
4. Brand PW: Repetitive stress in the development of diabetic foot ulcers, in Levin ME, O'Neal LW, editors: *The diabetic foot*, ed 4, St Louis, 1988, Mosby–Year Book.
5. Brodsky JW, Kourash S, Stills M, et al: Objective evaluation of insert material for diabetic and athletic footwear, *Foot Ankle* 9:111–116, 1988.
6. Cavanagh PR, Sanders LJ, Sims DS: The role of pressure distribution measurement in diabetic foot care, in *Rehabilitation R&D progress reports*, Baltimore, Md, 1987, Department of Medicine and Surgery, Veterans Administration.
7. Cavanagh PR, Ulbrecht JS: Plantar pressure in the diabetic foot, in Sammarco GJ, editor: *The foot in diabetes*, Philadelphia, 1991, Lea & Febiger.
8. Coleman WC: Footwear in a management program of injury prevention, in Levin ME, O'Neal LW, editors: *The diabetic foot*, ed 4, St Louis, 1988, Mosby-Year Book.
9. Edmonds ME, Blundell MP, Morris ME, et al: Improved survival of the diabetic foot: the role of a specialized foot clinic, *Q J Med* 60:763–771, 1986.
10. Edmonds ME, Watkins PJ: Management of the diabetic foot, in Dyck PJ, Thomas PK, Lambert EH, et al, editors: *Diabetic neuropathy*, Philadelphia, 1987, WB Saunders.
11. Frykberg RG: Podiatric problems in diabetes, in Kozak GP, Hoar CS Jr, Rowbotham JL, et al, editors: *Management of diabetic foot problems*, Philadelphia, 1984, WB Saunders.
12. Frykberg RG: Diabetic foot ulcerations, in Frykberg RG, editor: *The high risk foot in diabetes mellitus*, New York, 1991, Churchill Livingstone.
13. Gould N: Shoes and shoe modifications, in Jahss MH, editor: *Disorders of the foot and ankle*, ed 2, Philadelphia, 1991, WB Saunders.
14. Habershaw G, Donovan JC: Biomechanical considerations of the diabetic foot, in Kozak GP, Hoar CS Jr, Rowbotham JL, et al, editors: *Management of diabetic foot problems*, Philadelphia, 1984, WB Saunders.
15. Harkless LB, Dennis KJ: The role of the podiatrist, in Levin ME, O'Neal LW, editors: *The diabetic foot*, ed 4, St Louis, 1988, Mosby-Year Book.
16. Janisse DJ: A scientific approach to insole design for the diabetic foot. Paper presented at the 14th International Diabetes Federation Congress, Washington, DC, 1991. (Submitted to *Foot*.)
17. Janisse DJ: The art and science of fitting shoes, *Foot Ankle* 13:257–262, 1992.
18. Johnson JE: Prescription footwear. In Sammarco GJ, editor: *Foot and ankle manual*, Philadelphia, 1991, Lea & Febiger.
19. Johnson JE, Janisse DJ, Kaczmarowski J: Modern pedorthic and orthotic management of complications in the foot and ankle, in Johnson JE, Brennan MJ, Gould JS, editors: *Complications of foot*

*and ankle surgery*, Baltimore, Williams & Wilkins (in press).

20. Kuncir EJ, Wirta RW, Golbranson FL: Load-bearing characteristics of polyethylene foam: an examination of structural and compression properties, *J Rehabil Res Dev* 27:229–238, 1990.

21. Leber C, Evanski PM: A comparison of shoe insole materials in plantar pressure relief, *Prosthet Orthot Int* 10:135–138, 1986.

22. Levin ME: The diabetic foot: pathophysiology, evaluation, and treatment, in Levin ME, O'Neal LW, editors: *The diabetic foot*, ed 4, St Louis, 1988, Mosby-Year Book.

23. Prescription Footwear Association: *Physician's desk reference and directory of certified pedorthists and orthopedic shoe technicians*, Columbia, Md, 1991, Prescription Footwear Association.

24. Riegler HF: Orthotic devices for the foot, *Orthop Rev* 16:293–303, 1987.

25. Rossi WA, Tennant R: *Professional shoe fitting*, New York, 1984, National Shoe Retailers Association.

26. Sammarco GJ, Scioli MW: Examination of the foot and ankle, in Sammarco GJ, editor: *The foot in diabetes*, Philadelphia, 1991, Lea & Febiger.

27. Sammarco GJ, Stephens MM: Diabetic foot function, in Sammarco GJ, editor: *The foot in diabetes*, Philadelphia, 1991, Lea & Febiger.

28. Sanders LJ, Frykberg RG: Diabetic neuropathic osteoarthropathy: the Charcot foot, in Frykberg RG, editor: *The high risk foot in diabetes mellitus*, New York, 1991, Churchill Livingstone.

29. Schaff PS, Cavanagh PR: Shoes for the insensitive foot: the effect of a "rocker bottom" shoe modification on plantar pressure distribution, *Foot Ankle* 11:129–140, 1990.

30. Schoenhaus HD, Wernick E, Cohen RS: Biomechanics of the diabetic foot, in Frykberg RG, editor: *The high risk foot in diabetes mellitus*, New York, 1991, Churchill Livingstone.

31. Schwartz RS: Foot orthoses and materials, in Jahss MH, editor: *Disorders of the foot and ankle*, ed 2, Philadelphia, 1991, WB Saunders.

32. Sinacore DR: Total-contact casting in the treatment of diabetic neuropathic ulcers, in Levin ME, O'Neal LW, editors: *The diabetic foot*, ed 4, St Louis, 1988, Mosby-Year Book.

33. Stephens MM: Amputations below the knee, in Sammarco GJ, editor: *Foot and ankle manual*, Philadelphia, 1991, Lea & Febiger.

34. Thompson DE: The effects of mechanical stress on soft tissue, in Levin ME, O'Neal LW, editors: *The diabetic foot*, ed 4, St Louis, 1988, Mosby-Year Book.

35. Ullman BC, Brncick M: Orthotic and pedorthic management of the diabetic foot, in Sammarco GJ, editor: *The foot in diabetes*, Philadelphia, 1991, Lea & Febiger.

# CHAPTER 26

# Foot Care in Minorities: Preventing Amputations in High-Risk Populations

**Stephen Rith-Najarian, M.D.**

**Melvin Price, D.P.M.**

**Dorothy M. Gohdes, M.D.**

Minorities in the United States, including blacks, Hispanics, Asians, and American Indians, are a significant and increasing proportion of the total population. The prevalence of diabetes mellitus in minority populations increased during the latter half of this century and has now reached epidemic proportions.[21, 49, 54] Recent surveillance studies suggest that compared with the U.S. white population, minority diabetic populations are at equal, if not greater, risk for major complications, including lower limb amputations.[42, 46, 53] This disproportionate burden of lower limb amputations may result from both high rates of diabetes and high rates of risk factors for amputation among the minority diabetic patients compared with the U.S. white population.[20, 43] The combination of an increased prevalence of diabetes and increased rates of major complications has created a "double jeopardy" for minority peoples in terms of the impact of diabetes.[53] Reduction of the burden of diabetes and its complications among minorities represents a major challenge to health care providers. This challenge ranges from the organization of effective preventive foot care to the development of culturally appropriate patient education. This chapter reviews the epidemiology of diabetes and lower limb amputation in certain minority groups and discusses strategies for reducing this tragic outcome.

## DIABETES IN MINORITY POPULATIONS

Diabetes mellitus has reached epidemic proportions among indigenous peoples throughout the world.[31] The predisposition for a "thrifty" metabolic gene places these populations at particularly high risk for the development of obesity and its attendant non-insulin-dependent diabetes mellitus (NIDDM) when they are exposed to a modern Western life-style.[41, 53] In the United States, the Second National Health and Nutrition Examination Survey (NHANES II) found that the prevalence of diagnosed and undiagnosed diabetes was 1.45 times greater in the black population than in the total U.S. population during 1976 to 1980 (Table 26–1).[28] Among Mexican Americans and Puerto Ricans who participated in the His-

The opinions expressed in this chapter are those of the author and do not necessarily reflect the views of the Indian Health Service.

**TABLE 26–1.**

Prevalence of Diabetes Among Selected Populations Aged 20–74 Years in the United States*

|  | Age-Standardized Rates (%) |
|---|---|
| White | 6.2 |
| Cuban | 9.3 |
| Black | 10.2 |
| Mexican American | 13.0 |
| Puerto Rican | 13.4 |

*From Harris MI: Diabetes Care 14(suppl 3):639–648, 1991. Used by permission.*

panic Health and Nutrition Examination Survey in 1982 to 1984, the prevalence rate of diabetes was 1.66 to 2.74 times higher than the rate observed among all U.S. races in the NHANES II study.[15] The risk for diabetes in Cuban Americans in these studies was intermediate between those of their other Hispanic counterparts and those of all U.S. races.[15] American Indians also have high rates of diabetes. Among Pima Indians, more than one half of the adult population is affected by diabetes and rates have increased markedly in recent decades.[32] Other American Indian tribes show varying but also high rates.[50, 56] Although national data on the prevalence of diabetes among Americans of Asian extraction are lacking, the rate of diabetes among Japanese American men living in King County, Washington, during 1983 to 1985 was 2.2 times the rate for all U.S. races.[18]

The predominant form of diabetes in minority populations is NIDDM.[31] This form of diabetes, which is generally associated with advanced age in whites, can manifest at a relatively young age in minority populations, leading to major complications during their productive years.[32, 53] In an 8-year follow-up study in San Antonio, Texas, the mean age at onset of diabetes in Mexican Americans was significantly lower than in non-Hispanic whites (46 vs. 52 years).[23] Among the Pima Indians, the incidence rate of new cases of diabetes was actually lower in older groups than in the middle-aged groups in the tribe.[32] This tendency for early onset of NIDDM in minority populations, combined with the clinically silent initial course, may contribute to the high morbidity from the disease.

# AMPUTATIONS IN MINORITY DIABETIC POPULATIONS

## Risk Factors Ascertained From Epidemiologic Studies

### Biomedical Risk Factors

There are few published reports on the risk factors for lower limb amputation in minority populations. The well-known risk factors, such as neuropathy, peripheral vascular disease (PVD), duration of diabetes, male gender, and a prior history of ulceration or amputation, appear to be risk factors among both minority populations and whites.[6] However, the prevalence of specific risk factors for lower extremity amputation may vary among individuals in particular minority groups and the white population.

**Neuropathy.**—Although few studies of diabetic neuropathy in minority groups have comparable methodologies, the reported prevalence of clinically detected neuropathy in the different studies is significant. Among diabetic Mexican Americans, 28% had clinical findings of distal symmetric neuropathy.[25] Among diabetic Chippewa Indians, 20% lacked sensation to a 5.07 Semmes Weinstein monofilament.[47] Based on nerve conduction testing, 46% of diabetic Japanese American males had findings consistent with neuropathy.[17]

**Peripheral Vascular Disease.**—Peripheral vascular disease also appears to be common among minority diabetic populations. Diabetic Mexican Americans who participated in the San Antonio heart study[24] were 1.84 times more likely to have an ischemic index less than 0.95 compared with non-Hispanic white participants, although this difference was not statistically significant. In Seattle, Washington, 17% of Japanese males had an ankle arm Doppler ischemic index less than 0.95.[17]

Medial artery calcification was detected in the feet of 40% of diabetic Pima Indian men and 28% of women.[13] Diabetic patients with medial artery calcification had 5.5 times the rate of amputation compared with diabetic patients without calcifications.[13] Medial artery calcification probably indicates significant neuropathy because impaired vibratory sensation was associated with an increased risk of medial artery calcification in this minority population.[13]

**Smoking.**—The contribution of tobacco use to the risk for lower limb amputation in minority populations is undoubtedly significant in some groups and may be associated with vascular and neuropathic changes.[8, 38] In the general U.S. population, smoking is only slightly more prevalent among adult blacks than among whites (32% vs. 28%).[19] However, among diabetic males, a history of current smoking among blacks is twice that of whites (55% vs. 27%).[16] In the Hispanic population, current tobacco use is reported as lower (24%) than the rate in U.S. whites and blacks.[19] Among Mexican Americans in San Antonio, overall smoking rates were the same as those of non-Hispanic whites, but Mexican Americans smoked fewer cigarettes.[24] American Indians nationwide reported current rates of tobacco use as 32%.[34] However, intertribal variations are enormous; for example, only 0.6% of Pima Indians compared with 32% of urban American Indians in Minnesota reported smoking at least one pack per day.[13, 20]

**Metabolic Control.**—There is a paucity of data on overall metabolic control in U.S. diabetic minority populations. Among newly diagnosed patients identified in health and nutrition surveys in the United States, no significant difference in mean fasting blood glucose levels was noted among Mexican Americans, Cubans, Puerto Ricans, whites, and blacks.[27] However, although mean glycohemoglobin values were similar among diabetic Mexican Americans and non-Hispanic whites residing in the San Luis Valley of Colorado, Mexican American diabetic individuals living in San Antonio had significantly higher mean fasting blood glucose concentrations than their non-Hispanic-white counterparts.[24, 25]

**Summary Studies.**—Detailed studies outlining the relative roles of various risk factors for lower limb amputation are lacking for most minority populations in the United States. However, risk factors have been examined in two American Indian populations. In a 12-year review[42] of first amputations among Pima Indians, amputation rates increased with increasing duration of diabetes. Pima men came to amputation more frequently than women. Significant risk factors for amputation among the Pima Indians included absent patellar tendon reflexes, impaired great toe vibratory perception threshold, presence of medial artery calcification, elevated fasting or 2-hour blood glucose levels, and the presence of nephropathy or retinopathy. Age was not a significant risk factor for amputation in this study when rates were adjusted for duration of diabetes. Among Chippewa Indians, a previous plantar ulceration or amputation indicated the highest risk for a subsequent amputation when patients were followed prospectively for 3 years.[47] Published studies suggest there may be variation in the major risk factors among minority populations. Although a retrospective review[43] of 104 black patients with diabetic gangrene associated the presence of hypertension with progression to above-knee and bilateral amputation, neither the presence of hypertension nor elevated serum cholesterol level was associated with amputation in Pima Indians, and systolic hypertension was not significantly associated with peripheral vascular disease in Mexican Americans.[24, 42] Studies of risk factors for ulceration and amputations among specific minority groups are needed to provide focus for prevention programs.

## Sociodemographic Risk Factors and Health Care Access

Socioeconomic status appears to have a variable influence on the prevalence of specific risk factors for amputation, but data on the role of socioeconomic status are lacking. Smoking prevalence is inversely related to socioeconomic status in both the general and diabetic populations.[16, 19] Although diabetic Mexican Americans living in low-income barrios were not at increased risk for either poor metabolic control or diabetic retinopathy compared with Mexican Americans who lived in the more affluent suburbs, barrio dwellers were less likely to be aware of their diabetic treatment regimens than their suburban counterparts.[22, 55] Lack of awareness could be a barrier to the regular practice of a preventive foot care regimen. Low income is a factor that can severely restrict access to professional health care. A study by Harris[26] reported that blacks with diabetes had 40% fewer visits to primary care providers than white diabetic patients. Lack of the special services needed by diabetic patients may compound the problem of access. A review[44] of urban health care facilities serving predominantly low-income black and Hispanic populations showed that only 9% of diabetic patients were followed in diabetes clinics, and only 60% of diabetic individuals seen by primary care providers on five or more occasions in 1 year had documentation of a foot examination.

### Amputation Rates

Although national data on the incidence of lower limb amputation for minority populations are limited, the findings of state and local amputation surveillance indicate that minority patients with diabetes are undoubtably at greater risk for amputation than diabetic patients in the United States as a whole (Table 26–2). Findings based on New Jersey hospital discharge rates for the diagnosis of diabetes and lower limb amputation between 1979 and 1981 showed that nonwhites had 1.4 times the rate of amputation in whites.[37] A similar methodology applied to national hospital discharge data showed the annual amputation rate for black diabetic patients ranged between 9 and 12 per 1,000 during 1985 to 1987, a rate 1.5 times greater than the rate for all U.S. races.[9] The age-specific hospital discharge rates for amputation among blacks in South Carolina in 1978 were higher than the rates for whites, particularly among the age group 65 years or more whose rate of 15 per 1,000 in blacks was more than twice the rate in whites (see Table 26–2). [39] The rates for first amputation for Pima Indians in the Southwest and Chippewa Indians in the Great Lakes region were 10.4 and 16 per 1,000 diabetic person-years, respectively.[42, 48] Estimated rates from hospital discharge data for all races in six states were 6.0 per 1,000 diabetic patients.

## PREVENTION STRATEGIES

### Patient Education

Patient education is fundamental to a program to decrease amputation in diabetic

**TABLE 26–2.**

Incidence of Lower Limb Amputation Among Diabetic Patients From Selected Ethnic Populations of the United States

|  | Incidence Amputation/1,000 Diabetic Patients | Comments |
|---|---|---|
| All U.S. races | 5.97 | Hospital discharge rates for LLA* and diabetes from six states, 1978[9] |
|  | 8.2 | Hospital discharge rates for LLA and diabetes from all states, 1980–1987[39] |
| Black | 9.0–12.5 | Hospital discharge rates for LLA and diabetes from all states, 1980–1987[39] |
|  | 2.2–15.0 | Hospital discharge rates for LLA and diabetes from South Carolina, 1978[9] |
| American Indians |  |  |
| Pima | 10.4 | First amputation, 1972–1984[42] |
| Chippewa | 26 | Any amputation, 1986–1988[48] |

*LLA = Lower limb amputation.*

patients. Informed patients can prevent or recognize very early the minor trauma that can initiate the cascade of events leading to amputation.[45] A 1-hour education session for high-risk patients followed in a Veterans Affairs hospital resulted in a subsequent decrease in major amputations compared with a control group followed in the same setting who did not receive the education.[35] However, for education to be effective, the teaching techniques must match the learning skills of the patients. This is particularly critical for patients with diabetes. In South Carolina a small study[36] demonstrated that one half of the participants in a diabetes education program could not fully understand educational materials at a fifth grade level. The National Health Interview Survey[40] showed that 50% of known diabetic patients aged 45 to 64 years in the United States had completed less than 12 years of school compared with 35% of the general population. The educational attainment of minority individuals as a whole was lowest among elderly blacks and Hispanics, who are of the age group likely to have diabetes.[57]

The techniques for developing appropriate educational interventions for low-literacy learners are well described and can be easily implemented.[10] In many cases, rewriting complex materials in simpler sentences that avoid three-syllable words results in a clearer message. Validation of text and illustrations by patients from the clinic where the materials will be used can provide invaluable input, and encouraging patients to ask questions can identify misunderstandings or a lack of clarity in a lesson.[30] Audiotapes and carefully structured videotapes can convey messages to people who cannot read English. Family members can play a critical and supportive role in a patient's self-care, and they should be involved in all self-care education. The importance of conveying the information to diabetic patients in a culturally and educationally appropriate way cannot be overemphasized. Simply handing out brochures without assessing the relevance, acceptability, and comprehensibility for minority patients does not constitute patient education and will not enable individual diabetic patients to recognize the importance of proper foot care and effectively perform the recommended practices.

## Podiatric and Footwear Issues

Among the issues surrounding podiatric and pedorthic interventions in minority populations, limited access to podiatric and pedorthic services because of financial and geographic barriers is a matter of special concern. A study[44] of urban clinics serving a predominantly black and Hispanic population found that less than 3% of diabetic patients had been referred for podiatry services. This referral rate contrasts strongly with the rate of 37% of patients referred to a podiatrist from an urban university referral center.[5] Podiatry services in rural areas in some regions of the United States may be very limited. Removal of such geographic and access barriers to adequate care will require extensive public health intervention. In the meantime, primary care providers in minority settings may need to expand the scope of the services they currently offer to meet the minimal diabetic foot care needs of the clientele they serve. These services include a careful physical assessment of the feet, footwear evaluation, and basic nail and callous care.

A critical period in the management of all podiatric interventions is the healing phase of a surgical or ulcerative wound. During the healing period, patients are typically faced with reduced mobility and function as they try to maintain a non−weight bearing status. The support an individual receives from his or her family or community is influenced by family dynamics and varies widely among various ethnic groups. A home assessment of the social support by a visiting public health nurse may enhance postoperative and wound care through family involvement. Many local public health agencies may also be able to assist by provision of direct services in the home.

The cost of prescriptive footwear can be prohibitive. Patients and providers faced with limited resources for footwear should consider lower cost alternatives when appropriate, such as running shoes, padded hosiery, or inserts, to modify existing footwear.[52, 58] These interventions can reduce plantar pressures and, in turn, protect the high-risk foot from incurring untoward events. Social services can sometimes help patients to obtain what they need when apprised of the importance of the protective footwear.

## Organization and Delivery of Foot Care

Minority populations are concentrated in urban centers or isolated rural areas where access to primary care providers who are experienced in the management of diabetes is problematic.[44] Moreover, minorities are typically underrepresented in the health care professions, and the services that are offered may not be culturally sensitive to a particular minority group.[4] Improvement of foot care and reduction of amputations in minority populations requires attention to both the systems of health care that serve minority communities and to the care offered to individual patients. This section focuses on public health strategies directed at improving delivery of diabetic foot care services in minority community settings.

Many facilities located in minority settings may care for a relatively large number of people with both diagnosed and undiagnosed diabetes. Health care delivery issues to be addressed by clinics in these settings include the following:

1. Identifying patients with diabetes who use the facility.
2. Recalling patients with diabetes for routine and preventive services.
3. Identifying patients with diabetes who are at high risk for amputation.
4. Providing special preventive services in a coordinated manner that is convenient for the patients.

The task of identifying patients with diabetes may be facilitated by developing a list of known diabetic patients who are followed by the clinic. This list is known as a "registry." Simple methods of identifying diagnosed cases by reviewing clinic billing codes are possible as computer-based billing increases.[44] For clinics serving small populations, a chart review for the diagnosis of diabetes may accomplish the same purpose. Systematic diabetes screening of high-risk adults may aid in the identification of new or undiagnosed cases,[3] who should then be added to the registry.

To ensure patient recall, the clinic or office staff can add a "date of next visit field" to the registry in a computer or tickler file system. Periodic review of this "field" can serve as a prompt to mail appointment reminder cards to patients for foot care or any other required services at the appropriate interval. Having public health nurses follow up on patients who miss appointments may help to identify unrecognized barriers to care and also facilitate appropriate medical referral.

When a registry has been compiled, efforts can be directed at stratifying the individuals into risk groups, so that resources can be efficiently directed toward providing intensive prevention services to those at highest risk. Guidelines for identifying high-risk patients for amputation have been published by the American Diabetes Association Council on Foot Care.[2] Diabetic individuals at high risk include those with the following:

1. Signs or symptoms of peripheral neuropathy (sensory, motor, or autonomic).
2. Signs or symptoms of PVD.
3. Presence of abnormal gait or shoewear.
4. Foot deformity.
5. Prior ulceration or amputation.
6. Poor understanding of diabetes or the need to follow self-care practices.

Providers are advised to follow high-risk patients more frequently, with additional examinations as clinically indicated. Conversely, low-risk individuals, those without demonstrable risk factors, can be followed with a complete foot examination and foot care instruction on an annual basis.[2]

A number of recent studies have focused on the use of the Semmes-Weinstein monofilaments as a simple and inexpensive clinical tool to identify high-risk patients with neuropathy. Several retrospective reviews have demonstrated that individuals who lack sensation to the 5.07 monofilament (approxi-

| DIABETIC FOOT SCREEN | Date: |
|---|---|
| Patient's Name (Last, First, Middle)_____ | ID No.: |

Fill in the following blanks with an "R", "L", or "B" to indicate positive findings on the right, left or both feet.

Has there been a change in the foot since last evaluation?   Yes_____   No_____

Is there a foot ulcer now or history of foot ulcer?   Yes_____   No_____

Does the foot have an abnormal shape?   Yes_____   No_____

Is there weakness in the ankle or foot?   Yes_____   No_____

Are the nails thick, too long or ingrown?   Yes_____   No_____

Label:  Sensory Level with a "+" in the circled areas of the foot if the patient can feel the 10 gram (5.07 Semmes-Weinstein) nylon filament and "-" if he/she can not feel the 10 gram filament.

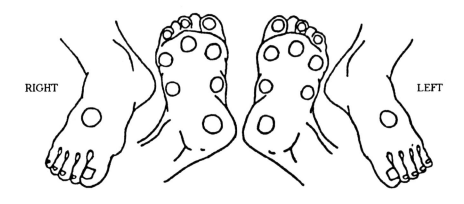

Draw in:   Callus ▨   Pre-Ulcer ▦   Ulcer ■   (note width/depth in cm.)

and Label:   Skin condition with R - Redness, S - Swelling, W - Warmth, D - Dryness, M - Maceration

Vascular:   Brachial Systolic Pressure   R_____  L_____
            Ankle Systolic Pressure      R_____  L_____
            Ischemic Index               R_____  L_____

Does the patient use footware appropriate for his/her category?   Yes_____   No_____

---

**RISK CATEGORY:**
_____ 0  No loss of protective sensation.
_____ 1  Loss of protective sensation (no weakness, deformity, callus, pre-ulcer or Hx. ulceration.
_____ 2  Loss of protective sensation with weakness, deformity, pre-ulcer or callus but no Hx. ulceration;
          or Ischemic Index < 0.45.
_____ 3  History of plantar ulceration.

---

Developed by the National Foot Treatment Center

**FIG 26–1.**
Foot screening format to categorize risk for ulceration, amputaion, or both. *(From Duffy JC, Patout CA: Milit Med 1990; 155:575. Used by permission.)*

mately 10 g linear pressure) are at higher risk for a history of plantar ulceration than those who retain sensation.[7, 29, 51] This simple method may be more sensitive in predicting risk than bioesthesiometry, a more expensive quantitative method.[33] Simple risk categorizations have been developed to stratify patients into four risk groups based on a history and clinical examination (Fig 26–1). The absence of sensation to a 5.07 Semmes-Weinstein monofilament, the presence of foot deformity, an ischemic index, and a history of plantar ulceration are easy to ascertain.[11] A recent prospective study[47] in 358 Chippewa Indians to evaluate the effectiveness of a risk categorization scheme found 74% of the patients were in the low-risk category, whereas only 8%, 5%, and 13% were in progressively higher risk groups. In terms of predicting patients at risk for complications, the study showed that more than 90% of ulcerations and all amputations occurred in the higher risk groups in the prospective 3-year follow-up period. Risk categorization schemes help providers in minority clinic settings to identify who among the many people with diabetes that they serve are at highest risk for ulceration and amputation. Scarce resources can then be directed efficiently toward high-risk individuals to prevent end-stage lower limb events.

Diabetic foot care, with diabetic care in general, is a complex task for both providers and patients with diabetes. Coordination of services to provide care in a logical and convenient manner to all patients is critical. At Kings College Hospital in London,[12] for example, the amputation rate among diabetic patients was reduced by one half after the implementation of a multidisciplinary high-risk foot clinic. In a study[14] of rural primary care clinics in southern Sweden, a significant reduction in amputations was observed in a community served by a clinic with a diabetes team compared with other communities served by clinics with conventional care. In primary care clinics serving rural American Indian communities, significant improvement in diabetes care practices was associated with organization of diabetes teams who had received education in diabetes care and who used defined standards of care.[1] Similar organizational practices have been associated with increased frequency of foot examinations in an urban diabetes clinic in New York.[5] The establishment of a diabetes team with coordinated delivery of care may be a logical first step toward improving the quality of diabetic foot care for clinics serving large diabetic populations.

## SUMMARY

The improvement of foot care and prevention of amputations for minority diabetic patients represents a major challenge to clinical providers and public health agencies serving minority peoples in the United States. Efforts to identify and track high-risk patients, reduce modifiable risk factors, provide culturally specific patient education, and improve access to foot care services all are needed. In many locations, resources to address many of these issues already exist, whereas in others, training and the development of programs and materials are needed. The complexity of these tasks at the clinic level may be facilitated by multidisciplinary team efforts. Public health agencies can interface with team efforts through coordinated referrals on home care. Nationwide and regional surveillance of amputation rates in minority populations will provide a window to monitor the effectiveness of combined intervention programs.

## REFERENCES

1. Acton K, et al: Improving diabetes care for American Indians [abstract], *Diabetes* 38(suppl 2):170A, 1989.

2. American Diabetes Association: *Diabetic foot care*, Alexandria, Va, 1990, American Diabetes Association.

3. American Diabetes Association: Screening for diabetes, *Diabetes Care* 14(suppl 2):7–9, 1991.

4. Anderson R, et al: Barriers to improving diabetes care to blacks, *Diabetes Care* 14:605–609, 1991.

5. Bailey T, Yu A, Rayfield E: Patterns of foot examination in a diabetes clinic, *Am J Med* 78:371–374, 1985.

6. Bild D, et al: Lower-extremity amputation in people with diabetes, epidemiology and prevention, *Diabetes Care* 12:24–31, 1989.

7. Birke JA, Sims DS: Plantar sensory threshold in the ulcerative foot, *Lepr Rev* 57:261–267, 1986.

8. Delbridge L, Appleberg M, Reeve T: Factors associated with development of foot lesions in the diabetic, *Surgery* 93:78–82, 1983.

9. Division of Diabetes Translation: *Diabetes Surveillance, 1980-87*, Atlanta, April 1990, Centers for Disease Control.

10. Doak CC, Doak LG, Root JH: *Teaching patients with low literacy skills*, Philadelphia, 1985, JB Lippincott.

11. Duffy JC, Patout CA: Management of the insensitive foot in diabetes: lessons learned from Hansen's disease, *Military Med* 12:575–579, 1990.

12. Edmonds ME, et al: Improved survival of the diabetic foot: the role of a specialized foot clinic, *Q J Med* 232:763–771, 1986.

13. Everhart JE, et al: Medial arterial calcification and its association with mortality and complications of diabetes, *Diabetologia* 31:16–23, 1988.

14. Falkenberg M: Metabolic control and amputations among diabetics in primary health care—a population-based intensified programme governed by patient education, *Scand J Primary Health Care* 8:25–29, 1990.

15. Flegal KM, et al: Prevalence of diabetes in Mexican Americans, Cubans, and Puerto Ricans from the Hispanic health and nutrition examination survey 1982–84, *Diabetes Care* 14(suppl 3):628–638, 1991.

16. Ford ES, Newman J: Smoking and diabetes mellitus: findings from 1988 behavioral risk factor surveillance system, *Diabetes Care* 14:871–874, 1991.

17. Fujimoto W, et al: Prevalence of complications among second-generation Japanese-American males with diabetes, impaired glucose tolerance, or normal glucose tolerance, *Diabetes* 36:730–739, 1987.

18. Fujimoto W, et al: Prevalence of diabetes mellitus and impaired glucose tolerance among second generation Japanese-American men, *Diabetes* 36:721–729, 1987.

19. Giebel HN, Mills S, Marcus S: Differences in the age of smoking initiation between blacks and whites—United States, *MMWR* 40:754–757, 1991.

20. Gillum F, Gillum BS, Smith N: Cardiovascular risk factors among urban American Indians: blood pressure, serum lipids, smoking, diabetes, health knowledge, and behavior, *Am Heart J* 70:765–777, 1984.

21. Gohdes D: Diabetes in American Indians, *Diabetes Care* 9:609–613, 1986.

22. Haffner SM, et al: Effect of socioeconomic status on hyperglycemia and retinopathy levels in Mexican Americans with NIDDM, *Diabetes Care* 12:128–134, 1989.

23. Haffner SM, et al: Increased incidence of type II diabetes mellitus in Mexican Americans, *Diabetes Care* 14:102–108, 1991.

24. Haffner SM, et al: Macrovascular complications in Mexican Americans with type II diabetes, *Diabetes Care* 14(suppl 3):665–671, 1991.

25. Hamman RF, et al: Microvascular complications of NIDDM in Hispanics and non-Hispanic whites, *Diabetes Care* 14(suppl 3):655–664, 1992.

26. Harris MI: Non-insulin dependent diabetes mellitus in black and white Americans, *Diabetes Metab Rev* 6:71–90, 1990.

27. Harris MI: Epidemiological correlates of NIDDM in Hispanics, whites, and blacks in the US population, *Diabetes Care* 14(suppl 3):639–648, 1991.

28. Harris MI, et al: Prevalence of diabetes and impaired glucose tolerance and plasma glucose levels in the U.S. populations aged 20–74 yr, *Diabetes* 36:523–534, 1987.

29. Holewski JJ, et al: Aesthesiometry: quantification of cutaneous pressure sensation in diabetic peripheral neuropathy, *J Rehabil Res Dev* 25:1–10, 1988.

30. Hosey GM, et al: Designing and evaluating diabetes education materials for American Indians, *Diabetes Educator* 16:407–414, 1990.

31. Jarrett RJ: Epidemiology and public health aspects of non-insulin-dependent diabetes mellitus, *Epidemiol Rev* 11:151–171, 1989.

32. Knowler WC, et al: Diabetes mellitus in the Pima Indians: incidence, risk factors and pathogenesis, *Diabetes Metab Rev* 6:1–27, 1990.

33. Kumar S, et al: Semmes-Weinstein monofilaments: a simple, effective and inexpensive screening device for identifying diabetic patients at risk of foot ulceration, *Diabetes Res Clin Pract* 13:63–68, 1991.

34. Lefkowitz D, Underwood C: *Findings from the survey of American Indians and Alaska Natives national medical expenditure survey*, research findings 10, Agency for Health Care Policy and Research, Rockville, AHCPR Publication no 91-0034, 1991.

35. Malone JM, et al: Prevention of amputation by diabetic education, *Am J Surg* 158:520–524, 1989.

36. McNeal B, et al: Comprehension assessment of diabetes education program participants, *Diabetes Care* 7:232–235, 1984.

37. Miller A, et al: Diabetes-related lower extremity amputations in New Jersey, 1979–1981, *J Med Soc NJ* 82:723–726, 1985.

38. Mitchell BD, Hawthorne VM, Vinik AI: Cigarette smoking and neuropathy in diabetic patients, *Diabetes Care* 13:434–437, 1990.

39. Most RS, Sinnock P: The epidemiology of lower extremity amputations in diabetic individuals, *Diabetes Care* 6:87–91, 1983.

40. National Center for Health Statistics: *Prevalence,*

*impact and demography of known diabetes in the United States*, Advance data from Vital and Health statistics, no 114, DHHS Publication no (PHS) 86-1250, Hyattsville, Md, 1986, Public Health Service.

41. Neel JV: Diabetes mellitus: a "thrifty" genotype rendered detrimental by "progress"? *Am J Hum Genet* 14:353–362, 1962.

42. Nelson RG, et al: Lower-extremity amputations in non-insulin dependent diabetes mellitus: a 12-year followup study in Pima Indians, *Diabetes Care* 11:8–16, 1988.

43. Ogbuawa O, Williams J, Henry L: Diabetic gangrene in black patients. *South Med J* 75:285–288, 1982.

44. Payne TH, et al: Preventive care in diabetes mellitus: current practice in urban health care systems, *Diabetes Care* 12:745–747, 1989.

45. Pecoraro RE, Reiber GE, Burgess EM: Pathways to diabetic limb amputation: basis for prevention, *Diabetes Care* 13:513–521, 1990.

46. Rate RG, et al: Diabetes mellitus in Hopi and Navajo Indians, *Diabetes* 32:894–899, 1983.

47. Rith-Najarian S, et al: Identifying diabetic patients at high risk for lower extremity amputation in a primary care setting: a prospective evaluation of simple screening criteria. *Diabetes Care* 15:1386–1389, 1992.

48. Rith-Najarian S, et al: Diabetes in a northern Minnesota Chippewa tribe: prevalence and incidence of diabetes, and incidence of major complications, *Diabetes Care* (in press).

49. Roseman JM: Diabetes in black Americans, in *Di-abetes in America*, NIH Publication no 85-1468, 1985, US Department of Health and Human Services.

50. Sievers ML, Fisher JR: Diabetes in North American Indians, in *Diabetes in America*, NIH Publication no 85-1468, 1985, US Department of Health and Human Services.

51. Sosenko JM, et al: Comparison of quantitative sensory threshold measures for their association with foot ulceration in diabetic patients, *Diabetes Care* 13:1057–1061, 1990.

52. Soulier M: The use of running shoes in the prevention of plantar diabetic ulcers, *J Am Podiatr Assoc* 76:395–400, 1986.

53. Stern MP, Haffner S: Type II diabetes and its complications in Mexican Americans, *Diabetes Metab Rev* 6:29–45, 1990.

54. Stern MP: Diabetes in Hispanic Americans, Diabetes in America, NIH Publication no 85-1468, 1985, US Department of Health and Human Services.

55. Stern MP, et al: Lack of awareness and treatment of hyperlipidemia in type II diabetes in a community survey, *JAMA* 262:360–364, 1989.

56. Sugarman JR, Gilbert TJ, Weiss NS: Prevalence of diabetes and impaired glucose tolerance among Navajo Indians, *Diabetes Care* 15:114–120, 1992.

57. US Bureau of the Census: *Statistical abstract of the United States: 1991*, ed 111, Washington, DC, 1991, US Bureau of the Census.

58. Veves A, et al: Use of experimental padded hosiery to reduce abnormal foot pressures in diabetic neuropathy, *Diabetes Care* 12:653–655, 1989.

# CHAPTER 27

# Diabetic Foot Clinic

M. Edmonds, M.D.

Althea V.M. Foster, D.Pod.M., M.Ch.S.

## INTEGRATED APPROACH

No single individual can handle every aspect of the prevention and treatment of diabetic foot problems. It is by combining the skills of podiatrist, diabetologist, orthotist, nurse, and surgeon in a team approach that the morbidity associated with diabetic feet can be reduced.[4] Since 1981, diabetic foot problems have been treated within a special Diabetic Foot Clinic at King's College Hospital, London, and this chapter is based on the work of this clinic. The crucial feature is a podiatrist and diabetologist working closely together to receive, diagnose, treat, and follow up in patients with diabetic foot problems. They are assisted by an orthotist who supplies insoles and shoes and by a nurse who also acts as technician to the clinic and carries out neurologic and vascular investigations. Patients with severe sepsis or ischemia who need admission are seen in joint consultation with a surgeon. The clinic has its own receptionist, who coordinates the work of the team and arranges emergency and routine appointments.

## ORIGIN AND DEVELOPMENT OF CLINIC

To understand better the working of this clinic, we describe its origins and development, because such information may be pertinent to hospitals trying to establish a foot clinic.

It is important to realize that all the members of the multidisciplinary team were present in the hospital when the foot clinic was set up. However, they were seeing patients at separate times, and it was difficult to coordinate a plan of care and apportion overall responsibility.

The foot clinic was born out of the desire of the podiatrist and diabetologist to work more closely together on a regular basis to both treat diabetic patients with active ulcers and provide long-term follow-up. Joint consultation and treatment seemed more efficient.

There was a need for a focal point that would be the base for regular treatment, as well as for the assessment and investigation of the diabetic foot. It would act as the administrative center for diabetic foot care to house patients foot notes and collate results of investigations, including microbiology and radiology reports. Diabetic patients also needed to identify a specific forum that was committed to the care of their feet and that would be easily accessible to them for urgent consultations and regular outpatient treatment. Furthermore, it would be a setting where they would be seen by all members of the team at one visit, and this would reduce frequent attendances at the hospital, which could be expensive on both their resources and time.

There was no funding for a specific new clinic, but the podiatrist agreed to allow it to take place in the podiatry clinic initially on one morning each week when the podiatrist would normally have been treating these patients. The diabetologist and nurse would usually have been seeing these patients in the diabetic clinic at this proposed time and thus were able to transfer to the diabetic foot clinic.

The orthotist was also treating diabetic patients in his own office in the hospital at this time. It seemed sensible to invite the orthotist to a joint consultation to formulate a single view about the type of insole and shoe needed for a particular foot and also to be able to monitor long term the value of both insole and shoe. Thus the orthotist was invited to the newly formed diabetic foot clinic. The surgeon was also conducting his own clinic at this time and offered to be available for consultation if there were difficulties in diagnosis or if a patient needed admission. However, it was not necessary for the surgeon to be in constant attendance.

Within the first few weeks of the clinic's existence, high-quality relationships that had developed in part before the clinic existed were consolidated between the various members of the team. The foot clinic became an active, successful focus of care for the diabetic foot, with its members continually learning from each other, supporting and trusting each other with openness and honesty, and there was no unhealthy competition or territorial boundaries. The members believed that their working together accomplished more than they could alone and achieved an involvement that was exciting, satisfactory, and enjoyable, and amputations quickly fell.

Initially foot investigations were carried out in the podiatry room, but in 1983 a further room was constructed adjacent to the podiatry room out of funds from the British Diabetic Association to develop an investigation room for the diabetic foot clinic. It also allowed space for the orthotist to carry out initial measurements on the patient within the diabetic foot clinic. Previously he had seen patients in the podiatry clinic and agreed a plan of insoles and footwear but had to take the patients back to his office to carry out this plan. In the investigation room, the orthotist had a grinder, convection oven, and facilities for taking plaster casts of the shape of the foot, with access to a sink with a plaster trap.

## AIMS AND PURPOSES

The aims of the diabetic foot clinic are as follows:

1. To diagnose the specific lesions of the diabetic foot by means of a full clinical assessment, which can be divided into two parts: a medical history and examination, followed by a structured foot examination.

2. To treat the lesions of the foot rapidly and appropriately with a combined approach by podiatrist, diabetologist, and orthotist.

3. To provide regular and close follow-up of all lesions of the foot and within this follow-up to provide an emergency service to receive patients without appointment if they are concerned that their lesion has deteriorated or a new lesion has formed.

4. To prevent the redevelopment of foot problems in the patient who has recently healed. The aim is to prevent recurrence and for the rest of the population to identify and educate those at high risk to prevent foot lesions from developing.

## DIAGNOSIS

### Neuropathic and Neuroischemic Foot

The diabetic foot can show two distinct types of problems: (1) those where neuropathy dominates, the neuropathic foot, and (2) those where occlusive vascular disease is the main factor (although neuropathy may also be present to a variable degree), the neuroischemic foot.[3] It is essential to differentiate between these two entities because their complications are different, and they require separate therapeutic strategies in the foot clinic.

Neuropathy results in a warm dry usually painless foot in which the pulses are palpable. It leads to three main complications: the neuropathic ulcer, the neuropathic (Charcot) joint, and neuropathic edema. In contrast, the ischemic foot has absent pulses and may be cold but not necessarily so, because there is often a coexistent autonomic neuropathy that causes vasodilatation of the skin capillaries in the ischemic foot. It is complicated by rest pain, ulceration from localized pressure necrosis, and gangrene. These two different entities, the neuropathic foot and the neuroischemic foot, and their complications must be thoroughly evaluated.

## Complications of Neuropathic Foot

### *Neuropathic Ulcer*

The neuropathic ulcer characteristically occurs at sites of high mechanical pressure on the plantar surface of the foot. The presence of neuropathy (even in its earliest stage, with relatively mild sensory defects) may itself disturb the posture of the foot and so predispose to local increases in pressure, which are also commonly caused by deformities such as claw or hammer toes, pes cavus, Charcot joints, and previous ray amputations. The situation is exacerbated by wearing tight, ill-fitting shoes, especially in the presence of edema. The high vertical and shear forces under the plantar surface of the metatarsal heads lead to the formation of callosities, of which the patient is often unaware. Repetitive mechanical forces lead to inflammatory autolysis and subkeratotic hematomas, which eventually break through to the skin surface, forming an ulcer. Occasionally frictional forces lead to bullae for-

mation, particularly over the dorsal surfaces of the toes (Fig 27–1).

### *Neuropathic (Charcot) Arthropathy*

The precipitating event is often surprisingly minor trauma, such as tripping, which results in a swollen, erythematous, hot, and sometimes painful foot. Initial radiologic examination is usually normal, but subsequent films show evidence of fracture, osteolysis, and fragmentation of bone, followed by new bone formation and, finally, subluxation and disorganization of the joint. Bone scans are more sensitive indicators of new bone formation than radiography and should be used to confirm the diagnosis. This destructive process often takes place over only a few months.

In its fully developed form, it manifests with considerable deformity and swelling; bony damage in the metatarsotarsal region leads to two classical deformities, the rocker bottom deformity, in which there is displacement and subluxation of the tarsus downward, and the medial convexity, which results from displacement of the talonavicular joint from tarsometatarsal dislocation. If these deformities are not accommodated in properly fitting footwear, ulceration at vulnerable pressure points often develops (see Chapter 7).

Early diagnosis is essential and is suggested by three features: (1) a history of trauma, often minor; (2) the presence of unilateral warmth and swelling, and (3) positive radiographic or bone scan findings.

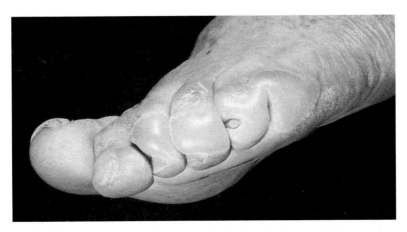

**FIG 27–1.**
Bullae over the third, fourth, and fifth toes from the frictional forces of a tight ill-fitting shoe.

## Neuropathic Edema

Neuropathic edema is fluid accumulation in the feet and lower legs, which is associated with severe peripheral neuropathy and is not explicable by other causes such as cardiac failure or hypoalbuminemia. It is extremely uncommon. Its pathogenesis may be related to abnormal vasomotor function after autonomic denervation, causing arteriovenous shunting and disturbances in hydrostatic pressure in the microcirculation.

## Complications of Neuroischemic Foot

The clinical features of ischemia are intermittent claudication, rest pain, ulceration, and gangrene. The ulcers manifest as areas of necrosis often surrounded by a rim of erythema. The most frequent sites of ulceration are the great toe, medial surface of the head of the first metatarsal, and the lateral surface of the fifth metatarsal.

## ORGANIZATION

### Space

The foot clinic consists essentially of three rooms on the ground floor of King's College Hospital. The first room, known as the podiatry room, consists of three podiatry chairs, each in a separate cubicle together with a small office area that houses the receptionist's desk, wall cupboards to store stationery, and filing cabinets to hold the patients' notes. The clinic phone is situated in the reception area and is a direct line into the clinic. All patients are given this telephone number and are encouraged to call if they are concerned about the progress of their feet. The room also contains all of the podiatry equipment and foot dressings, which are described in detail later on. The second room is known as the investigation room and contains three cubicles, each fitted with a conventional examination couch where vascular and neurologic examinations are carried out. It also contains two desks at which patient consultations can be carried out by the diabetologist or nurse. This room stores the Doppler stethoscope, Biothesiometer, and a digital skin thermometer. Part of

this investigation room is committed to the orthotist and contains the convection oven and grinder. The third room is a waiting room, which is adjacent to the podiatry room, from which patients can easily be observed, particularly for hypoglycemic episodes. This room also contains many wall-fitting cupboards to store excess podiatry materials. Free spaces on the wall are used for foot education posters, and education pamphlets are on show and readily available.

### Equipment

#### Podiatry Room

The basic equipment for the podiatrist includes disposable scalpel blades, scalpels, fine tooth forceps, nail clippers, nail drill, gloves, plastic aprons, clinical drapes, antiseptic agents, moisturizing cream, dressings, tape, and bandages. Dressings include simple nonstick dressings, dressings with a foam backing to use on weight-bearing areas, and cavity dressings for large ulcers. It is safe to use tape directly on the skin in the neuropathic foot, but it is avoided in the neuroischemic foot where bandaging is used to apply dressings. The podiatry room also contains an autoclave so that freshly sterilized instruments are used for each patient. A supply of wound swabs and transport medium are also kept in this room.

Total contact casting is also carried out in the podiatry room, and thus plaster and synthetic casting materials, cotton and other padding materials and bandages, together with a plaster saw, are available (see Chapter 13).

#### Investigation Room

1. Hand-held Doppler stethoscope.
2. Biothesiometer (Biomedical Instrument Company, Newbury, Ohio) to measure vibration threshold (Fig 27–2).
3. Nylon monofilament to a thickness of 5.07 to assess protective pain sensation (Physical Therapy Department, Hansen's Disease Foundation, Inc., Carville, La).
4. Digital skin thermometer (Hale Instru-

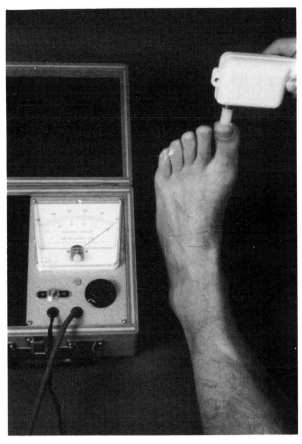

**FIG 27–2.**
Measurement of the vibration threshold at the hallux using the Biothesiometer.

ments, Ltd., Hale Barns, Cheshire, U.K.).

5. A pedobarogram (also housed in the investigation room but used for research projects).

Thus, only simple equipment is needed for the routine investigation of the diabetic foot. As mentioned previously, equipment for the orthotist, namely, convection oven, grinder, and plaster of paris, is also kept in stock.

## Access

The diabetic foot clinic is situated on the ground floor of King's College Hospital and can be approached through wide corridors providing easy access for patients, including those in wheelchairs. Patients use various forms of transport, including their own transport, public transport, and hospital ambulance. Transport by ambulance is arranged by the receptionist, who maintains a good liaison with the hospital ambulance control center to facilitate this service, which is invaluable for the elderly, frail ischemic patients.

At the inception of the diabetic foot clinic, patients were seen on a Thursday morning only, but since then, the clinic has grown steadily. At present there are two main diabetic foot clinics per week that patients with active foot ulceration attend. The main clinic takes place on Thursdays throughout morning and afternoon, and there is a further clinic throughout Monday. The nurse is in attendance on Monday and Thursday to cover these clinics and to provide a service for vascular and neurologic assessment. The orthotist attends the Thursday clinic on a weekly basis.

Podiatry clinics are held throughout the rest of the week. It was originally intended that these clinics should treat follow-up patients and high-risk diabetic patients but not those with active ulceration. However, it has been difficult to contain patients with active ulceration to the Monday and Thursday clinics because of increased number of referrals, and these patients are also seen on other days of the week in joint consultation with the podiatrist and diabetologist.

Patients in full-time occupation are offered preferential appointments either early morning or late afternoon to avoid missing excessive time off work.

Throughout the week, patients who have urgent foot problems are seen as emergencies, in addition to patients with standard appointments.

At weekends and evenings, patients with urgent foot problems are asked to go to the emergency room and are seen by a member of the diabetic service who can coordinate care in communication with the diabetologist and podiatrist, both of whom will come back to the hospital to treat these patients.

## PERSONNEL

### Role of Podiatrist[5]

The podiatrist fulfills several important roles:

1. To carry out routine care of the neuropathic foot, including debridement of callus.

2. To perform debridement of the neuropathic ulcer. The callus that surrounds an ulcer needs regular removal by the podiatrist to promote reepithelialization from the edge of the ulcer.

3. To apply the total contact cast. This is the most useful treatment for large indolent ulcers and is an effective way of keeping pressure off a plantar lesion while still enabling the patient to walk freely (Fig 27–3).[2] This technique is effective as long as the cast is applied with great care and the patient returns early if problems arise (see Chapter 13).

4. To take care of the healed neuropathic ulcer. The site of a recently healed neuropathic ulcer will continue to form callus very rapidly for several weeks and needs regular removal by the podiatrist.

5. To carry out after care of digital or ray amputations in the neuropathic foot. Large quantities of callus form around the edges of these wounds, and healing will be delayed if they are allowed to accumulate.

6. To carry out after care of skin grafts. Skin grafts on the plantar surface of the foot develop heavy hyperkeratosis that will break down if neglected. However, regular podiatry reduces callus and hyperkeratosis on grafts and will promote their survival.

7. To perform routine care of the neuroischemic foot. Nails are cut straight across; thickened nails should be carefully and gently reduced with scalpel or nail drill. Any defects in the skin, no matter how small, should be carefully cleansed and dressed, avoiding the use of tape directly on the skin. The diabetic foot clinic is an ideal forum in which the podiatrists can work in dealing with the neuroischemic foot, because constant assessment of the degree of ischemia in conjunction with the diabetologist and vascular surgeon is always needed.

8. To treat ulceration in the neuroischemic foot. Ischemic ulcers are debrided by the podiatrist and sloughy tissue gently cut away without damage to viable tissue. They are not usually surrounded by callus but are associated with accumulations of slough that are gently cut away without damage being caused to viable tissue.

9. To facilitate autoamputation of necrotic toes. In the ischemic foot it is often unwise to amputate toes, especially if the foot cannot be revascularized. Thus, a process of autoamputation is allowed. Debris and dried exudate and necrotic material are regularly pared away from the demarcation line by the podiatrist to facilitate this process.

10. To play an important part in the emergency service in conjunction with the diabetologist (see later discussion).

11. To educate the patients and their carers (see later discussion).

12. To advise on footwear. Podiatrists can advise patients that for everyday footwear, they should choose a shoe that fastens high on the foot with lace or strap, has an adequate toe box, and is sufficiently long, broad, and deep (see Chapter 23).

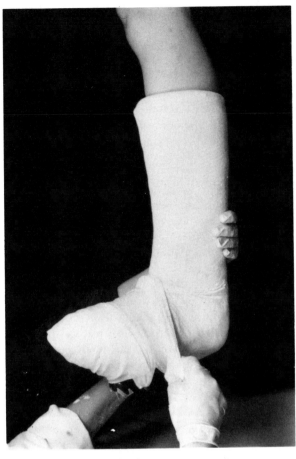

**FIG 27–3.**
Application of total contact plaster cast. Patient is being covered with stockinette to protect other leg.

## Role of Diabetologist

1. To perform an initial assessment of patient with full medical history and examination, including a foot examination.

2. To diagnose the diabetic foot syndromes, particularly the neuropathic and neuroischemic foot, and to examine the foot for deformities, edema, lesions, and signs of sepsis.

3. To diagnose the complications of the neuropathic foot and in cases of severe sepsis to arrange emergency admission and to start initial treatment with intravenous (IV) antibiotics and IV insulin, and to liaise with the orthopedic surgeons regarding operative drainage and local amputation.

4. To assess the degree of ischemia in the neuroischemic foot and to diagnose its complications.

5. To form a plan of treatment for ulceration in the neuroischemic limb. If it is not limb threatening, conservative treatment is employed. However, in cases of acute sepsis, it is necessary to arrange emergency admission, IV antibiotics, and IV insulin and to discuss management with the vascular surgeon. When there is worsening ischemia, admission is arranged for urgent angiography.

6. To take part actively in the intensive follow-up service and to assess progress of all lesions, if necessary by assessing area from tracings on sterile film or by photography. If progress is not apparent, to reexamine the foot and plan appropriate adjustments to treatment.

7. To be responsible for all aspects of the management of sepsis in the diabetic foot, particularly early diagnosis, follow-up of the results of swabs, and the prescription of antibiotics.

8. To diagnose the causes of edema in the diabetic foot and to prescribe appropriate treatment.

9. To achieve a wide experience in the manifestation and management of foot lesions such that the presence of surgeon in the actual diabetic foot clinic is rarely required on a regular basis, except to confirm the need for surgical intervention.

10. To take responsibility for all diabetic patients admitted from the foot clinic and to ensure continuity of care while the patient is on the ward in conjunction with the orthopedic and vascular surgeons.

11. To take part in the education program.

12. To be available to see and treat emergencies in conjunction with the podiatrist.

13. To make sure the patient is in good metabolic control.

## Role of Orthotist

1. To redistribute weight-bearing forces by special footwear. The orthotist supplies three main groups of shoes. Extradepth stock shoes are made in standard sizes but have an extra allowance in the depth dimension. They are fitted with sponge rubber insoles that can function as a cushion appliance or that can be replaced by purpose-made insoles of foot cradles. These shoes are available immediately from the orthotist and are suitable for patients with a history of ulceration but no great deformity. The second category is bespoke shoes for the deformed foot. The orthotist takes a plaster cast of the shape of the foot, and from this insoles or cradles, as well as the shoe itself, are fashioned. Often a rigid weight-distributing cradle is needed to relieve weight from high-pressure areas and to transfer it to other less vulnerable areas. The third category is temporary shoes made of felt or polythene foam. They are often supplied immediately to the patient while the bespoke shoes are constructed.

2. To follow up patients to check for patient acceptance of shoe and insole and to assess when new insoles and shoes are required.

3. To adjust shoes and insoles if new lesions develop.

4. To provide boots and special supporting braces to stabilize the ankle in the case of a Charcot joint.

Although the orthotist's formal visit is once weekly, it is possible to call him throughout the week particularly to supply temporary shoes when patients present as emergencies (see Chapters 24 and 25).

## Role of Nurse

Throughout the existence of the foot clinic, the nurse has had varying roles, partly depending on the interests of the individual nurse, although there has been a constant emphasis on education. In the early years, when there was one podiatrist only, the nurse assisted with foot dressings and education of the patients. When the number of podiatrists increased to two, the dressings were carried out by the podiatrists themselves after treatment of the foot ulcer. At present, the nurse manages the investigation room of the foot clinic, carries out neurologic and vascular investigations, and also assists in the education of the patients.

Community nurses are welcome to visit the clinic and discuss their patients because this maintains an important line of communication with the community.

## Role of Surgeon

It is not necessary for the surgeon to attend the diabetic foot clinic regularly, but to be available for consultation regarding difficult diagnoses or advanced foot problems that need to be treated in hospital. Thus it is desirable for the surgeon to be in the outpatient area at the time of the foot clinic and to visit the clinic when necessary.

The main reasons for calling the surgeon are as follows:

1. To confirm the need for removal of infected bone in cases of chronic indolent ulceration with osteomyelitis.
2. To discuss cases of severe sepsis and soft tissue destruction that need surgical debridement and possible local amputation.

3. In the case of the ischemic foot, to discuss with the vascular surgeon severe limb-threatening ischemia, including complicating sepsis; to organize an inpatient treatment plan for treatment and investigation, including urgent angiography.

## Other Personnel

Although they are not actually present in the clinic, it is important to mention other members of the wider diabetic foot team. They include interventional radiologists responsible for angioplasty, microbiologists who advise on antibiotic therapy, and dermatologists who in joint consultation give valuable advise about general skin problems as they affect the feet (e.g., psoriasis and vasculitic rashes), as well as advise on discrete lesions not typical of the diabetic foot (e.g., possible melanomas).

## PATIENT

### Source of Patient

The diabetic foot clinic takes referrals from many sources. The majority of patients come from the hospital diabetic clinic or are referred by local primary physicians who run their own diabetic clinics. Referrals are also accepted from other health care professionals, including physiotherapists, orthotists, and community nurses and podiatrists. The clinic also takes self-referrals of diabetic patients, although patients are encouraged to obtain an initial referral letter from their primary physician. Every effort is made to nurture close and friendly liaison with the primary physician, because he or she is often asked to prescribe oral antibiotics between foot clinic visits and to supply dressing materials.

### Presenting Lesions and Deformities

During the first 3 years of the foot clinic, 239 diabetic patients with foot ulceration were treated. There were 148 patients who were designated as neuropathic in that they had evidence of a peripheral neuropathy but

the foot pulses were palpable. There were 91 patients who were designated neuroischemic, again with peripheral neuropathy but also absent foot pulses.

## Ulcers

### Neuropathic Group

A total of 238 ulcers were treated. This comprised 169 ulcers as initial presentations to the clinic and 69 relapses after healing had been achieved in the original lesions. Apart from ulcers caused by direct mechanical or thermal injuries and 2 that appeared as spontaneous blisters, the ulcers in the neuropathic group were surrounded by callus tissue (i.e., areas of hyperkeratosis). In 64 out of 238 instances the ulcer was not obvious on examination but was recognized by an area of hemorrhage under thick callus. When the callus was removed, the floor of the ulcer was revealed. Thirty-nine of the ulcers (in 36 patients) were complicated by cellulitis, with erythema and edema of the ulcerated foot, and 28 patients complained of pain. Pain was not a feature of the uncomplicated ulcer in this group.

### Neuroischemic Group

A total of 148 ulcers were treated, consisting of 110 original presentations and 38 relapses. The majority of ulcers (139/148) manifested as areas of necrosis that were painful in 119 cases and had progressed to digital gangrene in 20. Callus was noted in only nine ulcers (in three patients). Seventy-three patients complained of pain and were taking analgesics; these included 23 patients in whom the ulcers were complicated by cellulitis.

## Site of Ulceration

### Neuropathic Group

One hundred sixty-one (67%) ulcers were on the toes. Seventy-one (30%) ulcers were situated on the hallux, and 90 (37%) ulcers were found on the remaining toes. There were 4 interdigital ulcers, 15 on the heel, and 58 on the metatarsal region, including 3 on the medial surface of the first metatarsal head, 4 on the lateral surface of the fifth metatarsal head, 48 on the plantar surface of the metatarsal heads, and 3 ulcers that developed on the dorsum of the foot.

### Neuroischemic Group

Eighty-eight (59%) ulcers were found on the toes. Forty-three were on the hallux, and 45 were on the remaining toes. There were 7 interdigital ulcers, 30 ulcers in the metatarsal region (14 on the lateral surface of the fifth metatarsal head, 12 on the medial side of the first metatarsal head, and 4 on the plantar aspect of the first metatarsal head), and 23 on the heel.

### Precipitating and Predisposing Factors
(Table 27-1)

Tight, ill-fitting shoes were the most frequent precipitating factor of ulceration. In neuropathic feet, these shoes lead to high pressures on the toes, resulting in hyperkeratosis, callus formation, and eventually ulceration. These were slip-on shoes with no laces and an inadequate toe box. In the ischemic foot, localized pressure from tight shoes results in direct epithelial damage and tissue necrosis, leading to ulceration in a different distribution from the neuropathic feet.

An important predisposing factor in both groups of patients was peripheral edema, which was associated with congestive cardiac failure in 40 cases, persistent proteinuria in 11, and neuropathic edema in 1 patient.[6]

### Clinical Assessment

#### First Visit

Initially the new patient is seen by the podiatrist and diabetologist in joint consultation in the investigation room. A medical history and examination are carried out, followed by an assessment of the neurologic and vascular status by the nurse or technician; finally, a full foot assessment is undertaken. When Charcot's arthropathy is suspected, skin temperature is also measured using the digital skin thermometer.

**Vascular Status.**—Vascular status is assessed by palpation of pulses and measurement of Doppler ankle-brachial systolic pressure index (see Chapter 15).

**Neurologic Status.**—Neurologic status is assessed by detecting sensation to pinprick, cotton wool, and vibration using a 128 cycles/sec tuning fork starting at the distal foot and moving proximally to confirm a symmetric stocking distribution of peripheral neuropathy. Knee and ankle jerks should be examined; their absence is proof of peripheral neuropathy, although knee jerks are retained until surprisingly late. It is difficult to examine the autonomic nerves

**TABLE 27-1.**

Precipitating and Predisposing Factors of Ulceration in Neuropathic and Neuroischemic Feet

|  | Ulcers in Neuropathic Feet (n = 238) | Ulcers in Neuroischemic Feet (n = 148) |
|---|---|---|
| Precipitating factors |  |  |
| Narrow shoes | 101 | 80 |
| Mechanical injuries | 7 | 12 |
| Thermal injuries | 4 | 0 |
| Bed sores (to heel) | 1 | 5 |
| Predisposing factors |  |  |
| Pedal edema | 20 | 32 |
| Claw toes | 19 | 18 |
| Pes cavus | 15 | 8 |
| Hallux valgus | 12 | 18 |
| Hallux rigidus | 11 | 1 |
| Hammer toes | 11 | 2 |
| Charcot deformity | 11 | 0 |
| Previous ray amputation | 13 | 2 |

except to note a dry skin with marked fissuring as indicative of a sweating autonomic deficit.

Having diagnosed a neuropathy, one must ascertain whether the patient has lost protective pain sensation that should render him or her susceptible to foot ulceration.

Two clinical investigations are useful: vibrometry and nylon filaments. Vibration threshold can be measured using a hand-held Biothesiometer (see Fig 27–2). The vibration threshold increases with age, and values must always be compared with age-adjusted nomograms.

Nylon monofilaments test the threshold to pressure sensation. There are various diameters, but the crucial filament is a nylon probe calibrated to a thickness of 5.07. Other thicknesses are available but not essential. The filament is applied to the foot until it buckles when the patient is able to detect its presence. Buckling of the 5.07 monofilament occurs at 10 g of linear pressure and is the limit used to detect protective sensations. If the patient does not detect the filament, protective pain sensation is lost (see Chapters 2 and 6).[1]

**Joint Consultation.**— At this stage, podiatrist, diabetologist, and technician converse to classify the diabetic foot into the neuropathic and neuroischemic entity and to diagnose its specific lesions. The *neuropathic foot* would involve callosities, ulceration, sepsis, digital necrosis, fissures, bullae, Charcot's joint, and edema. The *neuroischemic foot* would involve rest pain, ulceration, sepsis, digital necrosis, fissures, bullae, and edema.

The orthotist is invited to assess the patient, and in consultation with the diabetologist and podiatrist, a management plan is devised. It falls into three parts, namely, podiatric, orthotic, and medical treatment.

The patient then goes into the podiatry room and receives specific local treatment for the lesions of the foot. Callus is removed by the podiatrist using a no. E 11 scalpel blade. This may prevent the development of underlying ulceration, but until the callus has been removed, it is impossible to know whether the epithelium is intact below it.

Danger signs are small red or brown speckles within plaques of callus, which are tiny bleeding points where individual capillaries have been damaged by high plantar pressures that are leaking blood. Removal of callus may reveal ulceration and, indeed, sepsis (Fig 27–4).

During the course of treatment, the podiatrist initiates the education process, stressing the principles of foot care, which is backed up by written instructions available from the receptionist.

A culture specimen is properly obtained from all ulcers, stored in transport medium, and quickly sent to the microbiology laboratory (see Chapter 8 regarding techniques for taking cultures).

During this treatment, at which both podiatrist and diabetologist are present, a decision is made whether to perform radiographs of the foot, indications for which are as follows:

1. Deep indolent neuropathic ulcers to assess underlying bony involvement.
2. Cases of severe sepsis to assess the presence of gas in the soft tissues.
3. When there is a history of a possible foreign body in the foot.
4. To assess the hot, swollen erythematous foot with no obvious tissue breakdown for the possibility of early Charcot's bony abnormalities.

On return from the radiology department, the patient comes into the investigation room to see the orthotist, who then takes a plaster cast of the feet. The cast is sent to the workshop for construction of insoles and shoes.

Finally, the diabetologist checks on the patient's metabolic status and prescribes antibiotics if indicated for foot sepsis. If peripheral edema has been noted, a cause must be found, and this will entail an investigation of renal and hepatic function, initially by the measurement of blood urea and electrolyte and liver enzyme levels. Treatment of edema may necessitate diuretics and/or elevation of the foot. Compression stockings may be necessary but should not be used on the ischemic leg.

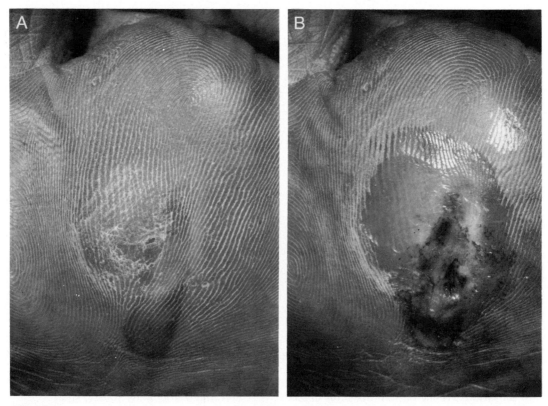

**FIG 27–4.**
**A,** callus over second metatarsal head showing discoloration and underlying hemorrhage. **B,** callus is removed to reveal ulceration.

If the patient has an acute lesion needing admission, the diabetologist arranges this. When there is severe cellulitis and sepsis, urgent admission is arranged in joint consultation with the orthopedic surgeon. When an ischemic foot has deteriorated either from sepsis or increasing ischemia, urgent admission is arranged after joint consultation with the vascular surgeon. In actual practice, the diabetologist and podiatrist can quickly reach a decision about the need for admission if the surgeon is not available, and in this case the surgeon will often review the patient on the ward after admission to the hospital.

If the patient is to be treated as an outpatient, he or she leaves the clinic with a follow-up appointment, and arrangements for transportation at this appointment are made. If the patient is frail or elderly, hospital transport is arranged for this visit.

Finally, the patient leaves with written instructions regarding foot care and care of the ulcer (see later discussion).

### Subsequent Visits

**Continuing Treatment.**—One of the most important functions of the diabetic foot clinic is to provide intensive follow-up of foot lesions with regular treatment and assessment of progress. At each visit, the ulcer is debrided by the podiatrist, and antibiotics are prescribed by the diabetologist until the ulcer has healed. Careful inquiry is made regarding possible side effects, and, if necessary, alternative antibiotics are substituted. The acceptability and value of footwear are also assessed at each visit.

**Assessment of Progress.**—Various techniques can be used to assess progress, including tracing of areas onto sterile transparent film and measuring the maximum diameter of the lesion. In the former, the area of the lesion can be measured from the tracing by counting squares when superimposed on graph paper, and the first measurement is defined as unity and subsequent areas expressed as a percentage. Percentage areas are plotted against time and the rate of healing assessed. Alternatively, photography is very useful. Polaroid photography is used to document large ulcers and to monitor their progress for the reassurance of both clinic staff and patients, photographs usually being taken at 2 weekly intervals. Standard color photography is used mainly to demonstrate specific features of the diabetic foot and their response to treatment for instructional purposes in the education of health care professionals. A 35-mm manual camera with a no. 105 macrolens and a flashlight unit is employed. Standard magnifications are used, for example, 1:2 for the hallux, to enable photographs to be standardized, especially when the same patient is photographed over a period of time (Fig 27–5). It is invaluable to have the assistance of the hospital medical photography department with regard to standard color slides and prints.

**Follow-up of Foot Lesions.**— If progress is not satisfactory, the cause should be determined and treated. If healing is not proceeding satisfactorily in an ischemic foot, sepsis may not be controlled, or, alternatively, ischemia may be worsening. The ankle-brachial pressure index should be repeated, and if this confirms deterioration in vascular supply and the ulcer is limb threatening, arteriography is indicated. If healing is not satisfactory in a neuropathic ulcer, there may be several reasons. There may be underlying osteomyelitis: surgery may be needed and antibiotics changed. Edema may have developed and may need treatment. The patient's footwear may need to be adjusted. The frequency of visits is determined by the severity of the lesion. However, on average, patients with ulcers are seen weekly during the initial phase of treatment.

The foot clinic also provides a suitable forum for follow-up of postoperative patients. It is useful for the foot care team to visit inpatients so that a plan for outpatient management can be discussed before discharge. Wound sites of toe and ray amputations need repeated careful debridement with pro-

tection of high-pressure areas by footwear and prevention of sepsis with antibiotics. Furthermore, the podiatrist can manufacture a toe prosthesis made of silicone rubber to fill the gap left by the missing toe and prevent displacement of adjoining toes (Fig 27–6). Plantar skin grafts also need careful follow-up, because they develop keratosis that breaks down if callus is not removed. A recent study at King's has shown that 10 out of 11 split-thickness skin grafts on neuropathic ulcers were still intact 1 year after operation.[8]

Furthermore, the foot clinic has become a forum to follow up ischemic patients who have had angioplasty or vascular reconstruction. Even after revascularization of the foot, ulcers still require regular podiatric treatment, and the pressure index needs measurement at 1, 6, and 12 weeks and then at 6-month intervals to detect restenosis or graft blockage at an early stage.

### Emergency Cover

An important part of the follow-up is to encourage patients to come to the clinic on an emergency basis if they are concerned that their lesion has deteriorated or a new lesion has formed. In a similar fashion, new patient referrals from podiatrists, physicians, and nurses are seen very quickly. The diabetic foot clinic at King's has an emergency service run by the podiatrist and the diabetologist where patients can be seen without an appointment as soon as they note a problem. In the first year, 107 patients were seen as emergencies. Eighty-three percent of these had skin lesions, 14% had acute nail and joint lesions, and 3% had rest pain. Treatment of 86 of these patients was conducted entirely in the foot clinic and had a 90% healing rate. Twenty-one patients with rampant sepsis were admitted without delay to achieve a 86% healing rate.

## PREVENTION

The ultimate treatment is prevention. In the patient who has recently healed, the aim is to prevent recurrence, and for the rest of the population the aim is to identify and ed-

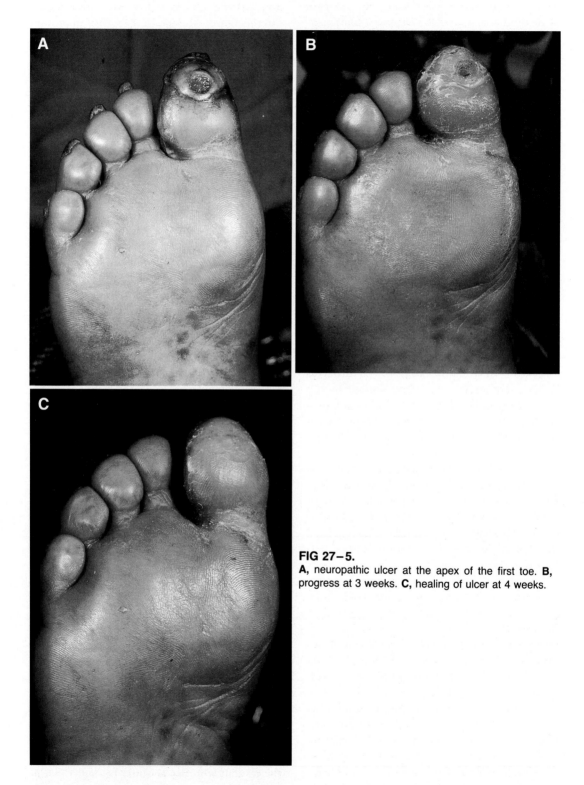

**FIG 27-5.**
**A,** neuropathic ulcer at the apex of the first toe. **B,** progress at 3 weeks. **C,** healing of ulcer at 4 weeks.

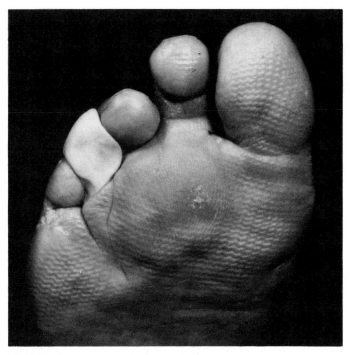

**FIG 27–6.**
Silicone prosthesis to replace amputated fourth toe.

ucate those at high risk to prevent foot le-sions developing.

## Screening

Screening technique is based on the foot examination described earlier, searching for the main risk factors, namely, neuropathy, ischemia, deformity, and edema. High-risk patients then receive routine podiatry in the foot clinic, as well as education in foot care, in which regular examination of the feet by the patient and caretakers is stressed.

## Education

The foot clinic has an important role not only in education of the patient but also in that of the health care professionals in-volved in foot care, including nurses, podia-trists, orthotists, and physicians. All pa-tients attending the clinic are instructed in basic foot care (see Fig 27–7), and further advice is given about danger signs and care of the patient's ulcer (Table 27–2). The spo-ken word should be backed up by written advice (see Chapter 2).

**TABLE 27–2.**

Danger Signs and Care of the Ulcer

Danger signs
  Check your feet every morning.
  Come to the clinic immediately if you notice:
    Swelling.
    Color change of a nail, toe, or part of a foot.
    Pain or throbbing.
    Thick hard skin or corns.
    Breaks in the skin, including cracks, blisters, or
      sores.
Care of the ulcer
  The aim of this clinic is to heal your foot ulcer as
    quickly as possible. To achieve this, we need
    your help. Please read these instructions and
    follow them carefully:
  Ulcers should have a fresh dressing applied
    every day.
  Rest as much as possible.
  If you think your ulcer is deteriorating, come to
    the clinic immediately. If the ulcer gets larger
    or begins to weep, the foot swells or becomes
    red, or any new ulcers develop, we need to
    see you at once.
  Ulcers need regular care in the clinic. If for any
    reason you have to miss an appointment,
    make another without delay.
  If you are given antibiotics, do not let them run
    out. Call the clinic if they cause any problems.

## KING'S COLLEGE HOSPITAL — DIABETIC DEPARTMENT

# CARE OF YOUR FEET

To help prevent complications:—

## DO

wash daily with soap and water.
dry well, especially between toes.
change socks/stockings daily.
see that your shoes are not too tight.
see a Chiropodist.

## DON'T

walk barefoot.
sit too close to a fire or radiator.
put your feet on hot water bottles.
neglect even slight injuries — see your Doctor.
attempt your own chiropody — see your Chiropodist.

**FIG 27–7.**
Education card of basic foot care.

### RESULTS

It is vital that there is close liaison between podiatrist, diabetologist, orthotist, nurse, and surgeon in the care of the diabetic foot, and the diabetic foot clinic is the optimal forum for this approach. The essence is continuous team care by podiatrist and diabetologist, with specific assistance from orthotist, nurse, and surgeon.

### Healing Accomplished

The foot clinic has achieved a high ulcer healing rate, and this has resulted in a reduction of major and minor amputations. Over a 3-year period in the neuropathic group of patients, 204 out of 238 (86%) ulcers were healed. Seventy-seven (32%) were healed within 4 weeks and 138 (58%) within 10 weeks; mean healing time was 10.3 ± 10.2 weeks (mean ± standard deviation). Ninety percent (161/178) of ulcers that had

been present for less than 4 weeks before the patient was seen were healed. Six of 12 ulcers that had been present for more than 50 weeks were not healed because of underlying osteomyelitis and septic arthritis. Forty ulcers were treated in hospital. Nine healed with conservative treatment, 9 healed after surgical drainage of pus, and 18 patients underwent drainage of pus and distal metatarsal amputations.

In the ischemic group (91 patients), healing was achieved in 107 out of 148 (72%) ulcers, and healing time was 14.0 ± 11.4 weeks. Nineteen ulcers (13%) were healed within 4 weeks and 54 (36%) within 10 weeks.

### Follow-up in Healed Foot

After initial healing, 121 patients in the neuropathic group were followed up in the foot clinic. Twenty-two out of the 86 (26% patients) wearing special shoes sustained further ulceration compared with 29 out of 35 (83% of patients) who developed ulceration while continuing to wear their own shoes against advice. Fifty of the neuropathic patients were in full-time employment when they developed ulceration. Forty of these were able to continue at their work throughout treatment. In the ischemic group, 52 (25%) who were wearing special shoes relapsed compared with 15 out of 18 (83%) who continued to wear their own shoes.

## Reduction in Amputations

The effect of the foot clinic on the number of major amputations and minor operations (which comprise drainage operations and ray amputation) was assessed by comparing the number of such procedures in both neuropathic and ischemic patients from the diabetic clinic for 2 years before the establishment of the foot clinic to those performed for 3 years after. In the 2 years before the clinic, there were 11 and 12 major amputations each year. This was reduced in the 3 years after this establishment to seven, seven, and five amputations, respectively. Similarly, the number of minor amputations was also reduced from 27 and 29 yearly before the clinic to 16, 21, and 15 per year after its establishment.

Several factors explain the reduction of amputations:

1. The foot clinic has facilitated optimum treatment of ulcers in both the neuropathic and neuroischemic foot by a combined approach from podiatrist, diabetologist, and orthotist.

2. Prompt diagnosis and treatment of infection have been important goals with very close liaison with the microbiology laboratory. Meticulous monitoring of ulcers with repeated wound cultures has facilitated this. Prophylactic long-term antibiotic treatment has also been used to prevent recurrence of sepsis.

3. The emergency service allows rapid access to the clinic, rapid diagnosis, rapid investigation, including angiography in ischemic patients, and rapid treatment, often before lesions become limb threatening. If the limb is threatened, rapid admission is arranged. It is necessary to throw everything at a small problem at an early stage to prevent it from becoming a big problem.

4. The foot clinic provides intensive follow-up of lesions, and this has been important in achieving high healing rates.

5. The foot clinic has provided a focus of care, interest, and responsibility for the diabetic foot that was difficult to achieve when its management continuously shifted between different disciplines. The foot clinic has taken over full responsibility for the outcome of the diabetic foot.

The reduction in amputation rate has been maintained throughout the last 10 years. Indeed, similar multidisciplinary clinics set up in the 1980s have achieved similar results.[7]

## REFERENCES

1. Birke JA, Sims DS: Plantar sensory threshold in the ulcerative foot, *Lepr Rev* 57:261–267, 1986.
2. Brand PW: The diabetic foot, in Ellenberg M, Rifkin H, editors: *Diabetes mellitus*, New York, 1983, Medical Examination Publishing, pp 829–849.
3. Edmonds ME: The diabetic foot: pathophysiology and treatment, *Clin Endocrinol Metab* 1986; 15:889–916.
4. Edmonds ME, Blundell MP, Morris HE et al: Improved survival of the diabetic foot: the role of a special foot clinic, *Q J Med* 1986; 232:763–771.
5. Foster AVM: The role of the chiropodist in diabetic foot care, in Bakker K, Nieuwenhvijzen Kruseman AC, editors: *The diabetic foot*, Amsterdam, 1991, Excerpta Medica, pp 137–149.
6. Lithner F, Tornblom N: Gangrene localised to the lower limbs in diabetics, *Acta Med Scand* 208:315–320, 1980.
7. Spraul M, Chamberlain E, Schmid M: Education of the patient, the diabetic foot clinic: a team approach, in Bakker K, Nieuwenhvijzen Kruseman AC, editors: *The diabetic foot*, Amsterdam, 1991, Excerpta Medica, pp 150–161.
8. Troman A, Foster A, Foulston J, et al: The value of skin grafts in the diabetic neuropathic foot, *Diabetic Med* 4:581A, 1987.

# CHAPTER 28

# Medicolegal Aspects of Care and Treatment of the Diabetic Foot*

**John J. Frank, J.D.**

**Joseph A. Frank, J.D.**

This chapter discusses the legal implications of the health care provider's care and treatment of the diabetic foot. We believe that this topic can best be addressed by what the personal injury attorney looks for when a client presents himself or herself with a potential malpractice case against a health care provider for the negligent treatment of the diabetic foot.

## PLAINTIFF'S CASE

A plaintiff in a malpractice suit must overcome five hurdles to satisfy his or her burden of proof:

1. Plaintiff and defendant were in a patient–health care provider relationship.
2. During the course of such relationship plaintiff had condition X.
3. There was a standard of care with regard to the care and treatment of condition X.
4. The defendant's care fell below that standard of care and was thereby negligent.
5. As a direct and proximate result of de-

fendant's negligence, the plaintiff sustained damages.

This chapter discusses each of these five elements as they apply to the care and treatment of the diabetic foot.

## Patient–Health Care Provider Relationship

In cases involving the diabetic foot, the patient–health care provider relationship issue can present itself in two ways. First, there is the scenario where the patient comes to the health care provider for care of the diabetic condition. Often the patient will come to the health care provider with a callus or a sore on the foot that will not heal. Second, there is the situation where the patient is under the care of the health care provider for a condition unrelated to the patient's diabetes, or the patient is receiving long-term care from the health care provider (e.g., the patient is a resident in a nursing home). Depending on which of these two scenarios is presented, the standard of care applicable to the patient will differ. Those differences are discussed later in the chapter.

The patient–health care provider relationship is based on contract. The patient promises that he or she will pay for the services of the health care provider. The health care provider promises that he or she will treat the patient with the best possible skill

---

*This chapter states general principles of law from a plaintiff's attorney's view point. The information provided in this chapter should not be considered as a substitute for independent research and independent counsel from one's attorney or insurer's attorney. It should also be noted that rules of law may vary from jurisdiction to jurisdiction.

and care. The contractual relationship is formed when the patient seeks a health care provider, engages the health care provider to render services, and the health care provider accepts the patient.

## Patient With Diabetes

The fact that the patient has diabetes is presupposed by the fact that he or she has come to our office with a potential malpractice claim for the amputation of a diabetic foot. One issue that arises in this area is whether the patient was already diagnosed with diabetes. If the patient had not, the attorney is concerned with whether the physician's failure to diagnose amounted to a breach of the standard of care.

If the patient had been diagnosed as having diabetes, the attorney looks to see if adequate preventive and curative steps were taken to prevent the necessity for amputation. These preventive and curative steps are discussed later in the chapter.

## Standard of Care

In nearly every medical malpractice action the plaintiff is required to present expert medical testimony as to the standard of care and whether the care provided by the physician was within the accepted standard. Cases involving care and treatment of the diabetic foot are no exception. After the attorney has been hired, he or she orders all of the medical records regarding the care of the client. Once all of the records have been gathered, the file is sent to an expert for review. On reviewing the file, the expert reports back to the attorney and gives his or her opinion as to whether the client has a case for malpractice against the health care provider.

The first thing that the attorney wants to know is if, in the opinion of the expert, the care provided to the patient fell below the standard of care. In most states the standard of care is defined as that degree of skill and learning ordinarily used under same or similar circumstances by members of that profession. In addition, in many states specialists are held to the degree of skill and learning ordinarily used under same or similar circumstances by members of the profession who practice that specialty. If the expert indicates that the care provided by the physician did not fall below the standard of care, the attorney will either withdraw from the case or seek another opinion. On the other hand, if the expert expresses an opinion that the care provided to the patient fell below the standard of care and that breach was negligent, the attorney will seek the expert's opinion as to whether the breach of the standard of care caused the patient's injuries. (Causation is discussed more fully later in the chapter.)

## Negligence

There are numerous ways in which a health care provider's treatment of a diabetic patient can fall below the standard of care. A discussion of the most common areas follows.

### Failure to Diagnose

A health care provider can be subject to liability on a claim for negligence for failing to diagnose the patient's diabetes or for failing to diagnose the patient's foot problem, for example, the existence of neuropathy or vascular disease. The standard that applies here is whether, in light of the circumstances presented by the patient's condition, the physician should have ordered appropriate tests.

Numerous "red flags" should alert the physician to the possibility that the patient has diabetes. Failure to recognize these red flags and conduct the appropriate tests will most probably be characterized as negligent and thus expose the physician to liability for failure to diagnose diabetes. Also, within the realm of negligent failure to diagnose is the situation where the diabetes mellitus is not noticed or is ignored. Again, the standard will vary depending on whether the patient is a diagnosed diabetic. If the patient is a diagnosed diabetic and has a foot problem, a physician will most likely be found negligent for failure to control the diabetes and properly examine the patient. If the patient has not been diagnosed as having diabetes, the standard referred to earlier will be applied to determine whether the physician was negligent.

### Failure to Prevent Decubiti

When a diabetic patient is under the care of a hospital or nursing home, that facility and the patient's attending physician have a duty to take all reasonable measures to prevent the development of decubitus ulcers on the patient's feet. This duty may require the physician to order protective apparatuses such as heel protectors and air mattresses. The physician may also be required to order daily examinations of the patient's feet to discover the development of erythema or ulcers. Regular turning and movement of the patient may also be required to prevent the development of ulcers. Regular visits by the attending physician may also be required. When a diabetic patient is admitted for long-term care, a complete physical, neurologic, and vascular examination should be performed to identify the patient's risks of decubitus ulcers.

A diabetic patient admitted for long-term care is at high risk for development of decubiti. In some situations, even when the highest degree of care is expended, the patient can develop decubiti. In such cases the health care provider is not guilty of medical malpractice. A legal cause of action for medical malpractice is not based on a bad result but on bad care. The errors and omissions just described all can be characterized as bad care.

To adequately defend a claim for negligent failure to prevent development of decubiti, the health care provider needs to show adequate documentation of the precautionary procedures. The medical record is the most critical piece of evidence in cases brought under this theory. The attorney bringing the action and his or her expert will look to the attending physician's orders and the nurses notes to make sure that due care was taken to prevent pressure sores. When reasonable preventive measures had been taken and documented, the patient's case is not likely to receive a favorable review from an expert. It must also be kept in mind that the patient's claim for damages must also be

"sold" to a jury. A health care provider's best defense is that they did everything in their power to prevent this type of injury to the patient. Without adequate documentation of the measures taken, this defense is not likely to be believed (see case study no. 1).

### Failure to Adequately Treat Ulcers

Because the patient has come to an attorney, he or she, in all probability, has already had an amputation. This amputation can be the result of severe peripheral arterial disease. This is not rare in diabetic patients, particularly in those who smoke, and have a large number of vascular risk factors. The most common cause for amputation in the diabetic is a foot ulcer complicated by infection and peripheral arterial disease. Substandard treatment accounts for approximately 50% of these amputations. In these cases the attorney will review the records of the physicians and the hospital and look for the following information: Was the patient adequately educated in foot care to prevent the development of ulcers? Has the physician routinely examined the patient's foot and done at least yearly neurologic and vascular examinations? If vascular insufficiency has been documented, was adequate consultation obtained? If an ulcer had developed, was it adequately treated? Was proper debridement carried out? Were both aerobic and anaerobic cultures obtained? Was the antibiotic selected a proper one? Because the outcome of infection can relate, at least in part, to the degreee of hyperglycemia, were routine blood glucose levels obtained, and were the appropriate changes made in insulin and oral hypoglycemia agents' dosages? Was hospitalization carried out at the proper time? If the lesion was not responding to treatment, did the treating physician have the expertise? If not, were proper consultations obtained (e.g., from an endocrinologist, diabetologist, infectious disease expert, vascular surgeon)?

A serious error in omission in many cases has been lack of proper inspection and prophylactic treatment to prevent decubitus ulcers of the heel in diabetics confined to bed. Failure to document orders to use heel protectors or special mattresses and to do daily inspection of the heels can be considered a significant error of omission. It has been shown in many cases that patients who have not been properly managed have developed pressure necrosis of the heels and ultimately have come to amputation. Settlements out of court in these situations have been sizable (see case study no. 1).

Another situation resulting in amputations has occurred in patients treated at home for foot infection who have not been carefully instructed to watch for signs and symptoms of worsening infection. It is very important that these patients be instructed in the signs and symptoms of worsening infection (see Chapter 2). Patients who have not been so instructed and who have not been informed to contact the physician at once, should any of these signs or symptoms develop, can make the physician liable for substandard care. Because patients frequently forget what they have been told, one of the ways to help the defendant in these cases is to document carefully in the chart the instructions that were given. The physician's best chance for successful defense is adequate documentation in the medical record, careful patient education, and proper use of consultation with experts in the field.

Because all amputations cannot be prevented, the lay jury, with the help of the defendant's attorney and experts, realize that the serious situation presented by a diabetic patient's extremities cannot always be successfully treated. Thus, the health care provider's best defense is that everything that could be done was done to prevent the tragic results suffered by the patient.

A glaring example of very superficial treatment and lack of follow-up can be noted in case study no. 2.

### Abandonment

A claim brought under an abandonment theory is based on the assertion that the physician knew or should have known that the patient's condition required continued expert medical attention and that the physician's failure to provide this care, or to at least ensure that such care was rendered by another qualified person, exacerbated the patient's condition. This theory can be presented in several different situations. The most common situations that give rise to a claim of abandonment are when the physician unilaterally withdraws from the care of the patient and when the physician has performed a procedure on the patient and fails to follow up with the patient for postoperative complications.

A physician who has a diabetic patient with an ulcer or a traumatic injury to the lower limbs should not withdraw from the patient's care or leave town and so forth, until such time as that patient has obtained another physician. That physician would not likely get much sympathy from a jury, especially after the patient's attorney argues to the jury that his or her client was in grave danger of developing infection and gangrene and the defendant physician left the patient "out in the cold" with no one to treat the condition (e.g., went on vacation; see case study no. 2). A defense to a claim of abandonment may be successfully based on an assertion that the patient, after repeated urging from the physician, refused to follow the orders and advice given.

Another example of abandonment is failure to treat because of unpaid bill. The physician is not likely to succeed if his or her defense is based on the patient's failure to pay the bill. A physician's duty to the patient cannot be excused for nonpayment of the bill. In addition, such an assertion is not likely to evoke much sympathy from a jury.

Once a successful operation or procedure has been performed, the physician has a continuing obligation to the patient. Unless the physician-patient relationship is mutually terminated by the parties, the physician's obligation to the patient continues until ended by the cessation of the necessity that gave rise to the relationship. A physician performing an operation on the lower limbs of a diabetic patient should continue to monitor the patient's surgical wounds until these wounds have completely healed. Otherwise, the patient will have a very strong case of abandonment against the operating physician.

### Informed Consent and Surgical Battery

A patient is entitled to full disclosure of the risks involved in a procedure that is to be performed on him or her. A physician's failure to so inform may give rise to a claim by the patient that the procedure was performed without his or her informed consent. A related cause of action is that of surgical battery. A claim for surgical battery is based on an assertion by the patient that a procedure was performed on him or her without consent or that the procedure performed exceeded the scope of the consent that he or she gave.

Surgical procedures performed on the lower limbs of a diabetic patient pose great risks of infection and postsurgical complications. It is imperative that all of these risks be explained in detail to the patient. It would be wise to prepare a pamphlet outlining these risks that could be left with the patient for his or her consideration. Finally, the physician should have the patient sign a consent form after the patient has been given sufficient time to review the material and discuss the options with the physician and the patient's family. The form should indicate that the physician has discussed the risks of the procedure with the patient (the physician may also want to enumerate what these risks are) and that the patient has been given time to weigh his or her options and has chosen to proceed with the procedure.

### Failure to Educate Patient

A physician may be found negligent for failing to educate a diabetic patient with regard to foot care. The patient should be informed of the serious and possibly tragic consequences of infection in the foot area. A physician should instruct the patient as to the proper footwear (shoes, socks, stockings, etc.). The patient should be instructed to inspect his or her feet regularly for cuts, blisters, calluses, and so forth (see Chapter 2) and to recognize the warning signs of infection. The physician should instruct the patient to seek medical treatment at the first signs of infection.

A common defense of physicians in cases involving amputation of the diabetic foot is the patient's own negligence. Depending on the jurisdiction, a patient's own negligence may reduce the amount of recovery or bar his or her recovery altogether. The defense of contributory fault can be very effective if the patient had been adequately educated regarding foot care. A physician cannot assert that the patient should have sought treatment sooner if the physician had not warned the patient of the serious consequences of infection and had not instructed the patient as to the warning signs of infection. Contributory fault of the patient may be the physician's best defense to a patient's claim for negligent treatment of the diabetic foot. However, this shield may be used as a sword against the physician if he or she had not adequately educated the patient (see case study no. 2).

### Causation

Once it has been established that the physician's care of the patient fell below the standard of care and was negligent, the patient's attorney must prove with a reasonable degree of medical certainty that the physician's negligence caused or contributed to cause the injury to the plaintiff. Again, this requires expert testimony on behalf of the patient. In medical malpractice cases involving the care and treatment of the diabetic foot, causation is one of the most difficult elements for the patient to prove. In almost every case the physician can raise the defense that even if he or she were negligent in the treatment of the patient, the patient would have suffered the same result if the highest degree of care had been exercised on the patient's behalf. A diabetic patient with an ulcer or a traumatic injury to his or her feet is at great risk of infection and gangrene. Often no matter what the physician does, the patient will suffer amputation or serious infection. Unless the patient's expert can testify that the negligence of the physician caused or substantially contributed to cause the patient's injury, the patient will not succeed on his or her claim for malpractice.

## DEFENDANT CASE

Attorneys who represent patients in medical malpractice cases anticipate the defense that the physician will raise before filing the claim. There are several defenses that are raised routinely that the experienced attorney can defeat and even possibly turn against the physician. These common defenses are as follows:

1. Judgment defense
2. General practitioner defense
3. "Patient would have lost his leg anyway" defense
4. Informed consent
5. Comparative fault/contributory negligence
6. "Empty chair" defense

A detailed discussion of the defenses follows.

### Judgment Defense

This defense is based on the physician's assertion that several courses of treatment could have been taken, but, in hindsight, another course of action should have been taken. In most states this is a valid defense. The patient's attorney will try to counter this defense by establishing that there was only one proper course of treatment for the patient and that the physician was negligent for failing to follow that course. What usually results from this defense is a battle of experts and authoritative texts. The side with the most convincing expert and the most authoritative texts will usually win.

### General Practitioner Defense

It has been estimated that approximately 80% of all diabetics are treated by general practitioners as opposed to diabetes specialists. Therefore, it is a common defense in these cases that the treating physician, as a general practitioner, should not be held to the same standard as a diabetes specialist. This defense is rarely effective. The patient's attorney will argue that all physicians have medical training and that even a general practitioner should be able to identify the serious consequences of traumatic injury or pressure sores on the diabetic foot. The physician will also be questioned as to why he or she did not refer the patient to a specialist.

### "Patient Would Have Lost the Leg Anyway" Defense

The basis of this defense is regardless of whether the physician was negligent or not, the patient was going to require amputation. In cases involving pressure sores or traumatic injury to the diabetic foot, this is sometimes true. Because of these patients' poor circulation, there is always a risk of infection or gangrene. However, some states allow a patient to recover for the loss of the chance to save the leg, thus defeating this defense.

### Informed Consent

Another common defense raised is that the patient was advised of all of the risks involved in the procedure and signed a consent form indicating that he or she understands the risks and consents to the procedure. The first pitfall to this defense is that the physician is most likely to be perceived as more knowledgeable in the area of medicine than the patient. If the patient testifies that the risks were not explained to him or her or that the risks were explained to him or her but he or she did not understand them, the jury is likely to believe the patient. Also, most consent forms are preprinted forms with the name of the procedure written in. The signed form is not likely to sway the jury to the fact that the patient consented because most jurors can relate to the situation where they are asked to sign something they have not read by a person of authority, and, in reliance on that person, they sign it. For a physician to effectively use a consent form as a defense, the form should enumerate each of the risks involved in the procedure. The physician may also want to have the patient put his or her initials after each paragraph.

## Comparative Fault and Contributory Negligence

This defense blames the patient's condition on his or her own acts of negligence. For example, a physician would claim that the patient's foot had to be amputated because the patient did not practice good foot care. In some states the contributory negligence of the patient is not a defense to the negligence of the physician. Other states ask the jury to assess the percentages of fault attributable to the physician and the patient. The damages awarded to the patient are then reduced by the percentage of fault attributed to him or her. This defense is ineffective if the patient had not been adequately educated by the physician. In addition, the patient is not likely to be held to the same standard as the physician because of the physician's training and experience.

## "Empty Chair" Defense

Perhaps the most effective defense that can be raised by the physician accused of negligence is that someone else or some other entity caused the patient's injuries. The physician will want to show that he or she ordered the appropriate tests or prescribed the proper care. It is very difficult for the patient's attorney to counter such a defense when the accused party is not in the suit or present at trial. Attorneys who represent patients in response to the increased successful use of this defense have been joining all of the parties involved in the care of the patient and then eliminating the unnecessary parties once they have been cleared of negligence.

## Case Study No. 1

L.B. was a diabetic who had suffered a stroke in June 1988. On July 1, 1988, she was admitted to defendant nursing home on her release from the release from the hospital. L.B. suffered from left side paralysis and was in a leg brace. During her stay at the nursing home, she developed an ulcer on her left heel, which was first noted on October 19. On that day the ulcer was treated with povidone-iodine (Betadine) and whirlpool treatment. The next note in the record is from November 12, at which point the nurse noted a foul odor. On November 15, L.B.'s temperature spiked at 39.7°C. Her physician performed a culture. The following day she was admitted to the hospital, and her ulcer was described as gangrenous, 5 cm, and stage II. Extensive debridement was performed on November 19. L.B.'s condition worsened, and her left leg was amputated above the knee on November 28. In September 1989, L.B.'s right foot and leg were amputated above the knee.

After the amputation of her left leg, L.B. retained an attorney for a potential medical malpractice claim against the nursing home. L.B.'s attorney ordered all of the medical records and sent them to an expert for review. The expert found that the nursing home personnel were negligent in the following respects:

1. The nurses failed to notify L.B.'s physicians about the condition of her foot or heel on any regular basis.
2. There was a lack of daily observation or supervision of L.B.'s feet, heels, and legs.
3. The patient was not provided with heel protectors.
4. The patient was not provided with an air mattress or any other special mattress.
5. Inadequate bandaging of the ulcerated area after the ulcer had developed.

In addition to his findings of negligence on the part of the nursing home, the expert also found negligence on the part of L.B.'s attending physicians. L.B.'s attending physicians were, in the expert's opinion, negligent in the following respects:

1. After her admission, L.B. was seen by a physician only three times, and not for the first time until August 22, 6 weeks after her admission.
2. At no point in the record did it indicate that a physical examination or a neurologic examination was performed, even though L.B. had suffered a stroke.

3. There was no examination recorded of her heart, lungs, or peripheral circulation, nor was there an examination of her skin.

4. There were no notes regarding her brace.

5. No orders were left to the nursing home personnel to examine her lower limbs on a daily basis.

6. The physicians did not order special mattresses, air mattresses, or heel protectors;

7. Once the lesion developed, no culture was taken until the day before admission to determine whether or not it was infected.

8. On November 12, the nurses noted a foul odor, but nothing was done until 3 days later when L.B.'s temperature spiked at 39.7°C. At that point a culture was done, but it was too late.

9. Once the patient's temperature hit 39.7°C, she should have received intensive antibiotic treatment and should have been hospitalized, but only cefaclor (Ceclor) was given. No white blood cell counts or blood glucose levels were obtained either.

10. The patient's ulcer should have been debrided.

The defendant physicians' defense was that they did everything that they could to prevent the injuries suffered by the patient L.B. and that if there was any negligence, it was on the part of the nursing home staff. The nursing home's defense was similar in that they claimed they did everything they could and that if anyone was negligent, it was the defendant physicians. This case was not tried but was settled out of court for a substantial sum of money.

## Case Study No. 2

L.N. was diagnosed as diabetic in 1960. L.N. remained under the care of the same physician for 20 years until he switched to Dr. Doe for convenience purposes. On Feb 11, 1985, L.N. fell on a patch of ice and sprained his ankle. The ankle became badly swollen and discolored. Eventually, on March 9, L.N. saw Dr. Doe about his sprained left ankle. On examination of L.N.'s feet, Dr. Doe found an infected callus, he described a draining diabetic ulcer on the ball of L.N.'s left foot. Dr. Doe trimmed the callus and painted it with merthiolate. Dr. Doe told L.N. to soak the foot and to come back if it did not get any better. No other instructions were given to the patient. L.N. told Dr. Doe that he did not think he could walk with his swollen ankle, so Dr. Doe gave him an off-work slip for the next 3 days.

At no time did Dr. Doe instruct L.N. that the condition of his ulcer could deteriorate and quickly turn to gangrene, requiring amputation. Dr. Doe then went on vacation until April 4. No one answered the telephone at the physician's office while he was gone. During the physician's vacation, L.N. continued to have problems with his foot. On April 4 he returned to Dr. Doe. L.N.'s wife told the physician that she wanted him to put her husband in the hospital. The physician disagreed and made an appointment for L.N. to see a specialist that treated him in 1982.

The specialist diagnosed gangrene of the left foot. Despite efforts to save the foot, the patient's left leg had to be amputated just below the knee. After his recovery, L.N. retained an attorney for a possible malpractice claim against Dr. Doe. L.N.'s attorney ordered the entire medical record and sent it to his expert for review. The expert communicated to the attorney that the care Dr. Doe gave to L.N. fell below the minimum standard of care in the following respects:

1. Dr. Doe did not perform adequate tests to make sure that L.N.'s diabetes was under control.

2. Dr. Doe's use of merthiolate on the ulcer was wholly ineffective.

3. No cultures were taken of the wound to determine the nature and extent of the infection.

4. Dr. Doe did not instruct L.N. to stay off his feet.

5. Antibiotics were not prescribed.

6. Dr. Doe did not adequately instruct L.N. or warn him of the elementary damages inherent to his condition.

7. Insulin was administered improperly.

8. L.N. should have been hospitalized so that the wound could have been cultured, medicated, and brought under control.
9. Dr. Doe did not examine the patient for loss of sensation.
10. No radiographs or bone scans were performed.
11. Merely telling the patient to soak the foot was bad medicine.
12. Dr. Doe should have referred the patient to the specialist immediately.

The plaintiff's expert also testified that if Dr. Doe had met the minimum standards, the patient would have stood an excellent chance of not losing his leg. The expert who testified on behalf of Dr. Doe testified that L.N.'s own negligence was the cause of his infection, not the negligence of Dr. Doe. L.N.'s expert responded to this claim by pointing out that L.N. was not properly educated with regard to proper foot care, nor was he warned of the seriousness of infection and the need for regular foot inspection. L.N.'s case was never tried before a jury. His case was settled out of court for a substantial amount of money.

## DO

- Educate the patient with regard to diabetes and foot care.
- Refer to an expert in the field if you believe you may be getting in over your head.
- Document in the patient's chart all that is done on behalf of the patient.

- Use aggressive treatment for foot ulcers.
- Include regular patient follow-up.

## DON'T

- Do not treat if you are in doubt about the patient's condition.
- Do not treat a diabetic with foot ulcers if that is not within your field.
- Do not delay in your treatment of the diabetic foot.
- Do not let the patient go untreated for an extended period.

## CONCLUSION

There have been hundreds of cases brought against health care providers alleging negligent treatment of the diabetic foot. Most of these cases involve amputation of the patient's foot or leg. Because of the very serious injuries involved, settlements and verdicts in these cases are usually quite high. A survey of 30 jury verdicts and settlements in these cases revealed an average figure of almost $350,000.

Almost 80% of all diabetics are treated by general practitioners instead of diabetic specialists. Therefore, the general practitioner should be aware of the potential legal consequences of his or her care of the diabetic foot. Serious injuries to the patient and malpractice suits against the health care provider can be prevented by following the simple legal rules discussed in this chapter.

# Index